DOCTOR: ALL MEMBERSHIP EXPIRED DECEMBER 31st. SEE YOUR COUNTY SECRETARY.

THE JOURNAL

of the

Oklahoma State Medical Association

VOLUME XII, NUMBER 1   JANUARY, 1919   Annual Subscription, $2.00

Published Monthly at Muskogee, Oklahoma, under direction of the Council.

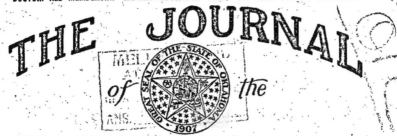

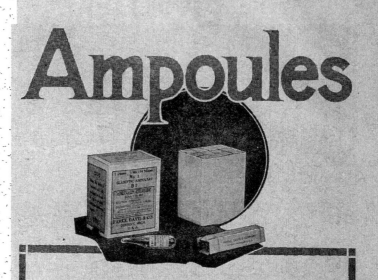

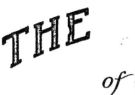

THE JOURNAL

of *the*

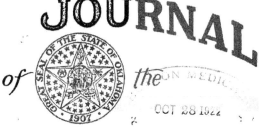

Oklahoma State Medical Association

VOLUME XII   MUSKOGEE, OKLA, JANUARY, 1919   NUMBER 1

THE ACCESSORY SINUSES OF THE NOSE.*

By R. O. EARLY, M. D., Ardmore, Okla.

I shall not bore you by going into the minute anatomy of the nose and will only refer to the anatomy of this part of the head when necessary in referring to some of the diseases of the sinuses.

Under normal conditions the accessory sinuses are capable of self drainage for the following reasons:

1st. The lining mucous membrane is composed of ciliated epithelium, the motion wave of the cilia being always directed toward the ostium of the sinus.

2nd. At every position of the body certain of the ostia are at the lowest portion of the sinus. Thus in standing or sitting the ostium of the frontal sinus is low, or lying down the maxillary sinus.

This accounts for the dissimilarity of the subjective symptoms often noted in affections of individual sinus, for instance a frequent symptom of chronic frontal sinus involvement is neuralgia over the orbital region, regularly appearing at a certain time in the morning, lasting several hours and ceasing suddenly. The explanation of this is that during the night the frontal sinus lies in an unfavorable position to allow the secretion to escape.

In the morning when the erect position is assumed the mucous membrane around the ostium is congested with resulting engorgement in the sinus; as soon as actual pressure occurs, neuralgia appears and continues until through pressure of the secretion the ostium becomes sufficiently patulous to allow escape of the secretion. Drainage is thus established and the neuralgia ceases. Of course the size of the sinus, the amount of secretion and virulence of the infection bears a direct relation to the severity and duration of the neuralgic attack.

The maxillary sinus under the same condition may exhibit totally different characteristics, for instance a patient may have all the classical symptoms of a maxillary involvement except no secretion is seen on examination, and still you get a history of profuse discharge from the nasopharynx. The explanation of this lies in the drainage mechanism; during the day the sinus secretes an amount that fills the cavity and as the ostium is situated at the superior portion, the secretion only escapes drop by drop, while the patient is in the upright position. When the patient lies on the sound side at night, the ostium is in the most favorable position for drainage and the secretion finds exit into the nose and is either hawked or blown out in the morning with the result that when one sees the patient no secretion is visible. The drainage of the ethmoid can either be simple or com-

---

*Read in Section on Eye, Ear, Nose and Throat, Tulsa, May, 1918.

plicated. Simple when the ostium is situated in the lowest portion of the cell and empties into one of the nasal passages. Complicated when one cell empties into another and into a second or third and finally into the nose. There exists several distinct processes by which the mucous membrane of the accessory sinus may become diseased.

1st.   Through direct invasion of the healthy sinus by pathogenic bacteria.

2nd.   As result of tuberculosis, syphilis, malignant tumors and latent empyema.

3rd.   Through traumatism—exposure to cold resulting in congested turbinates, with closure of the ostium.

4th.   Through contamination from pus from overlying sinus.

Under the head of non-bacteriological disease may be considered various chronic hyperplasias and hypertrophies of the nasal mucosa. Particularly is this true of the frontal and maxillary sinuses. This condition is accounted for by repeated attacks of colds or from other causes, certain portions of the mucosa in the neighborhood of the ostium being left edematous. When reclining the blood pressure is higher in this locality with consequent swelling and temporary occlusion of the ostium. You are all familiar with swollen and congested turbinates with the resulting blocking of the ostium, the sense of fullness and the complaining of dull frontal headaches of your patients. This headache symptom taken alone is unreliable, but its presence or absence in the entire symptom complex is most important. Its mere absence means nothing, while its presence may be of inestimable value in making a correct diagnosis. Pressure on the septum from hypertrophies, which often co-exist with sinus inflammation, is one of the main causes of headache associated with this disease.

In a general way tenderness over the sinuses is of diagnostic value when present over the frontal, rarely over the maxillary; the point of tenderness generally being confined to a small area on the floor of the sinus directly above the inner canthus of the eye, this being the thinnest bony portion of the wall. And while this symptom is most indicative of frontal sinus inflammation, comparison should always be made of the sound side, for in neurotic individuals false impressions may often be obtained.

Gruenwald claims that pressure between the eyes will often elicit tenderness in ethmoidal diseases. This hardly seems possible when one considers the anatomy of the ethmoid region and I can only account for this symptom, if it is ever present —and personally I have never been able to demonstrate it—from the fact that where the ethmoid is diseased the frontal is also involved, and I believe if any tenderness is obtained it is from the latter.

In enumerating the above and following symptoms I have endeavored to speak of the sinuses collectively, as it would require too much of your time to take up each individually.

One of the chief symptoms of sinus disease is the presence of a purulent secretion in the nose. However, the mere presence of the secretion is no more indicative of sinus involvement than is absence proof that no sinus disease exists. If, however, secretion reappears in the same spot shortly after being removed, the evidence is positive that a reservoir of purulent material is underlying; it being impossible for a circumscribed inflammation of the mucous membrane to secrete pus so rapidly in such a short space of time. The classical symptom of sinus empyema is the presence or continued reappearance of pus. In a particular locality of the nose (beneath the anterior third of the middle turbinate for anterior sinus disease, in the olfactory fissure and above the posterior end of the middle turbinate in posterior disease), diminution is usually a sign of remission, but sometimes is due to occlusion with recurring symptoms.

Another symptom sometimes overlooked, and which is indirectly caused by the secretion, is the subjective appreciation of an offensive odor in the nose.

Edema of the tissue over the affected sinuses is not generally present until the disease is well advanced. Fever is generally present but exhibits no noteworthy characteristics; the sudden rise of temperature in chronic inflammation is indicative of toxic reabsorption through the sinus walls or of impending and severe complication, such as rupture into the neighboring parts.

In making a diagnosis of a suspected sinus disease, therefore, we look for free pus. If we see pus coming down between the bulla and middle turbinate we ascertain whether the secretion is an overflowing or merely due to a circumscribed inflammation of the mucous membrane.

Our next step is to ascertain which sinus of the first series is involved. We first turn to maxillary sinus for this reason: (1) More frequently affected than others; (2) It is situated at lowest portion, and (3) It is reasonably easy of access.

The one best method of ascertaining whether pus is present is by needle puncture. If pus is present, our next attempt is to find whether the inflammatory product has been secreted by the maxillary mucosa or has merely acted as a receptacle for pus from overlying sinuses. If after a wait of an hour or so pus is noted beneath the middle turbinate, we can definitely say that one of the sinus higher up (frontal or anterior ethmoid) is affected. We then proceed to wash out the frontal sinus if possible.

The differentiation between frontal sinus empyema and suppuration of the anterior ethmoidal cells is more or less of a rhinological nicety, both generally involved and the therapy in both instances being the same.

Of the sphenoidal and posterior ethmoidal group, pus from these sinuses must appear in either of two places: (1) In the olfactory fissure; (2) Above the posterior end of middle turbinate. Other methods of diagnosis are: (1) Transillumination; (2) Roentgen Ray, and (3) Suction.

At Killian's clinic in Berlin, patients with suspected sinus disease are routinely subjected to X-ray examination. As regards treatment, this depends on many conditions. The individual's symptoms are the keynote upon which to base our therapeutic or operative efforts. Take for instance two cases of acute sinus involvement, one presenting a mild course, the other presenting every evidence of impending cerebral or orbital complication: The first may be treated expectantly, but to the latter prompt and energetic means must be applied.

I have not gone into the complications resulting from accessory sinus diseases. I might mention the more important being those of the orbital cavity, the optic nerve and brain complications. In closing, I wish to say a word regarding vaccine therapy in these cases. The value, I think, in sinus diseases is questionable for the following reasons: (1) Acute cases have a tendency toward spontaneous recovery; (2) The majority of chronic cases are associated with mixed infection; therefore, when the culture is planted, how can one decide which particular organism is causing the suppuration? To make a vaccine of the mixed culture would lead to no satisfactory result. In cases where one could get a pure culture of the infecting micro-organism, this treatment might be tried, but I think the cases rare which are not ones of mixed infection.

A. E. Ewing, St. Louis (*Journal A. M. A.*, Dec. 14, 1918), fully reports a case of glaucoma which was treated with repeated postciliary trephining operations. The result was not good, as it left a blind eye, but the process, as used, demonstrated that the removal of vitreous to the extent that the tension is far below normal is no more a cure for glaucoma than is the removal of the lens. Drainage may be established by way of the vitreous chamber. A trephined wound in the sclera is closed by newly formed fibrous tissue, in the same manner as a trephined wound in the sclerocorneal margin, and is no more dangerous. The clouding of the cornea and vitreous, and the pulsation on the disk may be instantly relieved by vitreous drainage with immediate restoration of vision. The full feeling and pain of glaucoma are relieved by sclerocorneal trephining, even though the choroid is not disturbed and there is no apparent lowering of tension. The lens is not affected by the operation, and there need be no visible operative defect.

OPERATIONS ON THE NASAL SEPTUM.*

By HARRY COULTER TODD, A. M., M. D., F. A. C. S.

Associate Professor of Clinical Ear, Nose and Throat, University of Oklahoma School of Medicine;
Ex-President, Oklahoma Academy of Ophthalmology and Oto-Laryngology; Ex-Chair-
man of the Eye, Ear, Nose and Throat Section of the Medical Association of
the Southwest, The Oklahoma State Medical Association, etc.

Nine years ago I read a paper before the Ophthalmological section of the Medical Association of the Southwest, which met at San Antonio, Texas, on "Conservation of the Mucous Membrane in Intra-Nasal Surgery." Radical intra-nasal surgery prior to that date and for some time following that period, was very general with little consideration given to the preservation and care of normal tissues. Radical intra-nasal surgery had its beginning largely in the Vienna and Berlin schools, and was quickly taken up by American operators. Beginning in the early 90's it reached its ascendency about eleven years ago.

What called forth my paper in 1909 heretofore referred to, was the end results in many of these radical intra-nasal operations performed by myself and others, which I was permitted to observe. I found that serious atrophic changes had often taken place. Scar tissue had supplanted healthy mucous membrane and often normal and necessary functionating intra-nasal structures had been destroyed and serious and incurable conditions had developed, which far outweighed in gravity the original disturbing trouble for which relief had been sought.

My paper was received at that time kindly, but with no great amount of enthusiasm, and little if any discussion. It is a great satisfaction to me, however, to know that others at that time were making similar observations, and the fact that the *International Journal of Oto-Laryngology* published in Berlin, reprinted this paper almost in full, would suggest that its editor regarded my words as at least timely. I do not need to tell you of the change that has taken place with regard to radical intra-nasal surgery during the past six or eight years.

I make this rather lengthy preface to my remarks at this time a little in defense, perhaps, of the position I am about to take in regard to operations upon the nasal septum. It is my opinion, gentlemen, that, in surgical procedures anywhere about the human body, and especially in the nose, no normal, healthy, functioning tissue of any kind should be removed, unless it is found absolutely necessary to remove such tissue in order to restore the functions of more important tissues or organs. This, I believe, should be the law of all good surgery.

Up until a few years ago a distorted, twisted, thickened and deflected nasal septum, if not the bane of the rhinologist, was to say the least, often operated with results not wholly satisfactory to the patient or to the surgeon.

A big step was made towards the satisfactory relief of these conditions in the operation devised by Freer and others, the sub-mucous resection of the nasal septum, as it has been quite universally done by rhinologists for the past few years. This operation, as you are well aware, consists in thoroughly elevating the mucous membrane from the deviated septum and removing for the most part all the twisted bone and cartilage. It has been my observation that many of the septa operated on by myself, and by other much more skillful operators, having lost the stability and firmness given them by the bone and cartilage often bow towards one or the other nasal cavity, greatly enlarging one nasal chamber at the expense of the other. It is true that this rarely if ever interferes with the breathing, as the septum is rendered sufficiently movable to admit of air being inhaled and exhaled through the constricted side, and therefore the chief disturbance from your septal deformity has been relieved. There are conditions I believe, however, in which the wide open nasal chamber on the one side and the more or less constricted chamber on the other, may have a pathological bearing.

---

*Read in Section on Eye, Ear, Nose and Throat, Tulsa, May, 1918.

One of these conditions, and that which led me to a consideration of the operation, which I shall later describe to you, is where we have deflected septum with the development of atrophic rhinitis on the open side of the nose. This type of unilateral atrophic rhinitis is quite frequently met with. It occurred to me that what we needed is these cases, was not a thinning of the septum and a further increase in the intra-nasal space, but a reduction of the nasal chamber on the affected side where the turbinates were already partly gone, and the bringing about of a normal patency on the obstructed side. I found that the sub-mucous resection as ordinarily done did not obtain this result. The mucous membrane on the open and affected side necessarily becomes greatly thinned by the atrophic changes upon this side, while the mucous membrane of the other side becomes thickened by the constant hyperemia produced by the ever present negative air pressure, due to the restricted nares. Following the ordinary sub-mucous resection with the healing process, along with the fact that one side was much more open from atrophy of the turbinates, etc., the yielding septum always bowed towards the side of the thickened mucous membrane, that is to the side that had formerly been constricted. This is exactly what we do not want in attempting to relieve these conditions. You will find (and I want you to note this remark) that if you will greatly reduce the nasal chamber upon the affected side in these cases of unilateral atrophic rhinitis almost to the point of producing a negative air pressure, at the same time establishing free breathing space upon the side hitherto obstructed by your deflection, you can bring about complete relief and a practical cure in a large per cent. of these cases. I am not able to account for this fact unless it be that the constriction causes a hyperemia more or less constant, which is just the condition that we need in the treatment of these conditions. The operation that I devised for this particular condition, and which I have since come to use in a large proportion in all cases of deflected septa, is this:

I proceed with my incision and the elevation of the membranes on either side of the septum exactly as I do in an ordinary resection. If the cartilage is badly twisted or curled, I remove it. If it is simply deflected, I separate it freely from its upper or lower attachment, sometimes from both, and swing it into place. The cartilage is more often removed if it is badly misplaced. If the palatal process is greatly thickened, with a pair of bone cutting forceps I cut backward just above this ridge and remove this process. The same is done if there is a thickened ridge in the septal plates, but a great mass of the deflected ethmoid plate or vomer, or both, are not removed. These, as you know, are very thin plates of bone firmer, but not usually thicker than an egg shell. These I grasp high up with a wide blade forceps and fracture thoroughly and bring them into proper position. I then press the blades of my sub-mucous speculum together while it is in position and examine both nasal chambers to be sure that I have perfectly corrected the deflection. I remove any small pieces of septal bone that have been broken off, and may have dropped down into the bottom of the cavity—although I have never seen any ill results from leaving them behind, as I am sure I have done a number of times, and I proceed with my dressings as in an ordinary resection. If the deflection is high up and far back, one needs to be a little more careful that gentle pressure is brought to bear from your dressings over the entire surface of the septum operated.

The principal bad result that can come as I have found in this operation, is in not fracturing the bony septum high enough so that you leave the upper portion protruding to the deflected side or by not fracturing your curved bony structure sufficiently.

The after dressings must be worn longer and be introduced with a little more care than is the case in the ordinary resection, but only on the deflected side where they cause but little trouble and should be replaced daily for a week or ten days.

In cases of unilateral atrophic rhinitis, I always over correct the deflection so as to permanently reduce the breathing space on this side.

I do not claim the above as a universal operation—there are cases where it could not be done at all with success. Again, where you have both nasal chambers greatly reduced from lack of breathing, it is of great advantage to make a septum as thin as possible. However, the longer I follow the above method the less and less bone and cartilage I am removing from the septum with the result that I am getting a firmer septum which stays where I place it and does not tend to sag to one or the other side. Moreover I am leaving things a little more as evidently God Almighty intended they should be, and I question whether or not the surgeon ever improves very much upon His handiwork when it is as He intended it should be. In the class of cases of which I have made special mention, and they are quite numerous, I am sure you will find it profitable to yourself and very beneficial to your patients, if you will attempt to follow out the method as I have here outlined. As to the technique, it takes perhaps a little more time and care, but it is not any more difficult than the ordinary sub-mucous resection. If while thoroughly fracturing your septal plates, as will rarely happen, you should get your bony structure so badly misplaced that you cannot get a smooth septum, you may then do a complete resection and no harm has been done from attempting to do the operation as I have herein described.

CHRONIC FRONTAL SINUSITIS.

T. W. Moore, Huntington, W. Va. (*Journal A. M. A.*, Nov. 30, 1918), after noticing the various advances that have been made in the treatment of chronic frontal sinusitis, considers that the most important is the operation devised and advocated by Lothrop. Lothrop recommends first the removal of the anterior end of the middle turbinate and the breaking down of the anterior ethmoid cells with a curet, which frequently gives a free opening into the frontal sinus, and ten days or two weeks afterward he uses his radical operation if required. The drainage from this first procedure will alone cause a cure in a large percentage of cases. The radical operation is described in detail. It is done under general anesthesia with a pledget of cotton saturated with a 4 per cent. cocain in epinephrin solution inserted in each nostril. A curved incision about 1 inch in length is made through the eyebrow beginning at the superorbital notch and extending to the nose, the periosteum carefully elevated. "An opening is now chiseled through the bone into one sinus at the naso-orbital angle, or Ewing's point. The sinus is now carefully inspected and any pus, polpi or granulation tissue removed, care being taken to preserve as much of the mucous membrane intact as is possible. A probe is now passed into the naso-frontal duct and used as a guide, while with curet, rasps and burrs, the cells anterior to the naso-frontal duct are broken down, and the mass of dense bone at the root of the nose, formed by the nasal process of the superior maxillary, frontal and nasal bones, is removed. The partition between the sinuses is broken through and removed and the intranasal floor of the second sinus removed, whether it is diseased or not. At the same time the operator takes away the upper portion of the nasal septum, thus making a large passage from the now single sinus into the nose, which may be entered readily from either nostril. The external wound is now closed, without packing, and a pressure bandage applied and left on for twenty-four hours, when a dressing of cotton and collodion is applied and permitted to remain for five or six days, when the stitches are removed." We must never overlook the roentgen-ray pictures of these cases, and Moore does not see the validity of an objection to opening a healthy sinus for increased drainage. It does not or did not become infected in any of his twelve cases.

THE SIGNIFICANCE OF PAIN IN THE EAR.*

By J. H. BARNES, M. D., Enid, Okla.

Pain in the ear being so common and a warning to be on our guard either for an ordinary affliction or a very dangerous ailment, I thought a short paper on this subject would be timely.

I find it very difficult in some cases to locate the source of the pain, and in other cases to relieve the pain when we have diagnosed the case.

I will give only a few of the cases of pain in the ear that are most common and that have given us considerable concern and the cause of the trouble and the treatment of the same.

Furunculosis of the external canal is a very painful disease and often is quite hard to arrest. It is caused by an infection of the canal, often by using some hard instrument in the ear to remove the cerumen or for an itching in the ear. Hair pins and ordinary pins as well as ear spoons are very dangerous instruments to use in the ear. They are a frequent cause of abscess in the external ear.

For the removal of the cerumen in the canal, I will refer you to another paragraph in the study. For the itching of the ear, use a cotton mop made on a tooth pick or some soft wood. The treatment should be to cleanse the canal thoroughly with peroxide on a cotton applicator, then dry thoroughly and wash out with alcohol. Open all well formed abscesses early with a small knife—a cataract knife—then give the patient a solution of boric acid in 50 per cent. alcohol to use in the ear with instructions to churn it back and forth in the ear with a medicine dropper.

Chronic eczema of the canal gives us a great deal of concern when we try to cure these cases. They are often relieved for a short time but soon return as violent as ever, and the patient is often more irritable than the ear seems to you.

The acute form of eczema is easily arrested by mild antiseptics and if treatment is used for a short time there is no further trouble, but when it is allowed to continue until the epidermis is thick and the cerumenous glands are destroyed, then it becomes quite difficult to cure. The cause of this trouble is not well known. In certain conditions of the system, the use of arsenic is indicated to relieve the trouble. Dry infected cerumen and secretions from the middle ear are some of the frequent causes.

The itching and pain becomes almost unbearable at times, fissures are often present which give excruciating pain. The hearing is often bad on account of the swelling and the debris in the canal. The tympanic membrane is often involved in the process causing a loss of hearing.

The best treatment in my hands has been to first cleanse the canal of all the scales and crusts by the use of H_2O_2 on cotton applicators. If the epidermis is rough and thick, apply 5 per cent. nitrate of silver to the canal and let it remain a few days and then repeat the treatment as often as is necessary to get the canal clean and smooth. Apply trichloracetic acid to deep fissures. Keep the canal clean for a few weeks and then apply powdered calomel to the canal or better in persistent cases, a prescription for ointment of ammoniated mercury 5 gr., oxide zinc drachms 1; vaseline drachms ½. If the canal is moist and has small vesicles exuding watery fluid, add to this prescription 5 gr. of salicylic acid. This treatment if persisted in and the canal kept clean will always stop the pain and many times the canal will become normal with its usual amount of cerumen, which is necessary for a complete cure.

Foreign bodies in the ear become quite painful, especially when someone of the family tries to remove a grain of wheat or some object from the ear with a

---

*Read in Section on Eye, Ear, Nose and Throat, Tulsa, May, 1918.

hair-pin and injures the canal. It soon swells and the secretions of blood and pus will obscure the object so as to make the extraction very difficult.

Small bodies, such as grains of wheat, flies, etc., should be removed by irrigation of warm water, and using a two-ounce syringe.

Flies and bugs that cause great pain should first be killed. The best way is to use chloroform fumes. A small amount of melted vaseline should be poured into the ear so as to protect the ear drum and the skin of the ear from the irritating fumes of the chloroform. Then saturate a small pledget of cotton with chloroform and insert it into the ear. Then put a small piece of dry cotton over it so as to hold the fumes in the ear. In a few minutes the insect is dead. Then it can be picked out or washed out with a syringe.

Hard bodies, such as a bean or small stones, should not be grasped with forceps for they slip off and tend to push the body further into the ear. If the body is large and is pushed past the isthmus into the bony canal, it becomes very difficult to remove it by any method.

A small tenaculum may be used when it is possible to insert it into the body.

Queri's foreign body extractor is a very useful instrument in my hand, especially with small stones. If the patient is a child and will not hold still, give it a few breaths of chloroform before trying to remove the foreign body. The main object in removing all bodies from the ear is to keep from injuring the canal or ear drum.

Impacted cerumen is a very frequent source of annoyance and when it becomes infected it becomes very painful. This is caused by an excess of wax in the ear, by over-stimulation of the cerumenous gland, or by the canal becoming diseased and the wax not being carried off properly. This impaction should always be removed as soon as discovered. There is only one way to remove it and that is by syringing with lukewarm water with a 2-oz. piston syringe. The removal of wax should never be attempted with a spoon or an instrument of any kind. If the wax becomes very hard and dry, use a few drops of camphor oil in the ear for three or four days and have the patient come back when it can be easily removed with a syringe. The camphor oil is 5 gr. of gum camphor to one oz. of liquid petroleum. Five drops three times a day for three days.

In syringing, some precaution may be timely. Do not direct the stream directly into the ear, throw it against one wall so as to follow the wall back behind the impaction and it will be more easily dislodged. Sometimes it will be necessary to press away the impaction from the wall so as to let the stream pass. The canal should be dried thoroughly and camphor oil applied to the canal.

Pain in the middle ear is the first symptom of otitis media. It is called earache by the laity and to them it means but little if the family is not disturbed at night. To the doctor who studies the consequences of middle ear disease, it means a great deal. The pain, though it may be of short duration, is almost unbearable. It is deep seated, lancinating and tearing in character. It is worse at night when patient is in recumbent position.

Sleep is impossible. When coughing or blowing the nose, the pain is often increased. Tenderness is often felt just below the ear between the mastoid and the lower jaw, along the course of the eustachian tube. The pain may continue for several hours before rupture of the ear drum, then the pain is suddenly relieved. This is why we should be very careful about giving opiates in these cases, for the pain is nearly all relieved spontaneously when the drum is opened. If the patient is full of opiates we will easily get opium poisoning.

If the pain continues for twelve hours, we should aid nature by opening the ear drum by a free incision. If the pain is intermittent from twelve to forty-eight hours, it should be opened. Early opening and good free drainage will save the hearing and prevent complications, such as mastoid disease, brain abscess and meningitis.

The indications for opening the ear drum are: Continued or severe pain, bulging ear drum, symptoms of mastoid trouble, great loss of hearing. There will be very little pus when the drum is first opened, blood and serum is usually found. Pus occurs about the second day. The character of pus will depend upon the kind of infection. It is much better for the future of the ear drum and hearing to incise the drum with a sharp knife than to have it rupture, especially after long continued pain, for the rupture tears the drum to such an extent that it heals badly and in some cases not at all.

If pain continues after free drainage and quantities of pus, you have mastoid complications and the treatment should be changed to that of mastoiditis.

The treatment of earache is often satisfactory and the ear drum may never need opening. Either there is no pus or it has drained through the eustachian tubes. The patient should be given calomel, followed with a good free cathartic. The external ear should be cleaned thoroughly of all cerumen or debris with peroxide on cotton applicator. Use 10 per cent. phenol solution and glycerine on a small cylinder of cotton packed into the ear loosely against the ear drum. This is much better than to drop the solution into the ear. The glycerine acts as a hydroscopic and the phenol is an antiseptic as well as an anesthetic.

If the nose or throat is sore, attention should be given to that. Very often we have pain referred to the middle ear from disease or soreness in the naso-pharynx. The ear drum is not red or swollen nor the hearing disturbed in these cases.

Pain that continues in the ear or mastoid for two or three days after the ear drum has been opened well, is a very dangerous symptom. It is an indication to open the mastoid.

If there is tenderness over the mastoid for several days after ear has been drained, the mastoid should be opened. Tenderness over mastoid when ear first begins to discharge will often be relieved by antiphlogistic measures such as heat or cold. Continued cold ice pack to ear for two or three days has been the best treatment in my hands. If this pain should recur after a few days or a week, you will most surely have to open and drain the mastoid.

Some of the most aggravating pains we have in the ear are reflex pains. We have spoken of one pain in the naso-pharynx. We sometimes have very acute pain in the ear from disease in the adenoid or tonsil or ulceration in the pharynx. The condition of the eardrum will usually tell us that it is not in the ear. On examination of the throat we are sometimes able to locate the trouble. Cheesy masses in the adenoid or tonsils will cause this pain at times when the mass becomes very large or impacted and the parts swollen around the impaction. This can be seen by close inspection.

The worst reflex pain that I have had and the hardest to locate has been that from the teeth. The wisdom teeth are the most frequent cause and yet it is very hard to say exactly even with the aid of the X-ray whether to remove the tooth or not. The tooth is often not erupted, and the parts around it are healthy. I had a patient recently who had severe pain in the ear for three days and nights; had not slept. X-ray showed impacted wisdom tooth. The dentist did not want to remove a so badly impacted tooth, so he pulled the one in front. The patient was relieved in a few hours.

I had another patient who had severe pain over the mastoid. No symptoms of mastoiditis except the pain. X-ray showed mastoid clear. A film of the lower molar showed impacted wisdom teeth. After extraction the pain in the mastoid soon cleared up.

Another patient who had pain at times in his ear for a week. No other symptoms of an otitis. Examination of the teeth, found tender molar with a small filling. Had the dentist to remove the filling. He found a piece of broach in the root canal. He was instantly relieved when the broach was removed.

KERATOCONUS.*

By W. T. SALMON, M. D., Oklahoma City, Okla.

Upon no other subject so important as conical cornea is there such a dearth of information to be found both in our text-books and journals. This may be due to the fact these cases are so seldom seen, that the pronounced cases are so easily recognized that argument is dispensed with. The cause is yet undetermined, the treatment disappointing and the many proposed operations attended with poor results.

Demours recorded cases of conical cornea as early as 1747, since which time it has been described by many authors, none of which have furnished a satisfactory explanation as to its cause, neither have the many remedies and various operations met with approval.

Up until 1917 there had been an interval of seventeen years in which this subject had not been considered by the American Medical Association. It is remarkable how few cases have been recorded by the prominent oculists; possibly Dr. Edward Jackson has reported more than has come from any other reliable source. He has recorded forty-seven cases during thirty-five years of practice.

Conical cornea is a deformity in which the apex of the cone becomes thinner and projects at a point while the peripheral portion of the cornea may be flattened, thus rendering a portion myopic, decreasing from apex to the bases which may be hyperopic. The apex is usually located below and at the nasal side of the center of the pupil. The cornea is very thin at the apex and if a probe be applied the tissue will be found to yield readily to the pressure and a rythmic, pulsating movement may be observed. The apex may become opaque and there is danger of a rupture, but in the majority of cases remains stationary.

The conditions under which this process begins are often difficult to determine, as they are rarely seen at the beginning. The patients seek advice for visual troubles, short-sightedness and polyopia. At the beginning and during its progress there will be pain and marked symptoms of asthenopia. The pain may be intensified if an attempt is made to correct the near-sightedness by the use of glasses.

The sight is further impaired by astigmatism which produces a great distortion and confusion of the retinal images. Upon inspection of such an eye there is an appearance of a tear-drop suspended in its center which appears unusually glistening and bright, the profile showing the size and shape of the conicity.

However easy a diagnosis may be made in the pronounced cases a cursory observer may easily overlook a slightly developed case or confuse it with myopia or diagnose it as amblyopia. The opthalmoscope is of great assistance in diagnosing even the slightest cases. The light from the opthalmoscope reflects a bright red in the center of the cornea which gradually becomes dark toward the base. Besides a distortion of the retinal images, a considerable parallax may be observed by moving a convex lens in front of the eye.

Direct inspection with the opthalmoscope is usually unsatisfactory, as no lens will afford a continuous field; the vessels appear distorted and broken, the optic nerve shifts with the point of view and is irregularly elongated. The placedo disc gives striking exhibitions of deformity, which astigmatism is so irregular that the opthalmometer furnishes little valued information and with the skiascope the most varied condition of refraction is found to exist close together, in the center is myopia, which quickly changes to hypermetropia.

This process usually begins between the ages of ten and twenty-five, although it may set up much later or may be congenital; there have been instances in which it has occurred in more than one member of the same family.

*Prepared for Section on Eye, Ear, Nose and Throat, Tulsa, May, 1918.

There has been much controversy as to whether the disease was caused by increased intra-ocular pressure or interference with the corneal nutrition. It is difficult to understand how a close observer would attribute it to increased tension, as all cases of uncomplicated conical cornea show a decreased tension. Any condition that might have previously existed to increase the tension is only a speculative opinion without evidence for a premises. The theory of anatomical peculiarity seems to more rationally account for the thinning and bulging. There is an actual anatomical change in the early stage of the process as evidenced by lack of sensitiveness in the cornea.

Innumerable remedies have been proposed for the relief and cure of conical cornea, all of which have been disappointing.

Sir W. Adams removed the lens, and afterward advised breaking up the crystalline lens by needling. Tyrell was the first to make an artificial pupil and advised a peripheral iridectomy. Critchett went one better by allowing the iris to prolapse and tying a ligature around it, thus drawing the pupil to one side. Graefe caused ulceration by shaving off the surface of the apex and then cauterizing with nitrate of silver. Hirschburg advised touching the apex with actual cautery, which procedure has been variously modified by the number of radiating incisions made. L. Webster Fox combines or follows the cauterization with an iridectomy and tattooing the scar. Myer Wiener advocates an excision of a segment of the corneal tissue near the periphery and suturing the wound. The object of nearly all these operations is a reinforcement of the weakened cornea by cicatricial tissue. In other words, the best efforts are the results of an artificial keratitis.

Up to the time of the two cases of which this is a report the prognosis was so universally bad I dismissed the few cases, that sought my advice, without hope of relief from the unfortunate condition.

It is owing to the fact that I received two cases in such a short space of time that I am able to make this report. The first case I sent away with the request that she come to see me again at some future date. I immediately began a review of the literature in the hope that I might find something that would enable me to be of benefit to my patient. As stated in the beginning of this paper, I was disappointed. However, at this time there appeared an article in the *Ophthalmic Record*, by Dr. E. R. Carpenter, which was the only reasonable and hopeful article I was able to find. He advised the use of the high frequency spark applied often enough to produce an interstitial keratitis.

About the time I read this interesting article my second case presented itself. I was fortunate in having an intelligent patient to whom I explained the nature of her trouble and the application of the high frequency spark, to which she readily consented, as any condition was preferable to the present one.

It will be interesting to note the ocular conditions of six other members of the first patient's family treated, as mypoia is thought to play an important role as the cause of conical cornea.

The first of her relatives to consult me was an uncle, G. W. S., Jan. 9th, 1902. Diagnosis: Myopia; R. E. –3.50, L. E. –4.25, comb. –0.25, ax. 180. This patient was very near-sighted and having an inventive mind he suffered much pain from the continued use of his eyes. I saw him at various times during the interval of Jan. 9th, 1902, to 1916, when he died of Bright's disease. Sept. 9th, 1903, Miss Pearl T., sister of patient, consulted me. Diagnosis: Myopia, and the following prescription given: R. E. –1.25, L. E. –1.00. In May, 1908, she consulted me for pain in her eyes. I changed the lenses to R. E. –1.00, comb. –1.00, ax. 180, L. E. –1.00, comb. –0.50, ax. 180, which she is still wearing with comfort. Oct. 10th, 1909, Mrs. T., mother of patient, the following correction: R. E. plus 1.25, L. E. plus 1.25, reading plus 3 in each eye. F. T., her brother, May 25th, 1915. Diagnosis: Myopia; R. E. –3.25, L. E. –3.25. August 17th, 1916, K. S., son of G. W. S. and first cousin to patient. Diagnosis: Myopia; R. E. –2.25, comb. 0.25, ax. 180, L. E. –2.00, comb. –0.50, ax. 180. The latter patient was rejected from the army on account of his eyes. April 25th, 1916, J. S., brother of last patient. Diagnosis: Myopia; R. E. –0.50, ax. 180, L. E. –0.50, ax. 10.

Miss F. T., age 23, Feb. 8, 1915. The cornea of the right eye was thoroughly cocainized and the effluve from a needle point of a high frequency current applied, allowing the spark to strike the conical portion only, just for a second. This was repeated four times and notwithstanding I had instructed that the point not come in contact with the cornea, the warning was not heeded and quite a burn was made on this cornea which lasted for several months but is now only slightly perceptible.

There was considerable reaction and a hypodermic of morphine and atropine was given and the patient instructed to go to bed and apply ice compresses. As was expected, I found my patient suffering intensely next morning, but at the end of two and a half days she was resting easy. Three weeks later I repeated the treatment, managing the point myself so the cornea would not be injured. And again at the end of two months from the second treatment I made the application to the same eye. In the end the results were so beneficial the patient came back Dec. 4, 1915, to have the other eye treated in the same way which, however, was treated only once. March 18, 1916, I examined her eyes and gave the following lenses: R. E. −2.00, ax. 120, L. E. −0.50, comb. cyl. −2.00, ax. 10.

As previously stated, this patient was a teacher of expression and at the time I first saw her, her vision was so poor that she had to give up her position. The vision in the right eye at this time was a little better than counting fingers which was improved with the above lens to 20-100. At the time these lenses were prescribed there was a considerable scar on the right eye caused as mentioned above, and there was much disappointment. This, however, cleared away with fine results. In the left eye there was at first a vision of 20-100 which was improved to 20-40. The results were so satisfactory that she resumed her former occupation as teacher.

In the meantime I had written to my first patient, Miss M. S., requesting an interview at my office. March 16, 1916, her vision in left eye was 20-200, right eye 20-60. On this date I applied the high frequency spark to her left eye and repeated it April 10th and again June 2nd. August 2nd the right eye received one treatment. Sept. 7th I prescribed the following glasses: R. E. −1.75, ax. 135, which gave a vision 20-40; left eye −0.75, combined with cyl. −2.50, ax. 35, which gave a vision of 20-80.

This case moved into the state of Texas in a short time after the above examination was made and I have not been able to learn her address. I have a patient now in the western portion of the state that I am waiting with much expectation to apply the above treatment.

Just here I would like to have this report terminate, but in response to a request for another examination, the first case, Miss F. T., came to my office May 6th and upon examination I found that the great benefit that she had derived was not permanent. The right vision was 20-200 and the left 20-60. This was quite a disappointment but as the immediate effect was so beneficial I am in hopes that the high frequency spark will be the stepping-stone to a permanent cure for this unfortunate condition.

FAMILIAL MACULAR DEGENERATION.

Since its first observation and reporting by R. D. Batten in 1897, a few cases of this condition have been observed and two new ones of the type with dementia are reported by H. S. Clark, Minneapolis (*Journal A. M. A.*, Nov. 30, 1918). It is characterized by symmetrical affections in the two eyes consisting of dark spots in the macula and pallor of the optic nerve heads. It belongs to the type of degenerative diseases such as the amaurotic family idiocy of Tay and Sachs. Combined with this type of macular degeneration they find cases of dementia, the maculocerebral type, such as the cases here described. Summarizing the findings in the cases of macular degeneration with dementia they have been able to form a definite syndrome, though some cases vary in details. Clark is inclined to regard macular degeneration with and macular degeneration without dementia as the same disease. Etiology is unknown and syphilis is strikingly absent.

EYE STRAIN AS A FACTOR IN GASTRIC NEUROSES.*

By ALONZO C. McFARLING, M. D., Shawnee, Okla.

A neurosis may be defined as a functional disturbance of the nervous system dependent upon no discoverable lesion.

The etiology of neuroses in general may be ascribed to the various forms of irritation, either central or peripheral in origin, which are capable of deranging or confusing the normal co-ordination of those central nervous impulses which actuate and control the physiological processes of the body. Of the numerous examples of such irritation which may be cited, eye strain is one which figures largely in the production of neuroses in general and in some cases may be the exciting cause of a gastric neurosis.

In discussing the important role of eye strain in the etiology of gastric neuroses, it is not my purpose to delineate the various forms of heterophoria or refractive errors upon which eye strain is consequent, nor to describe at length the clinical manifestations of such gastric disturbances as may originate therefrom, but I shall attempt to discover the manner in which eye strain may operate through the medium of the brain, to disturb the functions of an organ so remote from the eye as is the stomach.

Since the brain, the great central station of the nervous system, whose complex function serves not only to generate and control the working forces of the body, but spans the chasm which would otherwise separate the spiritual from the physical aspect of the mind, and is the clearing house through which every organ of the body must receive its impulses, I shall therefore review briefly the anatomical and physiological characteristics of the nervous and mental processes by which we perceive those of the forces and forms of energy in the world with which we are cognizant, to-wit: sensation, perception, association, concentration and inhibition.

The fundamental element or unit of the nervous tissue is the neuron, a cell with many processes projecting from it, some short and branching, one, or sometimes two of which often extend a long way and usually becomes the axon of a medullated nerve fiber, and which in some cases gives off a few collateral branches. Both axons and dendrons are composed of delicate fibrillae which pass without interruption through the cell body. Of these neurons, varying in form and size and supported by the delicate frame work of the neuroglia, the entire nervous system is composed.

The fundamental physiological characteristics of the nervous tissues are excitability and transmission, the power of receiving an excitation and not only transmitting it from one end of the neuron to the other, but also, of transmitting it to other neurons with which the first is in anatomical and physiological relationship. By its dendrons the nerve cell receives nervous impulses and by its axons it sends out its own impulses. There is experimental evidence which tends to prove that the activity of a nerve cell is the result of chemical reactions, while the conduction along nerve fibers is mainly a physiological process. The transmission of energy from one neuron to another in contact with it seems to depend upon differences in the tension of this energy in the two neurons. The cellular activity is, therefore easily exhausted, while the activity of the nerve fiber is not easily exhausted. Thus it will be seen that a nerve fiber may continue to transmit impulses received from other cells long after its own cellular exhaustion would have precluded the possibility of modification of such impulse by inhibition or promotion.

When the various impulses have passed along the various tracts and have traversed and been interrupted by several masses of gray matter, they reach the

*Read in Section on Eye, Ear, Nose and Throat, Tulsa, May, 1918.

sensory area of the cerebral cortex, and there give rise to a new form of energy called sensation. That is to say, a physical force is converted in a terminal organ into nervous energy, and as such, having traversed the sensory tracts, reaches the cerebral cortex. It is there transmitted into a new form of energy, as for instance the sensation of light which takes place in the brain—not the eye— and has no similarity to the indulations of either from which it formally originates, and it may indeed be caused not only by these, but also may originate in perfect darkness—from mechanical irritation of the eye, or from the optic nerve. And the same is true of other nerves, thus: if we mechanically irritate the auditory nerve, the impulse will be interpreted in the brain as sound; or if the impulse be given to a motor nerve, we may likewise expect a muscular contraction.

Sensation is the simplest manifestation of consciousness or cognition, and like electricity, requires for its production a certain degree of intensity of the nervous impulses; below this point of intensity the cortex may be in activity, but sensation will not result—the activity will be sub-conscious. A series of these slight impulses may by summation cause sensation. There is, therefore, a minimum of intensity necessary for sensation, just as electricity passing through a wire must have a certain intensity before the wire glows, and light is produced. There is also a maximum, beyond which no matter how great the irritation, there is no increase in sensation, but rather a diminution from exhaustion of the nerve cells. Between this minimum and maximum point, sensibility increases or diminishes by little steps in definite ratio to the stimulus.

Sensation is thus a special individual force produced in the cerebral cortex, and which has its special individual characteristics. A complex manifestation of this force constitutes consciousness and personality. Sensation and all other forms of mental activity are absolutley dependent upon a fairly healthy cerebral cortex, and a fairly abundant blood supply. If the cortex be destroyed in large part, or the blood supply be cut off, then sensation, perception, memory, thought, ethics, association of ideas, etc., are all partially or entirely suspended until such time as the normal blood supply be re-established.

This brings us to the consideration of perceptions and concepts, of which, for the purpose of this paper, it will suffice to say that a perception consists of a combination of sensations, which are received from various sensory nerves and organs, but all of which proceed, usually simultaneously, from the same external object.

Passing to a study of association, we recall the essential physiological characteristics of nervous tissue which are: (1) Its excitability, its reaction to stimulation by the discharge of nervous energy stored within it; and (2) Its transmissibility. This energy when produced does not long remain localized, but tends to pass along nerve fibers throughout its own neuron, and to other neurons. The channels along which it will pass depend upon the anatomical arrangement of the fibers. In consequence of heredity and evolution, certain channels are easier for the passing of this nervous impulse than others. This is especially true of certain reflexes which are present at birth, such as breathing, etc.

When a perception occurs impulses radiate out along the association fibers from that portion of the cortex from which it is produced. If at the same time another perception takes place in another portion of the cortex, the association fibers connecting these two portions of the cortex, being acted upon at the same time, will convey impulses more readily than the other association fibers. The longer and more frequently the association fibers are traversed by these impulses, the better conductors do they become, and these two perceptions become more and more easily excited the one from the other. The activity in the cortex does not long persist, so that when the associated idea is in consciousness, the original perception which awoke it is already, or soon will be, subconscious. Yet they are so firmly associated together, that in the future when one enters into activity, it may excite the other.

At this juncture let us review the more salient features of the process known as concentration. It seems to be a general law in the physiology of the nervous system that when there is a strong activity in one part, the activity of the rest of the nervous system is inhibited. Thus reflex activity can be inhibited by strong pain, and the reflex activity of the spinal cord is more or less inhibited when the brain is in activity. In the brain itself, when a portion of the cortex, or a group of nerve cells is in activity, the activity of the other cortical areas, as well as that of the lower centers, is inhibited. The stronger the local activity, the greater and more extensive will be the general inhibition, and the more this active portion will have a free and uninterrupted field. Naturally, consciousness remains limited to this strong activity for a long time. When an unusual or very vivid perception is in consciousness, it occupies the center of the stage. Consciousness is limited to this one vivid perception or idea and its associations, so that milder activities occurring in the cortex at the same time, which should produce ordinarily, perceptions and associations, remain sub-conscious. This phenomenon is called concentration, and is a very important function in nervous physiology, since the laws governing the same are applicable not only to consciousness, but to the subconscious processes as well, many of which have to do with the regulation of those important physiological processes and functions, whose sum total constitute the physical aspect of the phenomenon we call life.

Before pursuing further and in connection with our study of inhibition, it will be remembered that our study of sensation discloses the fact that when a perception or sensation occurs at a given point in the cortex, the energy or impulse does not long remain localized, but travels along the fibers of its own neuron, and by the association fibers to other neurons. Hence, it will be seen that when a nerve cell, or cell unit, in sending out impulses to an organ of the body, or to a muscle, or group of muscles, over whose functions it is its duty to preside, does not possess the ability to limit such impulse to that particular muscle or organ for which it was normally intended; but on the other hand unavoidably transmits a portion of such impulse to those nerve cells, or cell units which are in anatomical and physiological relationship with it. This law of the transmission of impulses is an invariable one, which fact does not preclude the possibility of an impulse radiating from a given point in the cerebral cortex, to a contiguous cell or cell unit, which impulse, if elaborated and promoted by the synergic action of the contiguous cell, would be antagonistic or detrimental to the normal function of that muscle, or organ, over which such contiguous cell unit presides. It does not necessarily follow, however, that such association impulse would be promoted by the contiguous cell, but instead, would in the normal physiological course of events, be neutralized according to this same law of the transmission of impulses, by other impulses generated and sent out by the contiguous cell in the regular performance of its duty. This constitutes what we call inhibition, and may in some degree be likened unto the rights of citizenship under the laws of a democracy whose constitution accords to every citizen the right to follow the bent of his own mind in the pursuit of happiness and the acquisition of wealth so long as such pursuits do not interfere with the rights of others. Thus it may be seen that if two cell units in the cortex in anatomical relationship with each other be in simultaneous activity, their respective association impulses will, if they be of the same degree of intensity, exactly neutralize each other. But, if the impulse originating in one cell unit be abnormally strong, then that portion of energy which travels by the association fibers will be proportionately stronger, and will override the weaker associational impulse which it may meet, and will, therefore, succeed in reaching the other cell unit, and there register itself as a distinct impulse.

Now then, let us assume that the cell unit, from which this stronger impulse originates, is the organization of cells which controls the physiological functions of the eyes. Let us assume further, the existence of a muscular imbalance, or a refractive error, or both, in a degree approaching the maximum amount which can be corrected by the ocular muscles. It is a well known fact that the brain will not tolerate anything in such a case, save perfect, single, binocular vision. It is self-evident, then, that the exaggerated muscular contractions necessary to correct this visual defect must necessarily be actuated and maintained by correspondingly exaggerated impulses from the brain centers which control the musculature of the eyes.

It is also evident that by reason of this greater activity, more blood will be attracted to these oculomotor centers than would be demanded for normal work, in consequence of which there will be a diminution of the normal blood supply of the adjacent tissues and a proportionate reduction in the inhibitive influence which these adjacent centers would normally exercise toward the excited oculomotor centers. It is equally obvious that these exaggerated motor impulses, radiating in rapid succession from the oculo-motor centers, will, by association, reach and register themselves upon all the adjacent cells with which they are in anatomical and physiological relationship.

Since the gray matter possesses the inherent faculty of summation, it necessarily follows that when these impulses have been repeated a sufficient number of times, sensation will result—the nature of which will be determined in each instance by the normal function of the cell so affected. Thus, in case a motor nerve cell were so influenced, the result would be an involuntary contraction of the muscle which it supplies; if a sensory cell, pain may be excited; if a cell unit controlling a gland or organ, then we may expect some alteration in the nature or amount of the secretion of the gland, or a perversion of the function of the organ so supplied.

In view of the fact that the intensity of a sensation occurring at a given point is in a direct ratio to the stimulus, we may safely assume the existence of a ratio between the intensity of the sensation and the impulses which may go out from the central cell receiving the sensation.

Hence, if the exaggerated impulses radiating from the oculo-motor centers in their exaggerated effort at correcting the visual defects assumed in our hypothetical case be capable of transmission by association to all the adjacent cells with which they are in relationship, thus confusing and causing them to send out impulses, at variance with their normal functions, we may likewise expect their confusion and excitement to spread to still other cells.

Since the incentive to perfect vision is absolutely constant in the brain, and since this state of confusion and excitement does not depend upon the intensity of one impulse or sensation, but rather upon their frequent repetition over a long period of time, we may safely assume the possibility and probability of this excitement spreading from cell to cell until the entire working forces of the brain would be thrown into a functional discord. In consequence of this incoordination of the working forces of the brain which control and regulate the vital functions incident to life, will necessarily follow the incoordination of the functions themselves.

By way of condensing and summing up the foregoing arguments, we may conclude: First, the nerve centers which control the normal functions of the body exercise a normal inhibitive influence toward each other, which eventuates in the proper co-ordination of these functions; and second, any form of irritation, either central or peripheral in origin, whose intensity is of a degree above the minimum required for sensation in the particular cell involved, if sufficiently prolonged will derange the normal inhibition of the cells, as a result of which the impulses radiating from a cell subjected to such irritation, being of a much higher degree of intensity than normally required, will be super-imposed upon all the cells with which that cell is in anatomical and physiological relationship.

If at this point we recall the fact that the ocular muscles derive their nerve supply from the third, fourth and sixth cranial nerves, while the stomach is supplied by the pneumogastric nerve, all of which have their origin in nuclei situated beneath the aqueduct of sylvius in the floor of the fourth ventricle, we may in the light of the foregoing deductions reasonably conclude that in this manner eye strain, when present, may be instrumental in the production of, and in some cases may be the exciting cause of, a gastric neurosis.

JOURNAL OF THE OKLAHOMA STATE MEDICAL ASSOCIATION

VOLUME XII   MUSKOGEE, OKLA., JANUARY, 1919   NUMBER 1

PUBLISHED MONTHLY AT MUSKOGEE. OKLA., UNDER DIRECTION OF THE COUNCIL

DR. CLAUDE A. THOMPSON, EDITOR-IN-CHIEF

ENTERED AT THE POST OFFICE AT MUSKOGEE, OKLAHOMA, AS SECOND CLASS MAIL MATTER, JULY 26, 1912

THIS IS THE OFFICIAL JOURNAL OF THE OKLAHOMA STATE MEDICAL ASSOCIATION. ALL COMMUNICATIONS SHOULD BE ADDRESSED TO THE JOURNAL OF THE OKLAHOMA STATE MEDICAL ASSSOCIATION. 308 SURETY BUILDING, MUSKOGEE, OKLAHOMA.

The editorial department is not responsible for the opinions expressed in the original articles of contributors.

Reprints of original articles will be supplied at actual cost, provided request for them s attached to manuscript or made in sufficient time before publication.

Articles sent this Journal for publication and all those read at the annual meetings of the State Association are the sole property of this Journal. The Journal relies on each individual contributor's strict adherence to this well-known rule of medical journalism. In the event an article sent this Journal for publication is published before appearance in the Journal, the manuscript will be returned to the writer

Failure to receive the Journal should call for immediate notification of the editor, 307-8 Surety Building, Muskogee, Okla

Local news of possible interest to the medical profession, notes on removals, changes in address, deaths and weddings will be gratefully received.

Advertising of articles, drugs or compounds unapproved by the Council on Pharmacy of the A. M. A. will not be accepted.

Advertising rates will be supplied on application. It is suggested that wherever possible members of the State Associa tion should patronize our advertisers in preference to others as a matter of fair reciprocity.

EDITORIAL

"WHEN JOHNNY COMES MARCHING HOME."

In the next few weeks many scores of Oklahoma physicians will return to the homes they left to enter the Army as volunteers to take up the necessary work of whipping into shape the physical development and improvement of the men who comprised our army.

It goes without saying that most of them will be sincerely glad to get back t o the friends and life work they left behind them. The spontaneous answer of nearly thirty-five thousand American physicians to war service needs no comment as pointing to the calibre and ideals of the American doctor. No comment is needed to call the attention of the thinking and informed public to the fact that he was nearer "Preparedness" than any other branch of the army, that he mostly fitted into his assignment as comfortably and smoothly as a kind old shoe. All of this demonstrating his worth as a citizen of the greatest nation and his value to the people from whence he sprang. Clouds do have silver linings and from what is undeniably bad there often springs some good. These men, many of them, come home knowing more about system, appreciating more than ever otherwise would have been possible the value of promptness, two elements often utterly absent in our doctors, which will fit them better for the future. Many of them will come home better physicians than before for the reason that the advantages of assignment to special work along technical lines was given them and they were thrown into intimate contact with our best pacemakers. True, many of them have had little to do, and it is natural that they will have their "mouthings" over the fact that they were sent to some cantonment instead of right on over as they expected and proudly thought and announced on leaving home for the "front." But all could not go, some were needed here, others wholly unfitted for foreign service while they could do good work at home.

Two facts should be borne in mind. No returning physician should be put to the pain and injustice of realizing that in his absence his place has been usurped by some other physician. As far as possible his patients should at least be given every opportunity—and in the best of good faith—to know that he has returned, that he left as a rule at a sacrifice, that unlike every other branch of the service men could not be "drafted" to supply the need he filled, so be it he stepped into the breach without much urging, leaving at home to others the accumulation of wealth and the enjoyment of comfortable homes.

We have heard much lately of doctors' "trusts." There never was one, but now would be a good time to accentuate to the braying asses who assert there is a trust, the real worth and indispensibility of·the doctor to good, safe citizenship. These gentry who lurk around our legislative halls and make slanderous and unsupported statements about the medical profession should now be told where to head in, and while the enforcement of the telling with a good strong, right, military left hook to the mouth is not considered good form, we believe that when the stupendous and otherwise unavailable services rendered by our profession is shown the people, they will appreciate that ours is not necessarily a pacifist profession and will applaud the means to the proper end.

Suppose we make it our business in the next few months to see that our returning doctor is treated squarely, and that our profession be accorded its proper place, not as compensation for what has been done—we will do that and more again when necessary—but by reason of right and common sense.

PERSONAL AND GENERAL NEWS

Dr. E. H. Troy, Wilburton, was reported seriously ill in December.

Dr. R. E. Weller, Pawnee, writes an interesting letter to his friends from Hakodate, Japan.

Captain F. M. Sanger, M. C., Oklahoma City, has been discharged and returned to his home.

Dr. H. W. Doty, Watonga, has received his discharge from the army and returned to his location.

Dr. C. A. Hess, Idabel, received a German helmet from Dr. L. H. Hill who is with the A. E. F. in Germany.

Captain S. J. Fryer, Muskogee, visited his old home in December, while on leave from Camp Sheridan, Ala.

Dr. T. J. Colley, Hominy, underwent an operation in Oklahoma City recently for the reduction of a fracture of the arm.

Dr. Thos. T. Clohessy, formerly of Berlin, has been discharged from army service at Ft. Riley and will probably locate in Sayre.

Dr. E. T. Butler, a negro physician of Muskogee, was given a life sentence by the jury which tried him for murdering another negro physician, Dr. J. M. Davis.

On Duty Overseas. The Journal is advised that Drs. Walter W. Wells, Horace Reed and J. H. Maxwell reached France in November. It is not stated if they know when they are to return.

Dr. C. R. Hume, Anadarko, received news in November of the safe arrival in France of his son, Dr. R. R. Hume, Minco. Dr. Hume was detached from his command and delayed by reason of influenza.

Dr. Millington Smith, Oklahoma City, spent a month hunting in Southern Texas during November and December, incidentally attempting to regain much lost vitality from an attack of influenza.

Dr. J. T. Martin, city physician, Oklahoma City, secured several hundred doses of influenza vaccine on his trip to Chicago to attend the Health conference and placed the product at the disposal of physicians in December.

Drs. H. A. Lile and T. A. Rhodes, Cherokee, advise that they expect to be released from army duty soon and will return to open the Cherokee Hospital. Both are captains and stationed at Camps McArthur and Funston, respectively.

Drs. LeRoy Long, E. S. Ferguson, S. R. Cunningham, L. J. Moorman and J. F. Kuhn have been appointed an advisory committee to assist Dr. J. T. Martin in handling the health situation of Oklahoma City. Drs. N. E. Lawson and R. S. McCabe were named as assistant city physicians.

Dr. E. F. Lovejoy, Oklahoma City, was sentenced to 30 days in jail and a fine of $500.00 by an Oklahoma County jury. His attorneys gave notice of appeal. He was charged with causing the death of a young woman by the performance of a criminal operation. Verily the ways of our "Peers" are past understanding.

Dr. J. T. Martin, Oklahoma City, newly appointed Superintendent of Health, fully agrees with Commissioner of Public Safety, Mike Donnelly, that kissing is a fruitful source of spreading any contagion, "particularly Spanish Influenza;" but the sage of medicine, though much younger than "Mike," observes "What's the use—nobody will quit kissing."

DR. D. E. WILSON.

Dr. D. E. Wilson, Elmer, one of Jackson County's oldest physicians, died at his home November 29, 1918, from influenza, after an illness of eight days. Dr. Bob Wilson, his son, was with him at the time of death. Dr. Wilson was born in Marion County, Arkansas, May 4, 1849, moving to Oklahoma with his family in 1888, homesteading a farm a few miles from Hess where he practiced until his removal to Elmer a few years ago. He leaves a large number of relatives and behind him the reputation of a man who will be missed as one of his country's best citizens and a prince among men.

DR. ANDREW L. WAGONER.

Dr. Andrew L. Wagoner, Hobart, died at his home December 26th from cerebral hemorrhage after an illness of only a few hours.

Oklahoma loses a splendid man and physician by the demise of Doctor Wagoner. He had the rare attribute of always fearlessly deprecating shams and smallness wherever he encountered them and stood for high and ethical ideals in medicine.

He was born in 1868, coming to Oklahoma and locating at Hobart in 1908, where he had lived and practiced continuously since. Since the war he had been Chairman of the Local Board for Kiowa County and rendered unceasing labor to his country.

Oklahoma Medical Officers returning. The Journal is in receipt of the information that the following medical officers are returning to their homes by reason of discharge from the Army: R. R. Culbertson, Maud; A. S. Graydon, Idabel; H. A. Lile, Cherokee; T. A. Rhodes, Cherokee; J. C. Matheny, Lindsay; J. L. Fortson, Tecumseh; J. M. Nieweg, Duncan; H. W. Doty, Watonga; Thos. T. Clohessy, Berlin; Captain F. M. Sanger, Oklahoma City; Major A. L. Blesh, Oklahoma City; Captain A. L. Guthrie, Oklahoma City; Captain F. E. Warterfield, Oklahoma City; Captain G. A. Wall, Tulsa; Lieut. R. A. Douglas, Tulsa; Lieut. V. L. McPherson, Boswell; Lieut. W. A. Moreland, McCurtain; Captain Benton Lovelady, Guthrie; Captain D. M. Lawson, Nowata; Lieut. P. B. Myers, Apache; Lieut. Edw. Abernathy, Altus; Lieut. J. C. Luster, Davis; Captain J. H. Scott, Shawnee; Lieut. H. O. Bailey, Sulphur; Lieut. D. F. Coldiron, Perry; Lieut. S. H. Landrum, Altus; Lieut. E. L. Milligan, Geary.

Attorney General Freeling, in an opinion to Senator E. M. Kerr of Muskogee who is seeking means to enact legislation preventing the duplication of effort in public health matters where cities and counties are jointly concerned, advises that the legislature may not legally enact a law taking from cities the right to appoint and provide for their own health officers; that such a right is a constitutional one in Oklahoma and therefore not reviewable by the legislature. He holds, however, that the lawmakers may pass an act requiring to the minutest detail any reasonable services from employes of cities, specifying every duty usually required of health officers.

Tulsa County Medical Society elected 1919 officers December 16, as follows: President, Dr. G. A. Wall, who has just returned from Army service at Camp McArthur; O. F. Beasley, vice-president, A. W. Pigford, secretary, who is still in the army. The delegates are Drs. H. D. Murdock, retiring president, S. De Zell Hawley and J. Walter Beyer.

Pontotoc County Medical Society elected 1919 officers as follows: President, L. M. Overton, Fitzhugh; vice-president, B. F. Sullivan, Ada; secretary, S. P. Ross, Ada; Drs. C. L. Orr, W. D. Faust, Ada, and Fred Harrison, Stonewall, were selected as censors.

Dr. L. S. Willour, Major in the Medical Corps, stationed in France, has charge of the surgical work of a large hospital, getting there on time to participate in the final cleaning up and care of the casualties. He hopes to be home soon.

Lieutenant Frank H. McGregor, Mangum, who we noted some time ago had been decorated for distinguished bravery in action, has been promoted to a Captaincy. He is with the British forces in Flanders.

Dr. J. M. Alford, Oklahoma City, Captain, M. C., stationed at Camp Beauregard, was reported seriously ill in December.

CORRESPONDENCE

FROM CAPT. J. HOY SANFORD.

Camp Custer, Mich., Saturday, Dec. 28, 1918.

My dear Dr. Thompson:

If it is customary for the doctors in the service to send in their dues for the coming year, please let me know and I will forward the amount to you. I am located at Custer and have been for the last nine months. I was called for overseas on three eifferent occasions, but was held up each time, can you beat it? I have been Chief of the G. U. service here for the last few months and from the looks of things I will be here for some little time to come. Rumor is going around that I am to be sent to some big reconstruction hospital as Chief of the G. U. service, but there is nothing authentic. Have been doing some very interesting work here and gained a most wonderful experience. I personally do all of the bladder and kidney work and we make the following routine examination of every urological case: Cystoscopy, ureteral catheterization with x-ray catheters, examination of the catheterized specimen, x-ray with the catheters in situ, distention of the renal pelvis with opaque fluid (using 25 per cent. sodium bromide with success), renal functional test, and where indicated renal pelvic lavage. You can see that we give every case a pretty thorough examination. I have three doctors working in my service and we have things well systematized. Capt. Eisendrath of Chicago is here and is certainly a fine surgeon. He was talking of you to me some time ago and I told him I knew you very well. He will most probably be sent to some big reconstruction hospital as chief of the surgical service. I am anxious to return to my practice, but I suppose I will return when the Government sees fit. I have picked up physically in the Army and have been repaid for my sacrifice professionally as I feel like I have been wonderfully benefitted. I like the Army and were I single I surely would select the Army for the future. Give my best regards to all of the "Docs" and tell them some day I will be back.

Trusting to hear from you in the near future and hoping that you are well and happy and busy, I remain,   Fraternally yours,
                                                                              Capt. J. H. Sanford, M. C.

MISCELLANEOUS

STERILIZING THE NASOPHARYNX.

Evidence is accumulating of the value of Dakin's antiseptics for sterilizing the throat and nose of persons exposed or suffering from Spanish influenza and other diseases transmitted by the secretions of the upper respiratory tract. The simplest and most convenient of these remedies to use is Chlorazene, which is available in tablet form for the preparation of aqueous solutions, which may be used for spraying or gargling. Such solutions are convenient, can be made up by anyone with ordinary intelligence, and are exceedingly efficient.

When possible the aqueous solution should be supplemented by the oil spray of Dichloramine-T dissolved in Chlorcosane, a 1- to 2-per cent. solution being employed for this purpose. This should be applied at least twice daily, where possible by the physician himself or by the nurse. The use of Dichloramine-T assures prolonged contact with the mucous membrane of an exceedingly powerful germicide, which can be used without danger to the patient. The extensive experimental work conducted by The Abbott Laboratories, preliminary to placing the Dakin products at the disposal of American physicians, seems to be justified by the splendid results which are being obtained.

WARIZEL!

A friend in the War Risk Insurance Department, in Washington, sends Luke a few of the questions received by the department and some of the answers received to queries sent out by the Department. Here they are:

"I ain't got no book lurnin', and am writin' for inflamation."

"I have a four-months-old babay and he is my only support.

"I am his wife and only air."

"I received your insurance polish."

"I have a child seven months old and she is a baby and can't work."

"Caring to my condition which I haven't walked in 3 months from a broke leg whose number is 975."

"I was discharged from the army as I have goiter which I was sent home on."

"Both sides of our parents are old and poor."

"Dear Mr. Wilson: I have already written to Mr. Headquarters and got no reply. Now if I don't hear from you I will write to Uncle Sam himself."

"My son is in the middle of the Mediterranean Sea."

"I have another war baby. How much do I get."

"Please return my marriage certificate. My baby hassent eaten any for two days."

"I am a window with a wife and four children."

"I do not know my husband has a middle name and if he has I don't believe it is 'None.' "

"I need his assisatcne to keep me in closed."

"Please send me a wifes form."

"I have been in bed for 13 years with one doctor and I intend to get another."

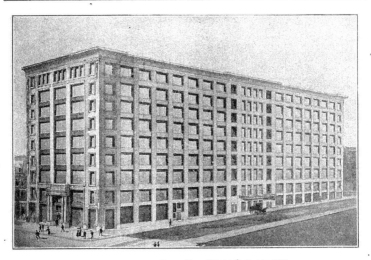

NEW HOME OF THE H. K. MULFORD COMPANY.

Having outgrown their present Pharmaceutical Laboratories, the H. K. Mulford Company have purchased and will soon occupy the modern building, located at Broad, Wallace and Fifteenth Streets, on Philadelphia's main thoroughfare, six blocks north from City Hall. The building is of modern construction, being fireproof throughout, of steel, concrete and stone, nine stories in height and has a total floor space of nearly ten acres.

All equipment is of the latest type used in building construction and includes four electric passenger elevators, four electric freight elevators, with a capacity of twelve tons; four enclosed fire towers for the safety of the occupants; electric generating machine; mail chutes; artesian wells, etc.

The structure will be further equipped with modern labor-saving devices and when occupied will house the general offices and the drug, chemical and pharmaceutical departments which are now distributed over a number of buildings in several locations.

This will be the largest building in the world devoted exclusively to the production of medicinal products. It will be a worthy peer of the Mulford Biological Laboratories, located at Glenolden, Pa., which are recognized as the largest and most complete in existence.

The rapidly increasing business at home and abroad has necessitated this expansion and the new premises will enable the H. K. Mulford Company to fulfill the long cherished aim of making the *Mulford Standard of Service* equal the *Mulford Standard of Quality.*

CAMOUFLAGE.

The call for volunteers in the medical service of the Army has brought out some stimulating examples of courage and patriotic loyalty; but it has also uncovered some cowards and unpatriotic slackers who are beneath the contempt of decent folk.

For instance: A man, so called, of the age of forty, able bodied and well equipped for good service, insofar as his preparation for the practice of medicine is concerned, with no dependents and with the medical needs of his community well provided for by reason of the presence of a good physician who cannot go into service, signs his application for membership in the Medical Service Corps and makes special mention of the fact that he prefers overseas service. As soon as his blank has been forwarded to Washington, he slyly proceeds to secure the services of several girls to circulate a petition among the people, begging the Surgeon-General to not deprive the community of the benefit of his invaluable and indispensable services.

Camouflage. Rotten camouflage!

And there have been others. The day of reckoning will surely come for all such.

—Tennessee Medical Journal.

This "coarse" work is not confined to Tennessee alone. Oklahoma has some rare specimens of the genus Assinus Medicus, who thought they were putting something over on the public when they applied for commissions, paraded the corridors and streets, sought scare head publicity by nauseating write-ups in local papers and then discovered they could not sacrifice their precious time to the Nation on account of pressing needs at home.

"CHIROS" AND APPENDICITIS.

Strange things do happen. The Chiropractors are trying to get favoragle legislation. Recently we saw some of the results of those "rubbing doctors" in two cases of appendicitis cited us by Dr. Border at the Hospital. Rev. Crumley had been treated by a "Chiro" for appendicitis. He came down here after his case became so awfully bad that death stared him in the face. When his appendix was examined there was silent proof of the violent rubbing, in its bursted and terrible inflamed condition. Rev. Crumley died because he had not had the right kind of attention at the right time, so the physicians report. A short time later Rev. Crumley's daughter took appendicitis and was at once brought to the Border Hospital for an operation. She is now well and in excellent health. We think there is small reason in giving more laxity to such methods above practised by the "rubbers."—Mangum Star.

COUNCIL ON PHARMACY AND CHEMISTRY
Articles Accepted

National Pathological Laboratories: Rabies Vaccine (Harris).

Schering and Glatz: Creosote Carbonate, S. and G.; Guaiacol Carbonate, S. and G.

NEW AND NONOFFICIAL REMEDIES.

Lutein Tablets-H. W. and D., 2 Grains. Each tablet contains 2 grains of lutein (the fully developed corpora lutea of the hog, dried and powdered). Hynson, Westcott and Dunning, Baltimore, Md. (Jour. A. M. A., Nov. 2, 1918, p. 1485).

Rabies Vaccine (Harris). An antirabic vaccine standardized by the method of Dr. Harris and stored in vacuo. Each package contains vaccine and apparatus for the administration of one complete treatment. One dose is given daily for ten days or more. National Pathological Laboratories, Chicago (Jour. A. M. A., Nov. 30, 1918, p 1825).

PROPAGANDA FOR REFORM
(Report in Part)

Digestive Absurdities. Scientific investigations have demonstrated beyond any doubt the irrationality of the combinations of digestive ferments which go to make up the various brands of aromatic digestive tablets, and all chemists and manufacturing pharmacists are familiar with these facts. The excuse for manufacturing them is that there is a call for them. It is a question whether the physician who ignorantly prescribes aromatic digestive tablets is not more morally culpable than the pharmaceutical house that supplies what such physicians demand (Jour. A. M. A., Nov. 2, 1918, p. 1489).

Value of Vaccination Against Influenza. There is no conclusive evidence that the Pfeiffer bacillus plays any greater role, if as great, in the present epidemic than any other bacteria found in the respiratory tract in this disease. Also, the influenza bacillus is a very poor antigen. There is, in fact, nothing to show that definite antibodies against this bacillus develop in the course of influenza. Animal experiments show that it requires prolonged immunization before any response becomes apparent. Again, there is no record of controlled experiments on human beings with influenza vaccine. From this it is evident that vaccination against influenza is in a wholly experimental stage (Jour. A. M. A., Nov. 9, 1918, p. 1583).

More Misbranded Nostrums. The following "patent medicines" have been declared misbranded under the U. S. Food and Drugs Act, and a "Notice of Judgment" giving an account of the prosecutions issued by the U. S. Department of Agriculture for each: Jacob's Liver Salt, an effervescent preparation consisting largely of soduim phosphate, sodium sulphate, and sodium chlorid. Lydia Pinkham's Vegetable Compound, containing 17.9 per cent. alcohol, and 0.56 gm. of solids to each 100 cc., with vegetable extractive material present. Maguire's Extract of Benne Plant and Catechu Compound, containing over 39 per cent. of alcohol and 1-10 grain of morphin to each fluidounce, besides camphor, catechu and peppermint. Hood's Sarsaparilla, a mixture of alcohol and water, containing about 0.9 per cent. of potassium iodid with sugar, vegetable extractives, which give indications of the presence of sarsaparilla, licorice, and a laxative drug resembling senna. Booth's Hyomei Dri-Ayr, consisting essentially of oil of eucalyptus, together with a small amount of resin-like solids and a mineral oil and a little alcohol. Hill's Kidney Kaskara Tablets, an iron oxid, sugar-coated tablet carrying emodin, caffein, acid resin, magnesium carbonate and talcum. Hancock Sulphur Compound, a calcium sulphid solution. Hancock Sulphur Compound Ointment, a petrolatum ointment containing sulphur, ash (chiefly lime) abd phenol. Palmer's Skin Whitener, containing amoniated mercury, mixed with a fatty base. Grossman's Specific Mixture, a balsam copiaba mixture (Jour. A. M. A., Nov. 16, 1918, p. 1681).

A Short Sighted Druggist. A correspondent writes: "I went to a nearby drug store and asked for twenty-five cents' worth of Liquor Antisepticus Alkalinus; I got one ounce! The druggist charged me fifteen cents an ounce, and ten cents for the container. Next time I fear I shall be forced to get Glycothymoline." To penalize a man who calls for an official product so as to drive him to ask for a "patent medicine" of the same general character is both poor pharmacy and bad business (Jour. A. M. A., Nov. 23, 1918, p. 1745).

Kennedy's Tonic Port. Kennedy's Tonic Port was booze sold as "patent medicine." Its conflict with the law came when a bottle of the preparation was sold at a Regina drug store in November, 1917, in that the sale of alcoholic beverages is prohibited in Saskatchewan. The Saskatchewan authorities proceeded against this concern, and the drug store proprietors were convicted and fined. They appealed the case, but the judge before whom the appeal was heard decided against the concern and increased the fine. Booze is booze in Saskatchewan (Jour. A. M. A., Nov. 23, 1918, p. 1763).

Compound Solution of Cresol. In an eastern institution where members of the U. S. hospital corps are being instructed, a bottle containing Liquor Cresolis Compositus is labeled "Lysol" so that doctors may recognize it. Comment is superfluous (Jour. A. M. A., Nov. 30, 1918, p. 1830).

Autolysin and Beer. Henry Smith Williams, who exploits "Proteal Therapy," also runs a publishing concern, the Goodhue Company, and has associated with him his brother, Edward Huntington Williams. Some time ago, complimentary copies of a book, "Alcohol, Hygiene and Legislation," written by Edward Huntington Williams, and published by the Goodhue Company, were sent broadcast to physicians with the compliments of author and publisher. The book championed the lighter alcoholic beverages and questioned the value of prohibition. Enclosed with the book was an advertising leaflet on the "Autolysin" cancer cure and a letter calling attention to a book by Henry Smith Williams on the Autolysin Treatment of Cancer. Now the secretary of the United States Brewers' Association has testified before a Senate Committee, according to newspaper reports, that a "Dr. Edward H. Williams" was employed to write articles "relating to the brewers' trade." Is the Dr. Edward Huntington Williams who wrote "Alcohol, Hygiene and Legislation" the "Dr. Edward H. Williams" who was employed by the brewers to write propagnda favorable to the brewing interests? Was the cloth-bound book, "Alcohol, Hygiene and Legislation," paid for, wholly or in part, by the United States Brewers' Association? (Jour. A. M. A., Nov. 30, 1918, p. 1846).

TONSIL INFECTIONS.

H. J. Nichols and J. H. Bryan, Washington, D. C. (*Journal A. M. A.*, Nov. 30, 1918), have studied the hemolytic streptococcus infections and are convinced that the tonsils play a part that should be emphasized. Swab cultures were made from various portions of the air passages, and the results pointed strongly to the tonsils as the foci of infection. Additional evidences as to their importance in carriers were found in the results of throat cultures taken after tonsillectomy. The removal of the diseased tonsil is, in their opinion, a necessity in carriers for the good of others, and they summarize their conclusions as follows: "1. The tonsils are the principal foci of infection in throat carriers of *Streptococcus hemolyticus*. (a) Cultures taken from different parts of the nose, mouth and throat show more streptococci in the tonsils than elsewhere. (b) Cultures from excised tonsils show streptococci in 75 per cent. of cases. (c) Crypt cultures show a higher percentage of positive results than surface cultures. (d) Excision of the tonsils renders the throat negative in nearly all cases. 2. The streptococci isolated from tonsils and throats show no cultural difference on sugar mediums from those obtained from empyema fluids. 3. Excision is the only radical method of curing carriers of the infection. (a) Dobell's solution, dichloramin-T and hot alcohol had little better effect than no treatment. (b) Silver nitrate, 25 per cent., gave the better results in negative throat cultures, but the crypts frequently remained positive. 4. The presence of hemolytic streptococci in pathologic tonsils is an additional reason for their removal."

INFLUENZA VACCINE

H. L. Barnes, Wallum Lake, R. I. (*Journal A. M. A.*, Dec. 7, 1918), reports his experience with the influenza vaccine furnished by Dr. Timothy Leary of the Tuft's College Medical School, at the Wallum Lake Sanatorium. The epidemic attacked the institution early in October and spread throughout the population, till there had been a total of eighty-two cases, or 25 per cent. of the total population. Counting all cases that occurred both before and after vaccination, forty-five, or 40 per cent. developed influenza. In computing the incidence of the disease for comparison between vaccinated and unvaccinated, no cases were counted that developed before the vaccine was given and no patient counted as vaccinated until he had received the three doses. Before the arrival of the vaccine eight cases that terminated fatally, had developed. Deducting children who were quarantined and so far as known not exposed, the influenza incidence was 20 per cent. The conclusion reached is that the morbidity was only slightly lower among the vaccinated, and the mortality from influenza was practically the same among vaccinated and unvaccinated patients.

OFFICERS OF OKLAHOMA STATE MEDICAL ASSOCIATION.

President—Dr. L. S. Willour, McAlester (A. E. F. in France).
President-elect—Dr. L. J. Moorman, Oklahoma City.
1st Vice-President,—Dr. E. D. James, Miami.
2nd Vice- President—Dr. H. M. Williams, Wellston.
3rd Vice-President,—Walter Hardy, Ardmore.
Delegate to A. M. A., 1919-1920—LeRoy Long, Oklahoma City.
Meeting place, Muskogee—May 20-21-22, 1919 Headquarters, Hotel Severs. For details address
Dr. A. L. Stocks, Barnes Building, Muskogee.

CHAIRMEN OF SCIENTIFIC SECTIONS.

Surgery and Gynecology—A. A. Will, Oklahoma City.
Pediatrics and Obstetrics—Vice Chairman, O. A. Flanagan, 305 Bliss Bldg., Tulsa.
Eye, Ear, Nose and Throat—R. O. Early, Ardmore.
General Medicine, Nervous and Mental Diseases—F. W. Ewing, Muskogee.
Genitourinary, Skin and Radiology—R. T. Edwards, Oklahoma City.
Legislative Committee—Dr. Millington Smith, Oklahoma City; Dr. J. M. Byrum, Shawnee;
Dr. W. T. Salmon, Oklahoma City.
For the Study and Control of Cancer—Drs. LeRoy Long, Oklahoma City; Gayfree Ellison,
Norman; D. A. Myers, Lawton.
For the Study and Control of Pellagra—Drs. A. A. Thurlow, Norman; L. A. Mitchell, Frederick;
J. C. Watkins, Checotah.
For the Study of Venereal Diseases—Drs. Wm. J. Wallace, Oklahoma City; Ross Grosshart
Tulsa; J. E. Bercaw, Okmulgee.
Necrology—Drs. Martha Bledsoc, Chickasha; J. W. Pollard, Bartlesville.
Tuberculosis—Drs. L. J. Moorman, Oklahoma City; C. W. Heitzman, Muskogee; Leila E.
Andrews, Oklahoma City.
Conservation of Vision—Drs. L. A. Newton, Oklanoma City; L. Haynes Buxton, Oklahoma
City; G. E. Hartshorne, Shawnee.
Hospital Committee—F. S. Clinton, Tulsa; M. Smith, Oklahoma City; C. A. Thompson,
Muskogee.
Committee on Medical Education—Drs. A. L. Blesh; A. K. West; A. W. White, Oklahoma City.
State Commissioner of Health—Dr. John W. Duke, Guthrie, Oklahoma

COUNCILOR DISTRICTS.

District No. 1. Texas, Beaver, Cimarron, Harper, Ellis, Woods, Woodward, Alfalfa, Major,
Grant, Garfield, Noble and Kay. G. A. Boyle, Enid.
District No. 2. Dewey, Roger Mills, Custer, Beckham, Washita, Greer, Kiowa, Harmon, Jackson and Tillman. Ellis Lamb, Clinton.
District No. 3. Blaine, Kingfisher, Canadian, Logan, Payne, Lincoln, Oklahoma, Cleveland,
Pottawatomie, Seminole and McClain. G. M. Maupin, Waurika.
District No. 4. Caddo, Grady, Comanche, Cotton, Stephens, Jefferson, Garvin, Murray, Carter,
and Love. J. T. Slover, Sulphur.
District No. 5. Pontotoc, Coal, Johnston, Atoka, Marshall, Bryan, Choctaw, Pushmataha
and McCurtain. J. L. Austin, Durant.
District No. 6. Okfuskee, Hughes, Pittsburg, Latimer, LeFlore, Haskell and Sequoyah. Vacant.
District No. 7. Pawnee, Osage, Washington, Tulsa, Creek, Nowata and Rogers. N. W. Mayginnis, Tulsa.
District No. 8. Craig, Ottawa, Delaware, Mayes, Wagoner, Cherokee, Adair, Okmulgee, Muskogee and McIntosh. J. H. White, Muskogee.

STATE BOARD OF MEDICAL EXAMINERS.

Melvin Gray, M. D., Durant, President; B. L. Denison, M. D., Garvin, Vice-President; J. J.
Williams, M. D., Weatherford, Secretary; O. R. Gregg, M. D., Waynoka, Treasurer; E. B. Dunlap, M.
D., Lawton; Ralph V. Smith, M. D., Tulsa; W. LeRoy Bonnell, M. D., Chickasha; Wm. T. Ray, M.
D., Gould; W. E. Sanderson, M. D., Altus; H. C. Montague, D. O., Muskogee.

Reciprocity with Georgia, Kentucky, Mississippi, Nevada, North Carolina, Wisconsin, Kansas,
Arkansas, Virginia, West Virginia, Nebraska, New Mexico, Tennessee, Iowa, Ohio, California, Colorado, Indiana, Missouri, New Jersey, Vermont, Texas, Michigan.

Meetings held second Tuesday of January, April, July and October, Oklahoma City.

Address all communications to the Secretary, Dr. J. J. Williams, Weatherford.

OFFICERS OF COUNTY SOCIETIES, 1919

County	President	Secretary
Adair		
Alfalfa		
Atoka-Coal		
Beaver		
Beckham		J. A. Norris, Okeene
Blaine		
Bryan		
Caddo		
Canadian		
Choctaw		
Carter		
Cleveland		
Cherokee		
Custer		
Comanche		
Coal-Atoka		
Cotton		
Craig		
Creek		
Dewey		
Ellis		
Garfield		
Garvin		
Grady		
Grant		
Greer		
Harmon		
Haskell		
Hughes		
Jackson	J. S. Stults, Olustee	W. H. Rutland, Altus
Jefferson		
Johnson		
Kay		
Kingfisher		
Kiowa		
Latimer		
Le Flore		Harrell Hardy, Poteau
Lincoln		
Logan		
Love		
Mayes		
Major		
Marshall		
McClain		
McCurtain		
McIntosh	S. W. Minor, Hitchita	W. A. Tolleson, Eufaula
Murray		
Muskogee	J. L. Blakemore, Muskogee	H. C. Rogers, Muskogee
Noble		Benj. A. Owen, Perry
Nowata	J. E. Brookshire, Nowata	J. R. Collins, Nowata
Okfuskee		
Oklahoma	W. J. Wallace, Oklahoma City	J. N. Alford, Oklahoma City
Okmulgee		A. R. Holmes, Henryetta
Ottawa	A. M. Cooter, Miami	G. Pinnell, Miami
Osage	A. J. Smith, Pawhuska	Benj. Skinner, Pawhuska
Pawnee		E. T. Robinson, Cleveland
Payne		
Pittsburg		
Pottawatomie		
Pontotoc	L. M. Overton, Fitzhugh	S. P. Ross, Ada
Pushmataha		
Rogers		
Roger Mills		
Seminole		
Sequoyah		
Stephens		
Texas		
Tulsa	G. A. Wall, Tulsa	C. A. Pigford, Tulsa
Tillman		
Wagoner		
Washita		
Washington		
Woodward		
Woods		

IN WRITING ADVERTISERS, PLEASE MENTION THIS JOURNAL.

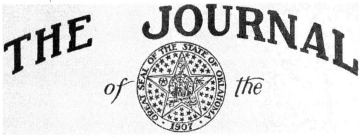

THE JOURNAL of the

Oklahoma State Medical Association

| VOLUME XII | MUSKOGEE, OKLA, FEBRUARY, 1919 | NUMBER 2 |

PYELITIS.*

By J. H. HAYS, M. D.

ENID, OKLAHOMA

Pyelitis is an infection of the pelvis of the kidney. Strictly speaking, I doubt if there is ever an infection of the kidney pelvis alone.

In the beginning there is undoubtedly some infection in the body of the kidney. During the process of many of the acute infectious diseases, as typhoid fever, pneumonia, tonsillitis, bacteria without pus is found in the urine and these organisms must have passed through the kidney without producing an infection. Similarly in the early stages of pyelitis, I am of the opinion that the calices and tubules are infected, but probably having a higher resistance, overcome the infection, and the disease becomes limited more nearly to the pelvis. In a pyelitis of a few days' standing there is a ureteritis and nearly always a cystitis, though the cystitis may be very mild.

Pyelitis in the adult is usually secondary to an infection in some other part of the body, or follows some acute infectious disease, as colitis, enteritis, lagrippe, tonsillitis, acute or chronic appendicitis, cystitis, salpingitis, etc. A renal stone may be the exciting cause of pyelitis. Any obstruction in the urinary tract, to the free outflow of the urine, as stricture in the urethra, enlarged prostate or stricture of the ureter, or any pressure on the ureter from without, as a pregnant uterus, ovarian cyst, or growth in the abdomen that prevents the free outflow of the urine may be an exciting cause of pyelitis.

The infecting organism in the order of their frequency, in my experience, is: First, the colon bacillus; second, the staphylococci; third, streptococci; fourth, gonococci; fifth, tubercle bacilli. I have found the colon bacillus to be the infecting organism in more than 80 per cent. of the cases. In about 10 per cent. of the cases there was a mixed infection of colon bacilli and staphylococci. I have had three cases of gonorrheal infection, two cases in which the tubercle bacilli was the infecting organism.

There is much discussion and great difference in opinion as to how the infecting organism reaches the kidney pelvis. I am of the opinion that in a majority of the cases, the bacteria reaches the pelvis by direct extension. I think this is particularly true of the colon bacillus, because on close questioning and securing a careful history, I have found that the patient has had some bowel disturbance, as constipation, colitis, or pelvic operation, or gives a history of some preceding bladder disturbance. Further, that the right kidney pelvis is more frequently in-

*Read in Section on Genito-Urinary Diseases, Skin and Radiology, Tulsa, May 15, 1918.

27

fected than the left, in about the ration of 3 to 1, and the ascending colon comes in very close contact with the right kidney.

In the three cases of gonorrheal pyelitis which I have had, two of them had severe gonorrheal cystitis; the other had a salpingitis. In these cases of gonorrheal infection, the two cases of severe cystitis, I obtained practically a pure culture of the gonococci from the kidney urine, while in the bladder urine, it was almost impossible to find the gonoccocci. The bladder urine was loaded with staphylococci, pus and mucus. These two cases gave a history of gonorrheal urethritis followed later by frequent and painful urination. One of the cases gave a history of a year's standing and the other a history of four years, and these cases have the appearance of a direct upward extension of the infection, as they gave no history of any other constitutional symptoms than pain in the back and an occasional chill; however, in the case of gonorrheal salpingitis there was not much disturbance of the bladder except some increased frequency of urination with little pain, and cystoscopic appearance of the bladder showed the trigone to be redder than usual and the ureteral openings were edematous. The infection in this case must have reached the kidney pelvis either through the blood stream or the lymphatics, and this patient had considerable constitutional symptoms, such as chills and fever, which however promptly passed away when the pyelitis was cured. In the two cases of tubercular pyelitis, they were in reality pyelonephritis, there being a direct extension of the ulcer from the pelvis into the kidney proper. In both of these cases a nephrectomy was done and the lesion was noted; no other part of the kindey was involved. In these two cases the original focus could not be located but were probably in the lungs and the bacillus undoubtedly reached the kidney through the blood stream. Both cases made a good recovery and are now in excellent health.

The symptoms of pyelitis are variable. The temperature is extremely variable. The height of the temperature does not necessarily indicate the severity of the infection. I have known cases with a temperature of 103 or 104 with but a small amount of pus in the urine. With one or two lavages of the pelvis, the temperature promptly dropped to normal and the patient made a rapid recovery. In some cases the temperature curve is like that of typhoid. In other cases it is remittent and in still other cases it is intermittent. There may be chills and high fever, there may be rapid rise and fall of temperature, without chills, and there may be chills with little or no fever, and there may be fever from day to day, for several days with only one or two degrees of variation in 24 hours.

The pain of pyelitis is as variable as the temperature, both as to location and severity. There may be pain all over the abdomen and the recti muscles rigid. In a right sided pyelitis, the pain is often in the region of the appendix or the fallopian tube and the right rectus muscles will be rigid. The pain may extend over to the region of the gall-bladder. There may or may not be tenderness over the kidney. If the kidney is well up under the ribs as on the left side it is difficult to elicit tenderness, while in other cases the pain is located in the back directly behind the kidney or kidneys and the kidneys are extremely tender on palpation. Many of the acute cases are nauseated, with vomiting and difficult to get a bowel movement.

It is practically impossible to diagnose pyelitis without an examination of the urine. In every case of pain in the belly, in every case of fever with abdominal symptoms, examine the urine. If the urine contains pus in large or small quantity, be suspicious of pyelitis. Go over the history of the case carefully, inquire closely as to previous illness, and if the patient does not improve in a day or two, and is old enough, have the patient cystoscoped.

Pyelitis is a very common disease, probably more often overlooked than any other infection. Many operations have been done for appendicitis, gall-stone and cholecystitis; had the surgeon taken the simple precaution to have the urine examined, he would have saved the patient an unnecessary operation and himself a keen disappointment. To be sure, pyelitis is frequently a complication of gall-bladder infection and chronic appendicitis. If circumstances will permit, it is better to cure the pyelitis before operation for the other condition, because the patient lying quietly in bed, with a lowered vitality following the anesthetic and operation, bowels not moving for two or three days, drinking little or no water for the same length of time, an infection in the kidney pelvis will become active and the patient will develop fever, and often pain, which will delay and greatly prolong and may even prevent recovery.

The prognosis in pyelitis is directly dependent on the infecting organism, the treatment, age, and vitality of the patient. If the infection is tubercular, the only treatment is a complete nephrectomy with removal of the ureter down as close to the bladder as possible. The amount of anesthetic and the time consumed in this operation is important.

If the infecting organism is streptococcus, the treatment must be energetic if you wish to save your patient. Direct pelvic lavage with 1-2 to 1 per cent. silver nitrate repeated every 24 to 48 hours, abundance of water, evacuation of the bowels, and anti-streptococcic serum give the best results. Fortunately there are not many of these cases. Unfortunately, the majority of them are in children and the pelvic lavage cannot be carried out and the patient therefore loses the most valuable form of treatment. These cases in children often become a pyo-nephrosis, which is usually fatal.

If the infecting organism is the colon bacillus or the staphylococci, the prognosis as to life is usually good, unless the patient is old and feeble or very young. However, these forms of infection are prone to become chronic with frequent exacerbations. The treatment in children is large quantities of water, urotropin in an acid medium, rest and good elimination. The disease is not always cured by this form of treatment but is checked and the patient apparently recovers but is likely to have a recurrence when indisposed from some other cause, as colds, lagrippe, etc. In the adult, pelvic lavage with 1-2 to 1 per cent. silver nitrate every 3 to 5 days, urotropin 20 to 40 grains daily in an acid medium, abundance of water, good elimination, is the most effective treatment. The lavages should be repeated until the catheterized urine contains no pus. The patient should then be requested to return at intervals from 2 to 4 weeks, for 2 or 3 months. If at the end of this time the urine is still free of pus the patient may be discharged.

To Summarize: Pyelitis is a very common disease, more frequent in women than in men, in about the ratio of 4 to 1. It occurs in all periods of life, from the 6 months babe to the octogenarian. It may be either unilateral or bilateral, more frequently bilateral in children than in adults. Pyelitis has no definite train of symptoms. It is frequently mistaken for appendicitis, cholecystitis, gall-stones or salpingitis. The most common infectious organism is the colon bacillus, the staphylococci, the streptococci, gonococci and tubercle bacillus.

The prognosis is good when diagnosis is made early and the proper treatment is instituted. The most effective treatment, except in the tubercular infections, is pelvic lavage with a weak solution of silver nitrate.

Discussion.

Dr. Julius Frisher, Kansas City, Mo.: The doctor has made no mistake when he says in his paper a pyelitis and a pyelonephritis are usually present and that the kidney proper is infected. Infection from a pyelitis, I believe, just as the doctor thinks, is usually due to a cold infection and follows some intestinal disturbance. In most instances the infection of the kidneys or the infection of the pelvis of the kidney, but if either takes place it is either a homatogenous infection or lymphatic infection or by direct ascension through the urethra into the pelvis of the kidney. Eisendrath has proved undoubtedly that the infection in the greater number of cases is lymphatic, passes up through the lymph channels outside the urine and infects the kidney proper and the pelvis of the kidney last. If the pelvis of the kidney alone is infected, why, if the patient has any resistance, the urine can carry off considerable of this infection and do away with it.

In regard to the treatment of this pyelitis or this pyelonephritis, we have received wonderful results in these cases, and especially in constipation, by doing away with intestinal disturbances, by taking care of the intestinal infection to begin with, that is by a buttermilk diet or whatever goes to the health of the patient, taken internally, to help out with intestinal diagnosis, in regard to a stasis of the bowel or infection of any certain part of the intestinal tract.

Cystocopy with kidney lavage once a week with one-half of one per cent. of silver nitrate (he used a two per cent., I use a half per cent. protargol in the pelvis of the kidney applied about once a week) gives us very nice results. The resistance of the patient is increased and in that way if the resistance of your patient is increased, the regulation of the diet will help those cases considerably.

Dr. Hays did not make reference in his paper to the vaccines. I see he does not use them. I think them to be of very uncertain value. My results with vaccines used in a great number of cases for different troubles of different character, proved them to be of very uncertain value.

Dr. F. K. Camp, Oklahoma City: While my experience has been very limited along this line, I did work in one of the largest clinics in Chicago, at the Cook County Hospital, this year for several weeks and I just wanted to confirm what Dr. Hays said here, that in that clinic we found about eighty-five per cent. of pyelitis was due to the colon bacilli. Cultures are made from the urine from the kidneys and that was the result. The treatment they are using there is one per cent. silver nitrate once a week.

A Voice: I would like to hear from the chairman.

The Chairman: We have such limited time I would rather give way to someone else. I would like to say this, I want to compliment Dr. Hays on this most excellent paper. This is a very important subject and it resolves itself into this fact, that I think all cases where we have symptoms of any kidney lesions, pyelitis or nephritis in whatever form, calls for a very careful differential diagnosis. The cystoscope must be used, catheterization and functional tests, so that we can know accurately the lesions we are dealing with. Whether it is one or both sides and then after we have located it in one or the other kidney or both, then of course we have to locate its cause. Usually there is focus somewhere in the body; find this trouble and try to remove this point, that is the teeth or from what source, tonsils, prostate, or bacillus colon, why of course, eliminate that trouble. For that condition we do that jointly in our treatment.

Now, as for the lavage, I have done but very little of that. I have used protargol in only a few cases, nitrate of silver, in say two or three, so I can't speak from personal experience.

I want to say this about the vaccines. I am a believer in vaccines. I think vaccines have a very important field and do not think they have any bearing whatever in acute gonorrhea, or things of that nature, but do think that in these older cases of this kind, the vaccines have given a cure. The reason why we do not get the results is because we go at it in a dilatory way, we give it today and skip two or three days and do not push it to the physiological limit. I usually give the stock vaccines and I give them each day until I feel that I have reached the physiological limit or until I throw the patient into some reaction and then of course we discontinue that. I do feel that the vaccines should not be discarded. They have their field of usefulness.

Dr. Hays, closing: I thank the gentlemen for discussing the paper. There is one point I tried to emphasize in the paper and that is, there are so many cases of pyelitis that were never diagnosed. I presume every one of you men that are doing this line of work have seen a great many cases that have been operated upon for chronic appendicitis, drainage of the gall-bladder, that were not cured, and you afterwards found that the patient would ultimately learn that he had an infection in one kidney or both and that the recovery was marked after they had been treated for this trouble.

There is one other thing that I should have mentioned in the paper relative to the treatment of pyelitis, and that is drainage of the kidhey. I don't lay all the cure of pyelitis to pelvic lavage. I use a large catheter when I find a case of pyelitis and I find a great many of them. I use as large a catheter as I can pass up the ureter. I have a number ten catheter and whenever I can pass this catheter up the ureter·I certainly do so. Why? Because it dilates the ureter and gives a better drainage to the kidney. I really believe that the drainage in these cases has as much advantage as the silver nitrate. I never use anything but silver nitrate, and before I inject the pelvis of the kidney with silver nitrate, I pass the catheter completely into the pelvis to try to draw off all the urine. I have found that in old chronic cases of pyelitis there is always some retention of the urine. I remember only last week that I drew off an ounce of urine from the pelvis of one kidney showing the beginning hydronephrosis which I think was due to an old chronic infection.

Dr. Wallace has brought up a very interesting question, the question of vaccine, and, doctor, I don't know about vaccine. I have used vaccines. Sometimes I think they help; sometimes I think they don't. I have used the stock vaccine and I have used the autogenous vaccine and I declare I don't know yet whether they have helped or not, but I do know this about the vaccines, that in every case of prostatectomy that I have had, I use the vaccines before I do the prostatectomy, and they helped in those cases. Just why, I don't know, but they did help, and if that is true that they do help in the bladder operations, they must help, of course, as the doctor says, in the pyelitis. Thank you.

CHANCRE OF THE FINGERS.

D. W. Montgomery and G. D. Culver, San Francisco (*Journal A. M. A.*, Jan. 18, 1919), call attention to the serious liability to syphilitic infection of the fingers of physicians, especially gynecologists and obstetricians. Nurses might be supposed to be similarly liable, but the authors have seen fewer cases among them. A paronychia-like chancre is especially hard to recognize, as it does not in any way resemble an intitial lesion. The nail and nail-fold obliterate the characteristics. An obstinate, long-enduring and exceedingly painful panaritium, occurring in a physician or nurse should excite suspicion and be examined for spirochetes. After five weeks the blood might be examined for the Wassermann reaction. An indolent bubo at the epitrochlea or in the axilla has diagnostic value, but any suppurative lesion of the finger might cause such a swelling. Any sore lasting longer than an ordinary infection and situated on the dorsal surface of the web, between the thumb and index finger, or between the index and middle finger of a gynecologist or obstetrician should excite the gravest suspicion, and one must not attribute too much importance to absence of the epitrochlear lymphatic nodule as some of its vessels pass directly to the axilla. A chancre, no matter where, usually ulcerates but this is not invariable. One should be always on the alert as regards the possibility of extragenital syphilis, and this is specially true nowadays when early treatment is so successful. The essential difficulty, however, of always recognizing these early lesions, is shown in cases the authors report, one of a nurse working with a physician, and the other two were in physicians in active practice. In none of these was the true nature of the disease recognized until the appearance of the secondary eruption.

WHAT THE SIMPLE EXAMINING CYSTOSCOPE MAY REVEAL TO THE GENERAL PRACTITIONER*

By F. K. CAMP, M. D.

OKLAHOMA CITY, OKLAHOMA

To the every day doctor with the every day practice, to whom comes every day puzzling problems in diagnoses, I present this every day paper. Such common manifestations as increased frequency of urination or retention of urine which, as a rule, present such accompanying symptoms that a clear diagnosis can be made, yet often many conditions present just such symptoms and still they do not yield to the usual treatment. The etiological factor in many conditions in which there is disturbance in urination or where pus or blood is found in the urine cannot be determined without some special means of diagnosis. In this class of cases the cystoscope is of the utmost value to the general practitioner. At once it may be determined whether the symptoms arise from intra-vesical or extra-vesical conditions.

While bladder symptoms in the female occur under the same conditions as in the male, yet let us not forget that in the female such symptoms are very often observed when the disease is in the female sexual organs or their neighborhood. Here a cystoscopic examination will show the bladder itself intact, and the bladder symptoms, as far as the bladder itself is concerned, will cease to worry us.

Let us enumerate some of the conditions that may give rise to bladder symptoms: Calculus, infection of any part of the urinary tract; tumors; ulcers; hysteria; diabetes; chronic interstitial nephritis; hypertrophy of the prostate, etc., while in the female we may have disease or displacement of the uterus and other adnexae. While it is true that many of these may be diagnosed without the cystoscope, yet even in such cases cystoscopic examination will be a benefit in confirming the diagnosis, one of the most satisfying things that can come to the true practitioner. We have in the cystoscope our most reliable diagnostic aid in determining the presence of a vesical calculus. It is far more reliable than the x-ray. A negative x-ray report does not mean that no calculus exists, but simply means that no calculus of a composition sufficient to make an x-ray shadow exists, as is the case in a large number of calculi where the predominant chemical constituent is uric acid and urates. Some investigators claim that fifty per cent. of vesical calculi are not shown by the x-ray, even in the hands of the most competent radiologist, owing to this fact; but there is no reason why a vesical calculus should be overlooked by the cystoscope and we are quite sure that it is only rarely missed. Infection of the bladder and the extent of it is easily determined by the cystoscope. As to tumors, while it may be impossible to diagnose absolutely the exact type of neoplasm encountered in the bladder, yet we know it is characteristic of growths in the bladder to pass quickly into malignancy. Therefore valuable results depend upon early diagnosis and efficient treatment. The mild symptoms manifested by the patient often lead both patient and physician to procrastinate, and complete examination may be neglected. It may be that a cystoscopist is not convenient. However, if the general practitioner with the simple examining cystoscope were to make an early examination, taking the diagnosis from the merely suggestive to the realm of absolute, what a service he would render his patient! If, upon examination, you should find the bladder and urinary passages intact, you have done no harm, and the other symptoms will probably disclose the etiology of the condition.

It is a matter of common experience now that immense light can be shed on pathological conditions of the bladder by a simple cystoscopic examination, and

*Read in Section on Genito-Urinary Diseases, Skin and Radiology, Tulsa, May 15, 1918.

we may go farther than this and say that no definite treatment, surgical or otherwise, should be undertaken in obscure conditions of the genito-urinary organs without making a cystoscopic examination.

One of the questions which often presents itself to the general practitioner is whether or not he shall refer the case to the specialist for operation or treat the case himself. A cystoscopic examination should give him such information. Of course, there are many conditions such as acute urinary retention, acute hematuria, calculus, anuria, and certain kidney affections calling for the immediate referring of the patient to the surgeon, yet there are many cases that can await the practitioner's diagnosis by means of the cystoscope. Certain bladder symptoms well known to us are caused by prostatic hypertrophy. In the majority of cases enlargement can be felt by rectal examination, but in many cases where the middle lobe is hypertrophied nothing abnormal can be felt, but the examining cystoscope will show a vesical projection. Stricture of the bladder neck is another fairly common condition which arises from a variety of causes and in which a correct diagnosis can only be made by a cystoscopic examination.

In diseases of the spinal cord in which the bladder is affected, what information can the cystoscope give us? If the urinary retention is due to inhibition of the bladder outer trabeculae formation is usually observed in the roof, and in the lateral walls of the bladder, while in ordinary obstruction, trabeculae are better developed in the neighborhood of the fundus. Thus we have a clue.

Simple cystoscopy may show clearly whether one or both kidneys are functioning. This may be determined by the urinary efflux from the ureters. Pus from the kidneys may be detected, if in definite quantities, as it passes from the ureter. It may also be suspected if after the first washing a clear medium should suddenly become cloudy—in this case it might be due to a fresh supply of pus being emptied from the ureter or kidney into the bladder. Of course the cystoscope would easily detect pus originating in the bladder as this could be easily observed. Simple cystoscopy will show the origin of a hematuria. It shows whether the bladder is dislocated by the pressure of an external tumor. It shows whether or not there are any abnormalities of the bladder or orifices of the ureters.

Most other pathological conditions of the genito-urinary organs are within the field of the specialist. That cystoscopy is a method that is indispensable is shown by the fact that it forms a part of the routine examination of all urological cases in every hospital of any importance, and even in cases where findings may throw light on other conditions.

It is not within the province of this paper to describe the technique of cystoscopy, but it can be said that the details can easily be mastered by any physician who has the desire and is willing to give the short amount of time that is necessary. There are different methods and many styles of instruments but the general principles are the same. To become fairly expert in the use of the simple examining cystoscope as well as in the interpretation of the pictures for the common conditions that are usually met with, is within the reach of every practicing physician and surgeon. The essential conditions for successful cystoscopy call for (1) that the caliber of the urethra must be sufficiently large; (2) that the vesical capacity be sufficient; (3) that the liquid contents must be clear; (4) good illumination must be had; (5) strict adherence to aseptic technique. Urethral dilatation under a local anesthetic may be required. If the capacity of the bladder is less than sixty cc. cystoscopy is difficult. For the third condition repeated lavages are necessary if there is pus or blood in the bladder. One should guard against producing trauma.

It is thus seen that a method of diagnosis which during the past twenty years has revolutionized our knowledge of the genito-urinary tract and inaugurated the specialty of modern urology is easily within our reach, at least in its simpler applications. Operative cystoscopy and catheterizing cystoscopy are still in the special province of the urologist, as well as the special tests for kidney functioning and the like and it is better that the general practitioner should refer such special matters to him.

There is still, however, an impression among many that cystoscopy cannot be done without great danger of infection. While this is true when it is a matter of an infected bladder and a careless practitioner, is it absolutely untrue when proper precautions are taken.

Galpi, of New Orleans, has recently reported that his last one hundred cystoscopies were done without a single serious result following, and his cases included pyelitis, hydronephrosis, pyonephrosis and cystitis, with and without ulcers. It is necessary for the strictest asepsis to be observed, but this is only repeating a truism which every practitioner admits. It can be obtained by the usual surgical precautions, and if one is not drilled in this he had better avoid even simple examining cystoscopy.

There is one other point concerning the value of cystoscopy to the general practitioner to which I wish to refer before closing; viz., its post-operative value. In many cases where a stone has been removed the cystoscope will detect whether or not fragments have been left behind, which may form a nucleus for a recurrence. The same remarks apply to cases of tumor, etc.

There are a few contra-indications to cystoscopy. These may be summarized as follows: (1) When the patient is very weak and infirm; (2) when the patient is in an emaciated or weakened condition; (3) when there is bilateral renal involvement of an intense degree; (4) when it is apparent that no surgical procedure would be of benefit; (5) during acute urethritis, acute cystitis and acute prostatitis.

In cases of extensive hypertrophy of the prostate gland it is best to refer the patient to the specialist.

The development within the last few years of so many new methods of diagnosis in diseases of the kidneys, ureters and urinary bladder—the Roentgen rays, the cystoscope, the segregator, the ureteral catheter, the endoscope and the research laboratory—has caused quite an advance to be made in this important field. The purpose of this short paper today is to call to the mind of the general practitioner that while a number of the above diagnostic aids may be necessary in many cases, yet there is a vast store of information that the simple examining cystoscope may furnish him, to the end that the practice of his profession may be less burdensome and that earlier diagnoses in these cases may be reached, to the ultimate benefit of the one we all try to serve—the patient.

Discussion.

Dr. Horace Reed, Oklahoma City: Mr. Chairman, for a goodly number of years I have been trying to use the cystoscope for the purposes of diagnosis. I have found that the trouble which I have had is being repeated by others who undertake it for the same purposes. The general practitioner, when he undertakes to take up cystoscopy, wants to do too much.

I remember very well that my ambition was to be able to introduce the ureteral catheter as soon as I was able to employ cystoscopy at all. As time goes on and as I use the cystoscope over and over, I find myself using the catheterizing cystoscope less and less. Understand, please, that my work is not genito-urinary surgery, but general surgery, and I have found that the simple examining cystoscope, in the great majority of instances, gives me the information that I want as well as the examination, which can be carried on just as easily at the same time, for functional capacity of the kidneys. I would go further than the essayist in recommending the simple cystoscope, which can be easily mastered and that the different tests for kidney function be taken up. I am very enthusiastic in the employment of indigo carmine as a test of kidney functions. I have been using it for years and I have yet to find a case where it does not give quite satisfactory results. I have, in addition, employed the phenolphthalein test to determine the functionating capacity of the separate kidneys, but there are so many cases otherwise in determining the tests in cystoscopy that I have virtually abandoned it where I wish to determine the functioning capacity of both kidneys as a whole.

The simple cystoscope can be used if a person will master the technique and it must be mastered in order to be used successfully. It can be mastered easily if a person will take a little time and use a little judgment. It can be used just about as easily as can the urethral sound. There is no need of getting infections following the use of the sound, indeed I cannot recall a single instance in which I have had any complications following the employment of the simple cystoscope. The only trouble that I have had in cystoscopy has been in those cases, in a few instances, where I tried to employ the ureteral catheter. There is this reason why we do not get complications with the cystoscope. I stated a while ago that one must master the technique. The technique which I employ is that really which one should employ in sounding the urethra; namely, cleanliness. It is absolutely essential, as the essayist brought out, that the bladder fluid, or the fluid in the bladder be clear. In order to obtain that he must irrigate the bladder. I go a little farther and after I get through with the cystoscope (this is a technique which I learned several years ago, and have been following it ever since), I use one to five hundred solution of nitrate of silver in the bladder, one hundred cc. drawing it in at one time: the first fifty I allow to pass out through the catheter and the second fifty I allow the patient to void. This is within a few minutes following the examination.

I have never had cystitis or the infection that I recognized as such following that technique. It was the technique as taught me by Capshammer some ten years ago. In using that technique in making simple cystoscopic examinations I find that a large number of my patients would be cured of bladder irritations. I think, by the thorough irrigation which I gave them and by the employment of silver nitrate as a prophylactic against infections. But I wish to emphasize this fact, that the simple cystoscope is so simple in the technique, which is very easy, that after it is completely mastered there is no reason why the average practitioner should not avail himself of so valuable an instrument and so valuable a method of diagnosis as there is in the cystoscope, and, as I said a while ago, for diagnostic purposes I can get along with the simple cystoscope plus indigo carmine, because indigo carmine does not add to the technique—the only means that he employs, about two and a half grains of indigo carmine in twenty cc. solution boiled just before it is injected. It aids one in locating urethritis; it gives one an idea of the relative capacity of the two kidneys, it makes this very easy, and, as I stated a while ago, I have found that the results obtained from that method has proved worthy of consideration.

The paper is a valuable one but I think the mistake we make is, we lay stress upon the fact of the value of these things in diagnosis, without telling the practitioner and insisting upon the fact that a certain very definite technique must be mastered or the man will fail. Just a little thing which seems so trivial is sometimes the thing which amounts to a great deal.

Take simply the adjusting of your instrument before you begin your examination. The awkward cystoscopist, and I hope I don't step on anyone's toes, will introduce his instrument and then say, "Now, turn on the light." The man who goes about it that way is going to continue to turn out his lights. This thing should be adjusted before the cystoscope is introduced, it should be just as much a part of the technique as the cleaning of the instrument, because it means success or failure. A man must adjust his light just as constantly as he performs the examination or the operation, that is the only way—a little point. I mean that to emphasize the fact that you must have a technique and there is no reason why the average general practitioner could not master this thing and use it just as easily as he uses the sound.

Just one more word about instruments. I use a Wolfe. Unfortunately we can't get that instrument any more, or at least they are very scarce in this country.

We have to give the devil his due and say that the Germans could beat us making cystoscopes. The man who undertakes to buy a cystoscope should get a simple examining cystoscope and master it before he ever goes any further. Just at this time it would be hard to get a real good simple cystoscope, at least so far as I know they are not being made in this country as satisfactorily as they were made by the Germans before the war. I hope that some company will be patriotic enough to take it up and see that they are manufactured.

Dr. Frisher: I consider the paper a very valuable one, especially for the general practitioner; that he should be more conversant in the fact that genito-urinary diagnosis can be made, and I do not agree with what Dr. Reed has said concerning the use of the cystoscope in the hands of any man, because one cysto-scope does not cover all purposes. That is one thing.

The next thing is that the American cystoscopes are as good if not better, than the German instruments. The Wappler Company, in New York, are putting out instruments at the present time that are as good, if not better, than any German instrument ever manufactured, and in fact the Germans, previous to the time that the war began, bought their instruments in New York, some of them did. Of course, their method of grinding lenses has not been as good as—is better than our method of grinding lenses, in fact they were masters in that phase, but the Wappler Company at the start had those lenses on hand and were furnishing them in their instruments. When I stocked with my cystoscopes I knew at the time that repair parts for German instruments were unavailable, and especially when one needed them most, the same as the automobile of today. An Italian car manufactured in Italy, you can have a broken axle or some other part broken on that car, and before you could send to Italy and get it repaired you might have to go to another patient. I mean with the cystoscope you might have to use it in the meantime.

Now you have to commend Dr. Camp on his paper on the fact that the genito-urinary diagnosis and functional test of kidneys are very essential to obtain a good urinary diagnosis, especially as to the functional capacity of the kidneys and the measuring capacity of the pelvis of the kidney and so forth, but to complete all that now we are estimating the retaining waste nitrogen in regard to the urea and so forth, and are doing better work by making our blood examinations in conjunction with our function and kidney tests and using one against the other in getting accurate information.

Dr. Camp, closing: Mr. Chairman and Gentlemen: I wish to thank you for your discussion but I do not believe there is anything that I have to add, except that I use a Brown-Buerger examining cystoscope. There may be others that are better, I do not know, but I know it is a very, very satisfactory instrument.

MULTIPLE CHANCRE.

J. C. Sargent, Milwaukee (*Journal A. M. A.*, Jan. 11, 1919), reports a case of multiple chancre of the penis. He has found only one complete case report of the kind in the literature of the last ten years, contrary to Osler's statement that such lesions were common. In the case reported, the first appeared after four weeks, and the second after eight weeks incubation. And it seemed probable that both are due to the same infection. Of the two possibilities of transplantation and second infection, the latter seems most probable.

CYSTOSCOPY.

Bransford Lewis, St. Louis (*Journal A. M. A.*, Nov. 30, 1918), publishes the description of several new instruments for use in operative cystoscopy. The first is a prostatic incisor, with a platinum blade, used for applying fulguration more effectively. A case is reported, showing its advantages. The after-effects, he says, are so slight that the case is ambulatory with the possible exception of a day or so of quiet. Other instruments devised and figured are a ureteral knife for opening a constricted ureter, forceps for differentiating phlebolith from ureteral stone, a ureteral dilator acting evenly for a given distance along the course of the passage.

A QUARTER OF A CENTURY IN EMERGENCY SURGERY.*
Some Observations of a General Practitioner.

By J. S. FULTON, M. D.

ATOKA, OKLAHOMA

In making a comparison of today's practitioner of medicine and that of the general practitioner of the early 90's, there is indeed a wide range, not only in the scope of their work, especially so when it is considered from the standpoint of the writer whose work largely was in a sparsely populated country. Nearly thirty years ago, the writer hereof located in the eastern part of the State, then Indian Territory, at Atoka, a small village, depending upon meagre farming enterprises, largely a cattle country, open ranges, and mainly inhabited by Indians. Travel was done principally on horseback and in some cases with buggy and team. Located on the main line of the M. K. & T. railway with a spur line running into Lehigh and Coalgate, mining towns. Just out of college, the writer began his professional life with no nearer colleagues than ten to fifteen miles away; the only graduate of medicine between old McAlester and Denison. There were plenty of would-be doctors at all the towns along the main line of the M. K. & T. and our early experiences with these fellows were very often as amusing as they were disgusting. One of the first evidences of confidence being extended to me was an appointment by Dr. E. F. Yancy, of Sedalia, Missouri, then Chief Surgeon for the M. K. & T. railway system, as Local Surgeon on the Choctaw Division, extending from old McAlester to Denison, Texas. Holding this appointment midway between these points, with no older or experienced assistants of any kind, the writer went forth to do emergency surgery and for some time many were the startling messages delivered similar to the following, which came within a week or ten days after receiving my appointment:

"Have Local Surgeon, Dr. Fulton, come on Yard Engine to Boggy Bottom to attend many injured in wreck of passenger train at Mile Post_____."

Every hair on our head was standing on its end. No one to assist, many injured, what could I do? We shall not attempt to tell you how we came out. One thing we do well remember, the very active secretion of the kidneys and the frequent desire to relieve same. During these early years and for many years following, wrecks were of most weekly occurrence, sometimes daily, and never more than a few weeks apart. The injured list mounted high during the year. The injuries were much the same as of today under such conditions, from the most trivial to the most severe, but every one must have attention, even though there be no injury but the feigning of injury preparatory to a claim against the company for a good fat judgment, which—if you will pardon me—has the medical and surgical fraternity skinned a city block in perfecting a cure. Being situated as we were and at a time when no one could render any assistance, having to act as surgeon, anesthetist, assistant, nurse and orderly, we think we learned early that very important lesson—*self-reliance, cool headedness, quick decision, and prompt command.* If a young surgeon doesn't know what to do, he can procrastinate by giving orders to some one else for something to be done, though it be a trivial matter—it gives him time to think. One of the greatest assets of the young physician during emergency service is to have the confidence of the injured party, his friends and bystanders. It helps wonderfully. Such gives the doctor self-assurance and thereby enables him to render better service.

In our early work, many times we have been called to lumber mills to attend wounded employees with no one to assist us, and sometimes an amputation of the thigh or lower limb. How keenly we have felt the responsibility of having to administer the anesthetic, do the amputation, dressings, etc., and on these occa-

*Read in Section on Surgery, Tulsa, May 15, 1918.

sions we have often wondered how a surgeon from the city who is accustomed to having assistance and hospital advantages would feel if called upon to perform such an operation, unassisted, under similar circumstances.

To recite a case or two: A big robust young man, with both limbs crushed, virtually dismembered, one below the knee, the other at the knee, was brought to our office from up the road some miles, and having lost a quantity of blood, was under severe shock. Stimulants had to be administered and hot packs applied for some time, with no assistant present—one called some ten miles distant, but could not be gotten—we administered the anesthetic, and to a kindly bystander the anesthetic was turned over and we made the amputation in as great haste as possible, having to handle every instrument, and sponges, and just about as we had all hemorrhage controlled and ready to close the flaps, our doctor friend came in. It was a dry, hot summer day, dust everywhere, and he came in loaded with it, having driven the distance in a buggy without gloves, and the first thing we knew he had his dirty hands into the wound, feeling of the thickness of the flaps, and making comment on the same. When I saw what he was doing and excitedly called his attention to the fact that he had not washed his hands, he good-naturedly said: "Why, my boy, don't get excited; don't you know about that laudable pus; they didn't get that out of your head in college, did they? You will have to have that laudable pus, and there will be plenty of it here, for you have mighty thick flaps to slough away." I guess they would have sloughed all right, but my patient beat its time and was buried the next day.

In traumatic surgery we have the greatest trouble in securing non-septic field. Many of these cases are found to have been rolled under a car with mangled bones and bruised and torn tissues, with coal dirt and filth of every kind ground into the wounds. To render the field clean is most impossible; in many cases even impossible to remove all of the foreign and dirty bodies.

The first consideration to be given the injured is to look after the proper control of hemorrhage, protect the wounds from further liable infection by applying sterile gauze, look after the shock which is usually great in traumatic injuries, especially so in railroad work. We have seen severe cases of shock from slight injuries in railroad employees where they have fallen between the cars or otherwise injured where they expected possible death, though their actual injuries were minor ones.

Hot water is the salvation of the country doctor doing emergency surgery. Everything can be made clean with boiling water. Soap, under certain conditions, is a great aid, but we do think it a great mistake to try to render sterile all tissues with antiseptic solutions by scrubbing, etc. In our early work, bichloride solution was used extensively, but we believe better results can be secured with an application of iodine and then removed with alcohol, or probably the cleansing of the tissues with gasoline or benzine will render traumatic tissues as clean and will give better results than too much handling otherwise. We suppose at this time that the Dakin's solution, now extensively used in army service, will give better results. However, our experience with such is very limited.

We think we have our greatest disappointment in the improper application of stitches. We believe that such mistakes are very common with the general practitioner doing emergency surgery. Traumatic tissues swell badly; stitches snugly applied bringing the parts together will, in many if not most cases, cause such irritation and cutting off of the blood supply as to create sloughing. Too much stress cannot be applied on this point; never put tight stitches in traumatic tissues.

Another very important fact to bear in mind—tight dressings must not be applied. The swelling which follows such injuries must be expected and arrangements made therefor, or much pain and possibly great damage may be done. Well do I remember a case in which I dressed an old man's foot and we had explained to him and his wife to loosen the dressing in case the foot should swell very much and give pain. I was assured in the strongest language: "Let it swell and pain; he can stand the pain all right."

We have seen some very interesting cases of mangled hands and feet recover and be useful members. We think we have made amputations of these in our early work that could have been saved. We believe other physicians and surgeons have made the same mistake. In fact, it now seems that we seldom have to remove a finger. These tissues seem to have mostly second life and will recover if given a chance.

In territorial times, when Indians were allowed full sway in this country, not being under state or government control, they would come to town and get plenty of bootleg whiskey and fight as much and as long as they pleased, no one to interfere; we have seen some remarkable cases in compound fractures of the limbs caused by gunshot wounds, and that with but little attention; while union has often been long delayed and usually with much deformity, in the course of time there has been perfect union.

We do not believe in too perfect immobilization of fractured bones. While we have used the plaster-of-Paris cast largely in lower limbs, not because we believed it the best or that better results can be had from its use, but because it is more convenient, takes less after attention; but in doing so, we have always made liberal allowance for the swelling and room for slight movements of the fractured bone. Have never used plaster-of-Paris on the upper extremities for the reason we think that better dressings and better results can be had, even though it takes more after attention, but as the patient can usually come to the office, they can be looked after nicely.

Bearing out the idea that there should be some motion provided for in fractured bones, we may call to mind whether or not we have ever seen an ununited fracture in the lower animals. We do not call to mind a single case.

Discussion.

Dr. W. J. Jolly, Oklahoma City: I have had a little experience somewhat like the doctor's in the country and in town. I have had to do considerable surgery. However, I have never felt very comfortable when I had to give the anesthetic and do the operation at the same time. About the treatment of dirty wounds: For several years I have used no water. I have used tincture of iodine or nitrate solution, but I know from experience that alcohol answers the purpose. I use thick saturated cloths of alcohol. I was in the Mayo's once and I saw them use alcohol and I concluded to use it on my dirty wounds and I found it very satisfactory. I am still using that treatment and I do my dressing once a day. It is very seldom I have an infection.

Dr. LeRoy Long: I would like to have Dr. J. N. Jackson of Kansas City discuss this.

Dr. Jackson: I must say that in recent years I have not had much experience in emergency cases. In my early days my living was made out of emergency surgery for a large insurance company. Nearly all our emergency cases in the large cities go to city hospitals. About six months of the year I have a great deal, but in my private work I have little of it to do. It is about the best we can have in a surgical way. A man who is able to do these emergency cases and to adjust himself to them and to manage them successfully, is a real surgeon. This brings to my mind that a great many men have come to me and have asked me about going to war, what need they have for us who are not specialized in surgery. It is just this sort of men, the men in the small communities, who have done emergency service and done it well, who are valuable in this war. I want to speak of the infrequency of infection and amputation. I remember that one of the first cases I had in which I made a little point in my surgery was where a negro had been crushed. His leg had been crushed in a rock crusher. The skin was all torn up and he had three fractures, with the dirt all in it. I took him to the hospital, gave him an anesthetic, and cleaned this off the best I could and called for a splint. The injury had not at all involved the main blood supply of that limb. The whole question was that of an adequate blood supply. No matter how it is mashed up if you have a good blood supply. Another thought is the infection. I believe in the efficiency of moist heat in the early stages to prevent infection. Infection can be controlled by moist heat if you have an adequate blood supply. Another case in my early experience: a man working on a press had his hands caught in the press and burst his fingers. He would not consent to have his fingers removed. The doctor did the next worse thing—sewed them up. He came to me and they looked like gangrene. He told me to see what could be done. I cut out the stitches and immersed the hand in hot water for five days and nights, and he did not lose a single digit.

THE MODERN TREATMENT OF BURNS.*

By O. W. Rice, M. D
ALDERSON, OKLAHOMA

In treating burns we must always keep in mind the anatomy and the physiology of the skin, for it is this organ which suffers most in all degrees of burns. I say organ; for the skin is not simply an envelope that covers the body, but a complex and vital organ with complex and vital functions. The physiological functions of the skin are protective, respiratory, heat regulating, sensory and secretory. An absolute suppression of the functions of the skin is followed sooner or later by death. It is one of the emunctories of the body, and if it is unable to functionate must be made up for by compensatory activity of the other three, the intestinal tract, the kidneys and the lungs.

So, in treating a burn of any degree, especially if it approaches in extent anything like one-half of the body surface, we must give the unburnt surface, as well as the intestinal tract, kidneys and lungs, a good portion of our attention. The bowels and kidneys must be kept active, the ventilation must be good so that the lungs can functionate to their fullest capacity, and the unburnt skin must be kept free from all medication and scrupulously clean by one or more daily baths.

Burns are usually divided into three classes, according to the depth of the tissue involved. A first degree burn is one in which the outer layer of the epidermis only is involved. In the second degree burn the entire thickness of the epidermis is involved, and with this we have vesication. A third degree burn involves the entire thickness of the skin, with or without the underlying tissue. I mention these classifications for the reason that burns of different degrees require, in many cases, different treatment. A first degree burn, if not too extensive, will get well in a few days under almost any treatment: all that is required is to relieve the pain.

When I first began treating burns in this district, now nearly twenty years ago—and I might add that there have been few weeks in all of this time that I have not had one or more on my hands—the old "Carron Oil" was used almost exclusively, and when it was used properly the results were usually very good. It was discarded some years ago for the reason that it had a disagreeable odor and that it was almost impossible to limit it to the burnt area. Usually it got all over the body, as well as the bed and bedding, which made its use very unsatisfactory in an extensive burn.

When the use of "Carron Oil" was discontinued various watery mixtures came into use, these consisting of solutions of picric acid, aluminum acetate N. B. diluted ten times, boric acid two per cent., sodium bicarbonate two per cent.,

---

*Read before Pittsburg County Medical Society, Nov. 21, 1918.

lime water, magnesium sulphate five per cent., potassium permanganate, and potassium sulphate. I have used almost all of these at one time or another, and I am convinced that a one per cent. picric acid solution will give the best results. I always add enough glycerine (one or two per cent.) to keep the solution from drying too quickly, and I usually add a small amount of creolin, which enhances the moral, and possibly the physical, effect of the solution.

During the last few years the paraffin treatment has come into great prominence, it being used somewhat at that particular spot on the map where the eyes of the world have been focused. By that means it has gained great notoriety, as also by the clever press agent of the patent nostrum, Ambrine, which cost ten cents and sold for four dollars per pound, this patent having received more valuable space free in high class magazines and papers than any nostrum that has ever been before the American public. One would suppose from reading these articles that it was possible to heal up and hair over a third degree burn over night. There is nothing very new about it after all, as it has been advertised to the American doctor under one name and to the American public under another for years. By adding a little white vaseline and benzoated lard to paraffin we have the old simple cerate, which has always been an official preparation, both here and in England, for the reason that it was used in the treatment of burns and skin abrasions.

I have treated ten burns with the wax paraffin film treatment, but I have never been able to contiune this treatment very long on the third degree burn. They invariably become infected, and if a large infected wound is sealed up the patient will soon show symptoms of sepsis, and the plan of treatment must be discontinued, temporarily at least. On most of my cases all three degrees of burns were represented, and on the first and second degree burns it gave as good a result as any dressing that I have used. The two main objects of a dressing for a burn is to relieve the pain, and to prevent infection. The wound is usually a sterile one, and we should endeavor by all means to keep it sterile. The paraffin will invariably come loose at the edge, or break, and the wound become infected, and if infection occurs at one spot it soon spreads over the entire wound. In nearly all of my cases I have used Stanolind. It contains no antiseptic, deodorant, or coloring, any one of which may be added if so desired. They will do no harm, but neither will they be of any benefit. It has been proven by a number of investigators that it is useless to incorporate any drug in the paraffin, for the reason that it is sealed up and can have no effect at the body temperature. It has also been proven that an antiseptic is not necessary. If the wound is covered over with a moist dressing and kept moist, the leucocytes will play out on the surface and are the best antiseptic. I have never used the paraffin gauze, but I believe that it will prove to be the ideal way of using this remedy.

Burns will heal no faster under paraffin than under other dressings. I have never seen a third degree burn, no matter how small, heal in less time than six weeks under any treatment. As to the resulting scar, there can be no difference. If the true skin is destroyed the end result is scar tissue, or an ulcer; if scar tissue replaces the destroyed tissue, it performs as does scar that develops under any and all forms of treatment, and as scar tissue has performed since the beginning of time. We can prevent further destruction of tissue from infection, and replace destroyed skin by grafts, and that is all. It is also difficult, if at all possible, to prevent contractions, since they occur in part weeks after the wound has healed.

In conclusion I will say, that dressing a burn is a surgical procedure, and as in all other surgical procedures more depends upon the technic—upon the thoroughness with which the work is done—than upon what you do it with. It is a time-consuming occupation. If an extensive third degree burn is dressed in less than two and one-half hours, it is not dressed properly. The paraffin dressing requires still more time.

The wax paraffin film is the cheapest dressing that I know anything about, and will give as good results as any on first and second degree burns. It is especially good on shallow burns of small area and brush burns. In my hands, at least, it is not a suitable dressing for a third degree burn.

There is no protection for a wound quite as good as gauze, old linen, or cotton, and moistening it with the picric acid solution has done more toward relieving the pain and preventing infection than any dressing that I have used on burns. Where these dressings are used over and over the expense is not very great.

At my first dressing I clip off all tags, but open no blisters, nor do I wash the burn. At my subsequent dressings, which may be in one or several days, where I find gauze firmly attached, I trim around and leave it and apply the new dressing over all. I have had several thicknesses of gauze four or five inches wide and over a foot long attached firmly to a back or an arm for two or three weeks, at which time it would look very much like a piece of leather. I trim off the edges as they become loosened, and this is the first portion of the deep burn to heal. Granulations do not bud out through gauze, as some would have us believe, and where it is firmly attached there is no occasion for removing it.

THE USE OF THE DICTAPHONE IN CASE HISTORY IN HOSPITAL AND OFFICE.

By FRED S. CLINTON, M. D., F. A. C. S.

TULSA, OKLAHOMA

The Oklahoma Hospital, in its desire to meet the increasing demands of efficiency, took one of the longest strides toward solving the case history problems by introducing, in the latter part of the year 1918, the dictaphone as the medium through which records may be made at the time and place and by parties who might give the most information concerning the patient.

As everyone of experience knows, the irksomeness of longhand records both to the one who secures as well as the one who endeavors to read the same, has not only been time consuming but quite unsatisfacotry.

The dictaphone is available any time of day or night, is always in the proper mood, and, if intelligently managed, will accurately record your findings. It will enable you to observe the usual privacy found necessary in securing the information concerning a given case, information which is not always available in the event a third party is present.

When one considers the interest awakened in industrial medicine during the last few years, it would appear quite necessary to avail ourselves of all the mechanical expedients which will enable us to get necessary information and present it in the most attractive form in the shortest possible time. Proper records are going to be required and those who make these records will not have the time to write them in long hand or be sufficiently skilled to type them.

It is necessary for the interest of the patient to have an accurately kept record. It is a great labor saver for the doctor, and the systematic examination of patients tends not only to improve the efficiency of his work but spares both parties many times great embarrassment.

Anything which will encourage and expedite this is worthy of the support of the profession and is more than worth the little extra money for its installation.

DIABETIC COMA.

By LEA A. RIELY, CAPTAIN, M. C.

OKLAHOMA CITY, OKLAHOMA

Osler has said that if one knows syphilis in all of its protean manifestations of pathological changes and complications, all else in a diagnostic way would be added unto him. I might add that if I knew the chemistry of the human body during all the changes of metabolism, physiological as well as pathological, the realm of the unknown in medicine would not be such a big factor. The study of diabetes is a study of the metabolism of the food to its proximate principles; and the study of diabetic coma is the study of the acetones, diacetic, beta-oxybutyric, lactic and phosphoric acids.

Futcher says: "Without qualification we can at present say that the acid intoxication of diabetic coma, or acidosis as Naunyn calls it, is due to the action of the beta-oxybutyric acid," thus endorsing Stadelman's dictum that diabetic coma occurs only when the urine contains oxybutyric acid.

McCashy reports a case of fatal diabetic coma without diacetic or beta-oxybutyric acid but had acetones in abundance. Albertoni says that acetones are faintly hypnotic but cause much dyspnoea and that they are decidedly toxic. Rhamy produced drowsiness, or even stupor, and other toxic phenomena and fatty changes in the liver and kidneys by hypodermic injection of acetones in guinea pigs. High grades of acetonia in diabetes are often associated with lipaemia (or better lipoidemia). An ingenious theory. Reicher postulates that the acetones, like other narcotics, leech the lipoids out of the cells and thus produce some of the narcosis phenomena of coma and precomatous stages.

A characteristic of human coma is that the cerebral centers are anesthetized while the respiratory center is stimulated. It may be taken as a general rule that dogs lose consciousness less readily than man and this applies to their diabetic coma. They begin by showing weakness, drunken gait and dyspnoea on slight exertion. The corneal reflexes are never lost and even attending surroundings may be preserved until the last, i. e. dogs not humans.

Breathing.

KUSSMAUL BREATHING—ALCOHOLIC TYPE.

Typical dyspnoea coma or Kussmaul's air hunger type, the kind Kussmaul described and most frequent:

Premonitory symptoms may be lassitude, headache, epigastric pain and occasional vomiting. Patient becomes restless and excited and tosses about in bed; his speech becomes thick and eventually incoherent; he grows dull and eventually passes into deep coma. A characteristic form of dyspnoea develops. It is inspiratory at first but later expiration is also involved. When fully developed the respirations are full and voluminous; they are loud and can be heard a considerable distance although they are not stentorian as in apoplexy; they are quite regular and greatly increased in frequency. Volume of the chest is greatly increased with each inspiration, hence called air hunger.

Alcoholic type with headache and symptoms suggesting alcoholic intoxication; the speech becomes thick, pulse rapid and without dyspnoea coma supervenes and patient soon dies.

Diabetic collapse: The patient suddenly begins to suffer from drowsiness and great weakness; the extemities become cold, hands and feet livid, pulse small and thread like; respiration is quickened but not dyspnoeic. Drowsiness develops, coma supervenes and patient dies in 24 hours. A large percentage of deaths in diabetes are due to coma and it is almost invariably the cause in children.

Certain factors tend to predispose to development of coma such as constipation, excessive fatigue, onset of various complications, such as carbuncle and pneumonia, subjection to an operation and sudden changes in diet.

Diarrhea may occur in the human coma but is invariably present in dogs.

Alkalinity of the blood, the buffer substance, i. e. $NaHCO_3$ is hard to maintain in man but easy in the dog. Many may die of coma with alkalinity of urine. Decreased hydrogen ion concentration (Explains).

Lowering of CO_2 alveolar tension. Marriett's apparatus shows 40 per cent. normal, below 20 per cent. should be careful, have seen it as low as 14 per cent. Riesman low blood pressure and subocular tension.

Physical symptoms: Nausea, anorexia, increased cerebrospinal fluid, substernal oppression and ringing in the ears.

Coma may come slowly or abruptly or intermittently.

Acetone intoxication: Anorexia, coated tongue, excessive thirst, nausea, vomiting, diarrhea, abdominal pain, tachycardia and other circulatory disturbances, dyspnoea, aromatic odor of breath, pallor, pruritis, haemoglobinuria, increase of temperature, headache, restlessness, vertigo, somnolence, convulsions and coma. Dr. Bladgett says pathognomonic sign is soreness on deep pressure over pancreas.

Dr. Yandell Harrison of Yale in 1914 said degree of acidosis is proportionate to length of time breath can be held. Advises against general anesthesia unless holds breath for 20 seconds.

Deaths from coma are due to: diabetes untreated; obesity high fat, low carbohydrate; patient abandoned treatment; imperfect supervision; ether anesthesia.

Treatment.

Bed: Warm, flannel night clothes, allay nervousness and discomfort.

Care of bowels: Enema not cathartic because of danger of diarrhea.

Liquids: 1000 cc. within 6 hours slowly, coffee, tea, broth and water. If nauseated given by rectum or intravenous.

(Joslin says it will seldom be necessary to give more than 1000 cc. liquids—thanks to avoidance of alkalis).

Diet: If fasting or used to fasting continue fast, but if on full diet give carbohydrate, orange juice, etc.

Heart: Digitalis.

Alkalis: Joslin. By former methods of treatment in which alkalis were generally employed to combat acidosis, 64 per cent. of all fatal cases succumbed to coma but with the partial adoption of the present method the total figures for my cases have already fallen to 60 per cent. and for the fatal cases during the year, 44 per cent.

Allen in his Harvard lecture: "Aside from the possible very brief rise in blood pressure sodium bicarbonate intravenously or otherwise brings no visible benefit to a dog dying of acidosis. Shows coma can be dispelled. Let up on alkalis. may stop acidosis as it eliminates it."

"Great loss of weight. Obviously it is due to a dessication of the body and in conformity to it can be placed my experience of not having seen a patient who has edema develop coma."

Vomiting at the onset of coma presages death because it is deprived of fluids with which to eliminate acids.

REPORT OF A CASE OF TRAUMATIC INFECTION RESULTING FROM INFLUENZA.

By M. H. NEWMAN, B. Sc., M. D.

OKLAHOMA CITY, OKLAHOMA

It is generally recognized that one infection, even of a mild nature, may have a deleterious influence on another infection with which a person may be afflicted. I could not find any similar case reported in medical literature to illustrate that B. influenza was the cause of infection entering through a simple cut on the face.

Miss B., age 19, family history unimportant except one sister had the "flu" in the same house a week prior to the accident. While scuffling with another girl in the office, Miss B. slipped and struck her face on the sharp edge of a chair, making an ugly wound about half an inch long between the eye and ear on left side. She washed the blood off and dressed it and did not pay any further attention to it. On the third day she had a chill, then fever came up and her left eye began to swell. She had a terrific headache. She came to my office November 11th with a temperature of 104, pulse 110, respiration 30, the left side of face red and inflamed and left eye partially closed. I made a larger opening and cleaned the wound out thoroughly, applying a bichloride dressing, and sent her home to stay in bed. I went out to see her the following day and I found her still with a fever of 104 and swelling over the left eye and nose. However, after three days of ordinary treatment I succeeded in getting the fever down and also the swelling. On the 16th of November she had another chill, temperature came up to 106 and the right side of her face began to swell. The soreness and swelling extended over the mastoid bones, first on the right side and in twenty-four hours over the left side, too, and both eyes practically closed. The wound, however, looked clean and healthy. In spite of all I could do she kept on having chills and fever, though the swelling of the neck gradually subsided. On the 21st of November, I took several smears of the wound for bacteriological examination. The three chief organisms found were streptococci, B. influenzae (Pfeiffer), and a few of the pneumococci. Those germs are rather unusual in a wound infection. But considering that her sister just got over a bad attack of influenza and they used the same room, it is easily explained how those germs influenced the cause of infection. I gave her three injections of 1 cc. mixed of serobacterin in three consecutive days; the temperature went down in twenty-four hours of the first injection and she made a good recovery.

The case is interesting in that it started from a simple cut and turned out to be so serious that she almost paid with her life. The germs which produced the seriousness were the same of the present epidemic, and they alone undoubtedly were responsible for the chills, fever and extreme prostration. It also shows that care should be taken in our surgical work to prevent contamination of the epidemic germs. It shows, in this particular case, the happy results of serum treatment. I thought my experience was worth while reporting as the epidemic is still raging in the country.

KIDNEY INFECTIONS.

Granville McGowan, Los Angeles (*Journal A. M. A.*, Dec. 7, 1918), says that frequent observation has shown him that infections of the kidneys and bladder persisting and unyielding to treatment, are always due to colonic stasis, usually in the cecum, and due to adhesions to surrounding organs immobilizing it. From this stasis, a constant supply of colon bacilli enter the circulation through the lymphatics of the kidney capsule or directly by the blood stream, and primarily infect the kidney pelves, in case there is any interruption to the free exit of urine. Once established, the condition can be cured only by surgical measures. Two cases are reported, illustrating the author's views.

JOURNAL OF THE OKLAHOMA STATE MEDICAL ASSOCIATION

VOLUME XII   MUSKOGEE, OKLA., FEBRUARY, 1919   NUMBER 2

PUBLISHED MONTHLY AT MUSKOGEE. OKLA., UNDER DIRECTION OF THE COUNCIL

DR. CLAUDE A. THOMPSON. EDITOR-IN-CHIEF

ENTERED AT THE POST OFFICE AT MUSKOGEE, OKLAHOMA, AS SECOND CLASS MAIL MATTER, JULY 28, 1912

THIS IS THE OFFICIAL JOURNAL OF THE OKLAHOMA STATE MEDICAL ASSOCIATION. ALL COMMUNICATIONS SHOULD BE ADDRESSED TO THE JOURNAL OF THE OKLAHOMA STATE MEDICAL ASSSOCIATION, 308 SURETY BUILDING, MUSKOGEE, OKLAHOMA.

The editorial department is not responsible for the opinions expressed in the original articles of contributors.

Reprints of original articles will be supplied at actual cost, provided request for them s attached to manuscript or made in sufficient time before publication.

Articles sent this Journal for publication and all those read at the annual meetings of the State Association are the sole property of this Journal. The Journal relies on each individual contributor's strict adherence to this well-known rule of medical journalism. In the event an article sent this Journal for publication is published before appearance in the Journal, the manuscript will be returned to the writer.

Failure to receive the Journal should call for immediate notification of the editor, 307-8 Surety Building, Muskogee, Okla

Local news of possible interest to the medical profession, notes on removals, changes in address, deaths and weddings will be gratefully received.

Advertising of articles, drugs or compounds unapproved by the Council on Pharmacy of the A. M. A. will not be accepted.

Advertising rates will be supplied on application. It is suggested that wherever possible members of the State Association should patronize our advertisers in preference to others as a matter of fair reciprocity.

EDITORIAL

IN DEFERENCE TO TEXAS.

The Oklahoma State Medical Association will this year meet in Muskogee on May 20, 21 and 22, a week later than usual. This change is made to give those Oklahoma physicians, formerly Texans, an opportunity to attend the Texas meeting and the Oklahomans now residing in Texas an opportunity to attend a real meeting of a real medical association. The change was made after consultation with and suggestion from the officers of the Texas Association.

TUBERCULOSIS LEGISLATION.

Elsewhere is a complete copy of proposed anti-tuberculosis legislation. This law is backed by the State Anti-Tuberculosis Association and, in essence, should have the support of every citizen of the State. The day is past when intelligent people should longer submit to the ravages of this controllable disease. So important is the matter that we deemed it of enough importance to reproduce the entire proposed measure. If the physicians of the State have any suggestions looking toward improvement of the proposal they will be welcomed by the Association and its Secretary, Mr. Jules Schevitz, Oklahoma City.

YOUR DUES, DOCTOR.

They are now due. If you have not a neat little 1919 certificate of membership you are possibly likely to be loser in the future. You will especially be loser should you be so unfortunate as to incur the displeasure of some worthless ex-patient, who only discovers your unworthiness after you have rendered him service, dismissed him cured, and you then seek to collect your fee. Some of these gentry, you know, find themselves permanently injured on account of your alleged unskilfull treatment when you go to collect, seek a lawyer and proceed to air your deficiencies in court.

Another phase of the matter, a costly one to your Association, and that means cost to you, is the work and expense incident to mailing you notices of delinquency. Every notice costs money, more money than ever before, and they are unnecessary if you will heed the first notice sent you, or this, and remit at once to your county secretary. It also costs a great deal of money comparatively to move your name from mailing lists, etc. The printer must be paid for his labor, and when your name is reinstated, as it invariably is, it costs more money, for he charges us again for his labor. Help yourself and your Association out by attending to this today.

THE VENEREAL AND OTHER LEGISLATION.

The question of control and suppression of venereal diseases has assumed such importance on account of war disclosures and findings at army contonments, that throughout the United States steps are being taken in an effort to suppress these controllable infections as far as may be. The United States Public Health Service is cooperating with all health authorities in this movement. In Oklahoma Dr. John C. Mahr, formerly State Commissioner of Health, has been commissioned to look after the matter. He is working in cooperation with the State and Federal authorities. His previous experiences as a Captain in the Army more than fit him for the task, and his acquaintance with the people of the State and their environment makes his appointment a good one. The only suggestion we have to make is that now is also a good time to consider practical legislation looking toward the control of other preventable infectious diseases. The people have never before had more examples of the meaning of control of infections before them; they have been shown by army experiences, where as far as could be strict observance of quarantine and prompt treatment produced results heretofore unknown to a civilian population. We can see no reason for not also requiring more strict observance of cases of tuberculosis and typhoid. The latter can be largely controlled and the tremendous death rate incident to it reduced a great deal. Some system should be devised by which the people surrounding every case could be advised of their danger and how to avoid it. If they will not, they should be forced to follow directions. It is just as sensible to require them to protect themselves against one death dealing disease as another. It seems it ought to be as legal to strictly supervise one as the other. As for typhoid; if it is legal to vaccinate our soldiers and sailors against it, the civilian population should be accorded the same treatment. None of our soldiers were hurt by it, certainly none of the others will be hurt by it.

THE PROSPOSED TUBERCULOSIS LAW.

HOUSE BILL NO.____

An Act Creating a Bureau of Tuberculosis in the State Board of Health, Fixing the Salaries of Officers and Employees, Providing the Duties of the State Board of Health and Bureau of Tuberculosis in the Prevention, Treatment and Cure of Tuberculosis, and Providing Penalties for Violation Thereof; Providing for the Location, Construction and Operation of Six State Tuberculosis Sanatoria and Making Appropriations Therefor; Requiring the Treatment of Tuberculosis Patients in Said Sanatoria, and Authorizing County Excise Boards to Make a Levy for Tuberculosis Fund, and Declaring an Emergency.

Be It Enacted by the People of the State of Oklahoma:

Section 1. Tuberculosis is hereby declared to be an infectious and communicable disease, dangerous to the public health.

Section 2. There is hereby created a Bureau of Tuberculosis in the State Department of Health, consisting of a Chief Physician, Assistant Physician and

Secretary, which shall supervise the prevention, treatment and cure of tuberculosis and the collection and dissemination of statistics, information and instruction in regard thereto, as hereinafter provided for, and shall perform such other duties as may be fixed from time to time by law.

Section 3. The State Commissioner of Health shall appoint, with the consent and approval of the Governor, the Chief Physician in the Bureau of Tuberculosis, who shall have direction and supervision thereof, under the State Commissioner of Health, and who shall receive a salary of $4,000.00 per annum, payable monthly, out of the State Treasury. The Chief Physician shall be an expert in the prevention and treatment of tuberculosis, and shall be subject to removal at any time by the State Commissioner of Health. The Chief Physician shall appoint an Assistant Physician at a salary of $3,000.00 per annum, and a Secretary at a salary of $2,400.00 per annum, payable monthly, out of the State Treasury, and such other clerical and stenographic assistants as may be provided by law.

Section 4. It shall be tye duty of every physician, owner, agent, manager, principal, superintendent or other officer of each and every public or private institution and dispensary, hotel, boarding or lodging house, in every town, city or county, and of every city and county health officer to report to the County Board of Health and the Bureau of Tuberculosis of the Ssate Board of Healjh, in writing, or to cause such report to be made by some proper and competent person, the name, age, sex, occupation and latest address and such other facts as may be required by the rules of the State Board of Health, of every person afflicted with tuberculosis, within one week of the discovery of such affliction.

Section 5. The State Board of Health, upon the request and recommendation of the Bureau of Tuberculosis, shall have the power to provide and enforce all necessary rules and regulations for the prevention of the spread of tuberculosis.

Section 6. In case of vacation of any apartment, or premises, by death or removal therefrom of a person having tuberculosis, it shall be the duty of the attending physician, or in the absence of such physician, of the person having charge of said apartment, or premises, to notify the County Superintendent of Health, and such apartment or premises, so vacated, shall not again be occupied until duly disinfected, and cleansed under the direction of, and in conformity with, the requirements of said County Superintendent of Health.

Section 7. Any person violating any of the provisions of sections 4, 5 and 6 of this Act, or any rule or regulation promulgated hereunder, shall be deemed guilty of misdemeanor, and on conviction thereof, shall be punished for each offense by a fine of not less than $5.00 nor more than $100.00, or by imprisonment for not less than ten days nor more than ninety days, or by both fine and imprisonment.

Section 8. For the purpose of treatment of patients afflicted with the disease of tuberculosis, there are hereby established six state tuberculosis sanatoria to be located, constructed and operated as hereinafter provided.

Section 9. Within thirty days after the passage and approval of this act, the State Commissioner of Health, upon the recommendation of the Bureau of Tuberculosis, shall district and divide the state of Oklahoma into six districts as nearly equal as may be in population, and shall certify such districts to the State Board of Public Affairs. Within sixty days after the receipt of boundaries of such districts, the State Board of Affairs shall select in each district a location for a state tuberculosis sanatorium, which shall be as near the center of the district as possible, with due regard to accessibility from all parts of the district, and shall be in, or contiguous to, some incorporated town or city, and shall consist of not less than ten acres of ground suitable therefor. The State Board of Public Affairs is hereby authorized to accept in the name of the State a grant or conveyance of suitable lands for such sanatoria, and any other gifts or endowments for the support thereof; and if such suitable lands cannot be secured by grant or donation, shall have the power to purchase the same or to condemn the same in the name of the State, with the approval and consent of the Governor.

Section 10. For the purpose of purchasing of sites, construction of six district sanatoria, equipping and furnishing the same, there is hereby appropriated out of the Public Building Fund not otherwise appropriated the sum of $600,000.00 as follows: $300,000.00 to be available out of the taxes and revenues levied, or to be levied, for the fiscal year ending June 30th, 1920; and $300,000.00 to be available out of the taxes and revenues levied, or to be levied, for the fiscal year ending June 30th, 1921. The State Board of Affairs is hereby empowered to let the contracts and arrange for the construction of said six district sanatoria upon plans and specifications approved by the State Commissioner of Health, and for the equipment and furnishing thereof, and shall promulgate necessary rules and regulations for the control and management of said sanatoria, not inconsistent with this act.

Section 11. Said state tuberculosis sanatoria shall be under the joint supervision of the State Board of Public Affairs and the State Bureau of Tuberculosis; the State Board of Affairs shall have supervision of the fiscal and business affairs of the said institutions; the State Bureau of Tuberculosis shall have supervision of the admission, treatment and discharge of the inmates thereof.

Section 12. There shall be appointed by the State Commissioner of Health, upon recommendation of the Bureau of Tuberculosis, a superintendent of each sanatorium, who shall be a qualified physician and who shall receive a salary of $2,400.00 per annum, payable monthly, together with rooms and board while residing in said institution. Such superintendent of each sanatoruim shall appoint such assistant superintendents, nurses and help as may be necessary and authorized by law, including a public health nurse who shall visit tubercular patients in the various counties within the district, and shall perform such other duties as provided by the sanatorium superintendent.

Section 13. Said sanatoria herein provided for shall be open to the treatment of all residents and citizens of this state, afflicted with tuberculosis; such patients as shall be financially able shall pay for board and room in such amount as may be fixed by the Bureau of Tuberculosis; all other patients shall be admitted upon request of the County health physician, public health nurse of the Sanatorium, or State Bureau of Tuberculosis; and the County Commissioners of the county from which such patient is admitted, or sent, shall pay to such district sanatorium the sum of not less than $10.00 nor exceeding $15.00 per week for board, care and treatment of each patient, payable monthly, until discharged; provided, this act shall apply to all bona fide residents of the State of Oklahoma at the time of the taking effect of this act, and as to all others, a bona fide residence of at least six months in the state shall be necessary to constitute a resident within this act.

Section 14. It shall be the duty of the county health physician in each county of the state to commit to the district tuberculosis sanatorium in the district in which such county is located all tubercular patients requiring nursing or medical treatment or attention, excepting such as are being treated in institutions conforming to the requirements of the Bureau of Tuberculosis of the State Board of Health.

Section 15. For the purpose of defraying the expense of transportation, and treatment of patients afflicted with tuberculosis at the district sanatoria herein provided for, the Excise Board of each county is authorized to make an annual levy upon all property in the county, subject to taxes, on an advalorem basis, of not exceeding one mill per annum, which is hereby declared not to be a current expense and to be for a special purpose, known as "tuberculosis fund," in addition to the maximum levy for current expenses not provided by law.

Section 16. The State Commissioner of Health is hereby authorized in the event that the capacity of any district sanatorium is not sufficient to accommodate tuberculosis patients of that district to admit patients therefrom to any other district sanatorium, and to change the boundaries of any district.

Section 17. The Superintendent of each district sanatorium is hereby authorized to arrange for the establishment of free tuberculosis dispensaries at centrally located places within the district, where patients may come for examination by the district superintendent and public health nurse.

Section 18. For the purpose of defraying the salaries and expenses of the Bureau of Tuberculosis in the State Department of Health, there is hereby appropriated out of any funds in the State Treasury, not otherwise appropriated, the sum of $_____ for the fiscal year ending June 30th, 1920, and the sum of $____ for the fiscal year ending June 30th, 1921; and for the purpose of defraying the salaries, maintenance and operating expenses of the district sanatoria herein provided for, there is hereby appropriated out of any funds in the State Treasury, not otherwise appropriated, the sum of $75,000.00 for the fiscal year ending June 30th, 1920, and the sum of $75,000.00 for the fiscal year ending June 30th, 1921.

Section 19. *Emergency Clause.* For the preservation of the public peace, health and safety, an emergency is hereby declared to exist, by reason whereof this act shall take effect and be in force from and after its passage and approval.

PERSONAL AND GENERAL NEWS

Dr. E. S. Milligan, Geary, is moving to Oklahoma City.

Dr. and Mrs. P. S. Mitchell, Yale, are visiting New Orleans.

Dr. J. L. Darrough, Pleasant Valley, Okla., has located in Perry, Okla.

Dr. T. T. Clohessy, formerly located at Berlin, is moving to Clinton.

Dr. J. B. Chastain has moved from Davis to Broken Bow, his old home.

Dr. C. B. Barker, Guthrie, spent the month of January at the Mayo clinic.

Dr. A. T. Dobson, Hobart, has been appointed county physician for Kiowa County.

Dr. L. T. Strother, Holdenville, accompanied by his family, is visiting New Orleans.

Dr. J. O. Hudson, Copan, seriously ill with influenza in January, is reported as recovered.

Capt. L. A. Hahn, Guthrie, now stationed at Ft. Bowie, Texas, spent a ten-day furlough at home.

Dr. H. K. Speed, Sayre, suffered severely from illness while on a visit to Ft. Worth, Texas, in January.

Dr. J. J. Clark, Tishomingo, who was recently operated upon for appendicitis, is reported as doing nicely.

Dr. and Mrs. R. D. Williams, Idabel, are visiting New Orleans where Dr. Williams is doing postgraduate work.

Dr. W. G. Woodward, State Representative form Kiowa County, was one of the earliest members to appear for the preliminary work in organizing the Legislature.

Dr. Joseph H. Stolper, Muskogee, according to press dispatches, has been court martialed and sentenced to dishonorable discharge from the United States Army. The specific findings are not obtainable at this time.

Dr. Calhoun Doler, Bokoshe, spent several days in Oklahoma City in January and February attending the Wesley Hospital Clinics and incidentally feeling the pulse of the legislature on medical and public health matters.

Dr. Claude Thompson and Miss Alva Coulter, Muskogee, were married in that city January 16th, to which place they returned after a short trip. Dr. Thompson will resume his practice, having received his discharge from the Army.

Dr. H. C. King, Ft. Smith, Ark., recently had a thousand dollar judgment assessed against him in the District Court of Muskogee County. The plaintiff alleged that he had exceeded an agreement between them and in operating removed organs without her consent.

DOCTOR THOMAS J. HORSLEY.

Dr. T. J. Horsley, Mangum, was found dead in his office by his Secretary Friday morning, January 3rd. The cause of death was presumably heart disease from which he had been a sufferer. Before death he was able to write a short note to his wife in which he stated he was very sick and believed he would never see her again. Dr. Horsley was 46 years of age at the time of his death and is survived by a wife and one child. He had practiced in Greer County for several years, was a member of the Masonic fraternity, under whose auspices interment was had. He served actively as a member and secretary of the Medical Advisory Board for Greer County during the war.

Dr. E. D. Jeter, Velma, and his little son Paul narrowly escaped death when a machine driven by Dr. Jeter skidded over an embankment into the bed of a creek 18 feet below. Dr. Jeter was badly bruised while his son received a compound fracture of the leg. They were removed to the Long-Bartley Sanitarium, Duncan, where they received treatment.

Oklahoma Academy of Ophthalmology and Oto-Laryngology, meeting in Oklahoma City January 2, elected the follow-ing officers: President, Dr. E. S. Ferguson; Edward S. Davis and D. D. McHenry, Vice-Presidents; A. L. Guthrie, Secretary. A board of directors was chosen consisting of Drs. W. T. Salmon, H. Coulter Todd and D. D. McHenry, all of Oklahoma City.

Tulsa Hospitals Organize. On January 18, 1919, representatives of all of the hospitals of Tulsa met and organized the Council of Hospitals and elected the following officers: Dr. Fred S. Clinton, President; Dr. C. L. Reeder, Vice-President; Mrs. D. I. Brown, Treasurer; Dr. W. E. Wright, Secretary. The following hospitals participated in the Council as charter members: The Oklahoma Hospital, Tulsa Hospital, Physicians and Surgeons Hospital and Morning Side Hospital. Other institutions, by conforming to proper standard, may be admitted to membership upon proper application. The purpose of the Council of Hospitals shall be to promote the efficiency of, and co-operation between, the various hospitals, to the end of better meeting the hospital needs of the community.

Discharged from the Army: H. E. Stecher, Supply; M. L. Lewis, Ada; E. N. McKee, Enid; R. B. Oliver, Bokohoma J. L. Dorrough, Perry; T. D. Rowland, Culbertson; Lea A. Riely, Oklahoma City; C. W. Heitzman, Muskogee; C. A. Thompson, Muskogee; Benton Lovelady, Guthrie; A. S. Spangler, Pauls Valley; K. R. Rone, Elk City; John Fewkes, Alva; R. K. Goddard, Supply; G. L. Johnson, Pauls Valley; A. E. Martin, Marietta; J. H. Scott, Shawnee; S. H. Landrum, Altus; P. B. Myers, Apache; J. C. Luster, Davis; E. W. Abernathey, Altus; D. M. Lawson, Nowata; W. A. Moreland, McCurtain; R. A. Douglas, Tulsa; V. L. McPherson, Boswell; F. E. Sadler, Coalgate; F. E. Rushing, Coalgate; R. C. McCreery, Erick; F. H. Norwood, Prague; J. S. Vittum, Muskogee; E. K. Allis, Shawnee; W. H. Aaron, Pawhuska; Roscoe Walker, Pawhuska; J. H. Thompson, Kusa; R. L. Baker, Wynnewood; M. C. Comer, Weatherford; J. R. Phelan, Oklahoma City; Reed Wolfe, Hugo; L. H. McConnell, Altus.

CORRESPONDENCE

A GOOD OPENING.

Skiatook, Okla., Jan. 21, 1919.

Dr. Claude A. Thompson,
Muskogee, Okla.

Dear Doctor:

I have decided to retire from the practice of medicine. I have been in active practice for 31 years, and feel now that I want to retire. So this leaves an excellent opening here for a live man who is not afraid to work. Can't you send me a man to take my place? I have a very good 2-room office over the drug store he can use. I have nothing to sell, he can just step into my place. This is a good monied community, town of 1,500, large territory, oil fields, Osage payments, etc. There are only two other physicians, and one of them has become so rich that he is figuring on retiring soon; in fact, I don't think he makes any night calls. I think I have collected 95 per cent. of all my accounts. This is no place for a kid, but a man of some experience and willing to work, can make himself some money.

Hoping to hear from you, I am,

Fraternally yours,
A. J. Butts.

MISCELLANEOUS

EPIDIDYMITIS.

A study of twenty-four cases of epididymitis as a complication of meningitis is rather briefly reported by J. R. Latham, (Belhaven, N. C.), Camp Jackson, S. C. (*Journal A. M. A.*, Jan. 18, 1919). Heretofore this has been little noticed, he says, among the complications of meningitis, but in the past year it has taken rather an important place. During the sporadic ourbreak of the epidemics of the past year, in one it occurred in more than 3 per cent. and in another more than a third of the thirty-six cases developed epididymitis as a complication during their convalescence. So far as can be determined there was no orchitic involvement. If it occurred at all it must have been slight and transient. The picture is that of a hard, sharply demarcated epididymitis, with the globus major as the primary focus, the process quickly extending to the body of the epididymitis. The tunica vaginalis testis usually contains a little fluid. The cause of the condition is in doubt. All cases occurred in men between 20 and 30 and all were treated by massive intravenous doses of antimeningococcus serum. The nature of the lesion would point to its being septicemic in origin. The records show that seventy per cent. of the cases had a positive blood culture; twenty per cent. showed a negative blood as well as a negative spinal fluid, and in the other ten per cent. the meningococcus was present in the spine, that is, the organism had reached the stage of localization and was no longer a systemic invader. From these data one would expect the onset of epididymitis to be a danger signal which was not the case. No relapses followed the condition and there was no apparent relation between the severity of the clinical features of meningitis or of sepsis, and the occurrence of epididymitis as a complication. The epididymal involvement was most severe in some of the mildest cases of meningitis. Apparently venereal disease was not a factor in causing this complication. None had active gonorrhea. The morbid anatomy of the condition is not known as no case has gone to necropsy. The inflammation quickly extends, but there is practically no pain or fever, and it lasts only a few hours. The diagnosis is usually self evident but a few cardinal points are mentioned: The preference in the locality for the condition, the absence of venereal infection and the absence of pain and constitutional disturbance, and lastly the lack of atrophy and the gradual return to normal of the inflamed organ, in this differing decidedly from the condition when it appears due to mumps or chronic syphilis or tuberculosis. There is no evidence of concurrent renal or bladder trouble and the prognosis is very good. The treatment consists mainly in leaving the patient alone and quiet and if the dragging pain is annoying a small pillow placed to relieve the tension will be found to be sufficient. The emunctories should be kept working. A tabulated statement of the laboratory data and clinical features in ten cases is given.

CHLORAZENE IN GENITO-URINARY CASES.

Dr. E. Styles Potter, visiting surgeon of the West Side Hospital, Genito-Urinary Department, New York City, has the following to say of irrigation in the treatment of urethritis:

"Irrigation has long been known to be a useful method of applying locally the various remedies that have from time to time been considered favorably in the treatment of the simple and septic varieties of urethritis. After an experience extending over many years and thousands of cases and including the use of permanganate of potash, hydrargyrum bichloride, boric acid, carbolic acid, protogal, argyrol, tr. iron chloride, infusion of common drinking tea, zinc chloride, normal saline solution, etc., I now wish to call attention to the fact that Paratoluene-sodium-sulphochloramide (Chlorazene) used as an irrigation remedy seems to possess most unusual curative effects. It has the advantage of not being irritating, is evidently a powerful germicide and appears to have a slight astringent effect as well. I have been using this remedy in acute simple and septic anterior urethritis for some months and really the results obtained have led me to regard it as a very satisfactory remedy in the treatment of these conditions.

"I have become to regard Chlorazene superior to permanganate, protogol, or other irrigating solutions in general use, and now use it exclusively."

COUNCIL ON PHARMACY AND CHEMISTRY
New Articles Accepted (Abridged Report).

During December the following articles have been accepted by the Council on Pharmacy and Chemistry for inclusion with New and Nonofficial Remedies:

Non-Proprietary Articles: Benzyl Benzoate; Emetine Bismuth Iodide.

Abbott Laboratories: Emetine Bismuth Iodide-Abbott.

Hynson, Westcott and Dunning: Benzyl Benzoate-H. W. and D.; Solution of Benzyl Benzoate, Miscible-H. W. and D.

H. K. Mulford Company: Bismuth Emetine Iodide-Mulford; Cachets Bismuth Emetine Iodide-Mulford, 2 grains.

E. R. Squibb and Sons: Chlopirated Eucalyptol-Squibb.

NEW AND NON-OFFICIAL REMEDIES.

Emetine Bismuth Iodide. A complex iodide of emetine and bismuth containing from 17 to 23 per cent. of emetine and from 15 to 20 per cent. of bismuth. It has the action of emetine, but when taken by mouth, it is less likely to cause vomiting than the soluble salts of emetine administered orally. It has been used with apparent good results in the treatment of chronic cases and carriers of amebic dysentery, even where the hypodermic administration of emetine has failed. The commonly used dose has been 0.2 gm. (3 grains) daily for four days, either in a single dose at the midday meal or in divided doses.

Emetine Bismuth Iodide-Abbott. A brand of emetine bismuth iodide complying with the N. N. R. standards. The Abbott Laboratories, Chicago.

Bismuth Emetine Iodide-Mulford. A brand of emetine bismuth iodide complying with the N. N. R. standards. The H. K. Mulford Co., Philadelphia.

Cachets Bismuth Emetine Iodide-Mulford, 2 grains. Each cachet contains 2 grains of bismuth emetine iodide-Mulford. The H. K. Mulford Co., Philadelphia.

Benzyl Benzoate. The benzyl alcohol ester of benzoic acid. It lowers the tone of unstriped muscle and has been suggested as a remedy against renal, biliary, uterine and intestinal colic and other spasms of smooth muscle, including angiospasm. Its clinical use is in the experimental stage. The dose is from 0.3 to 0.5 cc. (5 to 7 minims). Benzyl benzoate is a liquid at room temperature, insoluble in water, but miscible with alcohol, chloroform and ether.

Benzyl Benzoate-H. W. and D. A brand of benzyl benzoate complying with the tests and standards of N. N. R. Hynson, Westcott and Dunning, Baltimore, Md.

Solution of Benzyl Benzoate, Miscible-H. W. and D. A solution of benzyl benzoate-H. W. and D. in 78 gm. ethyl alcohol emulsified with 2 gm. castile soap. It has the actions and uses of benzyl benzoate. Hynson, Westcott and Dunning, Baltimore, Md.

PROPAGANDA FOR REFORM.

Leonard Ear Oil. This is an alleged cure for deafness, sold by A. O. Leonard, New York City. Formerly it was sold on the mail-order plan as an accessory to Leonard's Invisible and Antiseptic Ear Drums. Now the "Ear Oil" is sold in drug stores. The Department of Health in the city of New York found it essentially to be liquid petrolatum with camphor, eucalyptol and alcohol emulsified by a soft soap, prosecuted Leonard, and prohibited the sale of the "Ear Oil" in New York City. The sale of the "Ear Oil" has also been prohibited in Cleveland (*Jour. A. M. A.*, Dec. 7, 1918, p. 1932).

Emetin Bismuth Iodid. The Council on Pharmacy and Chemistry reports that because of the apparently good results obtained with it, emetin bismuth iodid has been accepted for New and Non-official Remedies. Emetin bismuth iodid is insoluble in water and dilute acids, but is decomposed by alkalis, and thus should pass the stomach unchanged but exert its action in the intestines. Those who have reported on the use of the drug in amebic dysentery report that the disappearance of ameba from stools was generally complete and apparently permanent even in chronic cases of carriers and in cases where the hypodermic administration of emetin has failed. Purging and vomiting, however, are not entirely avoided. The drug is usually given in a single dose of three grains at the midday meal for twelve days (*Jour. A. M. A.*, Dec. 14, 1918, p. 2013).

Fact and Opinion on the Influenza Epidemic. At the recent meeting of the American Public Health Association the discussions relative to the etiology of the present epidemic resolved themselves into the belief that the bacillus of influenza is not the primary etiologic factor and that the actual cause is as yet unknown. In the argumentation for and against the face mask as a means of preventing the spreading of the disease, sight was lost of the fact that definite evidence has been presented to show that the wearing of a mask prevents the diffusion of pathogenic organisms of which we have definite knowledge. A paper was presented which indicated to the satisfaction of most listeners that a significant factor in the spread of the epidemic in army camps was the inadequate washing of mess kits (*Jour. A. M. A.*, Dec. 21, 1918, p. 2074).

The Goldwater Ordinance. In 1914 the Department of Health of the City of New York revised the Sanitary Code so as to require that no "patent medicine" should be sold in the city of New York unless the names of the potent ingredients are declared. The ordinance was bitterly fought by the "patent medicine" interests, the fight being led by E. Fougera and Co., E. N. Crittenton Co., and H. Planten and Son. Now the Appellate Court of New York has decided that the ordinance is void, but has upheld the principle that a disclosure of the formula of medicines may be required. The underlying principle of the ordinance was the right on the part of the city to require disclosure of ingredients, and that right the Appellate Court upholds (*Jour. A. M. A.*, Dec. 21, 1918, p. 2093).

Influenza Vaccine. So far but two definite reports of adequately controlled experiments on the use of influenza vaccine appear to have been published. That of Barnes concerned the use of the Leary vaccine, composed of strains of the influenza bacillus, and indicated that the vaccine was not of prophylactic value. The second report, by G. W. McCoy and co-workers, concerned a carefully controlled experiment on the use of a mixed vaccine similar to that brought out by Rosenow, and indicated that this vaccine was not efficacious as a prophylactic against the present epidemic (*Jour. A. M. A.*, Dec. 21, 1918, p. 2094).

OFFICERS OF COUNTY SOCIETIES, 1919

County	President	Secretary
Adair	D. P. Chambers, Stilwell	J. A. Patton, Stilwell
Alfalfa		
Atoka-Coal	F. E. Sadler, Coalgate	W. T. Blount, Tupelo.
Beaver		
Beckham		
Blaine		J. A. Norris, Okeene
Bryan	H. B. Fuston, Bokchito	D. Armstrong, Durant
Caddo	P. H. Anderson, Anadarko	C. R. Hume, Anadarko
Canadian		W. J. Muzzy, El Reno
Choctaw		
Carter		Walter Hardy, Ardmore.
Cleveland		D. W. Griffin, Norman.
Cherokee		
Comanche	A. H. Stewart, Lawton	E. B. Mitchell, Lawton
Coal-Atoka	F. E. Sadler, Coalgate	W. T. Blount, Tupelo
Cotton		
Craig	C. B. Bell, Welch	F. M. Adams, Vinita
Creek		H. S. Garland, Sapulpa.
Custer		Ellis Lamb, Clinton.
Dewey		
Ellis		
Garfield		L. W. Cotton, Enid.
Garvin		N. H. Lindsey, Pauls Valley.
Grady		J. C. Ambrister, Chickasha.
Grant		
Greer		
Harmon		
Haskell		R. F. Terrell, Stigler.
Hughes		
Jackson	J. S. Stults, Olustee	J. B. Hix, Altus
Jefferson		
Johnston		H. B. Kniseley, Tishomingo.
Kay		A. S. Risser, Blackwell.
Kingfisher		C. W. Fisk, Kingfisher.
Kiowa		A. T. Dobson, Hobart.
Latimer	E. L. Evins, Wilburton	C. R. Morrison, Wilburton
Le Flore		Harrell Hardy, Poteau
Lincoln		
Logan		O. E. Barker, Guthrie.
Love		
Mayes	J. L. Adams, Pryor	L. C. White, Adair.
Major		
Marshall		
McClain		
McCurtain		
McIntosh	S. W. Minor, Hitchita	W. A. Tolleson, Eufaula
Murray		W. H. Powell, Sulphur.
Muskogee	J. L. Blakemore, Muskogee	H. C. Rogers, Muskogee
Noble		B. A. Owen, Perry.
Nowata	J. E. Brookshire, Nowata	J. R. Collins, Nowata
Okfuskee		H. A. May, Okemah.
Oklahoma	W. J. Wallace, Oklahoma City	J. N. Alford, Oklahoma City
Okmulgee		A. R. Holmes, Henryetta
Ottawa	A. M. Cooter, Miami	G. Pinnell, Miami
Osage	A. J. Smith, Pawhuska	Benj. Skinner, Pawhuska
Pawnee		E. T. Robinson, Cleveland
Payne		
Pittsburg	L. C. Kuyrkendall, McAlester	W. H. McCarley, McAlester.
Pottawatomie	E. E. Rice, Shawnee	G. S. Paxter, Shawnee.
Pontotoc	L. M. Overton, Fitzhugh	S. P. Ross, Ada
Pushmataha		
Rogers		J. C. Taylor, Chelsea.
Roger Mills		
Seminole	W. T. Huddleston, Konawa	W. L. Knight, Wewoka.
Sequoyah		Sam McKeel, Sallisaw.
Stephens		H. C. Frie, Duncan.
Texas	W. H. Langston, Guymon	R. B. Hays, Guymon
Tulsa	G. A. Wall, Tulsa	C. A. Pigford, Tulsa
Tillman		J. E. Arrington, Frederick.
Wagoner		
Washita		A. S. Neal, Cordell.
Washington		
Woods		J. A. Bowling, Alva.
Woodward		Arthur Bowles, Woodward.

OFFICERS OF OKLAHOMA STATE MEDICAL ASSOCIATION.

President—Dr. L. S. Willour, McAlester (A. E. F. in France).   G. F. Border, Mangum, acting.

President-elect—Dr. L. J. Moorman, Oklahoma City.

1st Vice-President,—Dr. E. D. James, Miami.

2nd Vice- President—Dr. H. M. Williams, Wellston.

3rd Vice-President,—Walter Hardy, Ardmore.

Delegate to A. M. A., 1919-1920—LeRoy Long, Oklahoma City.

Meeting place, Muskogee—May 20-21-22, 1919 Headquarters, Hotel Severs. For details address Dr. H. C. Rogers, Phoenix Building, Muskogee.

CHAIRMEN OF SCIENTIFIC SECTIONS.

Surgery and Gynecology—A. A. Will, Oklahoma City.

Pediatrics and Obstetrics—Vice Chairman, O. A. Flanagan, 305 Bliss Bldg., Tulsa.

Eye, Ear, Nose and Throat—R. O. Early, Ardmore.

General Medicine, Nervous and Mental Diseases—F. W. Ewing, Muskogee.

Genitourinary, Skin and Radiology—R. T. Edwards, Oklahoma City.

Legislative Committee—Dr. Millington Smith, Oklahoma City; Dr. J. M. Byrum, Shawnee; Dr. J. C. Mahr, Oklahoma City.

For the Study and Control of Cancer—Drs. LeRoy Long, Oklahoma City; Gayfree Ellison, Norman; D. A. Myers, Lawton.

For the Study and Control of Pellagra—Drs. A. A. Thurlow, Norman; L. A. Mitchell, Frederick; J. C. Watkins, Checotah.

For the Study of Venereal Diseases—Drs. Wm. J. Wallace, Oklahoma City; Ross Grosshart Tulsa; J. E. Bercaw, Okmulgee.

Necrology—Drs. Martha Bledsoe, Chickasha; J. W. Pollard, Bartlesville.

Tuberculosis—Drs. L. J. Moorman, Oklahoma City; C. W. Heitzman, Muskogee; Leila E. Andrews, Oklahoma City.

Conservation of Vision—Drs. L. A. Newton, Oklanoma City; L. Haynes Buxton, Oklahoma City; G. E. Hartshorne, Shawnee.

Hospital Committee—F. S. Clinton, Tulsa: M. Smith, Oklahoma City: C. A. Thompson, Muskogee.

Committee on Medical Education—Drs. A. L. Blesh; A. K. West; A. W. White, Oklahoma City.

State Commissioner of Health—Dr. John W. Duke, Guthrie, Oklahoma.

COUNCILOR DISTRICTS.

District No. 1. Texas, Beaver, Cimarron, Harper, Ellis, Woods, Woodward, Alfalfa, Major, Grant, Garfield, Noble and Kay. G. A. Boyle, Enid.

District No. 2. Dewey, Roger Mills, Custer, Beckham, Washita, Greer, Kiowa, Harmon, Jackson and Tillman. Ellis Lamb, Clinton.

District No. 3. Blaine, Kingfisher, Canadian, Logan, Payne, Lincoln, Oklahoma, Cleveland, Pottawatomie, Seminole and McClain. G. M. Maupin, Waurika.

District No. 4. Caddo, Grady, Comanche, Cotton, Stephens, Jefferson, Garvin, Murray, Carter, and Love. J. T. Slover, Sulphur.

District No. 5. Pontotoc, Coal, Johnston, Atoka, Marshall, Bryan, Choctaw, Pushmataha and McCurtain. J. L. Austin, Durant.

District No. 6. Okfuskee, Hughes, Pittsburg, Latimer, LeFlore, Haskell and Sequoyah. Vacant.

District No. 7. Pawnee, Osage, Washington, Tulsa, Creek, Nowata and Rogers. N. W. Mayginnis, Tulsa.

District No. 8. Craig, Ottawa, Delaware, Mayes, Wagoner, Cherokee, Adair, Okmulgee, Muskogee and McIntosh. J. H. White, Muskogee.

STATE BOARD OF MEDICAL EXAMINERS.

Melvin Gray, M. D., Durant, President; B. L. Denison, M. D., Garvin, Vice-President; J. J. Williams, M. D., Weatherford, Secretary; O. R. Gregg, M. D., Waynoka, Treasurer; E. B. Dunlap, M. D., Lawton; Ralph V. Smith, M. D., Tulsa; W. LeRoy Bonnell, M. D., Chickasha; Wm. T. Ray, M. D., Gould; W. E. Sanderson, M. D., Altus; H. C. Montague, D. O., Muskogee.

Reciprocity with Georgia, Kentucky, Mississippi, Nevada, North Carolina, Wisconsin, Kansas, Arkansas, Virginia, West Virginia, Nebraska, New Mexico, Tennessee, Iowa, Ohio, California, Colorado, Indiana, Missouri, New Jersey, Vermont, Texas, Michigan.

Meetings held second Tuesday of January, April, July and October, Oklahoma City.

Address all communications to the Secretary, Dr. J. J. Williams, Weatherford.

THE JOURNAL

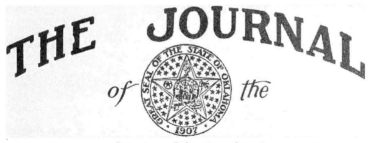

of the

Oklahoma State Medical Association

| VOLUME XII | MUSKOGEE, OKLA., MARCH, 1919 | NUMBER 3 |

SPASTIC COLITIS.*

By Arthur W. White, A. M., M. D.

OKLAHOMA CITY, OKLAHOMA

I have presumed in this paper to advance some ideas somewhat at variance with standard authority and to set down some conclusions reached from a rather careful study of a condition which is quite common and which, to me has been so far as I have been able to find, unsatisfactorily dealt with by writers.

While I have headed this paper Spastic Colitis, it is necessary to refer to most of the conditions of a chronic nature incident to the colon.

Much work has been done in the past few years on the study of the large bowel by surgeons, roentgenologists and internists. But almost wholly the premises on which the work started were arbitrary and accepted without question and an effort made to deduct conclusions with reference to distant organs or to better determine the presence of gross pathology of the organ itself.

The older writers and some few modern ones have recognized the existence of a condition of the colon, non-surgical but having definite anatomical changes and of different types—a common classification being ulcerative, mucous, spastic and membranous.

The ulcerative type is rare and is nearly always an incident in the course of some particular infection or disease elsewhere.

The other types we have come to believe are merely stages of the same condition, when the spastic type occurs; in other words, in every case of spastic colitis we have all the evidences (varying in degree) usually attributed to mucous colitis and there may occur such shedding of epithelium along with the mucous to amount to a (so-called) membrane. These conditions disappearing as the spasticity or tension of the bowel improves. There is another type that should be mentioned as the flaccid type, which probably is rare, at least, when not interrupted by spasticity.

We are prone to consider these cases as auto-intoxication, bowel stasis, etc., and the accompanying symptoms as those of toxemia and to force elimination by heavy cathartics, etc.; which may relieve the situation temporarily only to return worse than before. Just how much of the symptom-complex is due to toxicity I am unable to say, but I do believe that the greater part is reflex and is due much more to the disturbance of the nervous system than to any other cause, for in some subtle way there seems to be a close relationship between the nervous system and the large bowel.

---

*Read in Section on General Medicine, Nervous and Mental Diseases, Tulsa, May, 1918.

A spastic condition of the bowel affects the nervous system and the condition in turn is greatly affected by a disturbance of the sympathetic nervous system. Hence, I arbitrarily think of all cases of chronic colitis as spastic. for as soon as tension and spasm is controlled and the bowel relaxed to normal, all of the other evidences promptly disappear.

The condition varies greatly in degree; some cases are so mild that they amount to a little more than an irritable bowel, while others are so severe as to produce marked constitutional disturbance.

The majority of cases complain of a feeling of discomfort in the abdomen with pains varying in intensity and frequency a few hours after eating or just before defecation. There is a feeling of tension or bloating of the abdomen which may be relieved by the passage of gas. Occasionally the flatulence may become so severe as in itself to be responsible for other symptoms as shortness of breath, angina, palpitation, etc.; more often, however, it is merely sufficient to produce pressure against the stomach so that the patient interprets it as gas in the stomach and an effort is made to belch, which gives momentary relief. These patients mostly report belching of gas, but as they are observed one soon discovers that no gas is brought up, only the air that has been swallowed in the effort of belching.

The symptoms common to most cases are colicky pains in the abdomen, general sluggishness, variable appetite, sense of weight over the lower abdomen, tenderness of the plexuses of the abdomen and along the course of the colon, all or in the part depending upon the part of the colon involved, stools either mushy or formed, but of small calibre or alternating and an unsatisfied feeling after defecation as though the action were incomplete. Constipation may or may not be present, but was present in more than 60 per cent. of those I have recorded.

Loeper and Esmonet contributed rather extensively to the subject of abdominal tenderness in colon troubles and refer to the points of tenderness in bowel affairs.

Robert T. Morris lays special stress on the value of tenderness of the mesenteric plexuses in chronic colon troubles. Sippy considers it an important diagnostic point. For the most part the inferior mesenteric and the superior mesenteric plexuses are always tender on deep palpation and the ileo colic is sensitive if the ascending colon is involved.

One of the most interesting features of these cases is the fact that they rarely seek relief for a bowel condition. They consult the physician either because of a general lack of interest in life and feel they need a tonic or because of a reflex disturbance as of the stomach, or a lumbago. In a large proportion of all cases the subjects are nervous in greater or less degree. Some cases have had hysterical outbreaks, others are neurasthenics or mild melancholiacs. These patients are self-centered and easily worried. They complain of difficulty in getting to sleep after retiring and later dreaming all sorts of things. Some of them, especially business men, rather emphasize an inability to concentrate, "thick headed" being a common form of reference.

The diagnosis is as a rule not difficult if we are careful to note the character of the stools. The rule is a tendency to constipation with small formed stools varying with stools that are very soft or mushy (practically never a normal stool). This, together with the evidence referred to, will usually make a clear-cut case.

The final positive diagnosis, however, should not be made without first excluding all other suggested possibilities.

For example, a chronic appendix may produce a constipation, tenderness at McBurney's point and some of the other evidences of colon trouble so that it is often difficult to determine whether we are dealing with a simple bowel affair or a diseased appendix, or both, which incidentally is quite common and comprises that class of cases who continue to have their "appendicitis evidences" after removal of the appendix.

The stomach, being so susceptible to reflex effects, is almost always disturbed functionally; either a hyperchlorhydria or hypochlorhydria is present and may often produce, as a result, symptoms sufficient to focus the attention of the patient on it. Other conditions are to be remembered, although not common, as diverticulitis, Hirschprung's disease, intestinal infection, mesenteric aneurisms, adhesions, etc.

The treatment of these cases consists (in those cases which are primarily a bowel affair) in first bringing about a complete relaxation of the bowel until the stools become normal, and so educating the patient as to his diet and habits that he may live according to his physical demands. Complete relaxation of the patient is one of the first essentials, and one must remember that as the patient is irritable by virtue of his bowel condition so will the bowel condition be aggravated by any outside irritation affecting the nervous system of the patient. Hence rest in bed is of first importance if the condition is at all marked. The diet ranks almost with rest in importance. Foods that are stimulating or irritating to the bowel, as meat, yeast bread, fruit, raw vegetables, salads, etc., are not to be permitted. Only those foods having a non-irritating residue or no residue and are not stimulating to secretions are to be employed, as cereals, hot boiled milk, soft eggs, puree soups, and soft vegetables, frequent feedings in small quantities, being prone to allay peristalsis and encourage mass movement is much preferred.

In the more severe types it has been my habit to restrict the diet at first to strained cereal (or gruel), sometimes with a raw egg whipped into it, 3 to 5 ounces every two hours during the day, no feeding at night. Warm applications constantly to the abdomen seem to add relaxation.

In case of marked colonic spasm with constipation, heat at 140 degrees F. applied at hourly intervals for one hour gives better results. If the pain due to spasm is persistent, a warm enema given slowly and retained and repeated as often as necessary gives the quickest relief. This enema sometimes aggravates the pain momentarily, doubtless due to distention of the bowel, but it is followed in from 20 to 30 minutes by complete relief. Bismuth subnitrate and creta preparata given frequently may have a sedative effect on the bowel and aid somewhat in the treatment.

For constipation a retention enema of a vegetable oil at night and if necessary followed by a low water enema in the morning to insure a bowel movement. It is not probable that the oil has any positive healing effect. Its only value being a substitute for a laxative cathartic, either of which must not be given on account of the stimulating effect on the musculature of the colon. The stool should be inspected daily, as whatever might be the improvement in the symptoms no marked change in diet can be made with safety until the stool shows a form and consistency approximating normal. This occurs in from 7 to 21 days, depending on the severity of the case.

Following this the diet can be added to, daily, the patient may be encouraged to take an increasing amount of exercise and the intervals between feedings lengthened to 3 hours.

After the symptoms have disappeared and the stools have taken on normal form, if there is still a tendency to constipation, the laxative foods, that is, stewed fruits, rye bread, and honey, may be added to the diet. No yeast bread, meat or raw fruit, however, should be allowed for several weeks after the patient has seemingly regained his health. It is well, too, to advise the continuance of rather frequent feeding.

Sippy believes that the diet is the key to the treatment of all bowel affairs and emphasizes two things, frequent feedings, two hours intervals preferably, an abstinence from meat fiber and yeast bread, believing that they especially have an irritating effect upon the bowel, that is in the least, susceptible to irritation.

SIGNIFICANCE OF ABDOMINAL PAIN.*

By J. M. BYRUM, M. D.

SHAWNEE, OKLAHOMA

In assuming the responsibility of preparing a paper on the selected subject, it did not and could not enter my mind to attempt saying all the things that could be said. The field is practically without boundary and many of the real facts are yet to be discovered. I shall attempt only to recount a few of the every-day features of this subject and seek to excite a little more care and scientific consideration of the more prominent manifestations of abdominal pain.

The old term "colic" has, like that of "rheumatism," "malaria" and "congestion," served in the past among quite a percentage of so-called physicians to cover a multiplicity of ill-defined and misunderstood complaints. The old idea of an attack of "colic" treated by the conventional purgative and the soothing hypodermic has undoubtedly won the iron cross as a producer of surgical cases of peritonitis from a ruptured or gangrenous appendix.

To the discriminating physician, pain is the most important single symptom in the differential diagnosis of intra-abdominal disease and furthermore it is often the only symptom presented by the patient, and our ability as diagnosticians is frequently put to the test in making an early determination of the significance of abdominal pain. In this connection, I wish to emphasize the fact that the prognosis in several intra-abdominal conditions depends very materially upon an early diagnosis. Many hopeless cases of peritonitis sent to the surgeon might well have been a very simple, harmless operation for appendicitis, or for gall-bladder disease, or for intestinal obstruction in its various phases, and the undertaker could have been displaced in his last sad administrations. The Board of Health records of the state show numerous deaths caused by "congestion" which should have been reported peritonitis with predisposing cause "A doctor's carelessness or ignorance in studying his abdominal symptoms."

In the very beginning of the study of disease we learn that abdominal pain is a sensory manifestation of a pathologic state located usually within the region of the pain, but often in some other region served by the same nerves; or it may be in the very centers of that part of the nervous system. In other words, pain at one place within the abdomen may indicate disease elsewhere. What physician present has not made a diagnosis of acute appendicitis to return a few hours later to behold a pleuro-pneumonia? Gastric distress is often the overshadowing feature in a chronic appendicitis or gall-bladder disease. An acute abdominal pain in the region of the umbilicus is more often the beginning symptom of an acute appendicitis. Pain in the kidney may and often does mean disease in the other kidney, and who has not had the embarrassing experience of diagnosing renal or ureteral calculus as appendicitis, and what surgeon is there who has not opened more than one abdomen to find no pathology at all: Witness the crises of locomotor ataxia, or some other ill-defined neuroses. There is a reason for this seeming aberration of pain. That reason is found in the nerve supply of the parts.

It is, therefore, imperatively necessary in making a correct interpretation of abdominal pain, to retain a minute working knowledge of the origin and distribution of the nerve supply of the abdominal organs and the inter-relation of the various plexuses of the nerves within the abdomen. It is also just as important to know the histologic development of this part of the anatomy. For instance, if you do not know histology, how are you going to explain the pain in the testicle in renal calculus?

For convenience in the study of abdominal pathology and to segregate the various conditions confronting us, we have learned to group the anatomy of the abdominal organs. Thus we speak of the right and left upper quadrants, the

*Read in Section on General Medicine, Nervous and Mental Diseases, Tulsa, May, 1918.

epigastrium, the right lower quadrant, and the umbilical and the pelvic regions. The right upper and right lower quadrants contain by far a majority of the immediate danger signals of intra-abdominal inflammatory processes.

Here again our student-day knowledge of anatomy, which should be uppermost in our minds when presented with any of these abdominal pains, will bring to view the organs within these regions. Thus pain in the right upper quadrant usually means an involvement of the gall-bladder, the ducts, the pancreas, the duodenum, the pyloric end of the stomach, or perhaps the kidney. Pain in the left upper quadrant most frequently shows a pathology of the spleen, the cardiac end of the stomach, the splenic flexure of the colon or the left kidney. In this particular connection I wish to mention a case of obstruction of the splenic flexure of the colon which recently came under my observation. Mr. H., a robust young athlete of 25, was seized with pain in this particular region and was, on the second day, admitted to the hospital. A leucocyte count but slightly above normal was noted and a high enema was not returned. There was but transient nausea, a pulse of 80 and normal temperature. The next day the screen showed another picture. There was much nausea and vomiting. There was marked general abdominal distension and rigidity: Pain and tenderness were extreme in the right lower and left upper quadrants and severe pleuritic pain had developed in the lower left chest accompanied by respiratory distress and a rapid feeble pulse. The leucocyte count was now very high, the temperature became slightly elevated and a pneumonia of the base of the left lung was suspected. The nausea and vomiting were extreme, the emesis becoming more fecal as the case progressed. Another enema was not returned and at no time was there any flatus expelled. A tentative diagnosis of obstruction was made and operation advised. When the abdomen was opened, a markedly distended transverse and ascending colon, caecum and appendix were found. There were no other abnormal findings in the appendix to account for pain in that region. There was practically a complete obstruction of the splenic flexure of the colon. The left lung and pleura proved to be in a normal condition. A correct explanation of all the allied symptoms is found in a careful study of all the anatomy of the parts involved. The similarity of nerve supply and the mechanical gas disturbance of the appendix makes the picture clear.

Pain in the right lower quadrant usually brings to the receptive mind the appendix; yet renal or ureteral calculus, a ptosis of the colon and kidney, salpingitis, unrecognized adhesions and intestinal kinks, colitis and a varied collection of neuroses may, on opening the abdomen, prove the undoing of a carefully planned and well argued diagnosis.

Pelvic and hypogastric pain is almost in a class unto itself and a surgical condition if not an exact diagnosis is usually easily recognized because the female patient generally comes to the physician with an interesting story of the many diseases of her generative organs; yet this very prominence may lead to error. A slight spinal curvature or a sigmoiditis may be responsible for enough pelvic distress to tempt the active but not very discriminating surgeon. However, here again a careful examination and a proper analysis of the symptom-complex should and usually does lead to a correct diagnosis and a proper procedure. But there still may be exceptions. Witness this case:

Miss W., age 22, of prepossessing disposition and perfect physical development, called me in the middle of a cold night last winter for extreme pain rather low in the left pelvis. The temperature was 99, pulse 105, a leucocytosis of 17,-000. There was nausea and some vomiting. The history developed the old story of menstrual disorders and also two or three previous attacks of pain of like nature to this, but a venereal infection was strenuously denied. Such denials are usually expected, however. The picture was entirely that of appendicitis yet the location was abnormal. Operation next morning proved a left-sided appendicitis, a healthy tube and, for all I know, a virtuous young lady.

This case proves the necessity of taking into consideration the whole picture, not only the pain but the history, the general symptoms, the blood pictures and other laboratory findings.

After all, internal medicine, and surgery as well, are more and more dependent upon careful laboratory investigation. He who tries to practice scientific medicine or surgery without careful laboratory technique, will fall into shell holes at nearly every angle of his pathway. Let us have the whole truth and nothing but the truth, and further the affiant sayeth not.

In conclusion I wish to remark that what I have said on the subject of abdominal pain may have been prompted more by a limited experience in abdominal surgery than an internist; yet, I am frank to say that a great majority of abdominal diseases in which pain is a manifestation are medical cases. There is such a thing as "colic," there is such a disease as gastritis, as enteritis, as colitis; and in this connection I wish to say that the pain picture of these diseases, more particularly colitis, is so varied that I am going to ask our chairman to have it discussed by Dr. Fishman. The treatment of more than half of all the diseases manifesting abdominal pain comes within the sphere of the internist and that the careful study of the history and symptoms-complex of all abdominal diseases is wholly within such sphere.

Let us as general practitioners of medicine be up and busy delving into the ofttimes seeming mystery of abdominal disease, and even though the surgeon makes an enviable reputation and earns a comparatively fat fee, but returns to the family circle and our future care a living, happy patient, we shall possess the inner consciousness of having made a correct and early diagnosis; and have been the first efficient, responsible factor in his restoration to health and happiness.

If we do not get this just credit, mark my words, there is a screw loose somewhere in the surgeon's ethics or we have been lax in our own administrations.

EMPYEMA.

A paper on the bacteriologic control in the treatment of streptococcus empyema by A. L. Garbat (New York), Waynesville, N. C., appears in *The Journal A. M. A.*, Feb. 1, 1919. The importance of the subject has been recognized, and what is true of streptococcus empyema should also hold true for other organisms. "The technic of the culture method was that employed by the commission: Sterile Petri dishes are brought to the ward and each is placed from 0.1 to 0.2 c.c. of sterile decinormal soldum thiosulphate solution (the thiosulphate is kept in a test tube with a sterile pipet passed through the middle of the cotton plug, and is sterilized by boiling or by steam pressure). When the dressings and Dakin tubes are removed, the surgeon, a long platinum wire with a standard sized loop at its end is passed into the empyema cavity *without touching the walls of the sinus if possible*, and a loopful of secretion is removed. It is thoroughly washed off in the thiosulphate solution in the Petri dish. (Thiosulphate is employed so as to stop the action of any Dakin's solution that might be contained in the loop of secretion.) The plates can be kept until all the cultures of the ward are completed and then taken to the laboratory where the blood agar is poured; or, as was done at the General Hospital No. 12, the blood agar is poured directly in the ward, each plate being completed while the surgeon finished the respective dressing." For each plate 10 c.c. of melted neutral agar were poured under sterile conditions into a test tube containing 1 c.c. of sterile defibrinated human blood, and the mixture emptied into the Petri dish containing the loopful of secretion.

In making the reports to the ward surgeon, a division between the hemolytic and non-hemolytic organisms was made. Special attention has been given to their relationships although no definite conclusions have been reached. The cultures usually showed pure growths of hemolytic streptococci, with a very small portion of contaminating organisms. Cultures from cavities were made every one or two days, and if the gradual downward curve of the number of the bacteria does not occur, or if a sudden upshoot takes place, the cause is one of several conditions; either a secondary small pouch connecting with the main empyema cavity exists; the necrotic tip of a rib projects into the empyema cavity; a foreign body enters it from the operation, or the formula used needs changing. When sterile conditions began to appear cultures were made more frequently, but the wound was not allowed to close until the cavity was absolutely sterile, as well as the sinus connecting. Garbat's conclusions are: A bacteriologic control is of paramount importance in the treatment of empyema when the Carrel-Dakin method of disinfection is employed. Cultures should be made directly from the cavity, and not from the Carrel tubes. The cavity and sinus should be proved absolutely sterile before they are closed, and a persistent high bacterial count or increase means some complication in the healing. Citrated blood may be used in the blood agar medium.

ACNE.

Its Etiology, Pathology, Prognosis and Treatment.

By Charles H. Ball, M. D.

TULSA, OKLAHOMA

During the three years that I was a member of the staff and in charge of the out-clinic of the Barnard Free Skin and Cancer Hospital of St. Louis, we saw and treated from five to thirty patients daily, besides having in the hospital from 50 to 100 patients. This embraced all forms of skin disease, cancer and the cutaneous manifestations of syphilis. This was at the time when Parke, Davis & Co. first began the manufacture of the different varieties of vaccines, acne, staphylococcus, furunculosis, streptococcus, gonococcus, etc., and before they were distributed to physicians generally throughout the country, a number of physicians doing clinical work at different places in the United States were requested to join their experimental staff, to whom they furnished the vaccines in unlimited quantities for experimental work. It was my good fortune to receive one of these appointments, and it is largely on the reports received from the different workers that the present knowledge and use of these vaccines is based.

One of the diseases of the skin that for many years had been the least amenable to the ordinary methods of treatment, acne, was selected first for a try-out with the vaccines and some 125 cases were experimented with and results carefully notated and records kept, not only as to clinical data, but also by the Lumier or color photography, showing the exact pictures at different stages of the treatment. Practically all of the patients were benefitted, many of them apparently cured, but in a large percentage of the cases there was a recurrence in a shorter or longer period and repeated courses of treatment with the vaccines failed to effect a permanent or lasting cure. Therefore it was decided that we had not determined the precise etiology of the disease and further research was begun. Wherever it was possible to do so a portion of skin was excised of the papules, pustules, comedones and milia and sectioned, thereby enabling us to study with the microscope the exact pathological changes occurring in the skin. At the same time cultures were made of the germ contents of the pustules and we found present in most of the cases acne bacilli, the staphylococcus aureus, citreus and albus, with the staphylococcus albus butyricus predominating, and also a new form of bacilli, which, on account of its shape, we called the bottle bacillus.

Wright's opsonic index was also one of the methods we used in determining the antibody forming or bactericidal action of the vaccines. Then autogenous vaccines were made of these different germs and most of the patients were given injections of these vaccines, but with no better results as to permanency than with the stock vaccines. Therefore an intensive study was begun of the pathology of the skin itself and the following conclusions arrived at:

Acne begins at or shortly after puberty when all the functions of all the organs of the body are stimulated to increased activity, including the skin and all the appendages of the same.

The sebaceous glands of the skin secrete most abundantly at this period and become closely packed with the sebum.

As a general rule this period is also the age at which the boy's or girl's mother ceases to assist them with their toilet (in other words, scrub their face and neck) with the result that when they start out for themselves they do a poor job of it, their faces and necks are not cleansed properly and the openings of the enlarged sebaceous glands are filled with dirt and we have the so-called comedone or blackhead.

The sebaceous matter thus becomes imprisoned in the gland, the same being very much distended and enlarged by the constant secretion. We have therefore a splendid culture media for the propagation and proliferation of the different germs always present on the skin, followed by the invasion of the epithelial lining of the gland first and later the muscle fibers surrounding the same, with their resultant inflammatory reaction and proliferation, followed by the papule and pustule.

As you all know, when any long continued irritation from whatever cause acts upon the tissues anywhere in the body, the result is atrophy, destruction through sloughing or proliferation, or thickening.

The pathological sections all demonstrated a hyperkeratosis, atony and proliferation of the muscle fibers, the arrectores pili, sometimes the inflammation being limited to the gland, at others being periglandular, sometimes plasma (large fusiform), giant and mast cells present, and, when suppuration occurred, with leucocytes added. The lodgment for long periods of dirt in the gland openings had produced to a certain extent an atrophy of the muscles and a consequent permanent distension of the gland and an inability to empty itself, an occlusion of the same, therefore a gland continuously full of sebaceous matter makes it a permanent culture media for the development and proliferation of bacteria.

The question of diet, hygiene and other factors were considered in the study of the etiology, but, only so far as they disturbed the general and normal metabolic processes of the economy were they influential. While it is true that in cases of endometritis, cervicitis, leukorrhea, menstrual disorders, fibroid tumors, abortions as well as extreme errors of diet there is an aggravation of the existing trouble, still the original causative factor remains the same.

Therefore, first and foremost, vaccines are only indicated and effective when the disease has become periglandular as it is impossible to manufacture antibodies that will reach the proliferating bacteria in the inspissated sebum of the gland, when there is no invasion of the epithelial lining of the gland or the periglandular tissue.

To sum up, we have thus anatomical, physiological, pathological and structural changes in the skin and the only treatment that will be effective is one that presupposes a more or less complete desquamation of the epidermis, at the same time applying astringents to close up the glands and prevent the reforming of the comedones,

The plan of treatment carried out at the Barnard Free Skin and Cancer Hospital, and subsequently by myself since leaving there, is first to determine from a study of each individual case whether or not an autogenous or stock vaccine is indicated, and if so to push it to its full physiological effect, but in no instance depend entirely upon the vaccines, but always combine with it external applications and in some cases internal medication, diet and strict attention to hygiene.

The first requisite in the treatment is to cleanse the skin thoroughly and remove all the dirt from the opening of the glands. To do this I instruct the patient to scrub the parts thoroughly with hot water, brush and the official sapo viridis at least once daily, usually at night. After the parts have been dried I prescribe an ointment containing acid salicylic and sulphur in cold cream, instructing them to rub this in well, the object of these drugs being to act as a parasiticide and also assist desquamation. On arising in the morning the parts are washed with the same sapo viridis again, but not as vigorously as the evening previous, and then they are instructed to apply a lotion composed of resorcin in calamin and zinc oxid, allowing it to dry on the skin, the object of this lotion being to act as an astringent and also prevent the filling of the glands with dirt during the day. This program is repeated daily for one week, at the end of which time the strength of the ointment must be doubled because, of all the organs of the body, the skin adapts itself most quickly to medicinal treatment and a continuation of the same at the same strength would be of no value whatever. Each week, therefore, the strength of the medicine must be increased until a cure is effected.

After the first week the desquamation becomes very pronounced, fine branny scales, and must be encouraged by increasing the strength of the medicine until in a measure an entirely new skin has formed, which will have its anatomical and physiological characteristics more nearly perfect.

If at any time during the treatment there are any large, deep-seated pustules, they must be opened with a bistoury and the contents expressed, otherwise there would be scar formation from pressure necrosis.

The x-ray, violet ray and high frequency I have given also a thorough tryout, but am not very favorably impressed with any of them, although in acne necrotica or a tendency to keloidal formations the x-ray will arrest its progress and soften up the scar tissue.

WHAT CAN WE DO TO IMPROVE HUMANITY?*

By M. A. WARHURST, M. D.

SYLVIAN, OKLAHOMA

Degeneracy has increased in all nations. Fifty years ago the estimate of centenarians was six times as great as today. It is seldom that we meet with men one hundred years of age at the present time. There must be some reason for this. We all admit that human life is abnormally short. No exact estimate has been agreed upon as to the age to which life should reach. Flouren's estimate of animal life to us seems most logical: He states that animals live five times as long as their growing period. From this we conclude that man should reach one hundred fifty years, as his growing period is something near thirty years. A close study of the statistics of the causes of death shows at least ninety are from preventable causes. Seven of these causes, under suitable management and control, would reduce the death rate twenty-five per cent.; namely, broncho pneumonia, infantile diarrhea and enteritis, meningitis, typhoid, tuberculosis and acute pneumonia. When the human family realizes the benefits to be derived from hygiene and sanitation, the main factors in the prevention of diseases, the race will then begin to strengthen and improve physically and mentally. The generation will not be the old man afflicted with weakened memory and intellectual weakness, but will be able to apply his great experience and knowledge to the most delicate and complicated parts of social life. Our American people age prematurely; the vital organs fail early in life; organic disease is increasing; men weaken and die when they ought to be at their best. Physical degeneracy is common with many of our young men and women. A large per cent. of our school children are defective, dental decay, adenoids, diseased tonsils and eyes occur in something near seventy-five per cent. With proper care and attention most of these defects could be removed. Each county of this state should have a medical examiner of schools, with sufficient pay so he could afford to devote his full time to this work. Statistics show that practically 300,000 infants are yearly stricken by death, under one year of age, and that seventy per cent. of these were bottle fed. Bottle feeding alone should not ne held responsible for this death rate; in many cases the infant inherited its weakened vitality from degenerate, alcoholic, syphilitic parentage. Not a few mothers are rendered unfit to nurse their young from these causes. The loss to the state from the sterilizing influence of gonorrhea upon the productive system, and the blighting destructive effect of syphilis upon the offspring, are immense. In fact, it is the opinion of the foremost medical men of the world that venereal diseases are the main factor in the depopulation and degeneration of the world. I am sorry of the fact that these diseases are not reportable, so that we might have something near the true estimate of the havoc which they are responsible for. I cannot see any good reason why they should not be reported. If there is any disease more destructive to humanity I would

*Read in Section on Genito-Urinary Diseases, Skin and Radiology, Tulsa, May, 1918.

be glad to know what it is. Neglect and the fear of exposure are the causes of the spread of these enemies of man. With care, these loathsome diseases are preventable.

Venereal diseases are so prevalent that they are by many, especially the laity, considered as a matter of fact. There is no doubt that the extensive habits of cigarettes and alcoholism of the past thirty or forty years are manifesting themselves in the population of today. Any nation composed of syphilitics, alcoholics and tobacco users need not be surprised if their offspring are defective, either physically or mentally, or both. If the amount spent for alcohol and tobacco were placed in the national treasury the demands of the government could be met without taxation. If tea and coffee were discarded by our nation we would have less nervous troubles to contend with. A better and stronger race would be built up. This is essential for every nation, for, upon strength, power and vitality, all nations depend. Trace history as far back as we have any record, and it will be found that the loss of power through degeneracy was the cause of ·the fall of all of the great nations. No people that expects to hold their own can afford to neglect the health of their various governments. If the same amount of interest were taken in the health of our people as is given to financial matters it would not take many years to build a strong and efficient nation. We work along financial lines, take great interest in political affairs, but, health and social matters virtually take care of themselves.

The effects of venereal diseases in our army have cost thousands of dollars in money, beside other costs which cannot be estimated. The eradication of these diseases is no one man's problem. It concerns every man, woman and child of our country. We have become an extravagant, luxury-loving people, and for our extravagance we have paid the price, by the sacrifice of our health. We must get back to the same, simple life that nature intended us to live. Disease and poverty go hand in hand. Each is a source from which vice and crime originate.

One point which is neglected by us, as physicians, I will mention here. That is, we often overlook good means of cure because they are used by irregulars. Here we leave a loop-hole for the divine healer, osteopath, chiropractic and numerous other so-called healers.

In conclusion: I have brought out no new points. My intention is to place emphasis on those points which, in my opinion, would greatly benefit our people in the future, of which I give the summary:

Federal, state and municipal boards should be shown more appreciation, and better supported. Their power, especially administration and investigation, should be increased.

School hygiene should receive more attention.

Medical inspection of schools should be compelled by law. This is of more importance to the state than compulsory education.

Personal hygiene should be taught and encouraged. The multiplication of degenerates, epileptics, hopeless insane and criminals should be made impossible by the use of sterilization.

A higher standard of morality, heredity and environment should be encouraged.

Discussion.

Dr. L. W. Cotton, Enid: Mr. Chairman and doctors: I have been especially interested in social hygiene for a number of years, and especially since I have been honored by holding the place of superintendent of health and also being the medical member of the Garfield county draft board.

There are two features of his paper of which I want to speak. I hope that every physician will take upon himself the duty of insisting upon knowing something about what the candidates for election to the legislature stand for.

If you will examine the children in the schools throughout the state at any time, you will see the great necessity for doing just what the doctor suggested; you will feel like we ought to look more into the legislators who go from our several districts and represent us in that important department of the government.

It is appalling to know the ignorance of many of the men that we send to the legislature to make our laws along these lines. I not only would ask our own candidates, but I would inquire from my neighboring districts. I tell you we are very lax along that line. We ought to know that our men stand for what they should, and if they do not stand for those things we ought to say: "We are against you, you are against the very foundation that makes our country." There is but little politics to contend with just now, and I am sure that politics is not going to be what it has in the past, and people are going to say: "What can you do, can you deliver the goods? We do not care what your politics are but we want to know that you will do certain things and represent our district." It is going to be more and more so all over these United States, and I am thankful for it. We want men to do business and act, that is what we want.

I will pass that, and mention another thing we are doing which I think as doctors we should take a very decided stand against. I do not know who I may be tramping upon when I say this; you may be a cigaret fiend, I do not know, but you must agree with me in one thing, and that is that as a rule nicotine is detrimental, especially in the form of cigarets.

Only a few days ago in the last examinations I made, this was forcibly brought to my attention. I mention this because of the fact that I paid special attention to it. In the fourteen hundred men that I have examined in the last eight months I have found that the cigaret user in nearly every instance has more or less trouble with his heart. Dr. Hatchett, if you have been examining you will bear me out on that one proposition.

Dr. J. A. Hatchett, El Reno: That is right.

Dr. Cotton, continuing: A few days ago I had four men brought up; they were all fine looking specimens of humanity. There are four questions asked, and I will not take the time to run over them, I know them by heart. The first man was asked the four questions, and after answering he said: "Dr. Cotton, I am all right, but I take spells, I cannot get my breath, I have weak spells and I have got to stop. I have consulted a number of physicians but I have gotten no relief and I think I have got some kind of a bad stomach trouble or something of that kind." I examined the four. The last one was a farmer boy, he had never used coffee, tobacco or any of those stimulants. I said: "This first man is a confirmed cigaret fiend; I have not asked him a question but I know what I am talking about. This case uses tobacco, and this case uses tobacco." After I got through they took their turn examining this man that never used cigarets, never used anything; and his old heart was thumping away as regular as could be, it was just as regular as a clock. The others were confused, and they could easily see it, they did not have to be physicians. I told the first man: "You are just simply wrecking yourself with cigarets."

I just merely mention this because we make a great noise, and many of the best people in our religious circles all over the United States and more especially Oklahoma are going to break their necks almost to get cigarets to the boys. I had rather they would have the canteen so far as I am concerned. I think it is an awful mistake.

I think the physicians of this great state of ours ought to rise and rebel against it; whether users or not, you know it is wrong, and we ought to stand out firmly and emphatically against these things.

Those are the two points I was anxious to make. I do not think I am exaggerating this one iota when I say that I know the cigaret is doing more harm for our boys than any one thing, that is, outside of the social evil.

Dr. W. R. Joblin, Porter: I am on the school board. One thing which the doctor brought out in his paper is very important, and that is the medical inspection of the school children. I want to speak briefly of that.

One of the great benefits we are going to get out of this war is that it is going to teach the man what his constitutional rights are. Heretofore a man's constitutional right has consisted of anything in the world he desired, irrespective of the rights of others. Those are a man's constitutional rights now.

But we are beginning to teach and be taught that the government has some say, and the people have some say as to what a man's constitutional rights may be.

It is going to bring the medical inspection and it is going to teach the people that the government will have the right to control the health of the children as well as the health of the animal on the farm. And until we get that, until we get our legislators to understand the fact that the health of the school children and the neighbor children is of as much value as that of his stock and his neighbor's stock, then we will have school inspection and better general health, but not until then.

Dr. J. G. Smith, Bartlesville: I just wanted to mention one thing that Dr. Cotton spoke of, and that was the political side of it. If our representative is all right, then the medical inspection of school children and all of these other things are coming. But if we send men to the legislature who are opposed to everything that is good and opposed to everything that is progressive and opposed to everything that the medical men advocate, then we are handicapped and our hands are tied.

Now in this last election in Washington county, the medical society appointed a committee to see each candidate and find just where he stood; not what he said, but his history and his record so that we would know absolutely without question where he was. Not only that, but at least one of them came before the medical association at a regular meeting and he outlined his position and gave us a real genuine good talk on the medical law that we were expecting to pass and trying to pass during the last legislature. Last month's medical journal will show that he was right all the way through. We then threw ourselves behind him and he went to the legislature and he made good. That was Judge Craver.

If the medical association in each county, when these men come out and announce themselves as candidates for office, would find out where they stand and give them to understand that we are going to be behind the good man, I think that will do more than anything else we can undertake to bring about these improvements spoken of in this discussion.

Dr. M. A. Warhurst, closing: I thank the section for the interest taken in my paper; and I do not know that I can add anything important to it.

AN EFFICIENT SCRAP OF PAPER.

Those who talk of foreign red tape and of how we Americans cut it are invited by June Richardson Lucas to consider the British hospital telegram, which serves also as passport, railroad and steamer ticket, and hospital permit. She writes in the *The Modern Hospital* (Chicago, December):

"Englishmen can hurry with a skill and an efficiency that take even an American's breath away. When it comes to their fighting men they break all speed records. Thousands of men have died in the mud of Flanders—thousands have been wounded and sent home—but thousands have had to lie in those 'Halls of Glory,' the base hospitals behind the lines, and suffer—beyond the conception of any man—before the tide turns back toward life, or slips out in the gray dawn of Flanders, never to flow back. And the British fight to save those suffering men just as stubbornly as they fight to beat the enemy beyond the heavy cannonading a few kilometers away. . . . After the doctor's rounds, he sends a telegram asking her to come to such-and-such a base hospital to see Private _____. That very evening, perhaps in Devon, where the sun sinks low, a small boy comes running and puffing up the lane waving the precious paper; the door under the thach stands open. She is there, waiting as the women are waiting the world over today and the message says 'Come.' That is all she needs—that telegram is passport, railroad-ticket, Channel crossing, bus fare, entrance to the war-zone, space on troop-train, pass into that long, low building where her 'love lies bleeding.' Yes, it's a wonderful highway the British build from the aching ward in Flanders to the cottage in Devonshire. Just a telegram—no bewildering officials, no hours of waiting outside important doors—just a telegram; and the next evening, at sunset, she is sitting by her man in Flanders as he sleeps for the first time because the tide has turned. Just a thin bit of blue paper—just a telegram."—Penna. Med. Jnl.

FOCAL INFECTIONS OF THE GENITO-URINARY TRACT AS A CAUSE OF CONSTITUTIONAL DISEASES.*

By JULIUS FRISCHER, M. D.

KANSAS CITY, MISSOURI

This is an opportune time to discuss infections of the genito-urinary tract, especially those giving rise to various constitutional symptoms following genito-urinary infections. These constitutional disturbances take place in some instances years following the primary infection. There has been no development in medicine during the past few years that has been of greater influence in the pathology and treatment of disease than focal infections.

We have come in contact with a great number of cases that have traveled the round of physicians and specialists and who, in spite of careful examination on the part of these men, come to the urologist and genito-urinary surgeon complaining of various chronic ailments. Even after the removal of tonsils, teeth, and other infected areas of the body, we have disclosed primary foci of infection in the genito-urinary tract.

It is our opinion that the general practitioner or the genito-urinary man has been very lax in the discharge of patients who seem to be apparently cured, but who have been discharged before complete recovery. This has caused untold suffering to follow in many cases.

The internist has found that focal infections of the teeth, mouth, throat and alimentary canal are the most frequent causes of numerous chronic ailments of the human body. I am of the opinion that infections of the genito-uninary tract are secondary only in importance to those of the teeth, mouth and throat.

I wish to add the following: It has been quoted (and I don't believe in error) that 90 per cent. of our male population have gonorrhea at some period in their life. Our female population comes in for their proportionate share.

Keyes, Loree and others claim that 70 per cent. of all these gonorrheal infections in the male become posterior cases in spite of all treatment. Involvement of Cowper's glands, the prostate, seminal vesicles, vas and epididymis follow. A latent infection of any of these parts of the genito-urinary tract can cause grave constitutional symptoms to follow. We can say, without disturbing the equilibrium of our brother internists, that latent focal infections of the genito-urinary tract should be taken into consideration when hunting for obscure causes of disease.

The consideration of this vast subject of focal infections of separate parts of the genito-urinary tract involves so much time and space that the writer will consider only those which are the most frequent causal factors.

Acute gonorrheal rheumatism is the most important complication of gonorrhea in both sexes. It is present in about 1 per cent. of all gonorrheal cases and occurs at all ages, even children being prone to it. It usually appears within a few days of the onset of the urethral attack and joint involvement follows. The gonococci are carried through the circulation, and invasion of one or more joints occurs. The gonococci have been cultured and demonstrated in these infected joints. In studying the etiology of some cases of chronic rheumatism (using the term to cover arthritis, and pains in general) we have made detailed examination of the posterior urethra with urethroscope and examined the prostate and seminal vesicles by palpation and have found foci of infection which formerly had been overlooked.

Some of our best authorities and investigators claim that after a gonorrhea is of seven months duration, it is utterly impossible to culture, stain and demon-

---

*Read in Section on Genito-Urinary Diseases, Skin and Radiology, Tulsa, May, 1918.

strate the gonococci from smeared specimens expressed from the prostate or a centrifuged specimen of urine. All they could find, despite the fact that there was discharge or morning drop or sticky meatus, were different strains of staphylococci, streptococci, and some diphtheroids. So we have to look for these organisms as the causal factor in latent complications.

Rosenow in his work has laid great stress on the streptococcus and its various strains as the main cause of focal infections. His opinion of the selective action of these organisms on different tissues of the human body has been of great value to us. A type of streptococcus which caused an arthritis when injected into a rabbit produced uniformly an arthritis, an endocarditis, an abscess of the liver, etc. We can add to this the staphylococcus, tubercle bacillus, colon bacillus and spirochaeta pallida as playing no small part in the dissemination of diseases of the body.

I wish to make some case reports: Dr. L., age 52 years, weight 180 pounds, married, four healthy children. Chief complaint: Has a dull aching in perineum (as he describes it, a heaviness); also has pain between the shoulders. Previous history: Had a gonorrhea when 21 years of age, 16 weeks duration, cured. When 27 years of age had a second gonorrhea which infected posterior urethra and prostate, had an epididymitis of right side. Has a sticky meatus and slight discharge in the morning at intervals since, some burning on urination. Has to rise two times at night to void. Examination of prostate by palpation, boggy and large. Expressed specimen shows staphylococci present. Urethroscopic examination shows prostatic urethra inflamed, verumontanum engorged, and pus exuding from follicles. Leukocyte count 10,000. Centrifuged specimen of urine shows staphylococci present, otherwise negative. Wassermann negative. Treatment: Prostatic massage and D'Arsonval high frequency current on verumontanum and in prostatic follicles. Prostatic urethra swabbed with 2 per cent iodine. Pains in shoulders disappeared.

Mr. P. S., Photographer, age 43 years, single, weight 195 pounds. Chief complaint: Pains in thighs and limbs. Gonorrhea when 20 years of age, 8 weeks duration, cured. Gonorrhea again when 34 years of age, 4 years duration. Claims to have been cured. Has had burning on urination for years, denies any other venereal history. No discharge at present. Specimen of urine shows a number of shreds present. Examination of prostate by palpation shows prostate large and hard. Expressed specimen stained shows staphylococci present. Leukocyte count 11,000. Wassermann negative. Treatment: Massage of seminal vesicles. Prostatic massage and treatment of posterior urethra with 2 per cent. iodine through urethroscope. Pains in limbs disappeared. Leukocyte count, 7 weeks later, 8,000.

I wish to make reference to two additional cases referred to me for frequency and burning on urination and for rheumatism. In these two cases, on cystoscopic examination and analysis, a diagnosis of pyelitis and pyelonephritis with colon infection of the pelvis of the kidney was obtained. The kidney infection had its origin in a hematogenous or lymphatic infection and was secondary to intestinal disturbance. The rheumatism in this case was latent, and the result of kidney involvement. As may be judged from the foregoing, most infections that occur in rheumatism, nephritis, endocarditis, and lymphadenitis, are to be traced from a focus of infection in some other organ of the body.

Much can be done by prophylaxis. The general practitioner should make a greater endeavor to use the urologist and genito-urinary expert for a complete examination of a patient when the diagnosis is obscure. A plea to the genitourinary man; that the most thorough examination be made in this work, using all means at his command for diagnostic purposes. He should work with the internist, oculist, aurist, roentgologist and surgeon to obtain the best result for his patient. In a great number of cases I have found the employment of vaccines a measure of very uncertain value in the treatment of these cases, and after considerable experience I have abandoned their use with exception in a few cases.

Conclusions:—1. Rigid treatment of acute genito-urinary infections to prevent these cases from becoming chronic.

2. In obscure cases with a history of genito-urinary infection, a thorough examination of the genito-urinary tract should be made for a complete diagnosis.

Discussion.

Dr. J. H. Hays, Enid: Mr. Chairman, as the Doctor said, this is a timely paper. We have heard a great deal, I presume, over in the Medical Section today about focal infection. I would say about focal infection, you examine the teeth and examine the tonsils, they all think about the intestinal tract and then forget the genito-urinary tract. The cysto-urethroscope I regard as one of the most valuable instruments that I possess. I presume every neurologist who uses it has passed it down to the posterior urethra and after a thorough, gentle massaging of the prostate with the urethroscope in the place that the Doctor has stated, has often seen pus exuding. In every case of chronic gonorrhea, of course, we have an involvement of the posterior urethra. In every case of involvement of the posterior urethra we have an infection of the prostate or the seminal vesicle.

The Doctor spoke about overlooking the prostate. I think more or less of us overlook an infection of the seminal vesicle and overlook an infection of the prostate. An infection in the prostate is easily felt, because we all know where to feel for it. If you find nodules in the prostate you are sure it is infected, but we forget to go farther up into the side and feel for the seminal vesicle. Many, many times if you don't get a discharge or find pus after massaging the prostate, you may not find pus in the urine after massaging the prostate, but if you will go up and gently massage the seminal vesicle from the outside towards the inner and gently massage it in that way and have him pass urine, you will find pus, proving definitely that you have an infection in the seminal vesicle.

The treatment for infection in the seminal vesicle is very difficult. About the only treatment I know of for the seminal vesicle is massage. Whether that ever cures a cause or not I do not know, but I do use (which the Doctor says he does not use much) when I find an infection in the seminal vesicle, vaccine, and this, at the same time with the massage, gives excellent results.

Dr. McCallum, Kansas City: Mr. Chairman, this is one of the most interesting subjects in medicine. I have heard Dr. Frischer's papers quite frequently and I want to commend Dr. Hays for the addition of looking for seminal to the vesicles. If our infection is not in the prostate then in the seminal vesicle. You can wash out the bladder and wash out the urethra, massage the prostate, and you will get nothing to speak of, but if you will go up in those cases as described by Dr. Frischer, that is, the main tract here of the perineum, and will massage, you will get out of a lot of these case, almost pure pus, and very few spermatozoa. You will find gonococcus there. In the last three years, my assistant and I have done between two hundred and fifty and three hundred vasectomies. We did not drain the seminal vesicle as has been done by a lot of our friends. We did a vasectomy and that is the cure for seminal vesiculitis. We will have a paper out sometime in the near future, my assistant and myself, showing the history of those cases and it is so striking that it is almost unbelievable. As a point of infection, the seminal vesicle is greater, I think, than the tonsils or the teeth. For instance, I will cite to you two or three cases:

One of our oculists sent me a case of iritis. A Wassermann made was returned negative. He had his teeth ex-rayed and pulled out a bad tooth. For a few days the iritis cleared up and then it reappeared again. He came to us and we went over him pretty thoroughly and massaged the seminal vesicles; sent him out to the hospital; we did vasectomy under local anesthesia and in four days his eyes began to clear up. That was last November and he has had no iritis since.

I have two or three other cases almost identical and there is no doubt in my mind but what the seminal vesicles is where the focal point of infection is, but they can be cleared up, they can be greatly benefitted by a vasectomy but not by drainage of the vesicles.

A Voice: How do you do that, Doctor?

Dr. McCallum: It is very easily done, it is a very simple matter, picking up the vas, bring up the skin, injecting cocaine; that is, first bring it up with a pair of forceps. After you have scrotum folded up and taking the forceps and open it right around it, just like sticking a needle through the skin; then put on a small rubber clamp that only has a small surface where the vas goes down between the lip, so it is not pinched, and then over the end; then inject into the skin the cocaine, leaving of course the hemostat; then it is dissected down until you come to the vas, but be sure you get the last covering off of the vas and at the same time you have got to take the artery of the vas and the vessels; then with a very small, fine knife a small incision is made, just a puncture into the vas and a silkworm gut is then introduced; be sure to get it in the canal.

In a great number of these cases (one recently) we found when we got in there a block in the vas and by manipulation we got through. We had three or four of those cases just last winter. When we get thru we then inject fifteen per cent. argyrol, about twelve or fifteen cc. into the vas, then the skin is closed and the patient goes on back to bed and lies there two or three days, perfectly quiet. He has no pain, once in a while he has a little swelling but not a great deal. Some have no swelling at all.

It is a very interesting thing and I am very glad to have heard Dr. Frischer read this paper because it is a thing that the general practitioner and the general surgeon should pay a little more attention to.

Dr. J. C. Fishman, Oklahoma City: Mr. Chairman and Gentlemen, in my work I know very little on this specialty of genito-urinary, but in diagnosis it is a pleasure and refreshing to hear that there are some men thinking about focal infections away from the teeth, abscesses, and away from the tonsils. My contention in all my association with medical men and with medical societies has been for a broad view of examination and I say it is refreshing to hear that there are other men in other specialties who are looking for foci of infection, which result in general infections away from the teeth and away from the tonsils in which most of the men are inclined to think the disease is localized. The sooner the specialists forget that their studies should not be confined to their local organs the sooner the public will get what is coming to them, and that is attention, attention in a broad way. All they want is to get cured and they don't care whether the genito-urinary man finds a few threads in his urine when he is examined, if it has no relation at the time the patient suffers and complains of the troubles for which he goes to his doctor; if it has no relation to his general disease, the genito-urinary man has no right to tamper with his prostate or with his seminal vesicle. Neither has the dentist any right to pull teeth accidentally, or incidentally rather, abscesses are found around his teeth, if he can be fairly, morally certain that it has nothing to do with the disease of which he is complaining.

But I do want to comment that a thorough search and a thorough examination should be made for all possible troubles which may have a bearing in a particular case. Sometimes it is hard to decide; it is a question of judgment in one case, it is a question of chance in another case. By chance, I mean which is examined first, whether the patient is treated for one thing or another, but if we do examine patients thoroughly, and that is the way it should be done, when they come for a general condition and we get all the evidence in the last analysis it should be and surely is a question of judgment, which is the thing that probably had to do with the symptoms of which the patient suffers and of the symptoms which brings the patient to us for treatment and not because we find an abscess of a tooth or a little trouble with the tonsils that may or may not have anything to do with it, or a few threads in the urine, should we ask a patient to subject himself to treatment and, worst of all, advise him that because I, as a specialist, do this I will get results if he does what I tell him to do. That is the saddest part of all, because that brings medicine into disrepute, and we must not allow that to occur.

I am very glad to have heard this paper, I think it is timely and I wish it would be heard by more medical men.

Dr. R. T. Edwards, Oklahoma City: The only comment to be made from my standpoint on this paper is the addition that it is a most excellent one and most timely. In this respect I would like to cite a case or two:

One is a kinsman of mine who has been invalided for a period of ten years. Ten years ago he had an attack of acute-articular rheumatism. From that time on he has been afflicted, more or less periods of recurrence of rheumatism, partially recover and be able to resume a portion of his duties and would have a recurrence. He was operated upon for an infection of the nose; he was operated upon for infection of the tonsils; he had several teeth removed; he had his appendix removed; he had double pneumonia twice; he had an infection of the bowel; and partitally recovered from all of that' and had a recurrence of his rheumatism. He fell in my hands about ten months ago and I learned that he had had twelve or fifteen years prior to that time an attack of gonorrhea. I had an x-ray made of his teeth, I had a specialst on the throat examine his tonsils and nose; I had a Wassermann made and finally, as a last resort, I investigated his urethral canal. He had a normal meatus, a slight stricture of the urethra and upon observation through the urethroscope he had a mass of patches that closely resembled the old proud flesh that we used to see in _____. His tonsils showed that he had a small particle of infected tissue in each tonsil, perhaps on one side the size of a pea, on the other side the size of a small pecan. His nose showed normal. Upon repeated three or four examinations by x-ray of the teeth we found four infected teeth. Three of those teeth were removed; the tonsils were again removed; we could not remove the appendix any more, and still he suffered with repeated attacks of rheumatism; and then I began by clearing up and draining the urethra, and then by destroying the mass of tissue, by attempting to clear up the prostate glands and the seminal vesicle and after nine or ten months of effort, for the first time in ten years he was able to walk with a cane. He now has a position in which he is working twelve hours in the twenty-four, and has suffered more or less pain recently during thunder storms with his feet. His trouble was principally rheumatic trouble, principally in the knees and feet with some degree of pain and tenderness in the small of the back.

I cite that case for what it is worth.

I have another case that I wish to give a report of: A gentleman came into my office with the assistance of his son and his son's wife, a gentleman sixty-five years old. He came to me for relief from a chronic infection of the bladder. It was so intense that he was incapacitated in every respect. He was a minister of the gospel, as good a man, I think, as I have ever known, as good a Christian man. He was a circuit rider, he rode from community to community and preached and took up a little collection and managed to exist upon that small pittance that he received. He got in such a state that his kidneys moved involuntarily and, at the same time, his bowels moved regardless of where he was or under what condition. He came to me on a reference of some physician and after going over him carefully I commenced the treatment of the urethral tract. Some four weeks after I had begun the treatment he had gotten in such a state that he could control the bowel movement and to a certain degree could control the kidney action, and he asked me; "Doctor, what is the matter with me? Nobody has ever told me. Tell me what is the matter with me?" "Why", I says, "didn't you know that you had a severe inflammation of the bladder?" "Yes, but what causes it, Doctor?" I says, "Father"—he was a much older man than I am today—I says, "Father, if I told you what caused it, it will probably make you mad, and before I tell you I want you to prepare yourself for this." He says, "Tell 'what', I want to know." I says, "Father, you have the clap." And he tore his hair and screamed and says, "Liar! thief! hound! dog!" and everything. He says, "You are a damned liar." He says, "I am a preacher, I am a good man, I never did any wrong in my life, I was married when I was twenty-two years old and I have never had intercourse with but one woman, she was a good woman and she was my wife." I says, "Father, wait a minute, go back, calm yourself, control yourself. Where did you live? Where were you born?" He says, "I was born in Tennessee." I says, "Where, in the country or in town?" "In the country." I says, "Did your father own a plantation?" "Yes." "Did he have a lot of negroes?" "Yes." "Didn't you at some time in the course of your life have intercourse with a little yellow girl?" "No, no, no!" I says, "Wait, think, don't answer, think." And after a while he acknowledged that he did. At seventeen years of age he had intercourse with a little yellow girl. He remembers that he had some soreness or irritation. There were no doctors in the community and he went to a neighbor who had been a druggist, who owned the adjoining plantation, and the neighbor gave him some medicine. He did not remember that the attack lasted more than a few days and he went on and began the study of the ministry. His father during the war lost everything he had, he had to quit school before he had finished his studies and he went around preaching about the community and married at the age of twenty-two. His wife died at the age of forty-two under an operation for pus tubes. She had never had a miscarriage, nor an abortion and that man had carried gonorrhea from the time he was seventeen years old until he was past sixty-five.

I give you the history of this case for what it is worth. These infections must of necessity be cleaned up, and his trouble was a gonorrhea that he had carried for all those years, which was a focal infection, from what I do not not know. As to the seminal vesicles and the prostate gland I feel that my experience has been that you will find the infection all over the body and unless you clear it up the patient is going to have a return of this attack in the hands or feet or wherever it may be.

A Voice: We would like to hear from the Chairman.

The Chairman: Gentlemen, this is certainly a very interesting subject to me, dealing with this line of work each day, and after talking on this in school sometimes I would take it up and talk quite a while, but I am going to just mention my opinions now briefly.

This combines the posterior urethra, the ejaculatory duct, the prostate and the seminal vesicle, sometimes the vas, which at times becomes involved. In our treatment of this we are forced to the process of elimination. We want to eliminate, of course, the teeth, tonsils, and go through the general routine, and when it resolves itself down to our line of work, genito-urinary tract, then, of course, the cysto-urethroscope comes into play. We take the urine test, three glass test; that should be used in every case that comes into the office. The next thing following that, of course, is our massage examination, looking after the seminal vesicles, then the prostate, then the next thing is the meatus; and I want to say in passing in a great many of these cases before you can do very much you can do your meatotomy, then you make your examination of the posterior urethra, then you begin your treatment. Generally a meatotomy I think is necessary in a great many cases, and unless the condition of the patient will admit of examination by sound, and we must have a very large sound, because the posterior tract is a big tract. Sometimes we would have adhesions the same as we have in other portions of the body as in the posterior tract, also a contraction of the ejaculatory ducts; you will have circumscribed abscesses, renal or prostatic ducts included. You will have these little cavities of the seminal vesicles. Bear that in mind. And then we begin our prostate treatment. A sound is absolutely essential, a large sound at that. We must smooth out, iron out this tract. I think that at this time a sound should always be used first, which will considerably tone up the ducts, then do your massaging; then of course go over your prostate, to the seminal vesicle, and try to locate it; and if it is a case of this character usually you can palpate the seminal vesicle. It is usually large and sometimes pouchy and hardened, not sensitive. Your sound is easily introduced, and you can milk the secretions through the canal into the urethra; then you can have the patient void it. Then of course you have your choice as to the line of treatment. As to injections, sometimes we inject our argyrol, then nitrate of silver. Again, we make direct applications of nitrate of silver. I frequently do that, make an application, often as high as ten per cent., in the posterior urethra.

It is a very interesting subject and I would like to say more but the length of time will not permit and we have to hurry. Will someome else speak? If not, we will ask Dr. Frischer to close.

Dr. Frisher, closing: I have only one or two things to add here. We are very fortunate to have Dr. Fishman, an internist, make such broad statements. We should not confine ourselves to looking in the alimentary tract, mouth, throat and teeth; the infection may be in the genito-urinary tract.

Now in regard to the vasostomy; according to Belfield's method of opening up and injecting fluid into the vas, I use the fifteen per cent. argyrol as Dr. McCallum uses. My results have not been as gratifying as Dr. McCallum's. I will say this, the fact that he made one injection into the vas, obtained a cure, does not seem reasonable. If it is reasonable, I can make one injection into the urethra in the case of acute gonorrhea, or chronic gonorrhea, and obtain as good results. Of course we have to take into consideration the fact that the argyrol that has been put into the vas goes down into the seminal vesicle and is retained there for a certain period of time. We can dispose of considerable infectoin by having it retained in the vas and seminal vesicle; but that would be the only sufficient reason why we could get a good result from the operation.

Now in regard to sounding the posterior urethra; I use the sounds in the posterior urethra, also the Kohlman dilator.

In reference to meatotomy, I don't like to make too large an opening in the meatus for fear of future infections; that would be the only reason.

I wish to thank you for the discussion of the subject.

JOURNAL OF THE OKLAHOMA STATE MEDICAL ASSOCIATION

VOLUME XII   MUSKOGEE, OKLA., MARCH, 1919   NUMBER 3

PUBLISHED MONTHLY AT MUSKOGEE. OKLA., UNDER DIRECTION OF THE COUNCIL

DR. CLAUDE A. THOMPSON, EDITOR-IN-CHIEF

ENTERED AT THE POST OFFICE AT MUSKOGEE, OKLAHOMA, AS SECOND CLASS MAIL MATTER, JULY 20, 1912

THIS IS THE OFFICIAL JOURNAL OF THE OKLAHOMA STATE MEDICAL ASSOCIATION. ALL COMMUNICATIONS SHOULD BE ADDRESSED TO THE JOURNAL OF THE OKLAHOMA STATE MEDICAL ASSSOCIATION, 308 SURETY BUILDING, MUSKOGEE, OKLAHOMA.

The editorial department is not responsible for the opinions expressed in the original articles of contributors.

Reprints of original articles will be supplied at actual cost, provided request for them s attached to manuscript or made in sufficient time before publication.

Articles sent this Journal for publication and all those read at the annual meetings of the State Association are the sole property of this Journal. The Journal relies on each individual contributor's strict adherence to this well-known rule of medical journalism. In the event an article sent this Journal for publication is published before appearance in the Journal, the manuscript will be returned to the writer

Failure to receive the Journal should call for immediate notification of the editor, 307-8 Surety Building, Muskogee, Okla

Local news of possible interest to the medical profession, notes on removals, changes in address, deaths and weddings will be gratefully received.

Advertising of articles, drugs or compounds unapproved by the Council on Pharmacy of the A. M. A. will not be accepted.

Advertising rates will be supplied on application. It is suggested that wherever possible members of the State Association should patronize our advertisers in preference to others as a matter of fair reciprocity.

EDITORIAL

THE MEDICAL PROFESSION WINNER IN THE GREAT WAR.

For the first time in the history of our Republic we have fought a war, placing nearly four million men in the field, more than two million of them across three thousand miles of dangerous water, and in the final accurate analysis find that we have lost more men from actual combat than from disease. This triumph of the medical man is precisely shown in the official statement of the War Department issued February 25th. The report shows that we lost a total of 107,444 men from all causes at home and abroad. The Expeditionary forces lost 72,951. These are divided as follows; From disease 20,889; from injuries received in battle 48,768, and from all other causes 3,354.

This is a double victory in that our medical officers had to cope with the epidemic of influenza and at that under very adverse conditions incident to unavoidable exposure, delay often in transporting the sick, which could not be avoided on account of the pressing demands of actual conflict and advances into new territory, all of which necessarily operated against recovery.

These figures speak eloquently to the thinker and the thoughtless as well. They should everlastingly convince all that the medical profession is one which for all time should command the respect and admiration of all classes. But will they? Acquainted somewhat with the human habit of forgetting tomorrow the lessons of today, we shall not be surprised to see the profession assailed tomorrow, its every proposition for human betterment scrutinized with the idea that there is some self seeking, ulterior motive behind its advice.

INEFFECTIVE QUARANTINE.

Oklahoma has among its laws and regulations which have almost grown into law, one requiring quarantine against certain communicable diseases. Almost since the memory of man these regulations have not been altered a particle, notwithstanding exact means for combating the disease have been always at hand.

The time and money wasted on inefficient quarantine against smallpox when there is no necessity for it whatever seems not to appeal to either health officers or the tax payers. Certain well known facts concerning this disease are so firmly established that they are axiomatic and any step to control the disease not based on such facts is farcical, unscientific and useless.

Promptly on the appearance of a case in the schools, where of all places we have a right to expect some semblance of reason to prevail, the patient is sent home, the school board hurriedly gets together and orders the teacher to close out for the time being; the health officer orders a quarantine which is observed more or less, usually not at all. The law in its majesty allows the patient's family to use its own free will as to vaccination. If they are paupers, they call on the county to feed them while they are going through the process of acquiring the easily preventable disease and recovering from it. If the school authorities ignore the existence of the disease, a howl promptly sets up from everyone about. It seems never to occur to any authority to issue a statement about as follows:

"Smallpox exists in school number ____. Pupils attending will be vaccinated by their attending physician if they wish or by the health officer without charge. No exclusion from school will be made on account of this disease. Parents and guardians are advised that successful vaccination will postively prevent the disease. If one has been previously vaccinated and is now immune, vaccination now will not 'take', they do not need it. If it is needed, it will likely 'take', showing the need for it, and at the same time the pupil will not contract the disease. It is not deemed advisable to penalize children protected against this disease by having them lose valuable school time. Children who do not see fit to receive vaccination will be permitted to continue in school, but must assume all risk of infection. The school board issues this statement for the information of all concerned".

MUCK RAKING THE DOCTOR.

Physicians over the State acquainted with the superb management of the Enid Institution for Feeble Minded Children since its organization, Dr. W. L. Kendall, Superintendent, were amazed at the recent notoriety given Dr. Kendall by the Oklahoma City Times by what is said to be a "Staff" or special correspondent for that paper. Designated, apparently, for the sole purpose of investigating the institution and its management, this writer made the serious mistake of accepting as true statements made by two ex-employees who had been, according to Drs. Kendall and McInnis, the Assistant Superintendent, discharged for improper conduct. The net result of the whole matter is that the Times and Daily Oklahoman now have on their hands dangerous libel suits from Dr. Kendall's attorneys for large amounts.

The Enid Institution is one which every physician who ever visited it, attracted at once the admiration and pride of the visitor. Dr. Kendall built the Institution from nothing to its present delightfully clean and orderly organization all Oklahoma may may be justly proud of. It is not recorded by the "Staff" correspondent that Dr. Kendall, when the State could not appropriate sufficient funds for the purpose, employed Dr. McInnis for the nominal salary paid a clerk for clerical work. It is not recorded that McInnis not only did that work, but assisted in operations, treated the sick and operated a complete laboratory up under the roof in the garret, and has always since that time been a most efficient servant of the State and the unfortunate little charges under him. It is not recorded either that Dr. Kendall, in addition to being a psychiatrist of no mean ability, was by necessity Executive Officer for the Institution, that he made up estimates for food, clothing, drugs, operated the farm, besides attending to the unlimited detail surrounding such a position.

It is understood by the intelligent that unpleasant things occur about any institution having the care of defectives. It is difficult to know when they are seriously sick and they are most difficult to treat. Keeping them clean and orderly is next to impossible. The writer has had the privilege of visiting this institution on many occasions and observed minutely the handling of matters above alluded to. The hospital was found cleaner than most any private hospital of the State; the children were treated with uniform kindness; the wards were also in an immaculate condition, the grounds and all outbuildings were neatly attended. During the epidemic of influenza this good physician and servant of the State was terribly overworked, not having either sufficient medical aides or nurses, yet his death rate compares most favorably with the rest of the country. For all this efficiency he has now come to face what most public servants sooner or later face—the most outrageous charges of inefficiency and maladministration. Enid and Garfield County physicians are a unit in commending his handling of affairs, yet we have the spectacle of a "Staff" correspondent hunting for trouble, making a mountain of a mole hill in such a manner as to ruin the reputation of a good man if the charges are allowed to go unchallenged. The eager papers hashing up this delectable. mess will now have an opportunity to make good their statements in court. When his friends recall Dr. Kendall's good fighting chin and his clean face we have no doubt as to the outcome.

PERSONAL AND GENERAL NEWS

Dr. S. E. Gayman, Tyron, has moved to Okeene.

Dr. J. T. Wharton, Duncan, is moving to Miami.

Dr. R. E. Johnson, Bridgeport, is moving to Hobart.

Dr. F. S. King, Muskogee, visited Battle Creek in February.

Dr. W. I. Wimberly, Hammon, is moving to New Orleans, La.

Dr. W. G. Brymer, Dewar, is doing special work in New Orleans.

Dr. S. C. Davis, Oklahoma City, has returned from overseas service.

Dr. and Mrs. A. B. Leeds, Chickasha, visited New Mexico in February.

Dr. T. J. Nunnery, Granite, has been discharged from the military service.

Dr. F. B. Fite, Muskogee, was seriously ill with influenza in January and February.

Dr. T. S. Booth, Ardmore, seriously ill in February, is reported as improving slowly.

Dr. A. J. Smith, Pawhuska, has been appointed county physician for Osage County.

Dr. W. C. High, Maysville, was reported as seriously ill in a Texas hospital in February.

Dr. W. W. Brodie, Tulsa, has been discharged from the army and will soon resume his work.

Dr. H. L. Dalby, Wilburton, has returned to that city after living in California for some time.

Drumright Medical Society has approved the plans for a hospital to be erected in that city.

Dr. Fred S. Clinton, Tulsa, announces the removal of his office to 411-12 New World Building.

Sapulpa citizens are agitating the voting of bonds for the purpose of erecting a city and county hospital.

Dr. H. A. Scott, City Physician, Muskogee, resigned. Dr. J. I. Hollingsworth was appointed in his stead.

Dr. and Mrs. T. C. Sanders, Shawnee, are visiting New Orleans where Dr. Sanders is looking in on the Polyclinic.

Dr. Hugh Scott, Dustin, returned from the Army as a Lieutenant Colonel, has moved his location to Holdenville.

Dr. J. V. Athey, Bartlesville, who is in France, is remembering his friends by sending them cuttings of rare French roses.

Tulsa nurses and physicians returning from army service were tendered a ball February 11th by the Tulsa Nurses Association.

Dr. McLain Rogers, Clinton, who was severely ill in January and February, has regained his health and is back on the job again.

Dr. K. D. Gossam, Custer City, has been appointed health officer for Beckham county vice Dr. Ellis Lamb, whose term expires.

DISCHARGED FROM THE ARMY.

E. W. King, Bristow.
Ira Mullens, Hominy.
E. B. Thomasson, Velma.
S. J. Fryer, Muskogee.
W. G. Baird, Oakhill.
W. R. Clement, Tulsa.
M. H. Edens, Anadarko.
J. O. Bradshaw, Welch.
J. B. Shannon, Pauls Valley.
W. W. Brodie, Tulsa.
E. E. Rice, Shawnee.

R. E. Thacker, Lexington.
T. J. Butler, Weatherford.
S. C. Davis, Oklahoma City.
C. C. Shaw, Ada.
W. B. Newell. Hunter,
Hugh T. Scott, Holdenville.
A. N. Earnest, Muskogee.
E. P. Allen, Oklahoma City.
E. R. Askew, Hugo.
O. O. Dawson, Wayne.
J. A. Munn, Wilburton.

Dr. G. H. Phillips, Pawnee, who has been absent in the Government Indian Service at various western agencies, has returned to his home.

Dr. Chester L. Hill, Haskell, **and Miss Bertha Pauline Kennedy,** Muskogee, were married in the latter city February 26th. After a short trip they will be at home in Haskell.

Dr. E. E. Rice, Shawnee, one of the earliest physicians from Oklahoma to enter the military service immediately on the outbreak of the war, has returned to his home from foreign service.

Drs. I. B. Oldham, F. B. Fite and C. A. Thompson have been named as executive committee for the Muskogee County Medical Society to handle all phases of the annual meeting. They will name all subcommittees and have charge of details.

Smallpox had existed only since November, 1918, in the Baptist Orphanage near Oklahoma City before the manager concluded to have a physician see what the disease was. Thirty-one of the children were ill when investigation was made by Dr. A. K. West, health officer of Oklahoma County.

Dr. J. P. Cowman, Comanche, has returned to his home after army service. Dr. Cowman has the unusual and proud distinction of being accompanied home by his son, Captain John Cowman, who "Beat the Old Man" by getting himself overseas while his father was "Tinning" around Camp Logan.

Dr. A. L. Blesh, Oklahoma City, says there is more dirt in the streets of his city than in an American Army Camp of 150,000 men. Blesh has always been "swelled" up over his town—we are over ours—so if the Major is hunting competition we respectfully refer him to the streets of Tulsa and Muskogee. They are far richer in dirt than those of the Capitol City.

Dr. Thomas B. Dickson, Ramona, for many years located at Chelsea, was found dead in his room in a Kansas City hotel where he had been murdered, the motive supposedly robbery as his pockets and clothing had been rifled. No clue has been found to the crime. Dr. Dickson is said to have amassed a large fortune in the oil business. He leaves a large family and a circle of friends to mourn his tragic death.

Dr. Joseph H. Stopler, Muskogee, a Captain in the Medical Corps of the Army reported in the February Journal as having been, according to press dispatches, courtmartialed and discharged dishonorably from the army, arrived home in February with a complete refutation of the sensational reports as printed in a Muskogee and North Carolina paper. Through some error the name of Dr. Stolper was used in this connection and it is a matter of regret that he was given the undeserved notoriety.

Dr. G. Pinnell, Miami, Secretary of the Ottawa County Society, drew "First Blood" for 1919 honors, and received as his reward for being the first secretary to remit 1919 dues, certificate "Number One 1919". Dr. Pinnell was formerly secretary of Comanche County Society and carried with him on his removal to Ottawa County the same "Punch" and activity which characterizes secretaries of "Live" County societies. It is almost an axoim that a good secretary means a good society and Ottawa County is one of the livest in the State.

Police Chief Nichols, Oklahoma City, is the recipient of some active attention from the Oklahoma City medical profession. The Chief is reported to have said that "for the sum of $5.00 or $10.00 practically all physicians of the county would furnish 'dope' to drug addicts." He is invited by special resolution to furnish the evidence of prescribing or giving in violation of the law and is assured that the profession will unitedly assist in the prosecution of such violations. (We happen to know the "Chief" and believe he is far and away the best police executive in Oklahoma, and we cannot conceive of such a statement emanating from him.—Ed.)

Dr. Fowler Border, Mangum, recently won a damage suit against the Mangum Electric Company and other codefendants,. the verdict being for $62,000.00. The action grew out of charges by Dr. Border that the Light Company and others conspired to ruin and damage him by conspiring to induce him to perform a criminal operation. At the time of the occurrence Dr. Border was Mayor of Mangum and a bitter fight arose over a municipal light bond issue. Some of the parties in question and the women induced to go to Mangum were trapped by Dr. Border and arrested by the Sheriff of Greer County. The suit just terminated at Sayre on a change of venue resulted from this espisode.

Joint Influenza Committee. A Joint Influenza Committee has just been created to study the epidemic and to make comparable, so far as possible, the influenza data gathered by the Government departments. The members of this committee, as designated by the Surgeon General of the Army, the Surgeon General of the Navy, the Surgeon General of the Public Health Service, and the Director of the Census, are: Dr. William H. Davis, chairman. and Mr. C. S. Sloane, representing the Bureau of the Census; Dr. Wade H. Frost and Mr. Edgar Sydenstricker, of the Public Health Service; Colonel D. C. Howard, Colonel F. F. Russell, and Lieutenant Colonel A. G. Love, United States Army; Lieutenant Commander J. R. Phelps and Surgeon Carroll Fox, United States Navy.

CORRESPONDENCE

_____, Oklahoma, February 21, 1919.

Editor Oklahoma State Medical Journal,
Muskogee, Oklahoma,

Dear Sir:

Your editorial in the January number entitled "When Johnny Comes Marching Home" was of special interest to me because I was at that time one of the Johnnies, and had found on my return from the Army that my practice had been usurped by another doctor.

As there was no other doctor in this village I tried to secure one to take care of my practice while I was away in the Army, but because I intended to return to the location after the war was over I could make no satisfactory arrangements. I heard a rumor that a certain doctor of _____, Oklahoma, near here, was thinking of locating here after I left, so I wrote him stating that I could probably make arrangements satisfactory to both of us if he were thinking of leaving _____, but specified that I would want him to give up the location when I returned. He answered my letter and stated that he had never thought of coming here and could not consider leaving _____ because one of the Doctors there was preparing to enter the service and that he would be needed at home more than ever. On the evening I left home to report for duty I happened to meet up with this doctor on the train and he reiterated his statement that he could not leave home. One week later he appeared in my drug store and wanted to rent my office rooms, stating that he was going to move to _____. My wife told him that she would not rent the rooms because I would return to use them after the war was over. He replied that that would be satisfactory to him because he was moving to Enid after the war was over.

When I returned after being discharged from the Army, various rumors came to me—rumors that had their origin somewhere else than from me—chief of which was to the effect that the doctor was going to stay in my little village which had never before supported more than one doctor. Two or three days later I called upon him, having not seen him before this, to see what his plans were. He very pertly informed me that he was going to stay, that I should have not left in the first place and that the war would have been won without my going. He gave as his reason for coming here that he saw some doctor from _____ would have to go to the Army or leave _____ so he came here. By this time I had heard about all I could stand of such "patriotic" talk so I told him straight from the shoulder what I thought of him and his actions, and added that if he were still sticking around by a certain date that I would give his face a genuine punching.

Later, thru the action of the County Council of Defense, Medical Council and influential men I was asked to refrain from carrying into effect my promise to the doctor and advised that these men would be glad to handle the matter for me. This I agreed to. A few of these men also talked to the other doctor and tried to show him where he was wrong, that his actions were not patriotic and that he was making an ass out of himself by doing the way he was. But he was defiant, swore that he had never been run out of a place and didn't intend to be run out of here. At the meeting of the _____ held at _____ we met and acted upon the suggestion of the Chairman of the Oklahoma State Council of Medical Defense, we selected a committee of medical men to settle the matter. After hearing our testimony this committee decided unanimously that the location belonged to me and recommended that the other doctor move away. And he did move away after two or three weeks—not because of the advice and requests given him (he defied all such) but largely because "pickings" were very scarce for him after I returned from the Army.

Now why any doctor would stoop to such underhanded methods and thereby demonstrate his slackerism is hard to say. But with this particular doctor a glimpse into his record is sufficient explanation. As I recall he finished Medical school in 1911 and located in _____, Oklahoma, a town of 20,000 population. Maybe his health (?) grew bad in that city, anyway he moved to ,_____ a town of about 2,000 population in early 1915 and went into parternship there but the partnership did not last long. Maybe some more bad health overtook him about the time I went to the Army, anyway he moved to _____ a town of 250 population. The epidemic of "Flu" coming on, and most of the doctors of any prominence around here having gone to the Army, he made the first real money that he had ever made in his life. There's the reason he hated to leave. Having been a failure every other place he had been he naturally wanted to stay here. I understand that he has bought into a "game" near here and I hope he has and will get it in the neck when the proper time arrives. I recite this affair to show what some of the men have confronting them "When Johnny Comes Marching Home". I hope, however, that another doctor with such a low code of ethics and lack of patriotism is not to be found in our excellent State and grand profession. If there is another such, may God pity him—not me—he needs it worse than I do.

_____M. D.

MISCELLANEOUS

THE HARRISON ACT.

As amended by the new War Revenue Act, will be mailed postpaid to any druggist, physician, dentist or veterinarian who will send a postal request therefor to "Mailing Department, Parke, Davis & Co., Detroit, Mich." Please observe directions strictly.

EMPYEMA.

Observations on the empyema following influenzal pneumonia at Camp Grant, Rockford, Ill,. are reported by Major Max Ballin (Detroit) (*Journal A. M. A.*, Feb. 1, 1919). The pneumonia was grouped in three types and the empyema, similarly, (1) the empyema following hemolytic streptococcus pneumonia; (2) that following lobar pneumonia, and (3) that following influenzal pneumonia. In the winter of 1917-1918, when the streptococcus epidemic occurred, the method used following lobar pneumonia, as we know it, that is, that of early evacuation by drainage through wide incision, preferably by costectomy, was employed. The result of this treatment was so unfortunate, the mortality being about 50 per cent., that the Surgeon-General sent an Empyema Commission to investigate. Several points were brought out; First, not to operate until after the pneumonic process had subsided; second, to aspirate if respiration was interfered with; third, to operate only after pus had formed, and then by intracostal incision or better by rib resection. Following these rules there was only one death in twenty-three cases. The principles laid down for the streptococcus epidemic, however, do not apply for the influenza cases, in which the large amount of exudation in the chest calls for early and repeated aspiration, and costectomy was an error. The differentiation of the two forms is made by the later appearance of the empyema complication in the influenza cases, the lack of early exudate, the process requiring at least four weeks and the character of the exudate itself, which is at first a gray-reddish fluid with small flakes in the steptococcal cases. In the influenzal cases it is from the beginning thick and purulent, and sometines containing large fibrinous masses. This is unsuited for aspiration and requires a large opening for drainage. The influenza empyema also differs from that following lobar pneumonia, as does the influenzal pneumonia itself differ from the lobar cases. The following are the special characteristics of the influenzal type: "1. It is complicated more frequently by other metastic abscesses, and for this reason is accompanied by a greater mortality. 2. In roentgen findings, fluid levels are absent. The exudate takes in the whole chest or is encysted. 3. Large lung abscesses are found frequently complicating lobar pneumonia in roentgenoscopies as well as in necropsies. In influenzal pneumonia they are not found." The empyema is of a less favorable prognosis, the death rate probably running up to 20 per cent. The empyema is only one of the complications occurring. There is no fluid level, and the lack of abscesses is notable. The diagnosis of empyema should be based on the typical chart of such cases, exploratory puncture, and the roentgen ray. In treatment, only local anesthesia should be employed, and Ballin describes the technic fully. The operation has been followed by about 14 per cent. of fatalities. All the patients that died had some complication rendering the case more severe, either suppurative meningitis or cholecystitis, etc. The Dakin treatment did not seem to lessen the mortality. In the after-care proper attention to caloric feeding is important, and also to fresh air and early muscle exercise. Special care is to be taken to elevate the arm on the operated side at every dressing to prevent rigidity of muscles.

PROPAGANDA FOR REFORM.

Misbranded Nostrums. The following "patent medicines" have been the subject of prosecution under the Federal Food and Drugs Act: Paine's Celery Compound; Botanic Blood Balm; Owens' Wonderful Sore Wash; Lafayette Cough Syrup; Gilbert's Gravel Root Compound; Strange's Rheumatic Remedy; Baur's Diamond Brand Bromides; S. B. Cough and Consumption Remedy; Gowan's Preparation; Urol; Roxenbaum Discovery; Tablets Creavita; Old Lady Fulton's Comforting Pills; C. C. C. (Crownall Elastic Capsules); Victor Injection; No. 19 Compound and No. 6 Compound; Hemogenas Pills; Restorative Tablets—Fountain of Health; Denn's Strong, Sure, Safe and Speedy Stomach, Liver, Kidney, and Rheumatism Remedy; Dr. Navaun's Mexican Lung Balm; Dr. Navaun's Kidney Tablets; Dr. Chas. DeGrath's Electric Oil; Bovinine; Fritch's Vegetable Liniment; Perkin's National Herbs Blood Purifier, Kidney and Liver Regulator; Dr. Lemke's Golden Electric Liniment; Dr. Lemke's St. Johannis Drops; Mentholatum; Enteronol; Dr. Herter's Lung Balm; Dr. O. Phelps Brown's Herbal Ointment; Taylor's Horehound Balsam; Breeden's Rheumatic Cure; Sulphur Bitters; Dr. DeWitt's Electric Cure; Dr. DeWitt's Liver, Blood and Kidney Remedy; Payne's Sylak; Dr. Bell's Pine Tar Honey, and Lung Germine (*Jour. A. M. A.*, Jan. 4, 1919, p. 59).

"Aspirin" a Common Name. The claim of the Bayer Company to the exclusive right of applying the name "aspirin" to acetylsalicylic acid will be definitely set aside if the recommendation of the examiner of interferences of the United States patent office is upheld. The stand taken by the patent office is in line with the established principle that no one can have a monopoly in the name of anything. Since "aspirin" gas become the common name for acetylsalicylic acid, no one firm can have an exclusive right to it (*Jour. A. M. A.*, Jan. 11, 1919, p. 119).

The Quality of the Market Supply of Procaine. The local anesthetic procaine (first introduced as novocaine by the Farbwerke vorm. Meister, Lucius and Bruening, Hoeschst A. M. Germany) is now manufactured by the Abbott Laboratories, the H. A. Metz Laboratories and the Rector Chemical Company. The products of these three firms were accepted for New and Nonofficial Remedies after the A. M. A. Chemical Laboratory had reported specimens chemically satisfactory and the Cornell Pharmacologic Laboratory had determined that they were not unduly toxic. In accordance with its announcement to report from time to time on the quality of American made synthetics, the Council on Pharmacy and Chemistry now publishes a report on the quality of the procaine now supplied to physicians. The examination demonstrates that the three brands were of a satisfactory quality. Some of the specimens of procaine-Abbott and procaine-Rector had a yellow or light brown tinge (a specimen of procaine-Metz "novocaine" recently sent the Council also had a slight yellow tinge), but so far as the evidence goes there is nothing to indicate that the discolored specimens are seriously impure. The Council considers the use of the discolored product justified in the present emergency, but urges that for the future a colorless preparation be supplied (*Jour. A. M. A.*, Jan. 11, 1919, p. 136).

Pluriglandular Mixtures. The Council on Pharmacy and Chemistry reports that the following preparations put out by Henry R. Harrower have been found ineligible for New and Nonofficial Remedies: Caps. Adreno-Spermin Comp.; Caps. Antero-Pituitary Comp.; Caps. Placanto-Mammary Comp.; Caps. Thyro-Ovarian Comp.; Caps. Pepato-Splenic Comp.; Caps. Pancreas Comp., and Caps. Thyroid Comp. Each of the mixtures contained one ingredient or more which is neither recognized in the U. S. Pharmacopoeia nor admitted to New and Nonofficial Remedies. For obvious reasons the Council does not accept a mixture containing an indefinite ingredient; hence, it would be necessary as a preliminary for the consideration of any one of the mixtures that their unofficial ingredients be made eligible for New and Nonofficial Remedies, by the submission of evidence that such ingredient is of uniform composition and that it is therapeutically valuable when given by mouth. The mixtures were also ineligible because in the light of our knowledge the administration of gland mixtures in the host of conditions enumerated in the advertising circular of Harrower is irrational and on a par with the use of shotgun mixtures once in vogue (*Jour A. M. A.*, Jan. 18, 1919, p. 213).

Unsuccessful Attempts to Transmit Influenza Experimentally. Two extensive attempts have been made under the auspices of the U. S. Public Health Service and the U. S. Navy to transmit influenza experimentally. Inoculations were made of pure cultures of the influenza bacillus, of secretions of the upper air passages in the early stages of influenza, and of blood from typical cases of influenza, and other methods of transmitting the disease were tried. In no case was influenza developed (*Jour. A. M. A.*, Jan. 25, 1919, p. 281).

Evidence. The Cutter Laboratory advertises that a physician has used between 700 and 800 doses of its Mixed Vaccine—Respiratory Infections as a prophylactic without a single failure to "protect" against the disease. The Cutter Laboratory thinks this is evidence which "is convincing enough to satisfy even the most conservative . . . ." If a physician were to report that 643 of his patients who had used salt instead of sugar in their coffee had remained free from influenza, would this be evidence of the prophylactic value of sodium chlorid? The science of therapeutics is complex enough at its best; and with commercialism dominating the production of therapeutic agents, the liklihood of ever arriving at anything approximating a true science of therapeutics seems hopeless (*Jour. A. M. A.*, Jan. 4, 1919, p. 45).

Coca-Cola. Analyses made by federal chemists showed it to contain from 0.92 to 1.30 grains of caffein to the fluidounce. It would seem that in the interest of the public health the indiscriminate sale to children and adults of an alkaloid like caffein in the enticing form of a "soft drink" is to be deprecated (*Jour. A. M. A.*, Jan. 25, 1919, p. 299).

Some "Patent Medicines" Investigated by the Government. The following are the names of proprietary medicines which have been the subject of prosecution under the Federal Food and Drugs Act in the government's attempt to protect the public against fraudulent or misleadingly advertsed products: Royal Baby's Safety; Simpson's Cerebro-Spinal Nerve Compound; Constitution Water; Tweed's Liniment; Pulmonol; Crown Skin Salve and Pile Cure; King of the World and Family Liniment; Ka-Ton-Ka; Greenhalgh Diphtheria Remedy; Mountain Rose Tonic Tablets and Herbaline; Parmint; Sulphurro; "Liveon, The 90 Day Consumption Cure;" "Liveon Lung Discs;" White Beaver's Cough Cream and Wonder Work; Watkins' Vegetable Anodyne Liniment, Female Remedy, and Kidney Tablets; Nature's Creation Co.'s Discovery; Radium Healing Balm; Phuton Kidney Remedy; Palmer's Skin Whitener; Barnes Baby Relief; Sayman's Healing Salve; Sayman's Vegetable Wonder Soap; Humphreys' Pile Ointment, Witch Hazel Oil (Compound); Hill's Honey and Tar Compound; "La Franco Combination Treatment" and "La Franco Vitalizer No. 200." (*Jour. A. M. A.*, Jan. 25 1919, p. 297).

NEW BOOKS

Under this heading books received by the Journal will be acknowledged. Publishers are advised that this shall constitute return for such publications as they may submit. Obviously all publications sent us cannot be given space for review, but from time to time books received, of possible interest to Oklahoma physicians, will be reviewed.

INFORMATION FOR THE TUBERCULOUS.

By F. W. Wittich, A. M., M. D., Instructor in Medicine and Physician in Charge Tuberculosis Dispensary, University of Minnesota Medical School; Visiting Physician, University Hospital, Minneapolis. Cloth, 150 pages. Price $1.00, C. V. Mosby Company, St. Louis, Mo., 1918.

This is a timely little volume on a subject, which on account of war revelations is engrossing the minds of the physician, people and organizations who are hoping to successfully cope with tuberculosis in better and more sane fashion than heretofore. It is agreed by thinkers that one of the prime elements for successfully handling this disease is the intelligent attitude and cooperation at all times of the patient himself. Without that there can be no lasting benefit from any measure. This book undertakes to state in plain language to the patient, the fundamental causes and phenomena associated with various phases of the disease, then handles the manifold measures associated with treatment of it and its complications. It is preeminently a book for the patient and should be placed in his hands for his intelligent guidance.

MENTAL DISEASES.

A Handbook Dealing With Diagnosis and Classification. By Walter Vose Gulick, M. D., Assistant Superintendent Western State Hospital, Fort Steilacoom, Washington. Illustrated, 142 pages. Price $2.00. C. V. Mosby Company, St. Louis, 1918.

"Born of the wants we all have for concise, digested information, it institutes a response to that need. . . The physician in a court or conducting office or public examinations of the insane, or unexpectedly called upon for diagnosis in private practice, will accept this book with relief. . . Original, pleasing. . with much Anglo-Saxon directness" is a part of the summing up of the introducer. Little can be added to that description. It is a readable, remarkably concise discussion of mental troubles, said in such language that the harried practitioner should find it welcome.

SURGICAL TREATMENT, VOLUME I.

A practical Treatise on the Therapy of Surgical Diseases for the use of Practitioners and Students of Surgery. By James Peter Warbasse, M. D., Formerly Attending Surgeon to the Methodist Episcopal Hospital, Brooklyn, New York. In three large octavo volumes, and separate Desk Index Volume. Volume I contains 947 pages with 699 illustrations. Philadelphia and London: W. B. Sanders Company, 1918. Per set (Three Volumes and the Index Volume): Cloth $30.00 per set.

The author of this magnificient system of surgery states that it is his aim to write in the interest of the surgical patient, to place in the hands of the surgeon the means for rendering help in every surgical condition under all circumstances. He lays down the rule that there is an ideal course to follow, the highest possiblity of surgery and endeavors to present the maximun of treatment, which is the ideal. He assumes that the application of the ideal often requires unusual skill and knowledge, but that circumstances may surround both surgeon and patient which limit the application of the best. With that in mind, he presents alternatives in treatment wherever he deems them necessary or likely to be called for.

He holds that surgery is an art based on a complex of sciences, that it is always in the developmental stage—a statement that will doubtless be taken with a grain of salt or reservation by those of us who have reached that stage of perfection in technique, diagnosis and other procedure allied to surgical work, evidenced by a habit and attitude sometimes plainly, but painfully apparent interpreted that we are through, this has stood me well in "so and so", etc.

The work is beautifully and clearly illustrated, many of the cuts and drawings original to the author.

This issue contains the following subjects: General Principles, Asepsis and Antisepsis, Surgical Materials, Anesthesia, Wounds and Operations, Inflammations, Surgical Fevers and Infections, Fistulas and Sinuses, Nutritive Disturbances, Tumors, Blood and Blood-Vessels, Lymphatic System, Diseases of Bones, Fractures, Dislocations, Diseases of Joints, Operations on Bones and Joints, Muscles, Tendons, Fasciae and Bursae, Skin and Its Appendages and Nerves. There is an index of names and subjects.

A MANUAL OF GYNECOLOGY.

By John Cooke Hirst, M. D., Associate in Gynecology, University of Pennsylvania; Obstetrican and Gynecologist to the Philadelphia General Hospital. 12mo of 466 pages with 175 illustrations. Philadelphia and London: W. B. Saunders Company, 1918. Cloth, $2.50 net.

A MANUAL OF DISEASES OF THE NOSE, THROAT, AND EAR. By E. B. Gleason, M. D., Professor of Otology in the Medico-Chirurgical College Graduate School, University of Pennsylvania. Fourth Edition, thoroughly revised. 12mo of 616 pages, 212 illustrations. Philadelphia and London: W. B. Saunders Company, 1918. Cloth, $3.00 net.

A TEXT BOOK OF GENERAL BACTERIOLOGY. By Edwin O. Jordan, Ph. D., Professor of Bacteriology in the University of Chicago and in the Rush Medical College. Sixth edition, thoroughly revised. Octavo of 691 pages, fully illustrated. Philadelphia and London: W. B. Saunders Company, 1918. Cloth, $3.75 net.

MILITARY HYGIENE AND SANITATION. By Frank R Keefer, M. D., Colonel, Medical Corps, United States Army; Formerly Professor of Military Hygiene, United States Military Academy, West Point. Second edition, reset. 12mo of 340 pages, illustrated. Philadelphia and London: W. B. Saunders Company, 1918. Cloth, $1.75 net.

OFFICERS OF OKLAHOMA STATE MEDICAL ASSOCIATION.

President—Dr. L. S. Willour, McAlester (A. E. F. in France). G. F. Border, Mangum, acting.

President-elect—Dr. L. J. Moorman, Oklahoma City.

1st Vice-President,—Dr. E. D. James, Miami.

2nd Vice- President—Dr. H. M. Williams, Wellston.

3rd Vice-President,—Walter Hardy, Ardmore.

Delegate to A. M. A., 1919-1920—LeRoy Long, Oklahoma City.

Meeting place, Muskogee—May 20-21-22, 1919 Headquarters, Hotel Severs. For details address Dr. H. C. Rogers, Phoenix Building, Muskogee.

CHAIRMEN OF SCIENTIFIC SECTIONS.

Surgery and Gynecology—A. A. Will, Oklahoma City.

Pediatrics and Obstetrics—Vice Chairman, O. A. Flanagan, 305 Bliss Bldg., Tulsa.

Eye, Ear, Nose and Throat—R. O. Early, Ardmore.

General Medicine, Nervous and Mental Diseases—F. W. Ewing, Muskogee.

Genitourinary, Skin and Radiology—R. T. Edwards, Oklahoma City.

Legislative Committee—Dr. Millington Smith, Oklahoma City; Dr. J. M. Byrum, Shawnee; Dr. J. C. Mahr, Oklahoma City.

For the Study and Control of Cancer—Drs. LeRoy Long, Oklahoma City; Gayfree Ellison, Norman; D. A. Myers, Lawton.

For the Study and Control of Pellagra—Drs. A. A. Thurlow, Norman; L. A. Mitchell, Frederick; J. C. Watkins, Checotah.

For the Study and Control of Venereal Diseases—Drs. Wm. J. Wallace, Oklahoma City; Ross Grosshart Tulsa; J. E. Bercaw, Okmulgee.

Necrology—Drs. Martha Bledsoe, Chickasha; J. W. Pollard, Bartlesville.

Tuberculosis—Drs. L. J. Moorman, Oklahoma City; C. W. Heitzman, Muskogee; Leila E. Andrews, Oklahoma City.

Conservation of Vision—Drs. L. A. Newton, Oklanoma City; L. Haynes Buxton, Oklahoma City; G. E. Hartshorne, Shawnee.

Hospital Committee—F. S. Clinton, Tulsa: M. Smith, Oklahoma City: C. A. Thompson, Muskogee.

Committee on Medical Education—Drs. A. L. Blesh; A. K. West; A. W. White, Oklahoma City.

State Commissioner of Health—Dr. John W. Duke, Guthrie, Oklahoma.

STATE BOARD OF MEDICAL EXAMINERS.

Melvin Gray, M. D., Durant, President; B. L. Denison, M. D., Garvin, Vice-President; J. J. Williams, M. D., Weatherford, Secretary; O. R. Gregg, M. D., Waynoka, Treasurer; E. B. Dunlap, M. D., Lawton; Ralph V. Smith, M. D., Tulsa; W. LeRoy Bonnell, M. D., Chickasha; Wm. T. Ray, M. D., Gould; W. E. Sanderson, M. D., Altus; H. C. Montague, D. O., Muskogee.

Reciprocity with Georgia, Kentucky, Mississippi, Nevada, North Carolina, Wisconsin, Kansas, Arkansas, Virginia, West Virginia, Nebraska, New Mexico, Tennessee, Iowa, Ohio, California, Colorado, Indiana, Missouri, New Jersey, Vermont, Texas, Michigan.

Meetings held second Tuesday of January, April, July and October, Oklahoma City.

Address all communications to the Secretary, Dr. J. J. Williams, Weatherford.

OFFICERS OF COUNTY SOCIETIES, 1919

County	President	Secretary
Adair	D. P. Chambers, Stilwell	J. A. Patton, Stilwell
Alfalfa	E. L. Frazier, Jet	J. M. Tucker, Carmen
Atoka-Coal	F. E. Sadler, Coalgate	W. T. Blount, Tupelo.
Beaver		
Beckham		R. L. Edmonds, Elk City
Blaine		J. A. Norris, Okeene
Bryan	H. B. Fuston, Bokchito	D. Armstrong, Durant
Caddo	P. H. Anderson, Anadarko	C. R. Hume, Anadarko
Canadian		W. J. Muzzy, El Reno
Choctaw	C. H. Hale, Boswell	J. D. Moore, Hugo
Carter		Robert H. Henry, Ardmore
Cleveland		D. W. Griffin, Norman.
Cherokee		
Comanche	A. H. Stewart, Lawton	E. B. Mitchell, Lawton
Coal-Atoka	F. E. Sadler, Coalgate	W. T. Blount, Tupelo
Cotton		
Craig	C. B. Bell, Welch	F. M. Adams, Vinita
Creek		H. S. Garland, Sapulpa.
Custer		Ellis Lamb, Clinton.
Dewey		
Ellis		
Garfield		L. W. Cotton, Enid.
Garvin		N. H. Lindsey, Pauls Valley.
Grady	Martha Bledsoe, Chickasha	J. C. Ambrister, Chickasha.
Grant		
Greer		
Harmon		
Haskell		R. F. Terrell, Stigler.
Hughes		
Jackson	J. S. Stults, Olustee	J. B. Hix, Altus
Jefferson		
Johnston		H. B. Kniseley, Tishomingo.
Kay		A. S. Risser, Blackwell.
Kingfisher	Frank Scott, Kingfisher	C. W. Fisk, Kingfisher.
Kiowa		A. T. Dobson, Hobart.
Latimer	E. L. Evins, Wilburton	C. R. Morrison, Wilburton
Le Flore	C. H. Mahar, Spiro	Harrell Hardy, Poteau
Lincoln		C. M. Morgan, Chandler
Logan		O. E. Barker, Guthrie.
Love		
Mayes	J. L. Adams, Pryor	L. C. White, Adair.
Major		
Marshall	J E Reed, Madill	J L Holland, Madill
McClain	J. W. West, Purcell	O. O. Dawson, Wayne
McCurtain		R. H. Sherrill, Broken Bow
McIntosh	S. W. Minor, Hitchita	W. A. Tolleson, Eufaula
Murray		W. H. Powell, Sulphur.
Muskogee	J. L. Blakemore, Muskogee	H C. Rogers, Muskogee
Noble		B. A. Owen, Perry.
Nowata	J. E. Brookshire, Nowata	J. R. Collins, Nowata
Okfuskee	C. Bombarger, Paden	H. A. May, Okemah.
Oklahoma	W. J. Wallace, Oklahoma City	J. N. Alford, Oklahoma City
Okmulgee	Harry Breese, Henryetta	W. B. Pigg, Okmulgee
Ottawa	A. M. Cooter, Miami	G. Pinnell, Miami
Osage	A. J. Smith, Pawhuska	Benj. Skinner, Pawhuska
Pawnee		E. T. Robinson, Cleveland
Payne		J. B. Murphy, Stillwater
Pittsburg	L. C. Knyrkendall, McAlester	T. H. McCarley, McAlester.
Pottawatomie	F. E. Rice, Shawnee	G. S. Paxter, Shawnee.
Pontotoc	L. M. Overton, Fitzhugh	S. P. Ross, Ada
Pushmataha	H. C. Johnson, Antlers	Edw. Guinn, Antlers
Rogers		J. C. Taylor, Chelsea.
Roger Mills		
Seminole	W. T. Huddleston, Konawa	W. L. Knight, Wewoka.
Sequoyah		Sam McKeel, Sallisaw.
Stephens		H. C. Frie, Duncan.
Texas	W. H. Langston, Guymon	R. B. Hays, Guymon
Tulsa	G. A. Wall, Tulsa	C. A. Pigford, Tulsa
Tillman		J. E. Arrington, Frederick.
Wagoner		C. E. Martin, Wagoner
Washita		A. S. Neal, Cordell.
Washington		A. North, Bartlesville
Woods		J. A. Bowling, Alva.
Woodward		Arthur Bowles, Woodward.

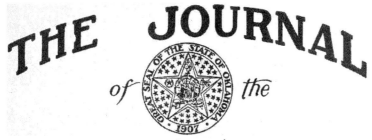

Oklahoma State Medical Association

VOLUME XII   MUSKOGEE, OKLA., APRIL, 1919   NUMBER 4

INFANT MORTALITY.*

R. M. Anderson, M. D.

SHAWNEE, OKLAHOMA

Since a high infant death rate is not only a stigma on the civilization of a country, but is a matter of vital importance to the existence of the nation among the powers of the world, no nation can wisely allow its vital resources to be continually drained by unnecessary and continued loss of life. The babies of this generation are the material out of which the citizens of the next are made, and they should be given every attention and protection.

The reduction of infant mortality is not merely a question of scientific value but it is a question of putting a value on human life above the commercial value of certain interests.

No better illustration of the cheapness of human life can be imagined than the past methods of civilized nations for investigating disease. The United States Government has spent untold thousands every year in official investigation of diseases of domestic animals, but has scarcely recognized the necessity for such work in human diseases.

I would like to say that last night I heard one of the medical officers say we are now getting anything we ask for. This situation I have just mentioned is possibly due to the medical profession and not the government, because we have not asked and demanded this from the government.

When extermination threatened the cattle in South Africa, the English government offered ten thousand pounds sterling, to a scientist, to investigate the matter and propose a remedy. But when sleeping sickness began to kill the natives by the hundred thousands, not a penny was appropriated. It might be put even stronger yet, for Anglo-Saxon democratic governments have opposed any appropriation of public funds for the investigation of human pathloogy. Life has been considered too cheap to waste money this way; if people died there were that many more positions to be filled by the unemployed, but when cattle died it was a serious matter. In a peasant family ,it was a far greater disaster to lose a pig than to lose the baby.

In discussing the causes of infant mortality, let us look at the subject from the three periods of time that relate to it: ante-natal, neo-natal, and post-natal. The strongest weapon which we have for fighting infant mortality may be used during the ante-natal period, in endeavoring to establish a high standard of physical motherhood by the education and care of the mother at the time. She

---

*Read in Section on Pediatrics and Obstetrics, Tulsa, May, 1918.

should know the importance of proper exercise, a well prepared and nutritious diet, and a happy and cheerful frame of mind. In fact, since the welfare of both the prospective mother and child depend in such large measure on the health of the mother, it might be well to consider the whole period of her life, under the ante-natal period.

I would like to say right here that I was glad to hear Dr. Fowler say this morning that in nearly every case, if not every case, he used the Wassermann. How many times in taking the history of our expectant mothers they will say: "I have lost several children at a certain month; I have never been able to carry a child to term"! What do we suspect right away? If we will take a Wassermann right there we would more than likely find out the condition and the reason why she was not able to carry her child to term.

As truly as the welfare of the ante-natal period is dependent on the common sense and judgment of the mother, the welfare of the neo-natal is dependent on the training and experience of those who attend her. And I should like to say something in regard to the midwives of today, since often there is only a midwife in attendance during confinement. Certainly there should be some law restricting the practice of midwifery to those who have been properly trained for the work. On this subject Clara D. Noyes, General Superintendent of Bellevue Training School, said:

"The more highly trained and educated the midwife, the less willing will she be to assume responsibilities which are not hers, and the more quickly will she recognize them, and the greater discrimination will she show in the type of physician she calls to her assistance."

It is very important that the one in attendance, whether midwife or physician, have an early knowledge of the position of the child, so that any change which may be necessary can be made before its life is endangered. It is also important that a too prolonged labor be guarded against, since the mentality, if not the life, of the child is often dependent on this. In such cases, the use of instruments is often necessary. While it is not a general practice to follow Crede's method of using the nitrate of silver solution for the eyes, nevertheless it is an excellent precaution against an infection that often results in blindness.

I wish to state here that I have delivered one hundred and thirty women since July 1st—that is the beginning of our medical year—and in no case have I failed to use nitrate of silver in the eye. I do not care what kind of a home it is, whether it is a preacher's home or a higher-up or a low-down, because syphilis knows no respect of persons—I mean gonorrhea knows no respect of persons—and I believe it will be required by law after a while. I think we just as well get down to it now.

In spite of the fact that some seem to regard the responsibility of a physician in confinement cases very lightly, the life of the child often depends upon his quick and sound judgment.

In considering the post-natal period, it would be well to quote from Dr. Holt, who in a few words strikes the keynote of the greatest dangers that threaten the early life of the infant:

"The fundamental causes of infant mortality, as we may call them, are mainly the results of three conditions: poverty, ignorance and neglect. The curve of diarrheal diseases is so important that it practically controls the curve of infant mortality; this group embraces acute gastritis, gastro-enteritis, all forms of acute diarrhea, dysentery, and cholera infantum, and makes up the largest part of the universal summer mortality. It is these diseases which cause, regularly, each year, the sharp rise in the death curve in July and August."

It is a well known fact that all these diseases are mainly caused by improper feeding, and in this way poverty, ignorance and neglect exert their greatest evil influence. It is a fact shown by statistics, that ten bottle babies die to one that is breast fed, and this is easily understood when we realize the sources and conditions under which the milk is obtained in the very poor districts. However, efforts have been made to correct this evil, by the establishment of pure milk stations for the poor in the crowded districts. Also trained nurses and doctors are employed to visit these homes in order to instruct the ignorant in the care of their babies. Naturally, the progress of such work is slow, but if persevered in, it will no doubt in time result in not only a great lessening of the death rate, but a wonderful improvement in the mental and physical makeup of our future generations. Ignorance and neglect are by no means confined to the poverty stricken districts, as we all very well know. How often, in well-to-do homes, are we obliged to combat wrong ideas in regard to the dressing of children, fresh air, etc.

Although gastro-intestinal disorders cause such a large per cent. of infant mortality, we should not forget the importance of respiratory troubles, under the head of which we might mention la grippe, measles, the pneumonias, whooping cough, etc. Just here let me lay stress on the importance of close attention to the baby suffering from whooping cough, for very often severe complications arise from this disease. It is needless to advise the early use of large doses of anti-toxin for diphtheria. Other diseases endangering the lives of infants could be mentioned, such as acute anterio-poliomyelitis, and cerebro-spinal meningitis.

The most that we can do is to guard, as carefully as posible, the infants that come under our care, and use all our influence to lessen the conditions that make the death rate so high; for as Dr. Wall, of Washington, so truthfully expresses it:

"Until that millenial dawn, when poverty ceases to exist, there will be an infant mortality which needs no electric emblazonry in the sky to flash out its startling message that a baby dies each minute throughout the land. So long as the grim reaper exists, just so long will there be the toll of death from the ranks of the new-born and the nurseling, and unless there be agitation and agitators to awaken the dormant sensibilities of those who have passed through and left in oblivion these early days of peril, and who in their blindness of ignorance, of apathy, or even of mercantile selfishness, neglect the problems of infant and child welfare, the sacrifice of the young will continue, and leave its impress of ignominy upon the human race."

Discussion.

Dr. H. M. Reeder, Shawnee: Dr. Anderson spoke of the three greatest factors that contribute to infant mortality as ignorance, poverty and neglect; I would like to paraphrase that and say "and the greatest of these is ignorance." I think there is more of this mortality that is due to ignorance than to any other cause, and many times not only the ignorance of the parents but of the neighbors. If the young mother does not know, she does not ask the advice of the doctor, some old woman, no matter how well the baby is thriving on the breast, will tell her it should be fed a little. I have seen them given coffee and say they think it is good for them. And yet that same mother will complain of her stomach and say she believes it is the coffee that is hurting her and she will quit it but she will feed it to the baby.

In other cases I have had trouble quite frequently in trying to teach the mother to have a separate bed from the child and separate the child from being in the bed between the mother and the father, where it would probably get too hot and then the cover would be thrown off of it. In one case I happen to know of, the mother rolled over on the child and smothered it to death. There is a sentiment about that, it seems they think it is cruel to the child to make it sleep by itself. If they go to bed with the child and they have respiratory diseases, the child is much more liable to have them communicated to him.

Dr. W. W. Wells, Oklahoma City: This is just as interesting as obstetrics, this discussion of pediatrics. The mortality you all know is great; we do not as a general rule pay much attention to the child. If he is lost, it is all right. It is like that old story about the young fellow who went out to take care of a confinement, and when he came back his wife asked him how he got along and he said he lost the child and mother but the father was doing well.

That is just about the way with this work. We are prone to let the child die or not try to relieve it and consequently the morbidity of childhood is great. We do not use the precautions that we should in taking care of the eyes. I have found in my work that a one per cent. silver solution gives better satisfaction than a ten per cent. argyrol solution. I have used them both in maternity and have had infection of the eyes following the use of the argyrol solution. Whether it was through neglect on the part of some of our nurses or the mother of the child or whether it was because we did not use a strong enough solution or whether silver nitrate is just a little bit better than argyrol, I do not know. I believe it is the latter because we all know that in our cases of urethritis when we cannot clear them up with argyrol, if we use a good strong silver solution they usually clear up. So I believe silver is much better; it seems that way. The doctor spoke of that point and I wanted to emphasize it.

Dr. L. W. Cotton, Enid: Just a word. I think that Dr. Reeder struck the keynote when he said that ignorance is the leading factor in the mortality of children. In treating people, especially in the country, and not only in the country but in the town, they often quote to you the old saying: "The Lord giveth and the Lord taketh away. He has given us our little baby and he has taken it away." You cannot prevail on them or get them to understand that it is their ignorance and carelessness and bad management that caused the loss of the child. That is one of the hardest tasks before the medical profession, to teach the people that we are not to blame for the large mortality in children.

In my mind there is only one good remedy to use on the eyes, and Dr. Anderson certainly struck the keynote there when he said he used it in every case in the last year—that is silver nitrate. On the birth service the question is asked, it is put up to our integrity and honesty to have regard for the rights of the children —"Did you use silver nitrate?" I want to impress upon you that one point. The profession at large, who know the use of silver nitrate and argyrol, certainly say that in a great majority of cases that silver nitrate is far superior.

Dr. O. A. Flannagan, Tulsa: There is just one point I wish to bring out, and that is with reference to the nursing. The nursing of the infant is the all important thing, it is the natural food for the child and whenever we put it on something else we are putting it on artificial food. One of the greatest dangers we have to children is for the mother to wean the baby and put it on some artificial food, and I think to some extent the physicians are responsible for that. With the least bit of a discouraging remark from the mother about inability to nurse the child, the physician or the mother will suggest the advisability of weaning the baby. That should be the very last thing attempted or the very last remedy suggested, especially in those cases where there is some difficulty in the digestive apparatus it is the last thing suggested. In some way, by examining the condition of the mother or by the analysis of the milk, some defective point will be brought out that in most cases can be remedied; and if the proper exercise and hygiene and food and the proper regulation of the life of the mother is looked into, these things can be mostly corrected.

Another thing that increases the infant mortality—I do not know whether the obstetricians brought it out this morning or not, but it seems to me it has a great influence on the infant mortality—that is the hastened delivery, pituitrin and the forceps delivery. If we really knew how frequently they were responsible for the death of the infant, I think they would be far less frequently used than they are at the present time.

Then we spoke about the children all being examined and looked after during the school age. As I said a moment ago, the most important time in the life of any organism is when that organism has its greatest time of development; and in the child's organism, particularly, that greatest time in the period of its development is the pre-school period, but this pre-school period is entirely neglected at the present time and left up to the intelligence of the mother. After the child begins to attend school, he comes under the supervision of the teacher and possibly of the school physician; but previous to that the mother is holding its care, and it depends upon her intelligence and how we as physicians teach her what knowledge she has in reference to the proper bringing up and development of that small organism which is so potentially subject to the infections and the disturbances, particularly at this period of life.

Dr. J. R. Burdick, Tulsa: I believe Dr. Flanagan brought out one of the most important things in the treatment of children. Very few physicians take the time to instruct the mother at all in the feeding of the baby. They are in a hurry to get away after the confinement and we very seldom give the mother instructions as to the feeding the baby.

There are only a few reasons or specific causes for taking the baby off the breast, such as syphilis, tuberculosis, and sarcoma. I believe the baby should be brought up on the breast. I have it put up to me so many times that they have not sufficient milk for the baby, but under those conditions I use some artificial food, but I absolutely refuse to take it from the breast unless there is some specific cause. I think that the doctors are too lax in instructing the mothers about how often and when to feed their babies and about taking care of their feed. I think this is very important right on the start but is too often neglected. And I will say that it is criminal neglect not to use the nitrate of silver in every case of confinement.

Dr. J. S. Hibbard, Cherokee: About infant feeding: Day before yesterday, before I came, I found two of my mothers, one with a baby fourteen days old and one seven days old, and both of them were weaning their babies. Both of them claimed they were short on milk; one of them was a very intelligent woman, one was of ordinary intelligence. Both of them had been advised by some neighbor women without consulting me about bringing up the flow of the milk.

I instructed them to put the babies back on the breast again and not to substitute a feeding of artificial milk, but to let the babies nurse at regular intervals just like they had plenty of milk and then top off with some artificial food. If you let the baby nurse at regular intervals, the mother will be more apt to have sufficient milk. It is only recently I got hold of that idea and I have found it makes quite a difference; where you substitute a food entirely, you won't bring back the milk like you will where you have your baby nurse regularly and top off with the artificial milk where you do not get enough.

Dr. Vest: I would like to hear from some men who have had experience in artificial feeding as to what they have found to be next best where it is necessary to take the child off the breast, what they have found to be next best in the way of artificial feeding.

Dr. J. R. Burdick, Tulsa: That is about all I am doing, is feeding babies. I want to say right here that until I came down to Oklahoma from Chicago I really did not know what Eagle Brand milk was; I never had used it, and I can say truthfully I never have prescribed it. I actually believe it would have to go out of existence if it was not for Oklahoma; it certainly is used a great deal in this state. I am using modified cow's milk entirely. I do sometimes use Mellin's Food with cow's milk and sometimes Horlick's Malted Milk; I never use Eagle Brand and I never have any trouble with modified cow's milk.

Dr. Vest: Don't you find you have so much trouble they won't use it?

Dr. Burdick: I do not find it so. I find some of the families who have found it was a good deal of trouble before I was called. But when I have been called into the family and explained the advisability of using it over the artificial food, I would not have any trouble. Of coures it is very often put up to me that the milk is bad, that they cannot get good milk; the poorest milk in the state is right here in Tulsa. But I get around that by insisting that in all of my cases they boil the milk. That is all I am using and I have splendid success.

Dr. Vest: Will you tell us how you modify it?

Dr. Burdick: That depends a good deal upon the patient. I figure out the caloric value of the milk. I believe that the baby should have an ounce and a half of milk per pound of weight and I get the weight of the baby and figure out the amount of milk it should have and then modify it according to the age and amount of feed each hour.

And I firmly believe that you will get better results from putting your baby for the first month on a four-hour schedule than you will on a three-hour schedule. I am doing that where I am using the cow's milk and I find that if I adhere to the four-hour schedule I can get better results than I can with the three-hour schedule.

We used to have the three hour schedule in Presbyterian Hospital in Chicago, and a year ago all their babies were on a three-hour schedule, and a record kept of each one of them. This last year every baby at the hospital has been on a four-hour schedule, and I am told that they have gotten better results and better gains throughout the year than they did on the three-hour schedule.

I believe the most trouble met with in feeding babies is feeding them too often. If you get the right balance in your milk so that the baby is satisfied at the time of feeding, he will sleep three hours and a half and sometimes sleep right through the next feeding, but I do waken them up at the feeding all during the day. I absolutely feed them by the clock.

Dr. Springer, over here, has had a little experience feeding babies, and I think he will bear me out. I would be glad to answer any other questions.

It is coming to the time when the future generation in this country as well as in foreign countries is dependent upon the development of our children; this is becoming more essential every day, and I think the time is comming when this feeding proposition will demand a great deal more attention.

I find that I have a great many cases here in the summer-time where they have been feeding Eagle Brand, and they are much more susceptible to stomatitis and summer complaint. You take the same baby on a proper artificial feeding and he will stand the heat much better; he has the punch to put him over the critical time. That is the reason I use modified cow's milk, and I always boil it. I demand the use of it and I have never seen any bad effects from it. They say it causes constipation and indigestion, but I do not find that to be true. I believe it is more easily digestible than if you have a foreign food, and will better take care of your baby.

Dr. Anderson, closing: All I have to say is that I want to thank you gentlemen who have waited here to hear the last paper at this hour, and I certainly appreciate the discussion. That is all I have to say.

THE MANIFESTATIONS OF SYPHILIS IN PREGNANCY AND THE NEW BORN.*

W. W. Wells, M. D.

OKLAHOMA CITY, OKLAHOMA

Syphilis is a disease which in the pregnant woman is often overlooked as the history is usually very indefinite. Perhaps the first sign we recognize is an abortion, or stillbirth. When a woman comes under our care bearing a history of repeated interrupted pregnancies, it would be well to have a Wassermann in the beginning of treatment. It is estimated that 40 to 80 per cent. of these cases are syphilitic.

Syphilis in the female does not show the marked manifestations of the nervous system, as paresis and tabes dorsalis as it does in the male. In the female, syphilitic ulceration of the cervix may be mistaken for cancer, as the most prominent symptoms of both is hemorrhage. Latent syphilis prevails more in the female than in the male.

The time and stage of the infection seems to have an important bearing on pregnancy, labor and the offspring. The manner of communicating the disease from the paternal side to the foetus-is still somewhat of a mystery. The spirochete is three times larger than the head of the spermatozoa, so unless the mother is infected, the only plausible way that the foetus could become syphilitic would be that the spirochete would be carried to the mother, through the semen. These women give a positive Wassermann, so they probably become infected through the semen, and actually have syphilis which is in turn communicated to the ovum.

Now, what may we expect, if a woman becomes pregnant and infected at the same time? First if the infection is located as a primary lesion on the cervix, the chancre would take on more malignant character and would be much larger, bleed more freely, destroy more tissue and would yield much more slowly to treatment. This applies not only to the lesion on the cervix, but anywhere about the female genitalia, as these are better supplied with blood and are edematous in the pregnant.

If the primary lesion, located on the cervix, heals, it leaves a dense scar which causes cicatricial stenoses of the os and will dilate, at the time of labor, very slowly.

The secondary stage comes sooner and with more virulency, often forming maculo-papular syphilide; these may become pustular.

The tertiary symptoms come on early and are more extensive, in the form of simple condyloma and gumma. In our work we see a good many cases where the vulva and floor of the vagina is a mass of flat condylomata; and when the head of the child begins to stretch the vulva, the skin and perineal body will tear like blotting paper. These cases when repaired do not heal by first intention, hence there is no use to put in sutures; we let them heal by granulation.

When a syphilitic woman becomes pregnant or a woman is infected with syphilis at the time of conception, interruption of pregnancy is the rule. A syphilitic woman may bear a living child that does not show symptoms of syphilis; but not the first pregnancy after infection; they usually have two or three abortions progressing further along in pregnancy each time, then one or two stillbirths, then a living child which dies soon after birth; and finally a living child which may show no symptoms of syphilis.

Here permit me to relate the history of a case which came under my observation. The patient, a girl of 18 years, became infected at the time of marriage. The primary lesion was located on the labia minora, and healed without specific

*Prepared for Section on Genito-Urinary Diseases, Skin and Radiology, Tulsa, May. 1918.

treatment. The secondary lesions came on in the usual time, and these she sought treatment for, and was found to be about two and one-half months pregnant, and aborted in a few weeks. Anti-syphilitic treatment was given immediately but was not continued successfully, owing to the indifference of the patient. About eight months later, another abortion at four months; and one year later, a seven month macerated foetus, which was sent to the laboratory for examination. The pathologist found live spirochetes in the placental blood. The blood of the cord, placenta and foetal heart gave a Wassermann. One year and a half later she delivered an eight month stillborn child. She has taken very little treatment, in fact none, since her second abortion. Her next child will probably live only a short time. If this patient would take treatment she could give birth to a living child; and even without treatment she may have a living child.

The cause of these abortions and miscarriages is syphilitic endometritis. The impregnated ovum is unable to develop. When it gets nourishment enough to go to term, we often have an adherent placenta. We may have infection and fever from retention of hypertrophied decidua. Acute nephritis occurring during pregnancy in some cases has been traced to syphilis. In labor the progress is usually slow, the pains are weak, and abnormal presentations are frequent. The child may be free from the disease, but may become infected at delivery in passing through an ulcerated syphilitic birth canal. The chancre is the mother colony and contains many organisms in an almost unkillable state.

The signs of syphilis in a newborn child are coryza syphiliticia (or snuffles), cutaneous eruptions, and mucous patches about the mouth and natal fold, as well as restless sleeplessness, marasamus and glandular involvement. If no symptoms develop in three months, we can be fairly safe in saying the child is not syphilitic.

With our modern methods of diagnosis, used intelligently in connection with our clinical findings, syphilis should net be overlooked in pregnancy.

TUBERCULOSIS AND CANCER.

A. C. Broders, Rochester, Minn. (*Journal A. M. A.*, Feb. 8, 1919), after quoting Rokitansky's views as to the incompatibility of cancer and tuberculosis and reviewing the literature of the negative side of the question to some extent, concludes as follows: "1. The theory prevailing among the majority of physicians for a number of years and still prevailing among a few, that tuberculosis and malignant neoplasia are antagonistic, has not been borne out by the facts. 2. The fact that some tissues or organs are, to a certain degree, immune from one or the other or both of these diseases does not prove that the two diseases are antagonistic. 3. If the observations of Naegeli are correct, in which he showed that in 93 per cent. of 420 necropsies on adults more than 18 years of age, either active, latent or healed tuberculosis had been present, then it is reasonable to believe that similar findings should prevail in an equal number of persons who have died with malignant neoplasia. 4. It would seem that the reason pathologists are not finding tuberculosis more frequently at necropsy in persons who have died with malignant neoplasia is that the pathologists are satisfied to find the malignant neoplastic condition, and therefore fail to make a thorough search for tuberculosis. 5. Since the surgical pathologist's examination is limited to the tissue removed by the surgeon, he is greatly handicapped in the search for the two conditions associated, while the pathologist doing a necropsy has access to a large part or the whole of the body. 6. The fact that active tuberculosis occurs most frequently in persons under 45, and malignant neoplasia, epithelial tissue malignant neoplasia, most frequently in persons over 45, does not prohibit the association of latent and healed tuberculosis with malignant neoplasia. 7. In our series of twenty cases the two conditions were associated in the same microscopic field seven times (35 per cent.)."

PRACTICAL THOUGHTS ON THE CARE OF THE PREGNANT WOMAN.*

MARTHA BLEDSOE, M. D.

CHICKASHA, OKLAHOMA

In this paper I do not hope to give any startling facts of recent output, or any radical treatment, but merely to clinch this thought: know what event is coming and prepare for it; and to educate our people in this as we should, that we can give them better care, and can protect ourselves from unpleasant happenings.

In these days we read and talk on preparedness, getting ready for the coming events, and I think it is safe to say that we all favor the plan. And so it is with the expectant mother, it is so arranged that Nature gives a warning, a notice, that some time soon we can expect just such a condition, so why not plan, and prepare, and get ready for it? For some time past it has been my custom to take only such cases as have engaged me at least two months before.

I believe that we, as physicians, should educate our people in this way and soon they will not call us without giving us a chance to be ready, posted and prepared for the case as we have found conditions from time to time. As soon as she is aware of her condition, or has a belief as to its probability, the expectant mother should place herself under the care of the physician of her choice, as a certain degree of medical advice and attention is required during the whole period of pregnancy.

While the conditions as a rule are weakness and unrest, the borderland between health and disease may very easily be overpassed. At any time disorders or complications may occur; these in all probability can be warned off or promptly remedied by physicians' watchful care.

We should take time to instruct the woman that her whole duty now is to herself and child; we should tell her of some things to expect, of other things that she should call our attention to at once if they do occur; in fact, I believe in taking the patient, in conversation, along the period of gestation.

The kidney I believe we all give more consideration to than we do almost anything else. We know how important it is to analyze the urine often, especially during the last three months.

Conditions of the bowels: Many women, perhaps most women, suffer from constipation during this period, due largely to the increased pressure exerted by the enlarged uterus upon the intestines and often it becomes a source of great discomfort during the last months of pregnancy.

It is very important that the bowels should act freely, at least once each day. This can be accomplished very often by the use of laxative foods, rather than by purgatives or enemas. Here it is that time must be taken and the physician explain that if they will do as you advise and follow your diet list, that in nine cases out of ten they will not be obliged to take medicine and that all will be well.

Give them a list of fresh fruits: oranges, apples, apricots, pears, figs, pineapples, grapefruit; cooked fruits, such as prunes, figs, apples. All food should be plain, nutritious, easily digested and taken at regular intervals. Bread, such as whole wheat, bran bread, graham bread, stimulates the intestines and increases their activity. Vegetables, those growing above the ground, are considered the most nutritious and most easily digested.

Exercise we should impress upon these women. I am in the habit of saying: "Go on with your work and habits very much as you would if you were not pregnant, except stop before you are completely tired out; stop short of fatigue. Spend a part of each day walking in the open air." Pleasant outdoor exercise

*Read in Section on Pediatrics and Obstetrics, Tulsa, May, 1918.

invigorates the muscles, and stimulates the sweat glands, and other excretory organs; strengthens and restores the nerve tissue; clears the brain and sends a supply of blood to all parts of the body, thus increasing courage, cheerfulness and general helpfulness.

With such advice we can help our pregnant women to look forward to delivery with confident cheerfulness. The pregnant condition often brings on a feeling of depression of spirits, and the delivery is looked forward to as a time of extreme suffering and peril, rather than one of triumph and joy.

Late hours, or excitement of any kind should be discouraged. An abundance of sleep is necessary, at least eight hours should be taken every night, and it is well to advise a nap after dinner; to those who cannot sleep during the day, advise them to lie down if only to relax and rest.

I have a few words only as a rule to say about their clothing, except to have loose comfortable clothes; the shoes and every piece of wearing apparel must feel comfortable. One thing I find in a great many cases is that they wear tight elastic garters which I order off at once.

Then we should advise about the care of the teeth, as the saliva is acid during pregnancy and the teeth decay more rapidly if neglected. We have all often heard it repeated: "For every child the mother loses a tooth too soon." So an alkaline mouth wash should be recommended.

Order daily massage of breast and abdomen with olive oil; this is often good.

When we have charge of these cases beforehand we can make examinations and order such care as needed, we can go into them with confidence, instead of fear and trembling.

INFECTION THROUGH THE EYE.

K. F. Maxcy, Fort Sill, Okla. (*Journal A. M. A.*, March 1, 1919), calls attention to the likelihood of infection through droplet spray in the eye. The fact of the spread of the disease by projection of droplet conveyed germs has been demonstrated, and this method of infection is most probable during active and waking hours. The infection through the nares, which are less directly exposed owing to the downward direction of their outlet, and the mouth, which is not liable to receive droplets except when held open, is practically less possible than that due to spray droplets on the directly exposed 600 sq. mm. of eye surface. When this is reached the germs can be carried into the lacrimal ducts to the nasal passages. Experiments are detailed by Maxcy showing how this process practically occurs. A suspension of B. *prodigiosus* could be instilled into the conjunctival sac and be recovered within from five to thirty minutes from the nasal passages. From this point the infective germs can be carried in to the larynx and to the respiratory tract, or into the gastro-intestinal tract through the esophagus as well as be discharged through the mouth in the sputum. The gauze face mask protecting the nose and mouth, therefore, is not a complete protection, and the frequency with which respiratory infections are conveyed from one person to another amply warrants this possible route of contagion as a formidable probability. It is impracticable, however, to use the gauze mask with very sick persons, and physicians and attendants should bear this fact in mind. Maxcy offers the following conclusions: "1. The eyes offer a relatively large surface area for the reception of droplets sprayed from the mouths of other persons. 2. An organism introduced into the conjunctival sac may be recovered from the nose in five minutes, from the throat in fifteen minutes, and from the stool in twenty-four hours. 3. The upper respiratory tract of a person wearing a properly constructed mask may be infected by exposing the eye briefly to direct droplet spray. 4. This portal of entry is of importance in the transmission of acute respiratory infections."

ACUTE FRACTURES OF THE SKULL.*

A. RAY WILEY, M. D.

TULSA, OKLAHOMA

Acute fractures of the skull are of such importance that any new or practical knowledge of the subject should at once be noted.   The mortality of this unfortunate condition as treated by the method of the recent past and the methods still in vogue in many localities is appalling.

During the year 1917 and part of 1918 it was my good fortune to be House Surgeon of the New York Polyclinic Hospital, and through the kindness and personal friendship of Dr. Wm. Sharpe, to improve my knowledge of the above subject.

The subject is too large for a single paper, so I will only attempt to take up some of the principal points in diagnosis and treatment.   The objects in diagnosis are: First and most important, the determination of the amount of intracranial pressure; second, localized pressure; third the after effects, or end results of the present condition and how they will be altered by operation or other treatment. In the order of their importance as aids in diagnosis are the lumbar puncture with the measurement of the pressure of the cerebro-spinal fluid, by a mercurial manometer whenever possible, the ophthalmoscopic examination of the fundi of the eyes, the pulse, the temperature and the blood pressure.   The diagnosis of a fracture is aided by a combination of history of accident, oozing of cerebral-spinal fluid from the ears, nose or mouth, localized ecchymosis, paresis or paralysis, disturbance of reflex, the x-ray and other clinical signs.

I cannot lay too much emphasis on the importance of the ophthalmoscopic examination in the hands of a competent oculist, being second only to the spinal puncture.· The fundus of the eye and particularly the retina, being an offshoot from the brain, is most intimately connected with the brain and intracranial cavity so that any lesion within the intracranial cavity which increases its normal contents would naturally tend to be shown in the fundus of the eye, especially the optic nerve head.   And an increased intracranial pressure sufficient to retard and even prevent the flow of blood in retinal veins would tend to cause a dilatation of these vessels with resulting edema and congestion.   So a thorough ophthalmoscopic examination should be made in all suspected cases of increased intracranial pressure.

The pulse is of importance, especially in the absence of other means.   A pulse of 48 or less with normal temperature or subnormal with other clinical signs, stupor, etc., demands a decompression.   If there is fever present, that will be taken into consideration in judging the pulse.   It is much better to operate on a declining pulse than on an ascending pulse.

The value of the x-ray lies in its ability to determine the amount of mechanical defect.   The x-ray will show practically all fractures of the vault, the fracture fissures, the position of bone fragments, etc., but it will not show fractures of the base of skull.   The x-ray will aid in diagnosing some borderline cases, especially where you are unable by palpation to determine whether or not there is bone depression of a pathologic degree.

After a diagnosis of increased intracranial pressure has been made and found that the patient will not be relieved himself through nasal or auditory leaks, or that there is localized pressure, then a decompression should be performed.

If the operator will limit himself to operate only in cases so diagnosed instead of operating all fractures of the vault, as Binnie advises in his "Operative Surgery", the mortality will be reduced from about 80 per cent to 30 per cent. or 35 per cent.   An infected decompression wound usually means a fatality.

---

*Read before Tulsa County Medical Society, February 10, 1919.

Do not operate within three hours following the accident, the only exception to this being excessive external bleeding. About 15 per cent. of all acute cranial fractures are moribund and will die within three to six hours whether operated or not. A large majority of the remaining 85 per cent. will die if operated while in shock.

The operation of choice is the subtemporal decompression, which was first used by Harvey Cushing about 1913. For this operation the entire head should be shaved, preferably by a barber, and a sterile field prepared; the evening before or in case of early operation, the head is shaved and painted with tincture of iodine. After the patient is under anesthesia, the dressing is carefully removed and the head again scrubbed quickly with sterile green soap and then 70 per cent. alcohol.

The anesthesia is of special importance in these cases. It is best to have an oxygen tank or compressed air machine and conduct a mixture of ether and oxygen or vapor ether to the mask, this with rubber tube connection as the head of the patient must be covered during the operation. While compressed air ether vapor may be used, I prefer the oxygen ether vapor.

Whenever possible the decompression is performed on the right side in order to avoid the motor speech area, which is situated in right handed persons in the posterior portion of the third *left* frontal convolution and vice versa in left handed persons. The head is slightly elevated with the grooved head block and sand bags. A faint skin mark or incision is made before the sterile drapings are placed. This permits you to correctly place your incision and gives clear view to all the landmarks before they are covered. Towels wet in 1-3000 bichloride mercury are clipped to the scalp parallel to the incision, then crosswise. By clipping the towels in place they will not become disarranged during the operation. The draping completed and incision made, beginning one-half inch anterior to the external auditory meatus and on a level with the upper border of the zygomatic arch, the incision is carried vertically upwards through the scalp to the upper attachment of the temporal muscle. Hemorrhage is controlled by manual pressure, using the ulnar edge of the hands until hemostats are applied. The temporal fascia is split, then the muscle is split and retracted, exposing the squamous portion of the temporal bone. One should be careful not to destroy the upper attachment of the temporal muscle, otherwise the closing will be greatly weakened. The periosteum is pushed to either side, and a Doyen perforator and burr are used until the bone is perforated to the dura, then rongeurs are used until the bony opening is sufficiently large. This method of attacking the bone is superior to the trephine method. The squamous portion of the temporal bone is the flattest portion of the cranium and should be the ideal place for the trephine, but due to the inequalities of the thickness of the bone, not only in this area but throughout the cranium, a trephine button too often injures the dura, the delicate cortical cells, or causes damaging bleeding by tearing dural vessels.

Remember that the dura is inelastic, especially in the adult, and unless the dura is opened the intracranial pressure will not be relieved, which relief usually is the primary object of the operation. All bleeding must be stopped before the dura is opened. The diploe and sinuses are stopped with bone wax.

The dura is picked up with a dural hook, a small pin point hooked instrument. The dura is incised or nicked and a grooved director slipped under the dura as it is lifted away from the cortical cells. The opening is enlarged, either a crucial or stellate opening being made. The blood vessels are avoided and if severed, the hemorrhage is best controlled by small v-shaped silver clips compressed on the ends of the vessel by means of special forceps. The hemorrhage, if small, may be controlled by simple compression with the hemostat, or small ligatures, although the ligatures are time consuming and danger of injuring the brain cells. If blood clots present themselves they should be removed, but prolonged searching and probing for clots should be condemned. Sometimes an extradural clot will give pressure symptoms, and on opening the dura the cerebral fluid is not bloody. The clot then should be located if possible. A rubber or gutta-percha drain one-fourth inch wide and several layers in thickness is inserted in the lower angle of the wound, inside the dura beneath the tempero-sphenoidal lobe as far as possible, draining the mid-cranial fossa and the operated area. If there has been much oozing, a like drain may be placed at the upper angle of the wound and removed at the close of the operation or a few hours after. All bleeding, no matter how small, should be controlled before closing. The temporal muscle is closed with two layers of sutures. Sharpe uses fine interrupted black silk throughout, including the skin. The temporal fascia is closed, the superficial fascia and then the skin. A pad of cotton dipped in vaseline is placed behind the ear and the entire head bandaged with gauze head rolls.

In the unoperative cases heavy doses of bromides, after recovery from shock and thorough purgation, will suffice. This applies to cases without severe pressure symptoms or those with ear or nasal leaks. If the ear is leaking it should be irrigated three to four times a day with solution of boric acid, alcohol and water. Mastoiditis, from infection through the ear and ruptureed ear drums is not infrequent and can best be avoided with the above treatment. Hematomas of scalp should all be incised and drained whether the skull is fractured or not, the strictest asepsis being used.

Conclusions: It is as important to know when and whether to operate these cases as to know how to operate them. Only 33 per cent. of fractures of the skull are operative cases. In the others, by treating the shock and then the use of ice caps or hemlets, bromides, purgation, etc., will suffice. Repeated lumbar puncture may aid in some cases where a decompression cannot be performed. An ophthalmoscopic examination of the fundi of the eyes and a lumbar puncture should be made in all suspected pressure cases. Patients should not be permitted to become blind or to reach the dangerous stage of medullary compression before a decompression is performed. The advantage over the subtemporal route is chiefly due to its anatomical relations. Not only is the squamous portion of the temporal bone the thinnist and therefore the least difficult to remove, but it exposes the portion of the brain most frequently involved in fractured skulls where the middle meningeal artery is torn. Also a permanent decompression here does not weaken the skull, in that the thick overlying temporal muscle most adequately covers the opening so that cerebral hernia need not be feared. It is also the route of choice in decompressions for tumors of the cerebrum, cerebral abscess, spastic paraplegia, hydrocephalus, and exploratory operations of the brain.

TUBERCULOUS ANORECTAL FISTULAS.

S. M. Hill, and A. A. Landsman, New York (*Journal A. M. A.*, March 22, 1919), report two cases of tuberculous anorectal fistula, in which the usual early accompaniments making diagnosis easy were absent. Ordinarily a tuberculous fistula has a flattened irregular opening, larger than that of the nontuberculous type. It is more or less insensitive, discharges a thin, dirty gray material, seldom thick or creamy, and the skin surrounding is bluish and undermined. In the cases reported the beginning was what appeared to be an ordinary abscess and fistula about the rectum, and for a considerable time it showed no pulmonary or other tuberculous indication. They were both followed by pulmonary involvement. They say: "1. Clinical signs that would serve to distinguish between specific and non-specific local lesions about the rectum are not dependable, because they may be late in making their appearance; consequently, laboratory examination should be resorted to as early as possible. 2. There may be a secondary pulmonary involvement from a tuberculous focus about the rectum, in individuals who lack resistance."

EPIDEMIC OR LETHARGIC ENCEPHALITIS.
Acute Infectious Ophthalmoplegia, Acute Encephalitis, Nona?

This unfamiliar disease, many cases of which were observed in England and France early in 1918 and in Vienna in the winter of 1916-1917, when von Economo suggested the name "encephalitis lethargica," now seems to be making its appearance in various parts of this country. In the recent discussion on influenza before the Institute of Medicine of Chicago, Bassoe[1] stated that during the last few weeks he had seen several cases which were characterized by marked drowsiness and paralysis of cranial nerves, especially the ocular, and which otherwise corresponded to the clinical picture of lethargic encephalitis, and that he knew of similar observations by other physicians. Last week Pothier[2] reported the clinical details of eight cases from Camp Lee, Va., and Neal[3] mentions the occurrence of cases in New York.

In previous editorial discussions[4] of the European, especially the English, reports on lethargic encephalitis, special emphasis was placed on its similarity to the cerebral and bulbar forms of epidemic poliomyelitis, and it was suggested that further investigations might show "the new disease" to be true epidemic poliomyelitis. In the meantime, the report[5] of an extensive investigation of lethargic encephalitis (168 cases) has appeared from which we learn that, while nothing by way of a causal agent has been demonstrated, intracerebral inoculations of monkeys with emulsions of diseased nervous tissue failed completely to produce any results. As the monkey is realyil susceptible to such treatment with similar material from cases of epidemic poliomyelitis, the present indications are that the two diseases are separate and distinct, and this conclusion is borne out also by certain clinical and epidemiologic differences to which attention has been called, by Netter in Paris, especially. It is noteworthy, however, that the anatomic changes in the two diseases are of the same general nature, and MacNalty[6] ventures the suggestion that the relation between epidemic poliomyelitis and lethargic encephalitis may be comparable to that between typhoid and paratyphoid fevers. The English investigators consequently regard lethargic encephalitis as due to an as yet unknown virus which causes inflammatory changes, especially perivascular infiltrations, in the basal ganglions, the upper part of the pons, especially in the gray matter of the floor of the fourth ventricle, and in less degree elsewhere in the medulla. It is distinctly a poliencephalitic disease: the outstanding clinical features are a more or less pronounced lethargy, often progressive, and paralysis of the third and less often other cranial nerves.[6]

Ophthalmoplegia was observed in about 75 per cent. of the English cases.

It is noteworthy that cases appear to occur with the general symptoms of fever, lethargy and weakness, but without paralysis, and hence are easily mistaken for the more common infections, though perhaps of the greatest importance in the spread of the disease, which now is notifiable in England and Wales. At present, however, no new cases seem to be occurring in these countries. The results of further and more complete observations of lethargic encephalitis as it occurs in this country will be awaited with special interest.

It is quite remarkable that while English and other Eruopean observers do not seem to place any special stress on the relation of the newly recognized disease to influenza, the American cases so far reported are associated by the observers, particularly Bassoe[1] and Neal,[3] more or less directly with influenza. Four of Pothier's[2] eight patients are said to have had influenza a few weeks before they came down with lethargic encephalitis. While the question thus raised cannot be answered at this time, the information we now have indicates that it is only in connection with epidemics of influenza that anything definitely resembling lethargic encephalitis is described in the older literature.

It is said that profound and prolonged sleep has been observed in connection with many epidemics of influenza since early times. Zuelzer[7] mentions that in the epidemic of 1712, somnolent conditions were so frequent and so marked that in Tubingen, for instance, the disease was known as sleeping sickness, and Longuet[8] gives a quotation from Camerarus which appears actually to describe ophthalmoplegia. Coming down to more recent times, we find that in the early nineties of the last century, at the time of the influenza outbreak of 1889-1881, quite a little was written about a since forgotten disease called "nona" (also "la nonna"), which is said to have occurred especially in northern Italy and Hungary, but also elsewhere, and of which lethargy and weakness were pronounced manifestations.[9] At about the same time cases of ophthalmoplegia with stupor and somnolence were described by Blanc, Mauthner and others,[10] and the question was raised then whether "nona," was not a kind of ophthalmoplegia. "Nona," however, failed to establish itself as a definite disease, and was soon forgotten completely.[11] —*Jour. A. M. A.* March 15, 1919.

1. Bassoe, Peter: J. A. M. A. 72: 677 (March 1) 1919.

2. Pothier, O. L.: Lethargic Encephalitis, J. A. M. A. 72: 715 (March 8) 1919.

3. Neal, Josephine B.: Meningeal Conditions Noted During the Epidemic of Influenza, J. A. M. A. 72: 714 (March 8) 1919.

4. Is Epidemic Poliomyelitis Prevalent in England and France? Editorial, J. A. M. A. 71: 1221 (Oct. 12) 1918; Encephalitis Lethargica: A new Disease? ibid. 72: 414 (Feb. 8) 1919.

5. Report on an Inquiry into an Obscure Disease, Encephalitis Lethargica, L. G. B. Rep. N. S. 121; reviewed in Brit. M. J. 1: 45 (Jan. 11) 1918.

6. For-more complete description of symptoms see p. 794, this issue.

7. Zuelzer: Influenza, Ziemssen's Handbuch der speziellen Pathologie und Therapie 2: 506, Part 2, 1874.

8. Longuet, P.: La nona Semaine med. 12: 275, 1892.

9. For reference to the literature on nona, which is well abstracted by Longuet, see Index Catalogue, Library of Surgeon-General's Office, Series 2, 7: 945, 1902 (Anomalous and Usual Forms of Influenza).

10. Cited by Longuet (Footnote 8).

11. The derivation and meaning of the word "nona" are obscure. It may have been a corruption of coma. Nona means literally ninth hour, and there is no evident connection between this meaning and the disease in question. "La nonna," a name also given the disease sometimes, means grandmother literally, and here again the connection is not evident. Nona is defined as follows in Foster's Encyclopediae Medical Dictionary (1894): "An alleged new form of disease reported in 1890 from northern Italy, Bavaria and Russia. It appears, however, that there is no foundation for the supposition that there is any such new disease, and that the reports are founded on cases of comatose typhoid fever, somnolence following influenza, and smallpox of an irregular and severe development."

MASTOIDECTOMY.

C. T. Perter (Boston), Camp Upton, Yaphank, L. I., N. Y. (*Journal A. M. A.*, Feb. 22, 1919), reports cases of operation for mastoid disease following influenza, with local anesthesia. "The method of administering was as follows: The patient was first given one-fourth grain of morphin subcutaneously, and in half an hour a 0.5 per cent. solution of cocain or procain, when the latter became available, was injected into the skin along the line of incision. The injection was then carried into the deeper layers and finally under the periosteum over the entire area of the mastoid. The insertion of the sternomastoid muscle and the posterior canal wall were injected at the last. About 15 c.c. of a 0.5 per ct. solution were used, in each case, although as high as 30 c.c. of a procain solution were used in one case—a double mastoiditis—and as low as 6 c.c. of a 0.5 per cent. solution of cocain were used in another case." After waiting for from five to ten minutes the operation was started and carried on in the usual manner. But little actual pain was complained of, though the pounding in removing the cortex was usually disagreeable. In only one case was general anesthesia necessary, and the total absence of any shock following the operation was remarkable. The incident of dry middle ears was 100 per cent., and there was no mortality. Several cases are reported, rather briefly.

JOURNAL OF THE OKLAHOMA STATE MEDICAL ASSOCIATION

VOLUME XII   MUSKOGEE, OKLA., APRIL, 1919   NUMBER 4

PUBLISHED MONTHLY AT MUSKOGEE. OKLA., UNDER DIRECTION OF THE COUNCIL

DR. CLAUDE A. THOMPSON, EDITOR-IN-CHIEF

ENTERED AT THE POST OFFICE AT MUSKOGEE, OKLAHOMA, AS SECOND CLASS MAIL MATTER, JULY 28, 1912

THIS IS THE OFFICIAL JOURNAL OF THE OKLAHOMA STATE MEDICAL ASSOCIATION. ALL COMMUNICATIONS SHOULD BE ADDRESSED TO THE JOURNAL OF THE OKLAHOMA STATE MEDICAL ASSSOCIATION, 308 SURETY BUILDING, MUSKOGEE, OKLAHOMA.

The editorial department is not re-ponsible for the opinions expressed in the original articles of contributors.

Reprints of original articles will be supplied at actual cost, provided request for them s attached to manuscr.pt or made in sufficient time before publication.

Articles sent this Journal for publication and all those read at the annual meetings of the State Association are the sole property of this Journal. The Journal relies on each individual contributor's strict adherence to this well-known rule of medical journalism. In the event an article sent this Journal for publication is published before appearance in the Journal, the manuscript will be returned to the writer

Failure to receive the Journal should call for immediate notification of the editor, 307-8 Surety Building, Muskogee, Okla

Local news of possible interest to the medical profession, notes on removals, changes in address, deaths and weddings will be gratefully received,

Advertising of articles, drugs or compounds unapproved by the Council on Pharmacy of the A. M. A. will not be accepted.

Advertising rates will be supplied on application. It is suggested that wherever possible members of the State Association should patronize our advertisers in preference to others as a matter of fair reciprocity.

EDITORIAL

THE ANNUAL MEETING, MUSKOGEE, MAY 20-22.

Local committees in Muskogee having charge of the annual meeting are perfecting arrangements and details for the event. All exhibits, and sections, so far as is now understood, will be held in one building, the County building at 2nd and Court streets.

Physicians contemplating attendance should make hotel reservations in advance as they are crowded. Requests for rooms should be mailed to the Hotel Severs. All hotels are operated on the European plan.

The May Journal will contain the program.

TUBERCULOSIS SANATORIA.

The State of Oklahoma is going into the business officially of combatting tuberculosis. The first step in that direction was the appropriation of $300,000 for the purpose of erecting three hospitals in different parts of the State. No locality was specified for these locations, though originally Talihina, the site of the United States Indian Service Tuberculosis Hospital, was named in the bill as one of the locations. That provision was eliminated. The management will be under direction of a branch of the Health Department created for that purpose.

THE NEW STATE COMMISSIONER OF HEALTH

The appointment by Governor Robertson of Dr. A. R. Lewis, of Ryan, to the position of State Commissioner of health will not only be welcomed by Dr. Lewis' many personal friends in the medical profession, but insures for Oklahoma a progressive and efficient State Health Department. Dr. Lewis is a trained and competent physician; he is in addition an able executive and a good business man—qualifications which are of importance in conducting a successful State Health Department.

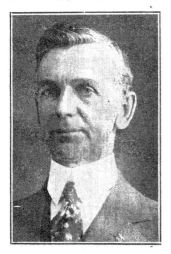

DR. ARTHUR RIMMER LEWIS
STATE COMMISSIONER OF HEALTH

Dr. Lewis is a Mississippian by birth, but has for many years resided in Oklahoma and is familiar with Oklahoma's needs from the viewpoint of public health. He was born in Kosciuszko, Miss., in 1872. While a boy he came with his parents to Mexia, Texas. He was graduated in pharmacy in Philadelphia in 1895, received his medical degree in St. Louis in 1900 and began the practice of medicine in Fleetwood, Oklahoma, the same year. He later practised at Terral, going to Ryan 17 years ago, where he has since resided and where he has for long been regarded as one of the best known and most valued citizens, as well as a leading physician.

Dr. Lewis was appointed a member of the State Board of Medical Examiners under Governor Haskell. For ten years he was surgeon for the Rock Island railroad. He is a 32nd degree Mason, a Shriner and a member of all the representative medical and allied associations in the United States.

Under the laws and appropriations passed by the recent legislature provision is made for greatly expanding the scope of the work of the State Health Board. The work of the department will be enlarged in many directions. Oklahoma has a well deserved reputation as being one of the most progressive states in the Union. It should have a Health Department adapted to this reputation and to the growing needs of the State. Dr. Lewis in our opinion as State Health Commissioner will give the State such a department.

THE VENEREAL LAW ENROLLED.
Senate Bill No. 43.
By Hill and Mayfield, of the Senate and Thomas of the House.

An Act to Prevent and Stamp Out Venereal Diseases; Prescribing Remedies Against the Spread of such Diseases; Providing Certain Regulations Affecting Such Diseases and Persons Infected Therewith: Regulationg the Ssle and Furnishing of Medicinal Remedies for Such Diseases; Forbidding Certain Practices and Customs in Connection with Such Diseases and the Treatment Thereof; Prescribing the Punishment for any Violation of any of the Terms of this Act; Repealing all Laws in Conflict with this Act, and Declaring an Emergency.

Section 1. For the purposes of this Act the words "venereal disease" shall include any and all diseases commonly communicable from any person to any other person of the opposite sex through or by means of sexual intercourse and found and declared by medical science or accredited schools of medicine to be infectious or contagious. All words or phrases using the male or female gender, in this Act, shall be construed to mean and cover the gender of the opposite sex. "Infected person", as used in this Act, shall mean and apply to any person, of either sex, who may be contaminated or afflicted with any venereal disease. The word "dealer", as used in this Act, shall mean and cover any person, firm or corporation who or which may handle, for sale, any medicinal remedies or supposed remedies for venereal diseases, and the agents, clerks, and employees of any such person, firm or corporation; and any person, firm or corporation who or which may profess or claim to treat or cure, by the use of medicine or otherwise, any such venereal disease, and their agents, clerks and employees. The word "physician", used in this Act, shall include reputable physicians who have complied with all the requirements of law regulating the practice of their respective schools of medicine, and duly licensed by such law to practice medicine in their respective schools, or surgery, or both, and no other person. The word "keeper", as used in this Act, shall mean and cover any person or persons in charge or control of any penal or eleemosynary institution whether public or private who may be authorized either by law or by the rules of such institution to receive or discharge any person into or from such institution. Wherever the words "Board of Health" or "Health Officers" appear in this Act they should be construed to include the Board of Health and Health Officers of the State, County or Municipality of the State.

Section 2. It shall be unlawful for any person, being an infected person to refuse, fail or neglect to report such fact to, and submit to examination and treatment by some reputable physician. Any person violating the provisions of this Section shall be punished by fine of not less than Twenty-five Dollars (\$25.00) or not more than Five Hundred Dollars (\$500.00) or by confinement in the county jail for a term of not less than thirty (30) days, nor more than one (1) year, or by both such fine and imprisonment.

Section 3. Any person who shall, after becoming an infected person and before being discharged and pronounced cured by a reputable physician in writing, marry any other person, or expose any other person by the act of copulation or sexual intercourse to such venereal disease or to liability to contract the same, shall be guilty of a felony and upon conviction shall be punished by confinement in the penitentiary for not less than one (1) year or not more than five (5) years

Section 4. Any physician who shall after having knowledge or information that any person is or may be an infected person, sell, give or furnish to such infected person or to any other person for such infected person a discharge from treatment, or written instrument or statement pronouncing such infected person cured, before such infected person is actually cured of such venereal disease, shall be guilty of a misdemeanor and punished by fine of not less than One Hundred Dollars (\$100.00) nor more than Five Hundred Dollars (\$500.00) or by confinement in the county jail for a term of not less than thirty (30) days nor more than six (6) months,.

Section 5. Any person who is not a physician, who shall undertake to treat or cure any infected person for pay, whether in money, property or obligation of any kind, unless acting under the direction and control of a physician, shall be guilty of a misdemeanor and upon conviction shall be punished by a fine of not less than One Hundred Dollars (\$100.00) nor more than Five Hundred Dollars (\$500.00) or by confinement in the county jail for a term of not less than thirty (30) days nor more than six (6) months or by both such fine and imprisonment; provided, however that any such person infected applying to any physician in this State shall receive treatment provided for in this bill, regardless of his ability to pay.

Section 6. It shall be unlawful for any dealer to treat or offer to treat any infected person or to sell, furnish or give to any infected person or to any other person whomsoever any medicine of any kind that may be advertised or used for the treatment of venereal diseases before requiring such person to produce and file with such dealer a proper prescription for such medicine issued and signed by a reputable physician, which said prescription shall be by said dealer kept on file for a period of one (1) year from the date of his receiving the same, and subject at all reasonable hours, to the inspection of the health authorities in this State. A violator of any of the provisions of this Section shall be punished by a fine of not less than One Hundred Dollars ($100.00) nor more than Five Hundred Dollars ($500.00) or by confinement in the county jail for a term of not less than thirty (30) days and not more than six (6) months or by both such fine and imprisonment.

Section 7.   Any and all institutions in this State, whether penal or eleemosynary and whether public or private and free or for pay, shall make and preserve for a period of at least one (1) year, a record showing the name, age, sex, color, nationality and place of residence of all infected persons of the inmates of such institution that may come to their knowledge and shall submit such record at all reasonable hours to the inspection of the duly accredited health authorities in this State.   All such institutions shall furnish a physician and all proper medicines, instruments and apparatus for the proper treatment of such infected person, and shall isolate and separate all infected persons from all other persons in such institution by causing such infected persons to use separate beds, rooms, lavatories and toilet rooms and facilities, from all other persons.   Any keeper, manager, guard, or other person in control of any such institution who shall wilfully fail or neglect to comply with the provisions of this Section or who shall violate any of the provisions hereof, shall be guilty of a misdemeanor and shall be punished by a fine of not less than Two Hundred Dollars ($200.00) nor more than One Thousand Dollars ($1,000.00) or by imprisonment in the county jail for a term of not less than thirty (30) days nor more than one (1) year or by both such fine and imprisonment.

Section 8.   The keeper, manager, guard or person in control of every prison or penal institution in this State, shall cause to be examined every person who shall be confined in such prison or penal institution after conviction for any offense against the laws of the State or any municipality thereof, to determine whether such person is an infected person.   Every such person found to be an infected person, after the expiration of his or her sentence, shall be kept in such prison or some other suitable place for treatment until pronounced cured by a physician and discharged by the health authorities of this State.   Where such infected person is unable to pay for such treatment the same shall be furnished and administered at the public expense by the State, County or Municipality in whose prison such infected person may be confined; provided, however, that where infected persons have served their full sentences to such prison, the Board of Health may permit such infected person to leave such prison and to stay at home, or other suitable place before being cured, if, in the judgment of said Board of·Health, such infected is able to do so, and will continue proper treatment for such venereal disease.   State, County and Municipal Health Officers, or their authorized deputies who are physicians within their respective jurisdictions, are hereby directed and empowered, when in their judgment it is necessary to protect the public health, to make examinations of persons convicted for sex offenses and ·to detain such persons until the results of such examinations are known. Any keeper, manager, guard, or other person on control of any such prison or penal institution who shall knowingly violate any of the provisions of this Section shall be deemed guilty of a misdemeanor and be punished by fine of not less than One Hundred Dollars ($100.00) nor more than One Thousand Dollars ($1,000.00) or by confinement in the County jail for a term of not less than three (3) months nor more than one (1) year, or by both such fine and imprisonment.

Section 9.   The prescriptions and records provided for herein to be filed and kept, shall not be exposed to any person other than the duly elected or appointed health authorities of the State, County or Municipalities, or when properly ordered by a court of competemt jurisdiction to be used as evidence in such court and no health authority shall be permitted to give any information whatever to any other person concerning any infected person except to appropriate persons for use in the proper courts of this State. Any person who shall violate any of the provisions of this Section shall be guilty of a misdemeanor and be punished by a fine of not less than Fifty Dollars ($50.00) nor not more than One Hundred Dollars ($100.00) and in addition thereto shall be liable in damages to any person who may be damaged by such violation.

Section 10. All Acts and parts of Acts in conflict herewith are hereby repealed.

Section 11. For the preservation of the public peace, health and safety, an emergency is hereby declared to exist, by reason whereof, this Act shall take effect and be in force from and after its passage and approval.

Passed by the Senate this 13th day of March, A. D. 1919.

M. E. Trapp,
President of the Senate.

Passed by the House of Representatives this 8th day of March, A. D. 1919.

Tom C. Waldrep,
Speaker of the House of Representatives.

Approved this 19th day of March, 1919.

J. B. A. Robertson,
Governor of the State of Oklahoma.

Correctly Enrolled.

J. S. Vaughon,
Chairman Committee on Engrossing and Enrolling.

PERSONAL AND GENERAL NEWS

Dr. W. H. Powell, Sulphur, visited the New Orleans clinics in April.

Dr. F. E. Rushing, Coalgate, has established a hospital in that city.

Dr. C. M. Pratt, Pauls Valley, is doing special work in New York.

Dr. W. D. Faust, Ada, is doing postgraduate work in New York and Boston.

Dr. Jesse M. Salter, Sulphur, has returned from army service and reopened his offices.

Dr. R. F. Cannon, Miami, has been discharged from the army and is taking up his work again.

Dr. N. H. Lindsay, Pauls Valley, has returned from a vacation of several weeks spent at Palm Beach, Florida.

Dr. R. H. Harper, Afton, who underwent an operation in St. Louis in February, has recovered and resumed his work.

Dr. C. L. McClelland, Miami, has returned to his home after several months postgraduate work in New York City.

Dr. G. N. Bilby, Alva, has returned from overseas service and is stationed at Debarkation Hospital No. 1, Hoboken, N. J.

Dr. C. J. Brunson, Adamson, has been discharged and returned from overseas service. He was stationed at Coblenz, Germany.

Dr. J. G. Waldrep, Claremore, has returned from a visit to Tennessee where he went to recoup his physicial losses after an attack of influenza.

Dr. L. A. Newton, Oklahoma City, has been discharged from the Army and returned to his Oklahoma City location, opening offices at 214 Colcord Building.

Captain H. M. Stricklen, Tonkawa, who is stationed at Ft. Jay, a few minutes out of New York City, expects to return to his Oklahoma location this month.

Dr. E. E. Shippey, Wister, who sustained a fractured skull due to a personal assault, is reported to be recovering. It is said his assailant struck him from the rear without warning.

Captain Arthur W. White, Olahoma City, after many months romping around and being romped on at army camps, is back on the job as a civilian. His new location is 221 State Bank Building.

Dr. Phil Herod, El Reno, one of the few Oklahoma physicians fortunate enough to secure foriegn service, is back at home, discharged from the army and has taken up the pleasanter duties of civilian life.

Dr. C. E. Putnam, Lieut., M. C., Cyril, Oklahoma, stationed at Coblenz, writes the Journal from Monte Carlo where he is taking a leave and vacation. He forgot to advise us the size of the chips they use in that haven of sports.

Dr. Charles E. Northcutt, Lexington, has been decorated for conspicuous bravery and distinguished service by the British Government. Dr. Northcutt is attached to the British forces and was one of sixty-six medical officers and men so decorated.

Dr. G. H. Clulow, Tulsa, Captain, M. C., U. S. A., stationed at Coblenz, and Mrs. Annie Anderson, Crossmyloff, Scotland, were married abroad February 18. Dr. and Mrs. Clulow were formerly fellow students in Western Reserve University, Cleveland.

Oklahoma Hospital Representatives will hold a meeting at the Severs Hotel, Muskogee, May 21 for the purpose of perfecting a State Hospital Association. Dr. Fred S. Clinton, Tulsa, Chairman of the State Committee on Hospitals, will call the meeting to order.

Captain William Patton Fite, M. C., U. S. A., Muskogee, who went overseas with the 36th Division, was signally honored recently when he received a special assignment in Paris, being the only man in his division selected for the work. He is a son of Dr. F. B. Fite.

Dr. P. E. A. Fling, Hugo, died suddenly from heart disease at his home March 16th. Dr. Fling was one of Choctaw County's oldest practitioners from the standpoint of residence, having practiced there eighteen years, but was in the prime of life at the time of death, being fifty years of age. He was a native of West Virginia and leaves to mourn his loss a wife and daughter and a number of brothers and sisters.

Dr. Geo. H. Wallace, Cheyenne, who has been stationed in the Philippine Islands during the war, has returned to his home. His home-coming is surrounded with some difficulties. During his absence a fire destroyed his library and instruments. Now would be a very good time for the people of Roger Mills County who he has so often befriended to "get back at him" with a "shower" of up-to-date medical literature and nickle plated paraphernalia.

Dr. A. B. Montgomery, Checotah, Lieut. M. C., U. S. A., has a service record which will always be a matter of pride to him and his many friends. In addition to the record he accumulated more than his share of bad luck, for when the record is noted we all agree that he should have long ago been promoted on the record alone without considering his many qualifications as an able practitioner and physician. Ordered into active service August, 1917, Ft. Sam Houston; August 26 to 13 Field Artillery; December 13 to Camp Greene, N. C.; March 14, 1918, to Camp Merritt, N. J.; sailed from Hoboken April 23, landed at Brest May 30; to nearby barracks until June 7; Camp de Songe until July 29 when he went to the Front via Paris to Chateau Thierry, arriving August 30; into action at Chery Chartreuse August 5 and constantly engaged until August 16; in action at St. Mihiel to September 12, rested from the 15th to 23rd then into Meuse-Argonne battle September 26th. While moving forward to Mountfacon September 28th, all other impediments having failed to stop him he fell to influenza, was evacuated to Base Hospital 3, not recovering he was ordered home from Bordeaux December 17; Newport News 30th; to Camp Kearney, Calif., January 15th where he has remained in the hospital until late in March when he was reassigned to active duty. This detailed statement of the happenings is given as an example of what occurred to many Oklahoma physicians. It is a record one may feel pride in and the Journal takes this means to congratulate Dr. Montgomery on his safe return.

DISCHARGES FROM THE ARMY.

Arthur W. White, Oklahoma City	J. M. Salter, Sulphur
T. J. Nunnery, Granite	W. W. Lightfoot, Thackerville
B. J. Plunkett, Duncan	Ed. D. James, Miami
F. L. Patterson, Woodward	G. H. Wallace, Cheyenne
W. A. Thompson, Kusa	T. H. Flesher, Edmond
L. A. Mitchell, Frederick	J. G. Harris, Muskogee
C. J. Brunson, Adamson	Phil. Herod, El Reno
E. H. Lain, Paoli	R. F. Cannon, Miami

MISCELLANEOUS

WHAT IS "PTOMAIN" POISONING?

The term "ptomain" poisoning has become a cloak for ignorance. Jordan says "ptomain poisoning is a convenient refuge from etiologic uncertainty." In fact, any acute gastro-intestinal attack resulting from a great variety of causes is apt to be called "ptomain" poisoning. Selmi, in 1873, first used the word ptomain (from Greek, a corpse) to include the poisoning products of putrefaction which gave the reaction then looked on as characteristic of vegetable alkaloids. From the time of Selmi, when ptomains were regarded as aminal alkaliods, our conception of these substances has changed markedly. The last attempt to give precision to the term was by Vaughan, who defined ptomains as intermediate cleavage products of protein decomposition. Rosenau and his associates at Harvard have been searching in vain for the past year and a half for ptomains that might cause gastro-intestinal or other symptoms. Split products of protein putrefaction are readily isolated. Some of these products have physiologic activity, but none of them thus far have been demonstrated to be poisonous when taken by the mouth. The so-called ptomains isolated and described by Selmi, Nencki, Brieger, Schmiedeberg, Faust and Vaughan were usually obtained from putrid organic matter that had decomposed past the point at which it would be used as food. Furthermore, most of these substances were tested by injecting them subcutaneously or intravenously into animals. Many substances are poisonous when thus introduced parenterally, though they may be harmless by the mouth. Again, many of the so-called ptomains isolated and described have since been shown to contain impurities. Chemists are now seldom confident of the purity of protein fractions, even when obtained in crystalline form. The chemical search for split protein products as the cause of "ptomain" poisoning has practically been abandoned. Most of these split products are amins, which are either not poisonous at all, or no more so than their corresponding ammonia salts. The chemical resemblance between muscarin and cholin has directed the work toward the phosphatids, but thus far this line of research has not helped solve the puzzle of "ptomain" poisoning. Chemists avoid the use of the word ptomains, for the reason that it lacks precision. This is a curious instance of the popular use of a technical term that sounds well, but means little. Only clinicians cling to it as a convenient refuge. Ptomain is a term for chemical substances of uncertain origin, unknown nature, and doubtful existence.—Jour. *A. M. A.*, March 8, 1919.

SOMETIMES YOU GET AN ORDERLY

Before I fell a victim
To the wiles of the Spanish "flu"
I'd gathered from the posters,
And certain movies, too,
That when it came to nurses
You always woke to view
Some peach from Ziegfield's Follies
Who slipped the pills to you.

I've read the artful fiction
About the angels fair
Who sat beside your pillow
And stroked your fevered hair,
And made you kind of careless
How long you lingered there
In the radiant effulgence
Of a lovely baby stare.

That may be true in cases,
The way it is in plays,
But mine was no white lady
Of lilting roundelays;
For while I was a blesse
The nurse who met my gaze
Was Private Pete Koszolski,
Who hadn't shaved for days.
—Lieut. John Pierre Roche,
87th Division, A. E. F., in *Saturday Evening Post*.

COUNCIL ON PHARMACY AND CHEMISTRY.

PROPAGANDA FOR REFORM.

B. Iodine and B. Oleum Iodine. The Council on Pharmacy and Chemistry reports that while B. Iodine (The B. Iodine Chemical Company) is said to be "Nitrogen Hydrate of Iodine" and B. Oleum Iodine a 5 per cent. solution thereof, the examination made in the A. M. A. Chemical Laboratory indicates that the first is a simple mixture of iodin and ammonium iodin, and the second a solution of iodin in liquid petrolatum. The Council declared these preparations inadmissible to New and Nonofficial Remedies because: 1. The composition of B. Iodine is incorrectly declared. B. Iodine is not a newly discovered iodin compound, but a mixture of iodin and ammonium iodid. B Oleum Iodine is not a 5 per cent. solution of B. Iodine as suggested by the statement on the label and in the advertising, but an 0.85 per cent. solution of iodin in liquid petrolatum. 2. Since the solution

, of B. Iodine in water will have the proprieties of other solutions of iodin made by the aid of iodid, the therapeutic claim made for it is unwarranted. 3. The names "B. Iodine" and "B. Oleum Iodine" are not descriptive of the pharmaceutical mixtures to which they are applied. 4. The preparations are unessential modifications of established articles. The first has no advantage over tincture of iodin or compound solution of iodin, and the second no advantage over extemporaneous solutions of iodin in liquid petrolatum (Jour. A. M. A., Feb. 1, 1919, p. 365).

Misbranded Nostrums. The following nostrums were declared misbranded under the Federal Food and Drug Acts because of the false, fraudulent or misleading claims made for them: M. I. S. T. (Murray's Infallible System Tonic); M. I. S. T. No. 2, Nerve Tonic; Imperial Remedy; "Japanese Wild Cherry Cough Syrup;" "Japanese Herb Laxative Compound"; Dr. E. E. Burnside's Purifico No. 1, 2; Dr. E. E. Burnside's Purifico No. 3: Emerald Oil; Bristol's Sarsaparilla; Dr. Belding's Six Prairie Herbs; Dr. Carter's K. and B. Tea; "Brazilian Balm"; "Renal Tea"; Las-I-Go for Superb Manhood; Blood Tabs; Dr. Miles Restorative Nervine; Kilmer's Swamp Root; Homenta; Hinkley's Bone Liniment; Kopp's Baby's Friend; Kopp's Kidney Pills; Reuter's Syrup; Garfield Tea; Di-Col-Q; Sloan's Liniment; Bannerman's Intravenous Solution; Cummings Blood Remedy; and Giles' Germicide (Jour. A. M. A., Feb. 8, 1919, p. 439).

Cerelene Not Admitted to N. N. R. Cerelene, a paraffin preparation for the treatment of burns, was submitted to the Council on Pharmacy and Chemistry by the Holliday Laboratories with the statement that it was composed of 84 per cent. paraffin, 15 per cent. myricyl palmitate stated to be purified beeswax, and 1 per cent. purified elemi gum, to which are added oil of sucalyptus, 2 per cent. and betanaphthol, 0.25 per cent. It was stated that on "special order" Cerelene has been made containing oil of eucalyptus and resorcin, oil of eucalyptus and picric acid, and picric acid alone. The Council declared Cerelene is inadmissible to New and Nonofficial Remedies because there was no evidence to show that this preparation had any advantage over simple paraffin of low melting point (Paraffin for Films—N. N. R. because there is no proof that the medicinal ingredients leave the wax when it is used, and because the constituent "myricyl palmitate" has not been accepted for New and Nonofficial Remedies (Jour. A. M. A., Feb. 15, 1919, p. 513).

Beef, Wine and Iron. So long as one of the largest mail order houses in this country continues to sell Vinum Carnis et Ferri, N. F. in gallon jugs, the drought from prohibition legislation may not be as noticeable as it might otherwise. Seriously however, is it not about time for the professions of medicine and pharmacy to heave into the discard such utterly unscientific combinations as "Beef, Wine and Iron"? (Journal A. M. A., Feb. 15, 1919, p. 498)

Misbranded Nostrums. The following nostrums were declared misbranded under the Federal Food and Drugs Act because of the false, fraudulent or misleading claims made for them: Hall's "Texas Wonder"; King's Liver and Kidney Alterative and Blood Cleanser; En-Ar-CO Oil; Lindsey's Improved Blood Searcher; White Eagle's Indian Oil Liniment; Aqua Nova Vita; Brown's New Consumption Remedy; Akoz Ointment; Akoz Rectal Suppositories; Akoz Powder; Akoz Dusting Powder; Akoz Plaster; Akoz Compound; Flenner's Kidney and Backache Remedy, and Wine of Chenstohow (Jour. A. M. A., Feb. 22, 1919, p. 591).

Styptics. Ordinary bleeding has a strong tendency to stop spontaneously with the formation of a clot, so that the benefit attributed to a drug that has been used as a hemostatic cannot easily be evalusted. Evidence of the current confusion of cause and effect in relation to local hemostatics has been furnished by P. J. Hanzlik. In general he finds that the local application of vasoconstrictor and astringent agents diminishes or arrests local hemorrhage, while vasodilator and irritating agents (without astringent action) increase local bleeding. The value of the newer thromboplastic agents of the kephalin or tissue extract type is considered as still uncertain. Epinephrin remains as the most efficient and desirable hemostatic agent. Tyramin and pituitary extracts were found efficient, and, unlike epinephrin, they do not increase bleeding later. Astringents were found variably effective, ferric chlorid and tannin standing highest, while alum was disappointing. The vaunted cotarnin salts (stypticin and styptol), antipyrin and emetin were found to increase bleeding on local application (Jour, A. M. A., Feb. 22, 1919, p. 577).

Wildroot Dandruff and Eczema Cure. Dr. Harvey W. Wiley, in his book "1001 Tests", thus characterizes this preparation: "Contains arsenic, and some phenolic body, probably resorcin; perfumed and colored. The trace of alkalodali material present was too small for identification. Contains 40 per cent. of alcohol, as declared, and less than one-half of 1 per cent. of nonvolatile matter. Claims that it is an herb compound and a positive remedy for eczema and dandruff obviously untenable" (Jour. A. M. A., Feb, 22. 1919, p. 594).

Benzyl Alcohol. While experience alone will tell whether or not the local anesthetic benzyl alcohol or phenmethylol will come up to the expectations of the discoverer of its action, it was deemed of sufficient promise by the Council on Pharmacy and Chemistry to warrant its admission to New and Nonofficial Remedies (Jour. A. M. A., Feb. 22, 1919, p. 594).

EMPHYSEMA.

H. K. Berkley (Los Angeles), and T. H. Coffen (Portland, Ore.), Camp Lewis, American Lake, Wash. (*Journal A. M. A.*, Feb. 22, 1919), describe an extensive subcutaneous and interstitial emphysema occurring in nine patients in Camp Lewis as a complication of bronchopneumonia. Two patients also developed spontaneous pneumothorax in the camp, and it seems to the authors likely that there is a relationship between the two conditions. One patient, indeed, presented both conditions at different times. In each case the bronchopneumonia was corroborated by roentgenography and in fatal cases by necropsy. The type pneumonia was comparatively mild, but different from that usually seen in robust young adults. It began usually with malise for twenty-four to forty-eight hours, diffuse body pains, aching joints, cough and chilliness. The patients appeared, as a rule, only moderately ill and the initial temperature was rarely over 101 F. Lung symptoms usually were present when they had been in the hospital twenty-four to forty-eight hours, and after three or four days most of the patients showed improvement and went on to uneventful recovery. In a few, however, the condition became critical and it was among these that the emphysema and pneumothorax developed. The authors describe the bacteriologic findings, but it was impossible to connect any special organism to the phenomena noted. The mechanism of the production of emphysema and pneumothorax is discussed, and the presumed routes, both intrapleural, and extrapleural, of the passage of air to the tissues of the chest wall are suggested. The article is illustrated.

COUNCILOR DISTRICTS.

District No. 1. Texas, Beaver, Cimarron, Harper, Ellis, Woods, Woodward, Alfalfa, Major, Grant, Garfield, Noble and Kay. G. A. Boyle, Enid.

District No. 2. Dewey, Roger Mills, Custer, Beckham, Washita, Greer, Kiowa, Harmon, Jackson and Tillman. Ellis Lamb, Clinton.

District No. 3. Blaine, Kingfisher, Canadian, Logan, Payne, Lincoln, Oklahoma, Cleveland, Pottawatomie, Seminole and McClain. G. M. Maupin, Waurika.

District No. 4. Caddo, Grady, Comanche, Cotton, Stephens, Jefferson, Garvin, Murray, Carter, and Love. J. T. Slover, Sulphur.

District No. 5. Pontotoc, Coal, Johnston, Atoka, Marshall, Bryan, Choctaw, Pushmataha and McCurtain. J. L. Austin, Durant.

District No. 6. Okfuskee, Hughes, Pittsburg, Latimer, LeFlore, Haskell and Sequoyah. Vacant.

District No. 7. Pawnee, Osage, Washington, Tulsa, Creek, Nowata and Rogers. N. W. Mayginnis, Tulsa.

District No. 8. Craig, Ottawa, Delaware, Mayes, Wagoner, Cherokee, Adair, Okmulgee, Muskogee and McIntosh. J. H. White, Muskogee.

STATE BOARD OF MEDICAL EXAMINERS.

Melvin Gray, M. D., Durant, President; B. L. Denison, M. D., Garvin, Vice-President; J. J. Williams, M. D., Weatherford, Secretary; O. R. Gregg, M. D., Waynoka, Treasurer; E. B. Dunlap, M. D., Lawton; Ralph V. Smith, M. D., Tulsa; W. LeRoy Bonnell, M. D., Chickasha; Wm. T. Ray, M. D., Gould; W. E. Sanderson, M. D., Altus; H. C. Montague, D. O., Muskogee.

Reciprocity with Georgia, Kentucky, Mississippi, Nevada, North Carolina, Wisconsin, Kansas, Arkansas, Virginia, West Virginia, Nebraska, New Mexico, Tennessee, Iowa, Ohio, California, Colorado, Indiana, Missouri, New Jersey, Vermont, Texas, Michigan.

Meetings held second Tuesday of January, April, July and October, Oklahoma City.

Address all communications to the Secretary, Dr. J. J. Williams, Weatherford.

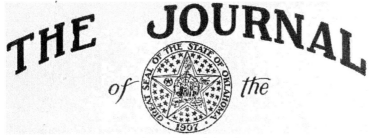

Oklahoma State Medical Association

VOLUME XII   MUSKOGEE, OKLA, MAY, 1919   NUMBER 5

FOCAL INFECTION AND ITS RELATION TO THE DISEASES OF THE EYE*

T. W. STALLINGS, M. D.

TULSA, OKLAHOMA

It is my desire in this paper to take up rather briefly a discussion of focal infection as an etiological factor in the production of inflammation of the structures of the eye. Focal infection may be defined as an acute or chronic localized area of inflamed tissue, harboring single or mixed strains of disease-producing organisms, the toxins and metabolic products of which are absorbed by lymphatic or capillary circulation and the clinical manifestations usually observed in the more delicate and highly specialized structures, often in distant and remote parts of the body.

The structures of the eye may become affected by toxins which have been absorbed from an area of focal infection. There may be all of the cardinal signs of a severe inflammation of any one or more of the various structures of the eye without the presence of any organisms in these structures. Such cases are considered toxic inflammations because they are not so acute in their onset and do not have an extensive exudation. They are not prone to involve the other structures of the eye and are often associated with the various forms of neuritis of the peripheral nerve endings in the eye. Toxic inflammations of the eye are observed with chronic infection in the pneumatic sinuses of the nose, the most important of which, with regard to eye conditions, are the posterior ethmoidal cells, sphenoidan, and frontal and maxillary sinuses. These toxic inflammations clear up very readily after removal of the foci of infection from which the toxic material is absorbed.

There are a number of pathological conditions of the eye which are more difficult to classify as toxic inflammation, or as infections, since it is more than probable that these lesions are caused by the direct effect of the bacteria. They are associated with focal infections and present a more severe chain of symptoms than the toxic inflammations. They are more often seen with general diseases such as rheumatism, syphilis and tuberculosis. It is my desire to speak of these particular lesions of the eye, as metastatic infections of the eye, since the organisms were derived from some other part of the body and no doubt carried to the eye in the blood stream. It is not, however, possible to prove the above assertions; but sufficient clinical evidence has been gathered by the various observers to warrant a classification of toxic inflammation and metastatic infections, and consider

---

*Read before Tulsa County Medical Society, March, 1919.

them as two separate and distinct pathological entities, which may be derived from focal infection. Because of the histological variations in the eye structures, some are more often involved by toxines, and others by bacteria. The cornea and sclera seem more resistant to the bacterial toxins of focal infection and this may be explained by the fact that these structures are of connective tissue origin.

The iris and ciliary bodies and choroid are very vascular structures and may easily become infected from the blood stream. They are not resistant to toxins and are very often inflamed by the toxins from a foci of infection.

The retina is of nervous tissue origin and it is most susceptible to toxic conditions; hence it is frequently absorbed by toxin absorption. It is well protected by the coverings of the eye-ball, but because of its extensive blood supply, it is very favorably exposed to metastatic infection. The conjunctiva may be affected by either toxins or bacteria. The conjunctiva is the glistening mucous membrane lining the lids of the eye and is reflected over the globe. It may be divided into: Palperba, that portion covering the lids; and bulbar, that portion attacheh to the globe. It is well supplied with blood vessels and receives its enervation from the ocular division of the fifth nerve. The importance of this will be seen in attempting to explain lesions of the conjunctiva and the cornea, caused by focal infections of the sphenoid, which is in close anatomical relationship with the gasserian ganglion. Acute or chronic conjunctivitis occurs very frequently with focal infection of the frontal or sphenoidal sinuses. It is rare to find a case of conjunctivitis derived from infected teeth or tonsils. Conjunctivitis associated with frontal sinusitis is subacute or chronic, is never severe and presents no marked clinical manifestations. When focal infection is located in the frontal sinus, because of its anatomical relationship, existing between the frontal sinus and the orbit, there is pain and tenderness over the inner margin of the orbit and slight tenderness in the eye-ball. Headaches may or may not accompany this conditoin. Sometimes headaches are not noticed nor the eye symptoms complained of until the sinus has become closed off. The inflammation may extend to the margin of the lids, less often the cornea is involved. After the focus of infection has been successfully treated, the conjunctivitis and other eye symptoms clear up readily without any further treatment, though it has a tendency to recur with acute colds and coryzas. It has been found that relief from symptoms is promptly followed by cocainization of the spheno-palatine ganglia. It is important to realize that conjunctivitis may be caused by foci of infection and when treating a case that apparcntly does not respond and for which there seems no definite cause, it is well to make a very complete nasal examination in an effort to find the foci of infection.

Scleritis and Episcleritis. Scleritis and episcleritis may be associated with a conjunctivitis or it may occur alone. Most of the lesions of the sclera are not traceable to sinus infection. Acute scleritis observed as a circumscribed swelling of pinkish color under the conjunctiva, forming a circular lesion tending to spread around the eye-ball, occasionally accompanies rheumatism; which in the light of our present knowledge, we know to be a disease of focal infection origin. In all probability this type of scleritis is a true metastatic infection by streptococcus, which has been carried to the sclera by some foci of infection. Scleritis and episcleritis of rheumatic origin, perhaps are more often derived from focal infection of the teeth and tonsils than from various sinuses of the nose, because the streptococcus is found more often a chronic invader of the teeth and tonsils. This form of scleritis and episcleritis does not respond readily to treatment. The sclera may be perforated and infection of the contents of the orbit with complete loss of the eye result. It is this fact which leads one to believe that scleritis and episcleritis of rheumatic origin is a direct infection of the sclera rather than a toxic inflammation. The scleritis is usually very chronic and acute exacerbations occur when the rheumatic symptoms are most severe.

Herpes of the Cornea. Herpes of the cornea may be understood to mean a toxic inflammation of the peripheral nerve endings of the ophthalmic division of the fifth nerve and also involving the cells of the gasserian ganglia. The lesion on the cornea is first seen as a small single or a group of vesicles on the cornea which later break down, forming a small ulcer. They are more often observed accompanying an acute, general infection with a severe systemic intoxication, of which pneumonia is a classical example. This same lesion of the cornea has been observed with a chronic infected post-ethmoidal sphenoiditis with neuritis of the fifth nerve. The involvement of the nerve usually occurs, however, without the herpes on the cornea. A neuritis of the fifth nerve is more often involved in focal infection of the ethmoidal and sphenoidal sinuses because of the intimate anatomical relationship of the ganglia to the sphenoidal sinus.

Keratitis Neuroparalytica. Keratitis neuroparalytica is an inflammation of the cornea which follows a paresis of the sensory endings of the fifth nerve in the cornea. The cornea becomes exposed to the action of extraneous substances because of the loss of sensation. Here again it will be found that chronic infections of the sphenoid and post-ethmoidal cells, with a consequent involve- of gasserian ganglia, is the real cause of the conditions found in the eye. In all cases of neuritis or symptoms of neuritis of the fifth nerve, an examination of the post-ethmoidal cells and sphenoidal sinus is important. Some of the best observers are now recognizing that operative procedure on the sphenoid with treatment of the ganglia, is more rational than the usual cranial operations and destruction of the ganglia, since the destruction of the ganglia relieves only the symptoms and not the cause of neuritis.

Corneal Ulcers. Corneal ulcers may follow infection of simple herpes previously referred to as a neuritis of focal infection origin, though in most instances ulcers of the cornea are caused by direct infection of the corneal tissue following wounds and abrasions. The cornea is of connective tissue origin, and therefore very resistant to toxins; but, as previously stated, the nerves in the cornea occasionally are affected by toxins derived from an area of infection. Ulcers of the cornea which have as their direct cause some area of focal infection are, no doubt, true metastatic infections and they do not differ from the usual corneal ulcer.

Iritis. Acute, subacute or chronic, either unilateral or bilateral. Iritis occasionally can be traced to a chronic infection of sinuses of the nose, infected tonsils or the gums. It is very often of streptococcal origin, in which case it should be considered a metastatic infection of the iris. This type of iritis is seen in rheumatism, endocarditis, septicemias, and all of the various infections caused by the streptococcus organism. The streptococcus viridans is the strain usually found, though the streptococcus hemolytic and nonhemolytic have occasionally been found in the focal infected area. The ciliary body and choroid may also become involved with the iris in this process and is particularly true of the metastatic infections by pyogenic bacteria. Iritis of rheumatic origin has long been known and described. There is nothing about it particularly new except the fact that the underlying cause of the iritis is also the cause of the rheumatism. In other words, they are both derived from focal infection. The toxic form of iritis has a chronic onset, a less severe course, and is manifested by congestion and inflammation, without extensive exudation. The focal infection, causing this form of iritis, may be located in any of the sinuses, teeth, tonsils, etc. In the last year many cases have been reported with post-ethmoiditis and sphenoiditis.

There are numerous other inflammatory conditions of the iris, retina and choroid which may be caused by focal infection and the cases reported at the present time demonstrate clearly that focal infection plays a most important part in lesions of the eye which previously were considered of unknown etiology. Some of the more frequent conditions seen in the eye associated with focal infection of the sinuses are retinitis, choroiditis, neuritis, optic neuritis descendens, blepharitis, tic douloureux, glaucoma, and some of the amblyopia. It is not within the limits of this paper to consider in detail the pathological changes of each structure of the eye brought about by focal infection. Though I do wish to emphasize the fact that the eye, being of delicate and highly specialized tissues and because of its susceptibility to toxins and organism of focal infection, may present the earliest and most convincing evidence of hidden focal infection.

The data for this paper was gathered from the works of the following authorities: Deaver's Anatomy, Howell's Physiology, Schaffer's Histology, Fuch's Ophthalmology, May's Ophthalmology, Week's Ophthalmology, Discussion of Sluder on Headaches and Diseases of the Sinuses, Leob's Diseases of the Nose, Dr. Dickerson of the New York Eye and Ear Infirmary, Prof. Burtsell of the New York Infirmary, Dr. H. W. Wooten, Manhattan Eye and Ear Infirmary, and a number of cases that have come under my own observation.

METASTATIC INFECTION*

Ross Grosshart, M. D.

TULSA, OKLAHOMA

Metastatic Infections as manifested in different forms of rheumatism, arterial sclerosis, ovarian cysts, thyroid glands, nephritis and various other secretory organisms that control the general metabolism of human economy.

The conditions enumerated above are not diseases but symptoms of a focal infection located elsewhere in the body and transferred to the point of demonstration through the blood or lymphatic system. The focal infection may be small and easily overlooked by the diagnostician, therefore, it takes close observation, blood examinations and x-rays with all the other available means at our command to locate the foci. The most prevalent foci are found in the teeth, sinuses of the nose, tonsils, urinary organs, gall-bladder, appendix, abscesses in various locations, puncture wounds, and syphilis, if we do not count it a focal infection when it is contracted before it becomes a blood condition.

The teeth and mouth may not show macroscopically any disease, whatever, and the only way to eliminate the mouth from being the focal infection is by the x-ray. Do not allow dentists to treat abscessed teeth with the known remedies of today; pull them, curette and drain the same as in osteomyelitis.

Tonsils may be overlooked by the general practitioner who is not accustomed to meeting with these buried tonsils, or one that gives a history of not having had a sore throat. Tonsils after having been affected and which do not return to a normal condition should be removed regardless of age and I do not believe there are many normal tonsils at the age of puberty so if they were removed early before the rupture of the ovum, the infection would not be transferred to the blood clot in the ovum nest.

The genito-urinary tract also may give trouble in regard to diagnosis, but the history and the microscope with physical and bi-manual examinations will generally give you a clear sight in regard to the organs.

The appendix as a rule, if giving any disturbance or acting as a focal infection, will give a history of indigestion or paroxysmal pains at intervals and tenderness upon pressure over the site of the organ.

Abscesses located in other parts of the body and excluding the other possibilities, can generally be diagnosed by the blood count.

Puncture wounds can be seen readily and diagnosed.

Syphilis in the chancre stage will give no trouble, but primary and secondary history may be absolutely negative and a Wassermann of the blood may also be negative. So do not exclude syphilis as being an impossibility until you have had a negative cell count and a Wassermann of the spinal fluid.

*Read before Tulsa County Medical Society, March, 1919.

The symptoms as enumerated above we call rheumatism, neuritis, arterial sclerosis, etc. The treatment is to locate the foci and remove it or drain it, allowing the patient to get well if this condition has not existed over a period of time long enough to destroy the parenchyma of the organ which has been infected. By the word parenchyma here, I mean the part of the organ that produces the symptom about which the patient consults the physician.

Rheumatism is a symptom that manifests itself in the organism in the form of pain.

Neuritis is of the same nature, causes pain and sometimes atrophy of the parts to which it supplies.

Arteritis manifests itself by causing pain, possibly swelling and fever.

Arterial sclerosis, and I am positive that here some of my colleagues will take issue with me, but I am of the firm opinion that arterial sclerosis is always due to infection whether it be that form called alcoholic or a form that is due to syphilis, or that form that is due to senility.

It is a trite saying that a man is no older than his arteries. To enter upon the discussion of the changes, and indicate the changes that take place in arterial sclerosis, it would be impossible to bring out in this paper, but enough to say that the arterial sclerosis is a conditon of a thickening of the walls of the vessels which you find in gummatic conditions following syphilis and in a lesser degree when due to other infections, but the principles are exactly the same; that the inflammtion that was produced upon the walls of the vessel by the infection, or toxins, was coffer-dammed as all infections whenever in the body, which resulted in a chronic thickening of the walls of the blood vessels, the coffer-dam causing arterial sclerosis which gives symptoms to which it will be necessary to explain to this society.

Goitre, or inflammation of the thyroid gland, to my mind are synonymous terms of the thyroid gland infection and are due to infections that are most generally found in the tonsil. This infection causes at first a congestion of blood into the organ and surrounding it and causes it to manufacture an overplus of the thyroid extract or internal secretion which results in the symptoms to the patient that we all know. The inflammation still exists in the thyroid glands and the process that goes on is the same as it is in the ovary, kidney, or pancreas or the other internal and external secretory glands until finally it destroys the parenchyma of the gland and we have what is known as a colloid degeneration of the gland, or tumor, changing the patient's symptoms from hyper- to a hypo-thyroidism.

The ovarian cyst is due to the infection in the blood stream and infects the blood clot that is formed in the corpus luteum and does not allow it to go through the stage of resolution normally and results in a cyst which continues to develop and pressure causes absorption of the organ and its parenchyma until finally we have left a shell or capsule filled with a watery solution.

Nephritis. The process of degeneration in the kidney is almost analogous to that of the thyroid gland. The pancreas and the other internal secretory glands (with the exception possibly of the pituitary body) undergo like degenerations with the ultimate results, the picture of which you all have seen ofttimes to your sorrow. This may not be a metastatic infection through blood or lymph, but direct from the bladder.

It would probably be a little far fetched at this period to make a declaration that I am about to make; that when we become more proficient in diagnosis of focal infections and the public realizes the many ailments and conditions that result therefrom, and their treatment instigated early, man's longevity will be increased many fold. As I have said heretofore, a man is no older than his arteries and what we have been terming arterial sclerosis, if my statement is right, when we eliminate focal infections, the causes of arterial sclerosis, the causes of the disturbances of the internal secretaion, man's pain and senility will be practically eliminated, but there is many a step and a great deal of research in the future to bring about these results. When we have obtained the active principles of the internal secretions of the different glands and can reproduce them in the chemical laboratory, or extract them from the animal, it will be possible after having eliminated the foci of infection, to administer the proper dosage of the active principle of the internal secretion that it is sufficient to bring about, or support the normal physical condition of our bodies to perpetuate life to any age, far beyond that of three score years and ten. We will also be able to take a new born infant and produce the size, habits and mentality to a uniform standard which may be set as being a perfect man or woman by the administration of the internal secretions, or the control of internal secretions, which are closely allied to each other. For example, ovarian and thyroid.

So the doctor of the coming age will not be the man of today who administers drugs to cure disease, but will be a scientific man to prevent disease and he will administer vaccines, serums and the excretions (or the chemical analogues thereto) from the internal secretions that now are necessities to a complete metabolism of a healthy body.

The druggist will not compound prescriptions but he will be a chemist, and a bacteriologist capable of making vaccines, serums, extracting from the glandular structure of animals, or producing that likeness in an extract, or chemical combination within his laboratory as per prescription of the medical man to his patient.

In summing up these few remarks to the present physician and surgeon of today, my advice is to make careful diagnosis and acute observation with the one idea in view that focal infection is the downfall and cause of the suffering of the human anatomy and it is his duty when consulted to use all the known elements at his disposal to locate the foci and remove the same or have it removed at the earliest possible moment and he will accomplish for his patients the enjoyment of good health and a reputation for himself and his profession and will redee 1 the wonderful science back to that pinnacle that it rightly deserves—to the elimination of the osteopath, chiropractor and Christian Scientist.

VARICOCELE.

W. A. Angwin, Philadelphia (*Journal A. M. A.*, March 29, 1919), says that varicocele is a frequent cause of disability in the navy, on account of the complaints of reflex or psychic nature attributable to it. Size alone is not an indication for operation, as it is frequently symptomless, while local plan or psychic disturbances, anxiety or worry over a possible defective genital condition may warrant an operation. The operation is divided by Angwin into six steps: the incision; the bringing the spermatic veins in view without disturbing the vas or its circulation; use of crushing hemostats to the veins; securing the cord with a nonslipping ligature; the further disposal of the cord; closing the supercial tissues, and providing suspension of the testicles. Most operative methods include the lifting the cord from its bed which increases the postoperative induration. Induration, itself, should be a rare sequel. The spermatic artery is excised with the spermatic veins without attempting to separate it. He quotes the authority of Bevan as to there existing two sources of blood supply for the testis, namely the spermatic vessels, and the other vessels accompanying the vas, either of which suffices. The article is fully illustrated.

FOCAL INFECTION*

A. W. FIGFORD, M. D.

TULSA, OKLAHOMA

During the last decade a new interest has been aroused in the subject of focal infection as an etiological factor of local and of general diseases. The wider discussion of the subject made it appear as a new principle. The wider and broader interest in the subject has been brought about by a better knowledge of bacteriology, of modes of infection, and by cooperative laboratory and clinical research.

A focus of infection may be defined as a circumscribed area of tissue infected with pathogenic micro-organisms. Foci of infection may be primary and secondary. Primary foci usually are located in tissues communicating with a mucous or cutaneous surface. Secondary foci are the direct results of infection from other foci through contiguous tissues or at a distance through the blood stream or lymph channels.

Site of Primary Foci.

Primary foci of infection may be located anywhere in the body. Infection of the teeth and jaws, with the especial development of pyorrhea dentalis and alveolar abscess, infection of the faucial and naso-pharyngeal tonsils and of the mastoid, the maxillary and other accessory sinuses are the most common forms of focal infection. Submucous and subcutaneous abscesses, including the finger and toenails, are occasional foci. Chronic infection of the bronchi and bronchiectasis; chronic infection of the gastro-intestinal tract and auxiliary organs of digestion, including cholecystitis, appendicitis, intestinal ulcers and intestinal stasis due to morbid anatomical conditions; chronic infection of the genito-urinary tract, including metritis, salpingitis, vesiculitis, seminalis, prostatitis, cystitis and pyelitis, are not uncommon forms. Infected lymph nodes, which are secondary to the primary foci named, become additional depots of local infection. The secondary lymph node infection may persist after the etiologic, distal, primary focus has been removed or has spontaneously disappeared. Other secondary foci may appear in various tissues as a part of the general or local disease which results from a primary focus. As we shall see, systemic and local disease may occur through infection from a focal point by way of the blood stream. This mode of infection is often embolic in character. The tissues so infected may constitute new foci, which in part explains the chronicity of many local and general infections.

Etiology of Focal Infections.

Focal infection, especially of the structures of the mouth and the upper air passages, is a very prevalent condition. The incidence of infection of the mouth is enormous everywhere. In addition to the presence of innumerable saprophytes in the mouth and pharynx, one may find in the saliva and pharyngeal mucus, streptococci and staphylococci, micrococcus catarrhalis, pneumococci, diphtheria and pseudodiphtheria bacilli, menigococci, tubercle bacilli and many other pathogenic bacteria. C. C. Bass[1] and others state that the endameba buccalis was found in the mouths of 95 and even 100 per cent. of all adults examined. The presence of these infectious mirco-organisms in the mouth and upper respiratory tract indicates unhealthful surroundings and individual uncleanliness. The individual carrier infects others by contact and by other means.

The character of focal infection in various parts of the body is so important that separate consideration should be given to each kind.

Pyorrhea Dentalis and Alveolar Abscess.

Pyorrhea dentalis and alveolar abscess (Rigg's disease) is a condition inci-

*Read before the Northern District Dental Society, Tulsa, Feb. 3, 1919.

dent to all classes of adults. It is much less prevalent in the young. It is a disease which fundamentally involves the periosteum of the root and neck of the tooth (peridental membrance). It is the chief cause of the loss of the permanent teeth. It may be associated with caries of the crown, and, on the other hand, the crown may remain normal. The infection first attacks the edges of the gum, which may be macerated by decaying food particles between the teeth, or the gum may be injured in masticating hard substances, by toothpicks, and other traumatic agents. Ill health and poor general nutrition make the gums less resistant. The endameba buccalis and various pyogenic bacteria which gain admission to the edges of the gums cause retraction of the soft tissues and the exposed peridental membrane of the neck and root of the tooth become involved in sequence. This periosteum injured or destroyed, there follows softening and ulceration of the soft parts with the end result of acute or chronic alveolar abscess.

Endameba has been known to be a parasite of the mouth for many years. Its relation to pyorrhea alveolaris was first described by F. M. Barrett,[2] in collaboration with Allen J. Smith in 1914. Without a knowledge of the work of Barret and Smith, C. C. Bass and F. M. Johns[1] had recognized the relation of the parasite to pyorrhea and had begun experimental treatment with emetin. The endamebas may be found in the gum lesions and they are numerous in the deeper abscesses where they live on the dead tissues. Bass and other investigators believe that the endameba buccalis is the chief etiologic factor in the development of pyorrhea alveolaris.

From the pus and dead material of alveolar abscess and the infected pulp of the teeth, with a proper technique, culture yields streptococci, chiefly streptococcus viridans and streptococcus hemolyticus, staphylococcus aureus and albus, fusiform bacilli and other less important bacteria. Doubtless the endamebas play an important part in the occurrence of pyorrhea alveolaris and permit infection with the pyogenic bacteria. The bacteria present in the infected areas are the important factors, however, in the causation of general infection from the focus.

Then we have another foci of infection such as acute and chronic tonsillitis and infection of lymphoid tissue in the nasopharynx; mastoiditis and sinusitis of the maxillary and other accessory sinuses; chronic bronchitis and bronchiectasis, focal infection of the gastro-intestinal canal, vermiform appendix, gallbladder and pancreas; and foci of infection of the genito-urinary tract.

Susceptibility to Systemic and Local Diseases From the Focus of Infection.

The high percentage of incidence of localized infection, especially about the head, has already been stated. The greater number of these infviduals affected, both young and old, do not develop acute systemic disease therefrom. A majority of children suffer from chronic infection of the tonsils and nasopharyngeal lymphoid tissue with occasional exacerbations, while the incidence of acute rheumatic fever and endocarditis is relatively small in youth. Nevertheless, rheumatic fever and endocarditis are unquestionably the result of focal infection of the mouth, throat and teeth.

A majority of civilized mankind, who are city dwellers, carry a latent tuberculous focus, usually infected lymph nodes of the mediastium, mesentery or elsewhere in the body. A comparatively small number develop clinically recognizable tuberculosis.

The marked prevalence of alveolar abscess is not generally recognized as associated with the frequent incidence of acute systemic infection. Probably the frequent relation of pyorrhea to rheumatic fever, heart disease, nephritis, and other acute local and general infections has not been given the etiologic importance it deserves.

The escape of a great majority of persons who harbor foci of infection from manifest clinical systemic disease, is the reason given by many thoughtful physicians for disbelief in the etiologic relation of foci of infection to systemic and local infection, especially of the chronic types.

Based upon the present knowledge obtained by clinical and laboratory research and experiments upon the lower animals, there can be no doubt now of the etiologic relation of localized infection of both acute and chronic systemic diseases. Many of the systemic chronic processes are sequential to primary acute diseases, etiologically related to focal infection. Other chronic systemic diseases are primarily due to infection derived from focal infection.

The relatively rare incidence of systemic disease as compared with the marked prevalence of focal infection may be answered, partially, at any rate, by well known facts concerning immunity both natural and acquired.

The natural defenses of the body, due to the bactericidal and antitoxic powers of the tissues, blood plasma and cells, especially the phagocytes, protect the majority of us from the acute infectious diseases. All individuals do not possess an equal degree of natural immunity; some more readily succumb to the invading infectious agents. When the animal body is invaded with the pathogenic bacteria, the natural defenses are increased by their presence in the tissues and blood. The processes are: first, the phenomenon of positive chemotaxis with resulting leukocytosis and the accumulation of leukocytes in the areas of infection of the tissues by the formation of local exudates, liquid (purulent) and fibrinoplastic, which may serve as walls of protection against further direct invasion; second, leukocytic phagocytosis with destruction of the invading bacteria; and third, the formation of protective antibodies in the blood and tissues.

Similar protective processes may be induced in the body by the injection of non-lethal amounts of living or of dead pathogenic bacteria into a healthy man or animal.

It is not improbable that the bacteria of a focal infection may excite the development of additional defenses in the host and prevent the evolution of a sequential systemic disease.

Bacteria may diminish in virulency and pathogenicity and exist as harmless parasites of the skin, mucous membranes and probably also as foci in the tissues (Kolle and Wassermann[7]), for it is known that the reaction of the tissues is influenced by the virulence of the bacteria. A non-virulent streptococcucs would be disposed of by the tissues with but little local or general reaction.

The Diagnosis of the Focus of Infection.

Usually a focus of infection is disregarded by the patient and physician unless it causes local discomfort. When a systemic disease occurs which present-day knowledge associates with a primary infectious focus, the site of the focus must be located. The character of the systemic disease may point to the most likely location of the primary portal of infection. The primary focus of acute rheumatic fever, endocarditis, chorea, myositis, glomerulonephritis, peptic ulcer, appendicitis and chronic deforming arthritis, as examples, is usually located in the head and usually in the form of alveolar abscesses, acute or chronic tonsillitis and sinusitis. One would look for the focus of ghonorreal arthritis in the genito-urinary tract. The failure to find a focus in the expected situation should indicate an extension of the field of examination until the primary infection should have been found. In a superficial and hasty examination the site of the focus of infection may escape detection or the focus may be assumed to be in unifected tissues and organs. Each patient should be carefully interrogated as to the past and present condition; a general examination should be made, including, if necessary, the services of specialists in diseases of the ear, nose and throat, the pelvic organs and the gastro-intestinal tract, and in all patients with evidence of pyorrhea and sinusitis the services of the roentgenologist is demanded.

Mode of Dissemination of Bacteria and Toxic Products from the Focus of Infection—Hematogenous.

Systemic infection and intoxication from a primary focus is usually hematogenous. The bacteria may be compared with emboli loosed from the place of origin and carried in the blood stream to the smallest and often terminal blood vessels. If virulent and endowed with specific elective pathogenic affinity for the tissues in which they will lodge, and if in sufficient number, the invading bacteria will excite characteristic reactions in the infected tissues and a sequential train of morbid anatomical lesions. The evolution of the anatomical lesions and the clinical phenomena aroused thereby are dependent on the type and virulence of the bacteria, the character of the tissues and the function of the organ involved. The specific tissue reaction consists of a local inflammation with endothelial proliferation of the lining of the blood vessel with or without thrombosis; blocking of the blood vessels; hemorrhage into the immediate tissue; positive chemotaxis with resulting multiplication of the leukocytes and plasma cells in the infected area, or fibrinoplastic exudate with local connective tissue overgrowth. We also have these infections going through the lymphatic as well as the circulatory system.

Focal Infection and Anaphylaxis.

Focal infection may be the cause of the condition known as anaphylaxis. The bacterial protein of the pathogenic micro-organism of the focus may sensitize the body cells.

If a foreign protein gains entrance to the body parenterally, via the blood stream or the lymphatics, the animal body always responds to the parenteral introduction of the foreign protein by the production of specific antibodies to that foreign albumen. The formation of the specific antibodies requires a certain period of time. After this interval a second introduction of the same protein, again by a parenteral route, results in a union of the newly-formed antibody with the antigen (foreign protein), which may excite physical phenomena of an explosive character. These phenomena, the so-called anaphylactic shock, differ materially with various species of animals and with man. In man the typical phenomena may consist of bronchial spasm, urticaria, vasodilitation, and fall of blood pressure, eosinophilia, physical weakness and arthoropathy. In some individuals urticaria or bronchial asthma may be the only expression of anaphylaxis.

Transmutation Within the Members of the Streptococcus-Pneumococcus Group.

Recent coordinate research on clinical medicine and bacteriology, fortified by animal experimentation, has made more evident the etiologic relation of focal infection to systemic disease. The main and fundamental principles which have been proved are:

The apparent confirmation of the transmutability of the members of the streptococcus-pneumococcus group in variations of morphology, cultural characteristics, biological reactions and also of general and special pathogenicity.

Just here I might mention the acquisition of pathogenic elective tissue by bacteria in foci of infection, in culture media and serial animal passage.

Clinical examples have been observed of acute appendicitis; cholecystis; acute gastric and duodenal ulcer; acute and subacute glomerulonephritis; rheumatic fever; erythema nodosum; herpes zoster; malignant endocarditis; simple endocarditis; myocarditis and other acute and chronic systemic diseases, associated with coincident focal infection of the tonsils, accessory sinuses, dental alveoli, the skin and its appendages, the fallopian tubes, the prostate and seminal vesicles and and other foci. Dominant pathogenic bacteria have been isloated from the tissues and exudates of patients at surgical operation; by blood culture; from the urine; from joint exudates and pieces of tissue (muscular, lymphoid, joint capsules and fibrous nodes), removed with the consent and often at the request of patients.

These cultures have been intravenously injected into laboratory animals and at the same time cultures of bacteria isolated from the primary foci of the patient have been likewise used to inoculate other animals.

The evidences of the specific elective tissue affinity of the pathogenic streptococci from the various tissues and likewise of the primary foci is very makred.

The practical application of the principles involved may serve to lessen the incidence and the recrudescence of many local inflammatory organic diseases, notably appendicitis, ulcer of the stomach and duodenum, cholecystitis, glomerulonephritis, acute and chronic arthritis and other abnormal conditions, by the removal of the primary focal cause.

I have seen some of the most severe cases of endocarditis traceable to apical infection. The first consideration and the most important to relieve such condition is the technical side of the˙ complete removal of infection. If we do these things there is no doubt but that the part may be replaced to a normal condition and the tooth or teeth be useful for many years.

The infection to be removed must be considered as not only being in the tooth root itself, but also in the surrounding area or granulation tissue and bone at the apex. Gentlemen, it is up to you as surgeons to apply your asepsis and make access to the infected tooth. In my profession I could not expect a necrotic bone tissue to magically disappear and be rebuilt by normal cell metabolism, without first surgically and asceptically removing each and evety part of the infected area. By this I mean to obtain free access to that part and eliminate all foci of infection. This has been thoroughly demonstrated on the battlefield of the European war. The surgeons go so far as to even cut back from a quarter to a half inch in good tissue in order to be sure they have removed all necrotic tissue, after which they are able to coaptate the edges of the wound and get union by first intention instead of having the wound heal by granualtion.

Realizing the difficulties of a dentist in obtaining such method of procedure to a tooth or teeth with all the surrounding bacteria such as are found in the mouth, requiring isolation from the part to be treated, it is your duty to plunge deeply in the line of surgical and aseptic technique. It has been thoroughly demonstrated to me in my profession that abscessed teeth—by that I mean those from the granuloma to the pus-producing kind—when properly opened through the nerve canal and treated in such a manner as to destroy the infected microorganism, that a goodly percent of these teeth repair in their surrounding tissue.

Allow me to state again that I have seen numbers of cases of desperate systemic condition as stomach troubles, indigestion, neuralgia, neuritis, persistant headaches, muscular rheumatism, joint affections of all kinds, and some of the most obstinate organic heart lesions that I have ever seen, traced to either apical infection, gingival infection or poorly constructed dental procedures; after which were corrected, a perfect cure was established. There are many other pathogenic conditions that one in the routine of practice could relate to you, but, gentlemen, you have heard these preached from all four corners of the books on research, of which there is a new author every day. Let us get busy as doctors, I mean dentists and physicians, work to one common fact and that is to eliminate and establish an absolute preventive and cure, and when she or he presents a condition, let us be capable of a correct diagnosis. If the field of operative dentistry is too˙ large for the dentist to accomplish, let there be separate fields of operation and each man select his field and get proficient. The man who is going to fight those mighty and millions of infective bacteria after they have gained their source of infection,.can only recognize one fact, that it does and must require an x-ray picture of the part beforé and after treatment.

Let us reflect in our mind an x-ray picture of a well-developed apical abscess. You see those cells globulin in type, surrounding the abscess. That is what is called dental granuloma. That is Nature's protective cellular outline. doing all in its power to overcome the infection. ˙X-ray interpretation is the first essential to a correct diagnosis. Every dentist and doctor should be able to read well all x-ray pictures of teeth. They should have x-ray pictures made by men who are experienced in x-raying teeth. I have seen some of the biggest blunders made on x-raying teeth by experienced x-ray men in other x-ray work, but not teeth.

I believe that every tooth should be saved where there is a possible chance but I do not believe in allowing one, two or three teeth to endanger a person's life. If the canal can be thoroughly cleared and all infection removed and incapsulating and filling will save the tooth, I believe it should be done, but if necessary remove a tooth or more, in order to establish free drainage—and last, but not least, all sockets should be thorouhhly curreted so as to remove all debris in the surrounding tissues and allow the granulation to take place from the bottom. These wounds should be kept open, if necessary, until they are healed from the bottom. Where it is possible, after thoroughly eliminating all necrotic tissue, I think the membrane should be sutured over, thereby giving you a much more rapid recovery. The teeth are necessary organs and are part of the digestive requirements to man. To protect and save these calcific formations God gave you, is as essential to your health as the other functionating organs of the body.

CALIPER TREATMENT

D. W. Crile, Edmonton, England (*Journal A. M. A.*, March 15, 1919), discusses certain points of the treatment of fractures of the femur by the caliper method, introduced into general surgery by Lieut.-Col. Besley, U. S. A., and recommends it very highly. The value of the caliper in these cases lies in the fact that a direct force can be applied to the bone without damaging it and without penetrating th ecortex. Penetration of the cortex implies misuse of instrument or a defect in its construction. The original instrument is better than some of its modifications. Penetration of the cortex depends on several factors, but chiefly on the shape of the caliper points. A long thin taper is the worst. The relative length of the handle arm is also important, and when the handles widely diverge the chance of penetration is greater. The arrangement of the cords at the handle ends has also much to do with the pressure. The position on the femur is another great factor. But the most important of all is the joggling or constant vibration, transmitted over the pulleys by the ropes and instigated by the body tone and movements. Gross movement is not referred to, but a constant fine vibratory one, such as that produced by boring, with a blunt instrument. In Crile's experience it has never been necessary to boer small holes into the bone to hold the calipers. The pressure on the points must be steady, and any variation of the pull of the ropes means pain, erosion or penetration of the cortex, or all three together. The most important points to be borne in mind are: (1) a short, broad tapering point, (2) the prevention of very slight joggling, (3) application to the hard portion of the bone, (4) low leverage (short handle ends not diverging too much), and (5) check appliances. There are several kinds of check appliances in use, the purpose of which is to check penetration by putting a stop betweent the handle ends of the calipers to prevent the points coming too close. This, however, does not prevent the one point from penetrating when the other is pushed away from bone and slips. Crile finds more satisfactory a screw locking both approximation and spreading. The question of corrosion of points does not apply to short heavy ones, which could not in many months corrode enough to do harm. The disadvantages in the use of the caliper are, Crile thinks, vastly outweighed by the improvement in length, early union good position and clearing up of sepsis, decreased number of cases of acute medullary osteomyelitis. stiffness and stiff ankles, and pressure paralyses of the external popliteal nerve. The drawbacks that cannot be avoided otherwise have been met by designing a caliper permitting the pull to be taken from the sides and allowing the knee to be fully extended. It has, however, the objection of being more expensive. Crile describes the method of applying the calipers which he has found most satisfactory. The fracture itself is an important factor in deciding the point of application, and much may depend on the direction of the pull. The rule is to pull in the direction of the long axis of the bone, except in duly considered exceptional cases. The amount of pull will vary according to the amount of shortening to be overcome, the strength of the muscles, the age and site of the fracture, the amount of swelling and tenseness of the deep fascia, and the degree of the infection. "It is my custom to apply 15 pounds directly. If this promises, after twenty-four hours, to stretch the fractures sufficiently, it is enough. If it seems not to perform its function, which can be from 1-4 to 2 inches per day, it is increased to twenty pounds, which is sufficient to stretch almost any fracture to full length, provided the apparatus is correct. One need not hesitate to use 25 pounds, or even 30 pounds for a few days, and often forcible reduction under an anesthetic may be resorted to. If the extra weight causes periosteal pain, it can be reduced. One finds that 10 pounds is the least that avails fully, although others can get results with only 5 pounds, I am told. However, one aims to get a little overlength inside a week and thereafter to hold this gain by tie-on fixed extension, which in reality takes very little pull once overlength is accomplished." The caliper will probably cause some discomfort the first forty-eight hours and perhaps at a later period. Relief can often be given by a little local anesthetic applied near the point of the caliper, such as a pinch of powdered procain on the dressing. Or a temporary reduction of the weight, if it can be done without slipping, will help. The method is applicable to bones other than the femur, such as the tibia, fibula and humerus, and others have had success in these cases. The illustrations are useful in making clear the description of the methods.

A BRIEF DISCUSSION OF TUBERCULOSIS IN CHILDREN WITH SPECIAL REFERENCE TO THE TRACHEOBRONCHIAL GLANDS.

L. J. MOORMAN, M. D.

OKLAHOMA CITY, OKLAHOMA

Our progress in the study of tubercolusis during the last few decades has been particularly illuminating; some long cherished theories have been converted into facts, and some significant facts have developed as if by accident, yet there are many recesses into which the light has not penetrated, and when we stop to think of "what we do not know about tuberculosis" after all the time and talent spent in its study, we are seized with a feeling of helplessness and an overwhelming consciousness of the need for further study and research in order that the missing threads may be gathered up and the riddle ultimately solved. .

When in 1882 Koch discovered the tubercle bacillus, it was thought by many that with a known specific cause, there would soon be an end to tuberculosis. But following this epoch-making discovery of Koch's and consequent upon the same, certain astounding facts developed which soon served to shake the faith of those who had foreseen the early eradication of the disease, However, before this disillusionment came, the whole world stood agog because of Koch's announcement of tuberculin as a possible cure for tuberculosis. Quite naturally tuberculin was soon employed for diagnostic purposes, and Pirquet in his attempt to find an easy and sure method of diagnosis, merely proved the almost universal presence of infection with the tubercle bacillus and thus shattered the hopes of those who predicted that tuberculosis could soon be wiped from the face of the earth. Through the stimulus which has grown out of the use of tuberculin for diagnostic purposes, post-mortem and x-ray studies have proven that anatomic tubercle is almost a constant finding, even in young children.

To state briefly the problem of infection, we may start with two fundamental facts, first, the tubercle bacillus is practically ubiquitous; it is to be found everywhere around us, and second, it may gain entrance into the human organism in a variety of ways. After disposing of the small number of cases in which infection takes place through other channels, there are two predominating ideas, the inhalation idea and the ingestion idea. In support of the inhalation theory we have to consider dust infection, championed by Cornet, and the droplet infection of Flugge.

By the ingestion theory we understand that the tubercle bacilli, bovine or human, enter by way of the gastro-intestinal tract. Without carrying the discussion further, we may say that one great fact is outstanding; with the few exceptions mentioned, the tubercle bacillus must pass the lips or the nostrils. After this is said we cannot be dogmatic about the portal of entry. Krause points out the fact that in support of the above theories, only the lungs and the bowels have been considered as portals of entry, and states that none of them give attention to the frequent probability of primary infection of the respiratory and digestive tracts, higher up than the lungs and intestines.

The Pirquet test shows that the greater part of mankind is infected first in childhood and yet pulmonary and abdominal lesions are relatively rare at this early age. After discussing this phase of the disease, Krause again points to the fact that superficial tuberculosis, especially of the lymphatic nodes of the neck, is perhaps the most common manifestation of the disease in childhood. He has called attention to the fact that about 50 per cent. of human beings receive their initial infection between three and seven years of age, just at the time they establish a more intimate contact with the outside world, or in other words, intimate contact with the material that carries the turebcle bacilli, whether food, droplets, dust or contaminated hands. In fact "hand to mouth infection" is given a prominent place in Krause's discussion.

Working with an attentuated strain of the tubercle bacillus, Krause has recently produced tuberculosis of the tracheobronchial lymph nodes in the guinea pig by means of the usual subcutaneous injection, thus upsetting the well known teaching of Gohn concerning the primary focus. This leads to a discussion of the frequency of tuberculosis of the tracheobronchial lymph nodes in children. Gohn attempted to prove all such cases as air borne with a primary focus in the lung, but his methods were such that his conclusions could not be accepted without question. Krause's recent experiments at least prove that the tracheobronchial glands may ultimately receive tubercle bacilli which have travelled from remote parts of the body and which have found no demonstrable lodgment in the lungs.

When we consider the peculiar tendency of lymph nodes to gather tubercle bacilli, and then give attention to the strategic location of the tracheobronchial glands, it is not difficult to understand why they are so frequently involved.

The tracheobronchial nodes become the converging point of all foreign particles that reach the lymphatics of the lungs and the lungs constitute the converging point for all foreign particles which reach the blood circulation. The other organs of the body receive only their own systemic blood supply, while the lungs receive all the blood from all the other organs of the body, and thus the tracheobronchial glands receive, not only the foreign particles which reach the lungs through the air, but also those which come through the blood stream. Though the portal of entry may be uncertain, and the primary focus not determined, the tracheobronchial glands are usually infected amd may be demonstrated during life by physical examination and the use of the x-ray.

We should ever keep in mind the fact that the great majority of children are infected and that infection may at anytime become clinical tuberculosis and that the first symptoms are those of toxemia, namely, weakness, undue fatigue, poor appetite, failure to gain, or loss of weight and nervous irritability. This group of symptoms becomes particularly significant when there is a history of contact with those who are suffering from tuberculosis, or when there are signs of local involvement, as cough, hoarseness and streaked sputum. The general appearance and the physical condition may or may not suggest tuberculosis. When it is impossible to find any other cause for the symptoms of toxemia, a thorough examination of the chest should be made with special reference to interscapular dullness and the presence of D'Espine's sign. In addition to the latter we may get certain changes in the breath sounds, the most frequent being a diminution in intensity on the side of greatest involvement, this probably is due to pressure resulting from enlargement of the hilus group of lymph nodes. Any attempt to diagnose tracheobronchial adenitis without the use of the roentgenray is incomplete, and yet roentgen findings must be interperted in the light of history and physical examination. The Pirquet test is of value, especially in children under four years of age. It should be repeated two or three times before considered negative. Pulmonary tuberculosis or involvement of the lungs proper, while comparatively rare in infancy and childhood, is not so very infrequent, and when present requires the same diagnostic procedure as that employed in adults.

At the Oklahoma City Tuberculosis Dispensary we have examined 135 children during the past year and the following interesting data has been gleaned from the more complete annual report of the dispensary. I have tried to gather up only those facts and symptoms which might have some relation to tuberculosis. Of the 135 children, 50 gave a history of exposure to open cases, 70 were exposed to suspected cases and 15 gave no history of exposure. 116 gave a history of measles, 50 had pneumonia, 34 influenza and 86 gave a history of whooping cough.

A history of the following symptoms was obtained: Cough 59, expectoration 29, pain in chest 24, pluerisy 14, hemoptysis 2, night sweats 11, loss of flesh 25, loss of strength 34, hoarseness 17, fever 19, loss of appetite 28, disturbed digestion 27. The physical examination revealed the following: Weight below standard 73, height below standard 17, general appearence good, 95 fair 48, poor 21. Type of chest normal 121, abnormal 14, superficial lymph nodes palpable 110 (some were not reported), tonsils hypertrophied 80, dullness elicited by percussion 89 (with few exceptions the dullness was interscapular), D'Espine's sign was present in ·35, rales in 29.

Every case examined was given a card for complete laboratory and x-ray of chest, but it has been impossible to get all the children to report for this work, consequently only 69 were x-rayed. The following interpretation was recorded in connection with these plates: Tuberculosis of the tracheobronchial glands alone, 11; tuberculosis of the tracheobronchial glands with peribronchial thickening, 29; tuberculosis of the tracheobronchial glands and peribronchial thickening, with involvement of the lung tissue, 19; non-tuberculosis infection, 3; negative 7.

The following gives the diagnosis as recorded in the 135 cases: Tuberculosis of the hilus alone, 34; tuberculosis of the hilus with peribronchial and lung involvement, 44; doubtful, 40; cases with non-tuberculous infection, 5; negative, 12.

The accompanying cuts show the x-ray findings in the various types of tuberculosis found in children. Figures Nos. 1 and 2 are particularly interesting because they represent two types in the same individual. This child, aged 15 years, was in school when she first came for examination. She was placed in the hospital for diagnosis December, 1917, and Fig. 1 shows the x-ray findings at that time. A large shadow representing a mass of enlarged glands at the right hilus with very slight tracings toward the periphery. At this time she was having a temperature of 100 to 104 and very rapid pulse. The physical examination revealed only enlarged cervical glands and interscapular dullness with diminished breath sounds on the right side. After a diagnosis of very active glandular tuberculosis predominating in the tracheobronchial glands, she was placed in the Oklahoma Cottage Sanatorium.

After four months management with absolute rest in bed, her temperature began to remain about normal and at the end of five months she had gained about 20 pounds and looked like a different girl. She was taken from the sanatorium against our advice and about 10 months later she returned in a pitiable condition with great emaciation, cough and fever, with tubercle bacilli in the sputum. Figure 2 shows the x-ray findings April 14, 1919. Extensive pulmonary involvement in the upper half of both lungs, predominating in the right.

Figure 3 represents a girl of 12 years in fairly good physical condition, who lived with an open case for several years. Typical hilus shadows are to be seen which are of the butterfly type and represent healed tracheobronchial glands. Her sister 10 years of age shows the same.

Figure 4 shows tuberculosis of the hilus with linear tracings toward periphery·with well defined calcified glands on the right. This represents the findings in a boy 14 with no history of exposure to tuberculosis, but whose living conditions have always been very bad. Four brothers and sisters show practically the same x-ray findings.

Figure 5 shows advanced pulmonary tuberculosis with positive sputum, in a boy of 12 years who had long continued exposure to open tuberculosis. In spite of the advanced stage of the disease, the boy manifested very little evidence of toxemia and was keeping up his school work and getting up at four o'clock A. M. to deliver papers.

Figure 6 shows an infant of five months with history of cough from the 10th day after birth, no known exposure. Physical examination revealed fine crackles in both lungs. A smear from the phlegm obtained by tickling throat with gause, showed tubercle bacilli. It is possible to see the indefinite shadows extending through both lungs.

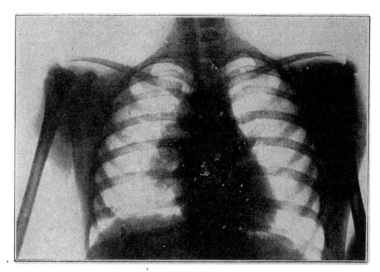

FIGURE 1

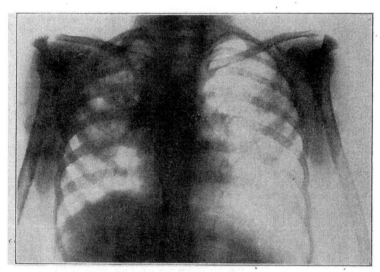

FIGURE 2

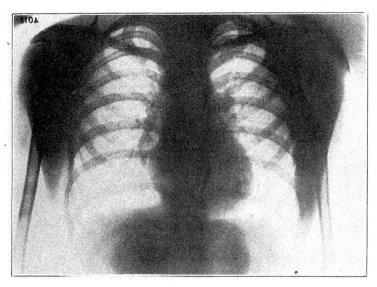

FIGURE 3

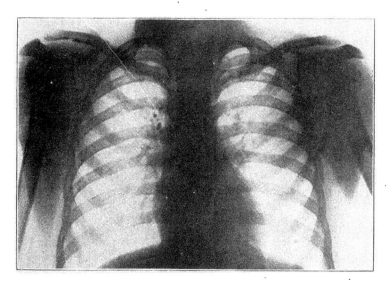

FIGURE 4

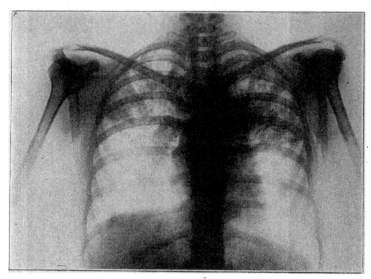

FIGURE 5

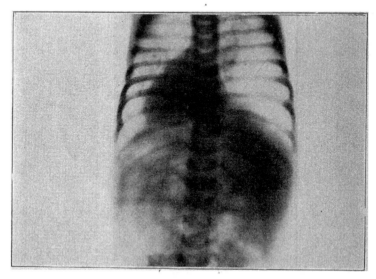

FIGURE 6

CASE·RECORDS.*

FRED S. CLINTON, M. D., F. A. C. S.

TULSA, OKLAHOMA

PRESIDENT AND CHIEF SURGEON OKLAHOMA HOSPITAL

Case records, like every other important part of a successful doctor's work, must have certain definite purposes in view and more or less systematized methods of procedure. So much has been written in the past and resurrected and discussed in the current medical literature that even an attempt to revise any considerable portion of the meritorious discussions would be imposing upon your good nature.

Surgery, Gynecology and Obstetrics, the *Modern Hospital*, and the *Journal of American Medical Association* have all carried numerous appeals and various methods of different individuals for the keeping of these records. One of the most satisfactory and comprehensible articles giving detailed description for action is the *Bulletin of the American College of Surgeons*, Vol. 4, No. 1, (January, 1919) by Dr. John G. Bowman, Director of the College, which may be read with pleasure as well as profit because it tells you what to do and in a general way how, to do it.

The important thing which has impressed itself upon the writer for a number of years is that all of these plans fail unless there is a personality behind it to make the wheels go round. The case and condition, together with the examiner's ability, time and opportunity, will determine the length of record.

The purpose of this paper is to emphasize the importance to all parties of a case record and to recommend the very careful reading of the plans as outlined in the above journals in the hope that each individual may be able to adopt sufficient amount of information from them to suit his individual needs and requirements.

The writer for a long time has kept some case records and from this experience, reading, observation and correspondence, the following points or suggestions are presented for consideration.

(*a*) From the business world we can easily draw some valuable lessons in efficiency. The changed economic conditions demand increased efficiency and require the saving of the doctor's time for other service than attempting to write case histories in legible long hand. The writer has for some time past been using the dictaphone with considerable satisfaction.

(*b*) The preparation of a case record should be approached with the same degree of thoughtful care one undertakes to perform a surgical operation. A useful case record cannot be obtained by a novice or one unskilled in this special line, so it must be someone's appointed work. It must be done regularly, orderly and after some acceptable plan or method. The constant repetition of the work improves the technic which not only gives a superior case history in a shorter time, but adds materially to the intelligent grasp of the salient points in the case.

(*c*) As the patient and his care is the unit about which the resources of the physician revolve, the responsibility must be fixed for every important step in this professional endeavor, and someone must be designated to secure and complete the case record unless the attending physician performs this duty himself. The physician must secure the personal history and patient's reasons for seeking medical aid, being governed by education, training and experience and guided by common sense, the case in hand, and the published requirements of the American College of Surgeons.

(*d*) The result of examination, laboratory reports, treatment, conduct, out-

---

*Read before Tulsa County Medical Society, April 14, 1914.

come, and other features of the case are recorded as soon as developed. The use of the dictaphone enables the physician to make this record at anytime during his convenience, such as completion of other work, investigation of certain details which would enable him to present it in a more orderly and intelligent manner.

(e) The record is then taken to the typist who transcribes it and at the close of the case this typed copy and any additional data is included with the charts in an individual envelope and filed at the hospital, if it has been a hospital case. The personal history and case records are at no time attached to the chart board where some curious or impolite person might read them, but are always kept as a sacred trust, which they really are, away from prying eyes.

(f) As a true case record reflects through its presentation the attendant's visualization of the patient, it is the time-keeper of professional progress. It encourages systematic study and education and safeguards the patient's interest and the physician against suits for damage or embarrassing situations due to the

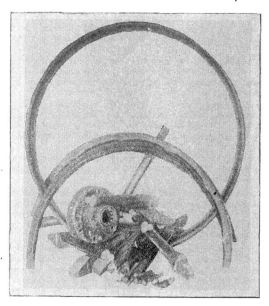

FIGURE 92*

request for or return of patient to obtain proper information relative to previous diagnosis, treatment or operation.

(g) The record, to be useful, must be true to the ascertainable history and condition of the patient, yet brief and systematic with proper headings so one may instantly refer to any feature. Dr. John G. Bowman, Director of the American College of Surgeons, says, "Novel writing under the guise of case records is a waste of time, energy and money."

(h) The writer has a loose leaf book for the office where a record of his cases is kept with such personal information as may be needed to facilitate the study.

*Courtesy Murphy's Clinic, Vol. 3, No. 2, April, 1914.

(i) The standardization of the modern hospital is a worthy ideal. However, the complex conditions now existing make it almost impossible, unless the various units which go to make up a hospital, such as patients, physicians, surgeons, nurses, dietitians, anesthetists, laboratory and social service workers as well as hospital administrators, are all standardized and correlated into one grand symphony of success. Yet by the constant use of known and approved procedures much good work may be done and continued progress made.

(j) The proper keeping of case records will force any person with pride to study the patient's welfare more thoroughly. Health is the greatest resource of any country, so why should the physicians be slovenly and unbusinesslike in their book-keeping methods with reference to this wonderful treasure?

(k) The true progress of medical education is largely dependent upon accurately chronicled case records. When these case records are made the stepping stones to professional reputation and medical men are to be judged by their diagnostic ability, then greater care will be exercised by conscientious persons in making of these records.

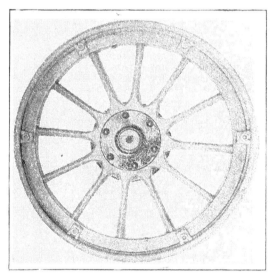

FIGURE 93*

(l) Diagnosis is the key-stone in the arch of medicine.

The late Dr. John B. Murphy, one of the greatest, if not the greatest all-round surgeons of his time, said of diagnosis;. "You must learn by a system of personal investigation of actual patients, and if you have such a system clearly in your minds, you will finally become diagnosticians and you will be capable of doing ably that thing on account of which the profession suffers most because it lacks the most; that thing through deficiency in which we have lost more people's confidence than through any other one, namely, diagnosis. People do not expect us to cure them of all their ills, because they all expect to die sooner or later. They all recognize in life so dangerous an undertaking that none of them

*Courtesy Murphy's Clinic, Vol. 3, No. 2, April, 1914.

expect to get through it alive. * * * * Success rests almost entirely on arriving at a diagnosis."

This distinguished teacher further says; "Failure carefully to examine cases is the most common cause of error. * * * * On what is the diagnosis to be based? The clinical course, the symptoms and signs, the physical and laboratory findings. I have often used the simile that a diagnosis is like a wheel, which is composed of a hub, spokes, felly, and tire, all in proper relationship to one another. These materials and parts separately do not constitute a wheel. They must be assembled to constitute it. The diagnosis of a diseased condition is the wheel, but is completed only by assembling all the details of the patient's illness in proper relationship to one another. First, there is the history—the story of how the disease began and when it began. It is the hub of your diagnosis. Second, the clinical course, the signs and symptoms, in chronologic order, represent the spokes and the felly. This practically makes the wheel, but you can often strengthen it or add finish by placing on it a tire, which is represented in our diagnostic wheel by the assistance we receive from the laboratory in the way of tests and microscopic examinations. A good diagnosis is a scientific construction. It must be built. Knowledge, perception, painstaking care, and the interpretation of clinical history, symptoms, signs, and laboratory findings are means needed to construct a diagnosic wheel no matter how mild or severe in degree the pathologic condition may be. The patient is entitled to the best service, and we must not only be prepared to furnish, but must render, it."

Properly kept case records will increase the intelligence, encourage the industry, and develop the integrity of any physician.

Let us use the means and measures at hand to improve ourselves in medicine and increase our usefulness to society. The case record is an individual, personal responsibility inseparably associated with the attending physician's effort to arrive at a diagnosis and proper advice and treatment. The gathering and grouping—the analyzing or putting together the symptoms and signs of disease—belong to the doctor, the recording may be done on dictaphone or by typist. The completed record is the written answer to the patient's prayer for relief.

IRRITABLE BLADDER IN WOMEN

C. A. L. Reed, Cincinnati, (*Journal A. M. A.*, Feb. 1, 1919), describes irritable bladder in women as being a condition in which severe pain in urinating and frequent desire to urinate make life miserable for the patient, and trying to the physician. The underlying condition is abnormal sensibility of the lining of the bladder itself which may be caused by conditions either external or internal. Those working from the outside usually act by pressure, such as in cases of pregnancy, uterine displacements or tumors. Among the conditions arising within the bladder and that have a causative bearing on the symptoms acute infection, generally gonorrheal, tuberculous infection, local growths, benign or malignant; calculi; diverticuli, etc., may be named. In a certain proportion of cases, circumscribed ulceration, the so-called Fenwick ulcer near the outlet has been found the essential condition. Another form of ulcer is specially mentioned, which might be designated as the Hunner ulcer, first described by Dr. H. L. Hunner; or, better, as the punctate ulcer of the bladder, as being more descriptive. Importance of differential diagnosis in these cases from the early thorough examination is emphasized, and three cases are reported. The symptoms are those of the irritable bladder first mentioned, and the urinalysis finidings are usually negative. Reed reproduces the description given by Hunner as he has found it most accurate and helpful. He calls attention to a glazed dead white appearance of a portion of the bladder mucosa as seen through the cystoscope. Sometimes there are small congested areas in the immediate neighborhood of this, which sometimes ooze blood and are often surrounded by an area of edema. In certain of these cases, Reed has observed a granular appearance suggestive of tuberculosis, but which we now know, from Hunner's research, is due to the development of minute cysts with mucous lining. The diagnosis of punctate ulcer is based on the history of the case, the existing symptoms and the urinalysis and cystoscopic findings. The causes have not yet been fully determined, but the possibility of focal infection is admitted, though longer observation is required. The pathology, so far as developed, seems to be that of a chronic interstitial nephritis, more or less involving the bladder wall. The treatment seems to be reduced to surgery, the complete excision of the ulcer-bearing area. The original method, devised by Hunner, was extraperitoneal, and was employed in the first of Reed's cases, while his other two were treated by a transperitoneal operation.

JOURNAL OF THE OKLAHOMA STATE MEDICAL ASSOCIATION

VOLUME XII   MUSKOGEE, OKLA., MAY, 1919   NUMBER 5

PUBLISHED MONTHLY AT MUSKOGEE. OKLA., UNDER DIRECTION OF THE COUNCIL

DR. CLAUDE A. THOMPSON, EDITOR-IN-CHIEF

ENTERED AT THE POST OFFICE AT MUSKOGEE, OKLAHOMA, AS SECOND CLASS MAIL MATTER, JULY 28, 1912

THIS IS THE OFFICIAL JOURNAL OF THE OKLAHOMA STATE MEDICAL ASSOCIATION. ALL COMMUNICATIONS SHOULD BE ADDRESSED TO THE JOURNAL OF THE OKLAHOMA STATE MEDICAL ASSSOCIATION, 308 SURETY BUILDING, MUSKOGEE, OKLAHOMA.

The editorial department is not responsible for the opinions expressed in the original articles of contributors.

Reprints of original articles will be supplied at actual cost, provided request for them s attached to manuscript or made in sufficient time before publication.

Articles sent this Journal for publication and all those read at the annual meetings of the State Association are the sole property of this Journal. The Journal relies on each individual contributor's strict adherence to this well-known rule of medical journalism   In the event an article sent this Journal fo publication is published before appearance in the Journal, the manuscript will be returned to the writer.

Failure to receive the Journal should call for immediate notification of the editor, 307-8 Surety Building, Muskogee, Okla.

Local news of possible interest to the medical profession, notes on removals, changes in address, deaths and weddings will be gratefully received.

Advertising of articles, drugs or compounds unapproved by the Council on Pharmacy of the A. M. A. will not be accepted.

Advertising rates will be supplied on application. It is suggested that wherever possible members of the State Association should patronize our advertisers in preference to others as a matter of fair reciprocity.

EDITORIAL

WILL THE CIVILIAN PROFIT BY WAR EXPERIENCES?

A very respectable number of Oklahoma's young manhood is back in civil life after varying degrees of service, experience and time spent in the army. We believe every one of them returns with new ideas as to the proper care of his body, his people and his surrounding neighbors and premises. Many of them are enthusiastic exponents of sanitation, prophylactic vaccination against disease and avoidance of those due to his own indiscretions. He comes home, as a rule, to paraphrase slightly "Unwounded by Woman", protected for years against smallpox, for a time against typhoid and her sister infections, paratyphoid. He knows the dangers of untreated water, of exposed waste and sewage, of crowded living conditions, of filth in all garbs, the value of regular living, good food and clothing. In practically every case he comes home a better man from all viewpoints. If he is of an investigative turn, analytical and retrospective, he will ponder shortly on the deaths during his absence. When he understands the civilian death rate from influenza, compares it with his army rate, he will mentally enter upon his approbation of prompt treatment on strict lines as a possible factor. If his kinsman died from typhoid or had it, he will promptly approve his vaccination.

In all seriousness, is it right to discriminate against our people? Why not apply the protective and harmless measures of the army, as far as practicable, to our citizens, cities and towns? Why not promptly penalize the grower of flies and mosquitoes? Is the soldier any better than his relatives? Why shall we not have inspection of his civilian relatives to discover and ward off incipient disease? In the face of the very obvious lessons of the war, Muskogee County sends to the Legislature a misrepresentative who would undo the practical effects of common sense by omission and opposition. This gentleman opposed inspection of school children on the ground that it would "Frighten" them, but finally, and there lies the serpent,—admitted that he was a Christian Scientist. Very likely had he been in the Draft age he would have objected to everything on "Conscientious" grounds. At the same time, due possibly to the same influence, school inspection in Muskogee was abrogated to all practical intents.

At the very time when the Nation was straining every effort to keep its energies at par we witness the amazing spectacle of a misguided portion of those at home reducing our force by every means.

In sincerity we suggest that now is the time to align all sensible people to the principle that a danger to the individual is a danger to the Nation. The returning soldier is a practical exponent of that. With his aid and that of intelligent people we should make long strides toward improvement of useless conditions. Necessity and enlightenment has greatly broadened the powers of the State Health Department. The legislation on tuberculosis and venereal control will prove of inestimable benefit. Why not make it unanimous?

TUBERCULOSIS SANATORIA LEGISLATION.

Oklahoma took a far step forward during the last legislature in providing for the establishment of three sanatoriums for the treatment of tuberculosis. The salient features of the law make the following provisions:

Supervision by the State Board of Health, the State Commissioner to immediately divide the State into three districts as nearly equal in population as may be, to select in each district a location suitable for a sanatorium, with due regard to accessibility from all points in the district.

Joint supervision is provided in that the Board of Affairs shall handle all matters of business, the State Board to handle admissions, treatment and discharge of patients.

A Bureau of Tuberculosis is provided for in the State Health Department, the Commissioner to appoint a Chief who shall be an expert in the prevention of tuberculosis, experienced in sanatorium management and construction.

Each institution is to have a superintendent residing at the sanatorium, who shall appoint necessary assistants and nurses, including a public health nurse who is required to visit tubercular patients within the district and perform other duties as prescribed.

Provision is made for acceptance of pay or private patients able to defray such charges as may be fixed by the superintendent.

Patients unable to pay shall be admitted on request of county superintendents of health, public health nurses and the county commissioners concerned, or the State Board of Health. County commissioners shall pay not less than ten, not exceeding fifteen dollars weekly for all necessary care of patients entered from their counties.

The law applies only to those resident in the State for one year.

Excise Boards are authorized to levy tax, not in excess of one mill, not to be held as current expense, but for a special purpose known as the "Tuberculosis Fund".

Each District Superintendent is authorized to provide for the opening of free tuberculosis dispensaries at centrally located points where patients may be properly examined by the designated officers.

CURRENT   MEDICAL   LITERATURE

Conducted by

DRS. LeROY LONG, CURT von WEDEL, Jr., and L. J. MOORMAN,
OKLAHOMA CITY

(Translated from original article in *La Presse Medicale*, February 24, 1919. Abstracted *in extenso*.)

LeRoy Long, M. D.
OKLAHOMA CITY

THE INTRAVENOUS INJECTION OF PEPTONE IN INFECTIOUS DISEASES.
(Les Injections Intraveinuses de Peptone dans les Maladies Infectieuses.)

Nolf, of Liege, speaking by invitation at a conference of the Paris Faculty of Medicine, January 21st, 1919, calls attention to a question which he says has greatly interested him for four years.

Before the war he had given much study to the action of peptone when introduced in various ways into the bodies of animals used for experimental purposes.

He had advocated, in the case of man, the subcutaneous injection of peptone in hemophillia, the various hemorrhagic states, paroxysmal hemorrglobinuria, etc.

For a long time he had believed such employment of peptone valuable in menacing abdominal meteorism, for he had proven on numerous occasions that there was energetic and persistent contraction of the intestines of the dog, which had had peptone by intravenous injection.

Practical application of the theory was put into effect in July, 1916, when, in the case of a woman who had pronounced meteorism as a result of a severe typhoid infection, three centigrams of dry peptone was used for each kilogram of weight. The total quantity employed was one and a half grams. This was dissolved in 200 c.c. of normal saline solution (solution saline isotonique). The injection (intravenous) was slowly made, the time employed being about thirty minutes. In about an hour and a half the patient had a violent and prolonged chill, followed by a temperature of 40.5 to 42 c. In an hour the fever began to subside slowly. The next morning the temperature was 36.6. At the same time there was an improvement of the general condition. Later the temperature went up again, but not to the height attained before the injection, and the patient, whose condition had been grave, progressed in a satisfactory way, the course of the disease being, henceforth, benign.

In time the meteorism disappeared, but this local result, which had been the reason for the intervention, disappeared after there was improvement in the pulse, the temperature and the general condition.

The author remarks that the reaction had been too distinct, the results too happy, not to warrant new trials. Since then he has treated a number of cases of grave typhoid by intravenous injections of peptone, and with success.

An analysis of the effects observed in the first case, and in those which followed, shows that the intravenous injections produce two very distinct results—one immediate and one more remote. A careful examination of both is interesting.

The immediate results depend upon the dose injected. If it is equal or inferior to one centigram per kilogram of the weight of the patient; that is to say, if in a patient of average weight one injects 5 to 6 c.c. of a 10 per cent. solution, one most often observes a rise in temperature, which takes one or two hours after the injection, and lasts a few hours. If the dose is increased a little, say 7 to 10 c.c., one observes the same initial rise, accompanied by a severe chill, and in the average case this takes place one hour after the injection. The chill lasts 20 to 30 minutes. It is followed by a fever which is usually succeeded by a sweating stage.

The temperature falls rapidly in the hours which follow, the sweating being profuse. Three or four hours after the beginning of the sweating stage the temperature is normal, or nearly normal, and remains there for a long time.

When the injection is made in the morning the lowest temperature is often between 4 and 6 in the afternoon. Usually the temperature remains down during the night, sometimes presenting a transitory rise, of little importance, in the first hours of the night. Sometimes the temperature goes down more slowly.

The author has observed that a typical reaction, that is to say, a fall of temperature notable and persistent, is more difficult to obtain during the first ten days of the typhoid than later.

It is believed that 12 to 15 c.c. of a 10 per cent. solution may be used in a subject of average weight and robustness, but it would seem that it is safer to fix the average maximum dose at 10 c.c., and this should be diminished from time to time in accordance with the improvement in the condition of the patient.

It is the custom of the author to make the injections early in the morning for the reason that the febrile stage will have been passed during the afternoon, and the patient be permitted rest and sleep at night during the febrile stage. He directs that the patient drink nothing but pure water, or sweetened water during the night before the injection.

It has been observed that the temperature does not rise again to the level before injection until the evening of the next day after the injection. It is advised therefore, to not repeat the injection more often than every two days for fear of demanding of the organism too great an effort to react.

The effect on the temperature is evidently not the result of action on the thermic centers, for it has been observed, in the case of those patients, in which the effect is not obtained, there is presented a high temperature instead of a drop. It seems, rather, that it may be an expression of a reaction more extended, which manifests itself by other signs. The patient feels better, is less excitable, and inclined to sleep. During a few hours he has a truce.

The author believes that the injection does not act as a simple "antithermique", but the "antithermique" effect seems to be the expression of an anti-infectious influence.

Attention is called to the remote effects (effects lointains). By repeating every two days there is obtained a persistent effect on the average temperature curve, but, in addition, the nervous excitement, the delirium, the insomnia, the prostration is relieved and finally disappears. After a few days the appetite returns, the diarrhea checks, the stools become more firm. If there has been meteorism it disappears. If the tongue has been dry it becomes moist. Even if the disease continues for several weeks, it runs a very benign course.

Often the benign influence of the injection may be proved by the disappearance of microbes from the circulating blood. Frequently there is a distinct diminution in number 48 hours after the first injection. In the case of many patients two injections render the blood sterile. Sometimes it takes longer, but the possibility of obtaining the result seems to prove that it acts as an anti-infectious agent.

The anti-infectious action is not specific. It occurs in various acute septicemias as well as typhoid.

Since the action of peptone is not specific, but consists probably in a stimulation of the means of general defense of the organism, it appears advantageous, a priori, to employ at the same time agents more or less specific. Thus, in typhoid, urotropin is given after the manner advised by Chauffard, sodium salicylate in polyarthritis, etc.

The author calls attention to certain dangers in the intravenous use of peptone, the first of which is a lowering of the blood pressure. This is noticed more particularly in those who have marked infections, and he is of the opinion that the infectious condition predisposes to this "hypotonie". This seems to be borne out by the fact that the subject in good health, or but lightly infected, has scarcely any inconvenience in this way.

When the reaction is marked the patient complains of headache, tumultuous beating of the heart, and often, also, arterial throbbing in the lumbar region, soon after the beginning of the injection. The face is injected, the pulse frequent, small and compressible. The respiration is accelerated, and in the case of those having pulmonary affections, there is a disposition to cough, and if it is not repressed it leads to nausea and vomiting.

When these phenomenae are not very marked they pass in a few minutes, But there may be more distressing symptoms such as difficult breathing and a very frequent pulse, even 140 to 160. After a little while there may appear on the trunk, limbs and face an eruption. The symptoms are like those in anaphylaxis from injection of horse serum.

In addition to the type of injection, the quality of peptone and the rapidity of the injection are other elements which bring about the above syndrome.

One should reject any sample of peptone which gives the least odor of decayed meat. It should be injected slowly and with extreme care—more so if there is any reason to believe that the patient is very sensitive to the product.

The injection should be made with a Luer syringe, armed with a fine Pravaz needle. An assistant should count the pulse, calling out in a loud voice the number each quarter of a minute. If it reaches 35 per quarter of a minute, the injections should be arrested until it slows. Usually several minutes should be occupied.

A safer way is to administer the same dose dissolved in 150 to 200 c.c. normal saline, taking 15 to 20 minutes, and this method is suggested as applicable to those physicians not accustomed to its use

If the blood pressure is low, adrenalin should be administered beforehand, and it is a good procedure to add one half milligram of adrenalin to the solution of peptone in pronounced cases of low pressure.

By taking these precautions one may employ the agent in the case of patients seriously ill.

Having described the effects of the treatment and its technique, the author remarks that it remains for him to say a few words about its rationale, so far as the immediate reaction is concerned.

He has not been situated so he could carry out extensive experimental work with animals, but he points out that there is a striking analogy between the immediate reaction of the patient to the peptone and the reaction that one observes after therapeutic intraventions, notably after intravenous administration of the preparations of the colloidal metals, such as gold and silver.

At first judging from the action, in vitro, it was supposed that the colloidal metals, introduced into the blood streams, would act, if not as germicides, at least in a way to inhibit germ activity.

As a matter of fact, good results have followed the intravenenous use of thel coloidal metals, but the author is of the opinion that their efficacity has not been due to the metals but to materials added by the manufacturers of pharmaceutical products in order to make the emulsions (suspensions) of the colloids more stable,—such as gelatin, serum, peptones, etc, for it is well known that the suspension of these metals in distilled water is very unstable. He refers to the experiment of A. G. Auld, an English physician, who administered to his patients these agents which were destined by the manufacturer to stabilize the suspension, without a trace of metal, the results being exactly the same, viz; chill and fever, followed by sweating, lowering of temperature and a more or less favorable condition of the patient.

The author endeavors to prove that even if the colloidal substances are completly exempt of the materials usually used to make them stable, still they produce the same kind of reaction, and he refers to the experiments of Contejean, Gley, Hedon and Delezenne, pointing out that the latter insisted that great numbers of substances, such as bacterial toxins and organic extracts, would produce the same kind of reaction observed after the intravenous use of peptone—a condition which the author aptly calls "shock peptonique". In reality, all substances having the qualities of an antigen produce like results (so far as the symptoms of reaction are concerned.)

Gley demonstrated that the fresh serum of the dog injected into the veins of the same dog produced the symptoms noted above, and Widal has demonstrated the same thing in the case of the human being, he and his pupils drawing blood from a patient, defibrinating it, and injected the serum into the same patient. In such a case it would be exact to say "shock produced by antigen", but since the effect of the intravenous use of peptone was first and more carefully studied, it would appear convenient to take it as a type.

The conclusion is reached that every substance, whatever its nature, will be able to produce the reaction effects of peptone, *provided it is introduced into the blood stream in such a way as to interfere with the protein composition or the colloidal equilibrium.* In fact even distilled water introduced rapidly may produce the effects.

It is necessary to make a clear distinction between the legitimate effect of peptone when properly administered and the condition of shock above described, which follows its rapid administration, or its administration in too large a dose.

The proper therapeutic dose properly given is followed in about an hour by a short chill which is succeeded by defervescence and abundant sweating.

It may be useful to recall that such a dose in a normal man in health does not produce any visible effect.

It remains to point out the cause of the efficacity and to determine the mechanism. Up to this time sufficient animal experimentation has not been done, but it is useful to recall that in the defense of the organism against microbes two elements are essential—the white blood cells and the antibodies in the blood. The introduction of peptone exercises a striking action upon the white blood cells, and upon the protein equilibrium of the plasma, and upon "certains appareils producteurs des albumines du plasma".

At present it is not possible to point out an exact infection in which peptone can be regarded as a specific, but, nevertheless, it presents certain practical advantages when a good preparation is employed.

It can be used in cases in which the causative germ is unknown.

It sensitizes the organism but feebly, there being but little danger of violent anaphylactic manifestations in cases of prolonged treatment, or the resumption of treatment after interruptions.

PERSONAL AND GENERAL NEWS

Dr. J. S. Rollins, Paden, has moved to Guthrie.

Dr. J. W. Craig, Vinita, visited Chicago in April.

Dr. D. Long, Duncan, is attending the Chicago clinics.

Dr. J. C. Dunn, Bartlesville, has been appointed county physician.

Dr. W. H. Powell, Sulphur, attended the New Orleans clinics in April.

Dr. J. F. Messenbaugh, Oklahoma City, visited the Chicago clinics in April.

Dr. R. M. Anderson, Shawnee, visited the Chicago clinics in March and April.

Dr. M. D. Faust, Ada, returned from the New Orleans clinics the last of March.

Dr. L. C. White, Alva, was reported in a very serious condition in April from pneumonia.

Dr. and Mrs. J. M. Workman, Woodward, are taking a two months vacation in California.

Dr. W. B. Newell, Hunter, announces his return from army service and relocation at his old home.

Drs. W. C. and Roy Pendergraft and W. G. Husband, Hollis, are establishing a hospital at Hollis.

Dr. T. L. Jeffress, Roff, has returned from New Orleans where he has been doing special work for a month.

Dr. W. B. Catto, El Reno, has returned from overseas service, received his discharge and will reopen offices in El Reno.

Bartlesville municipal authorities are planning the establishment of a bacteriological laboratory with a full time bacteriologist in charge.

Dr. M. C. Comer, Clinton, has completed a course of special work in Chicago eye, ear, nose and throat work and returned to his home.

Doctors S. H. Williamson and J. O. Wharton, Duncan; E. B. Thomasson, Velma, and J. A. Ivey, Marlow, are attending the New Orleans clinics.

Dr. W. B. Newlon, Tulsa, has been discharged from the army and has returned to his work. He will be associated with Drs. McCarty and Allison.

Nowata physicians have already begun action to establish a county hospital in conformity with an act of the last legislature permitting the voting of bonds for such purposes.

Dr. Jas. G. Harris, Muskogee, has been discharged from the army and has opened offices in the Flynn-Ames Building. He will devote himself to genito-urinary work exclusively.

Dr. C. C. Shaw, McAlester and Mill Creek, who prior to the war was physician to the State Penitentiary at McAlester, on being discharged from the army, decided to locate in Poteau.

Dr. Benton Lovelady, Guthrie, after trying to better himself in the way of a location, investigating Missouri points, decided that there was no place like home and Guthrie was good enough for him.

Dr. A. E. Davenport, Major, M. C., U. S. A., Oklahoma City, after a prolonged absence in army cantonments in the United States and Foreign service in France, has been discharged from the army and is at home.

County Hospitals may be established according to a law passed by the last legislature which provided that any county might vote a bond issue for that purpose. The exact text of the law is not obtainable as we go to press.

Drs. J. A. Hatchett and T. M. Aderhold, El Reno, announce that hereafter management of the El Reno Sanitarium will pass into the charge of Dr. Aderhold and that Dr. Hatchett will continue his association with the institution.

Hospital Management, an extensive publication of Chicago devoted to technical and special consideration of hospital problems, contains a most commendatory article on Dr. Fred S. Clinton, Tulsa, Chairman of the State Committee on Hospitals. The article concludes that Dr. Clinton is a "Southwestern Live Wire".

Dr. J. Hutchings White, Muskogee, Captain, M. C., who is oscillating over France and Germany, writes the *Journal* an interesting letter, accompanied by one of the very original French papers circulated among our soldiers overseas. He assures us that he will soon return and never again leave his native heath and Muskogee.

The Physicians' and Surgeons' Adjusting Association, of Kansas City, wishes to call the attention of physicians in this field to the fact that they do collect old accounts. This Journal has accepted their advertisement, which will be found on another page of this issue, and any business transacted with this company will no doubt be entirely satisfactory to those who have dealings with them.

Mr. C. C. Childers, Enid, has been appointed Superintendent of the School for Feeble Minded Children, vice Dr. W. L. Kendall, who resigned some time ago. Mr. Childers was formerly connected with the institution and rendered efficient services. His appointment is a radical departure from rule and custom. Heretofore a physician has always been appointed to be superintendent of that and similar instutitions of the State. The *Journal* is inclined to the opinion that the onerous duties of management may well be placed in lay hands. While the administration of Dr. Kendall is above reproach and very likely cannot be equalled by any successor, it is generally agreed that the multifarious duties of management of such institutions and the treatment of the sick should not be placed in one person.

DISCHARGES FROM THE ARMY.

W. B. Catto, El Reno.
A. E. Davenport, Oklahoma City.
C. H. McBurney, Clinton.
W. M. Stout, Oklahoma City.
W. H. Kingman, Bartlesville.
J. T. Lowe, Blair.
W. P. Rudell, Altus.
L. S. Willour, McAlester,

M. E. Stout, Oklahoma City.
E. T. Robinson, Cleveland.
W. T. Rowley, Miami.
F. R. Sutton, Bartlesville.
Benj. H. Brown, Muskogee.
L. E. Pearson, Reed.
W. Albert Cook, Tulsa.

MISCELLANEOUS

PROPAGANDA FOR REFORM.

Misbranded Nostrums. The following nostrums were declared misbranded under the Federal Food and Drugs Act because of the false, fraudulent or misleading claims made for them: Alkavis; Sulferro-Sol; Gonorrhea and Gleet 3 Day Cure; Old Indian Fever Tonic; Pain-I-Cure; Walker's Dead Shot Colic Cure (*Jour. A. M. A.*, March 1, 1919, p. 670).

Saccharin—After the War. Having satisfied a need during the sugar shortage, the manufacturers of saccharin appear not to be content to turn their talents and plants to better uses, but suggest that the great commercial sacrifices made in setting their works into operation to produce saccharin should be rewarded by premission to continue the traffic under post-war conditions. The referee board to which the saccharin question was referred in this country has by no means given a clean bill of health to the chemical, and the people need to be protected from the danger, or at least the deception, of a substitute for sugar which is in no sense a true food. (*Jour. A. M. A.*, March 8, 1919, p. 729).

Organo Tablets and Orchis Extract. The Organo Product Co,. Chicago, sells Organo Tablets as a cure for "lost vitality." The Packers Product Co. sold Orchis Extract until it was put out of business by the government in 1918 by the issuance of a fraud order. Even a superficial comparison of the circular letters and booklets used in exploiting Organo Tablets shows a close connection between this humbug and the government declared fraud—Orchis Extract. Has Orchis Extract of the Packers Product Co. become Organo Tablets of the Organo Product Co? (*Jour. A. M. A.*, March 8, 1919, p. 746).

Depilagiene. The A. M. A. Chemical Laboratory reports that "Franco–American Hygienic Depilagiene", a hair remover, essentially is a mixture of barium sulphate, barium sulphid, sulphur and starch. The amount of barium sulphid was found to be 22.6 per cent.: this is equivalent to about 45 per cent. of commercial barium sulphid. Depilagiene has no claim to originality, as practically all chemical hair removers are composed of some form of sulphid. Naturally, the preparation is likely to cause more or less irritation of the skin. (*Jour. A. M. A.*, March 8, p. 746).

Validity of Provisions Concerning "Patent" Medicines. In the proceedings instituted by E. Fougera and Co., Inc., against the City of New York et al, the Court of Appeals of New York holds that the provision of the sanitary code is not unconstitutional in that it prescribed the formula disclosure of medicines. The purposes and effects of the code were well within the police power and had the object of protecting the public. "No man has a constitutional right to keep secret the composition of substances which he sells to the public as articles of food" (*State v. Aslesen*, 50 Minn. 5, 52 N. W. 220). If that is true of food, it is even more plainly true of drugs. But there was one objection to the ordinance, though one that amendment might correct: that the ordinance did not except existing stores of merchandise in the hands of dealers, in that the board of health exceeded the powers delegated to it. (*Jour. A. M. A.*, March 8, p. 753).

The Victory Over Rabies. Amid the victories on the European battlefield, we may pause to contemplate man's conquest of rabies. During the year 1916, 1,008 persons in the district of Lyons received the antirabic treatment. A single death in this list places the mortality at 0.099 per cent. Since 1900, more than 9,000 persons have received antirabic inoculations, with a total of nine deaths, or 0.09 per cent. (*Jour. A. M. A.*, March 15, 1919, p. 800).

Nature's Remedy Tablets. A. H. Clark, of the A. M. A. Chemical Laboratory, reports that "Nature's Remedy" is claimed to contain ten ingredients; that the manufacturers declare seven of these—burdock, juniper, sarsaparilla, mandrake, rhubarb, dandelion and prickly ash; and that the manufacturers state they are "more proud" of the other three, but refrain from naming them for fear of imitators. Clark's analysis, supplemented by a microscopic examination by E. N. Gathercoal at the University of Illinois School of Pharmacy, indicated that the unnamed drugs are aloes (or a preparation of aloes), cascara bark and belladonna root. The microscopist stated that rhubarb, as well as all the other named drugs, if present at all are there in such small quantities that no evidence of their presence was seen.   As a result of the examination and a consideration of their powerful cathartic action, it is believed that Nature's Remedy is, essentially, aloes or aloin, cascara, and belladonna with, probably, resin of podophyllin (instead of mandrake)—a common cathartic mixture. (*Journal A. M. A.*, March 15, 1919, p. 815).

Misbranded Nostrums: A "Notice of Judgment" has been issued declaring the following nostrums misbranded: Chase's "Blood and Nerve Tablets," "Liver Tablets," and "Kidney Tablets," XXX Tonic Pills; Egiuterro; Uicure; Sweet Rest for Children; Beaver Drops Comp.; Blood Kleen; Heart and Nerve Regulator; Kidneyleine; Eye Powder; Tanrue Herbs and Pills, and 5 Herbs. (*Jour. A. M. A.*, March 22. 1919, p. 883).

Havens' Wonderful Discovery. The Council on Pharmacy and Chemistry reports that E. C. Havens, Sioux Falls, S. D., requested consideration of a remedy which he claims to have discovered for the cure of influenza. According to the label on a specimen, "This remedy is good for Coughs, Colds, Lung Diseases, LaGrippe, Influenza, Rheumatism; good for Pains, Cramps, Backache, Lumbago, Neuralgia; for severe pains soak your feet in hot water for 3 nights, add 3 tablespoons of baking soda in water and apply Anti-Flue Medicine to the affected parts." The "discovery" was stated to contain oil of wintergreen, oil of sassafras. oil of black pepper, spirit of camphor, spirit of turpentine, spirit of chloroform, tincture of arnica and alcohol, and was called Havens' Rheumatic Remedy before its supposed effect on "flue" was "discovered". The Council finds that Havens' Wonderful Discovery is an unscientific, irrational mixture, marketed under therapeutic claims which are unwarranted and without foundation. (*Jour. A. M. A.*, March 22, 1919, p. 883).

NEW BOOKS

Under this heading books received by the Journal will be acknowledged.   Publishers are advised that this shall constitute
return for such publications as they may submit.   Obviously all publications sent us cannot be given space for review,
but from time to time books received, of possible interest to Oklahoma physicians, will be reviewed.

GYNECOLOGY. By William P. Graves, M. D., Professor of Gynecology at Harvard Medical School. Second Edition, Thoroughly Revised. Octavo volume of 883 pages with 490 original illustrations, 100 of them in colors. Philadelphia and London: W. B. Saunders Company. 1918. Cloth, $7.75 net.

A TEXT BOOK OF PHYSIOLOGY: FOR MEDICAL STUDENTS AND PHYSICIANS. By William H. Howell, Ph. D., M. D., Professor of Physiology, Johns Hopkins University, Baltimore. Seventh Edition Thoroughly Revised. Octavo of 1059 pages, 307 illustrations. Philadelphia and London: W. B. Saunders Company, 1918. Cloth, $5.00 net.

CLINICAL MICROSCOPY AND CHEMISTRY. By F. A. McJunkin, M. D., Professor of Pathology in the Marquette University School of Medicine; formerly an Assistant in the Pathological Laboratory of the Boston City Hospital. Octavo volume of 470 pages with 131 illustrations. Philadelphia and London: W. B. Saunders Company, 1919. Cloth $3.50.

SURGICAL TREATMENT. A Practical Treatise on the Therapy of Surgical Diseases for the Use of Practitioners and Students of Surgery. By James Peter Warbasse, M. D., Formerly Attending Surgeon to the Methodist Episcopal Hospital, Brooklyn, New York. In three large octavo volumes, and separate Desk Index Volume. Volume III contains 861 pages with 864 illustrations. Philadelphia and London: W. B. Saunders Company. 1919. Per set (Three Volumes and the Index Volume): Cloth $30.00 per set.

NEOPLASTIC DISEASES. A text-book on Tumors. By James Ewing, M. D., Sc. D., Professor of Pathology at Cornell University Medical College, New York City. Octavo of 1027 pages with 479 illustrations. Philadelphia and London: W. B. Saunders Company, 1919. Cloth $10.00 net.

PATHOLOGICAL TECHNIQUE. A practical Manual for workers in Pathologic Histology and Bacteriology. Including Directions for Clinical Diagnosis by Laboratory Methods. By F. B. Mallory, M. D., Associate Professor of Pathology, Harvard Medical School; and J. B. Wright, M. D., Pathologist to the Massachusetts General Hospital. Seventh edition, revised and enlarged. Octavo of 555 pages with 181 illustrations. Philadelphia and London: W. B. Saunders Company, 1918. Cloth $3.75.

PRINCIPLES AND PRACTICE OF OBSTETRICS. By Joseph B. DeLee, A. M., M. D., Professor of Obstetrics at the Northwestern University Medical School. Third edition, thoroughly revised. Large octavo of 1089 pages, with 949 illustrations, 187 of them in colors. Philadelphia and London: W. B. Saunders Company, 1918. Cloth, $8.50 net.

THE ORTHOPEDIC TREATMENT OF GUNSHOT INJURIES. By Leo Mayer, M. D., Instructor in Orthopedic Surgery, New York Post Graduate Medical School and Hospital, with an introduction by Col. E. G. Brackett, M. C., N. A. Director of Military Orthopedic Surgery. 12mo of 250 pages, with 184 illustrations. Philadelphia and London: W. B. Saunders Company, 1918. Cloth $2.50 net.

SURGICAL TREATMENT.
Volume II.

Surgical Treatment. A Practical Treatise on the Therapy of Surgical Diseases for the use of Practitioners and Students of Surgery. By James Peter Warbasse, M. D., Formrely Attending Surgeon to the Methodist Episcopal Hospital, Brooklyn, New York. In three large octavo volumes, and separate Desk Index Volume. Volume II contains 829 pages with 761 illustrations. Philadelphia and London: W. B. Saunders Company. 1918. Per set (Three Volumes and the Index Volume): Cloth $30.00 per set.

This second volume of Surgical Treatment follows the high and correct ideals set by its predecessor. The reader is struck with admiration at the great care shown in handling the remoter and often slighted surgical subjects, those not often coming to the surgeons' notice, but when they do come resolve themselves into measures of prime importance. This issue contains treatments of injuries and diseases of the scalp, skull, eye, nose, nasopharynx and fauces, larynx and trachea, mouth, ear, spine, neck, salivary glands, thyroid; the throat, breast, abdomen, intestines, stomach and spleen.

PROGRAMME

TWENTY-SEVENTH ANNUAL MEETING, OKLAHOMA STATE MEDICAL ASSOCIATION,
MUSKOGEE, MAY 20-21-22, 1919.

(Subject to additions and modification.)

GENERAL INFORMATION.

MEETING PLACE: All meetings, unless otherwise announced, will be held in the Old Court House Building, Second and Court.

REGISTRATION: Every person attending any meeting or section, except those announced to be open to the public, is expected to register name, home and local address and telephone number, in order that they may be reached in emergency.

A roster of 1919 members made up from membership stubs will be found at the registration desk. Registrants on the list will be registered and provided badges and programs. Guests from other states will be provided registration and badges on application to the Secretary. Oklahoma physicians not members who wish to attend the meetings will apply to the Secretary who will arrange for their attendance and the courtesies of the meeting.

DELEGATES: Should leave their credentials with a member of the Credentials Committee who will be at the registration desk, after they have registered. Confusion and unnecessary duplication will be avoided by **not leaving credentials** with the Secretary.

YOUR PAPER: Papers on the program of this meeting **are the property** of this Association. No person should carry them home for any purpose. They should be carefully prepared in duplicate in the exact form the author wishes them to appear in the Journal. We suggest the following general arrangement of papers which, if followed, will save every one concerned much trouble.

First. Subject of paper.

Second. Name and address of author.

Third. The paper should be **double spaced, typewritten,** carefully punctuated. Authors are advised that proof will be sent them before the paper is published; with the proof quotations of prices of reprints will be furnished. If the article is to be illustrated, clear photographs or drawings must be furnished or suitable plates. It is requested that cuts, pictures or drawings be originals and strictly applicable to text of article unless it is obviously necessary to use others in order to properly illustrate the article.

Fourth. Papers should **postively** be left with either the reporter or Chairman of the Section when read or with the Secretary. If you carry them home you will cause unnecessary inconvenience and useless correspondence. Often such papers are not available for publication in the issue of the Journal to which they are best adapted, and discussion of them is lost.

HAND PROGRAMS: Will be furnished attendants at the meeting only. They will not be mailed to the membership as the following pages give a sufficient idea of the program.

SECTIONS: Will convene promptly at the time designated and will be continued until program is completed. Authors not present when their number is called, unless exceptional circumstances prevail, will have their papers placed at the bottom of the list to take their turn in rotation.

TUESDAY, MAY 20, 1919.

11:00 A. M. **Meeting of the Council.**

Matters pertaining to business of any character should be prepared in advance and submitted to this body. The House of Delegates should not have its time unnecessarily encroached upon by presentation of trivial matters. The Council is the business agent of the Association and first passes on matters of business. Appeals from constitutent societies or greviences of individual members should be presented to the Council.

2:00 P. M. **Meeting of the House of Delegates.**

4:00 P. M. **Meeting of Oklahoma Military Medical Men.**

8:00 P. M. **General meeting:**

Call to order by the President, Dr. L. S. Willour, McAlester.

Address of Welcome, Honorable N. A. Gibson, Muskogee.

Response on behalf of the Association, Major Hugh L. Scott, Holdenville.

President's Address, Dr. L. S. Willour, McAlester.

SECTION ON SURGERY AND GYNECOLOGY.

Dr. A. A. Will, Oklahoma City, Chairman.

WEDNESDAY, MAY 21, 9:00 A. M.

Chairman's Address.

1. Symposium on Pneumonia.
    (a) "Complications"—Dr. W. W. Rucks, Oklahoma City.
        Discussion opened by Dr. A. W. White, Oklahoma City.
    (b) "Surgical Complications With Special Reference to Empyema"—Dr. A. L. Blesh, Oklahoma City.
        Discussion—Captain F. M. Sanger, Oklahoma City.
    (c) "Etiology and Pathology"—Dr. L. A. Turley, Norman.
2. "Malignant Diseases of the Large Intestine"—Dr. LeRoy Long, Oklahoma City.
    Discussion opened by Dr. John Riley, Oklahoma City.
3. "The Use of Dakin Solution in Surgery"—Dr. M. Smith, Oklahoma City.
4. "Ovarian Function"—Dr. J. S. Hartford, Oklahoma City.
5. "Congenital Hypertrophic Stenosis of the Pylorus—Differential Diagnosis and Treatment"—Dr. G. A. Wall, Tulsa.
    Discussion—Dr. O. A. Flanagan, Tulsa.
6. "Gall-Bladder Infection"—Dr. McLain Rogers, Clinton.
7. "Exophthalmic Goitre"—Dr. W. H. Livermore, Chickasha.
8. "Treatment of Open Wounds in the War Zone"—Dr. W. M. Stout, Oklahoma City.
9. "Infection of Gall-Bladder—Etiology—Treatment"—Captain F. M. Sanger, Oklahoma City.
    Discussion—Dr. M. E. Stout, Oklahoma City.
10. "Blood Transfusion—Selection of Donors—Description of Technique"—Drs. F. L. Carson and R. M. Anderson, Shawnee.
11. "Important Procedure in Abdominal Surgery"—Dr. J. Clay Williams, Miami.

SECTION ON EYE, EAR, NOSE AND THROAT

Dr. R. O. Early, Ardmore, Chairman.

WEDNESDAY, MAY 21, 2:00 P. M.

Chairman's Address.

1. "Surgery of the Tonsil"—Dr. H. Coulter Todd, Oklahoma City.
2. "The Ear in the Recent Epidemic of Influenza"—Dr. L. C. Kuyrkendall, McAlester.
3. "Enucleation of the Eye Versus Mule's Operation"—Dr. J. D. Kiser, Bartlesville.
    Discussion opened by Dr. C. M. Fullenwider, Muskogee.
4. "Focal Infection from the Teeth"—Dr. J. H. Barnes, Enid.
5. "Causative Factors in Eye Conditions"—Dr. S. C. Davis, Oklahoma City.
6. "The Acute Infections of the Upper Respiratory Tract"—Dr. A. L. Guthrie, Oklahoma City.,
7. A Paper, Subject not announced—Dr. M. K. Thompson, Muskogee.
8. "Acute Glaucoma, Report of Case—Recovery Without Operation"—Dr. J. R. Phelan, Oklahoma City.
    Discussion opened by Dr. J. H. Barnes, Enid.

SECTION ON PEDIATRICS AND OBSTETRICS.

Dr. O. A. Flanagan, Vice-Chairman, Tulsa.

WEDNESDAY, MAY 21, 2:00 P. M.

Chairman's Address.

1. "Internal Gland Diseases of Children"—Dr. Winnie M. Sanger, Oklahoma City.
    Discussion opened by Dr. A. C. Hirschfield. Oklahoma City.
2. "Presentation of Case Histories in Children's Diseases"—Dr. J. Raymond Burdick, Tulsa.
3. "Mentality Measurements"—Dr. Bertha Margolin, Tulsa.
4. "Acute Miliary Tuberculosis Following Puerperal Infection"—Dr. M. H. Newman, Oklahoma City.
    Discussion opened by Dr. A. J. Sands, Oklahoma City.
5. "Pituitary Extract in Obstetrics"—Dr. C. Doler, Bokoshe.
    Discussion—Dr. W. W. Beesley, Tulsa.

SECTION ON GENITO-URINARY DISEASES, RADIOLOGY AND DERMATOLOGY.

Dr. J. H. Hays, Enid, Chairman.

WEDNESDAY, MAY, 21, 9:00 A. M.

Chairman's Address—"Some Studies in Pyelography".
1. "Venereal Control and Treatment in the U. S. Army"—Lieut-Col. Hugh Scott, Holdenville.
2. "Anent the Anti-Vice Crusade"—Dr. W. B. Pigg, Okmulgee.
   Discussion opened by Dr. F. K. Camp, Oklahoma City.
3. "A Paper"—Lieut. M. H. Foster, Alderson.
4. "Sporotrichosis"—Dr. E. S. Lain, Oklahoma City.
5. "Importance of a Thorough Urological Examination in All Cases of Obscure Abdominal Pain and in All Bladder and Kidney Infection"—Capt. J. H. Sanford, Muskogee.
6. "Operative and Diagnostic Cystoscopy" (Illustrated with lantern slides) —Dr. Bransford Lewis, St. Louis, Mo.
   Discussion opened by Dr. Jos. T. Martin, Oklahoma City.
7. "Gonorrhoea in the Female"—Dr. C. P. Linn, Tulsa.
8. "A Paper"—Dr. Rex Bolend, Oklahoma City.
9. "Some Obstructions at the Outlet of the Stomach" (Demonstrated Radiographically)—Dr. E. N. McKee, Enid.
10. "A Paper"—Dr. J. C. Mahr, State Health Department, Oklahoma City.
11. "The Relation of Focal Infections to Skin Diseases"—Dr. Chas. H. Ball, Tulsa.
12. "Chronic Urethritis"—Dr. T. B. Coulter, Tulsa.
    Election of officers for the Section

SYMPOSIUM ON SYPHILIS.

13. "Initial Lesion of Syphilis"—Dr. J. F. Gorrell, Tulsa.
14. "Skin Manifestations of Syphilis"—Dr. Curtis R. Day, Oklahoma City.
15. "Syphilis as We Find It, With Report of Fifty Cases"—Dr. R. A. Douglas, Tulsa.
16. "Syphilis and Mental Psychosis"—Dr. D. W. Griffin, Norman.
    Discussion—Dr. A. D. Young, Oklahoma City.
17. "Syphilis of the Gastro-Intestinal Tract"—Dr. Jos. T. Martin, Oklahoma City.
18. "Syphilis of the Eye"—Dr. A. S. Piper, Enid.
19. "The Fundamental Principles of the Wassermann Test"—Dr. A. J. Hinkleman, Oklahoma City.
20. "The Curability of Syphilis"—Drs. E. H. Martin and E. A. Purdum, Hot Springs, Ark.
    Discussion opened by Dr. Bransford Lewis, St. Louis, Mo., and Dr. L. S. Willour, McAlester.
21. "The Treatment of Syphilis"—Dr. J. W. Rogers, Tulsa.
    Discussion opened by Dr. W. J. Wallace, Oklahoma City.
22. "The New Treatment of Syphilis in the Various Stages"—Dr. W. J. Wallace, Oklahoma City

SECTION ON GENERAL MEDICINE, NERVOUS AND MENTAL DISEASES.

F. W. Ewing, M. D., Chairman, Muskogee.

WEDNESAY, MAY 21, 9:00 A. M.

Chairman's Address.
1. "Diagnosis of Pyelitis"—Dr. J. A. Hatchett, El Reno.
   Discussion opened by Dr. W. J. Wallace, Oklahoma City.
2. "Prevention of Influenza and Allied Diseases" —Dr. W. F. Dutton, Tulsa.
3. "Some of the Sequellae of Epidemic Influenza"—Dr. A. B. Leeds, Chickasha.
4. "Applications of Practical Methods in Health Conservation"—Dr. J. T. Nichols, Muskogee.
   Discussion—Dr. F. E. Warterfield, Muskogee.
5. "Insanity by Contagion"—Dr. John W. Duke, Guthrie.
6. "Nocturnal Enuresis"—Dr. W. A. Tolleson, Eufaula.
7. "Cardiac Arrhythmia"—Dr. Lea A. Riely, Oklahoma City.

8. "The Value of the Consultant in Medicine to the General Practitioner"—Dr. C. J. Fishman, Oklahoma City
   Discussion opened by Dr. J. A. Hatchett, El Reno.
9. "The Tuberculosis Dispensary"—Dr. H. T. Price, Tulsa.
10. "Diagnosis of the Pathological Heart"—Dr. Benj. H. Brown, Muskogee.
11. "Remittent Malarial Fever"—Dr. J. A. Haynie, Durant.
    Discussion opened by Dr. J. S. Fulton, Atoka.
12. "Concurrent Typhoid and Malarial Infection"—Dr. Sessler Hoss, Muskogee.
13. "Demonstration of the Value of Moving Pictures and Animated Diagrams in the Study of Percussion and Auscultation as Applied to the Diagnosis of Pulmonary Tuberculosis"—Colonel Wm. O. Owen, M. C., U. S. A., Washington, D. C., and Dr. John C. Breedlove, Muldrow, Oklahoma.
14. "The Prevention of Eclampsia"—Dr. David Armstrong, Durant.
15. Paper,   —Dr. F. K. Camp, Oklahoma City.
16. "Anthrax", with Report of a Case—Dr. W. R. Joblin, Porter.

COUNCILOR DISTRICTS.

District No. 1. Texas, Beaver, Cimarron, Harper, Ellis, Woods, Woodward, Alfalfa, Major, Grant, Garfield, Noble and Kay. G. A. Boyle, Enid.

District No. 2. Dewey, Roger Mills, Custer, Beckham, Washita, Greer, Kiowa, Harmon, Jackson and Tillman. Ellis Lamb, Clinton.

District No. 3. Blaine, Kingfisher, Canadian, Logan, Payne, Lincoln, Oklahoma, Cleveland, Pottawatomie, Seminole and McClain. G. M. Maupin, Waurika.

District No. 4. Caddo, Grady, Comanche, Cotton, Stephens, Jefferson, Garvin, Murray, Carter, and Love. J. T. Slover, Sulphur.

District No. 5. Pontotoc, Coal, Johnston, Atoka, Marshall, Bryan, Choctaw, Pushmataha and McCurtain. J. L. Austin, Durant.

District No. 6. Okfuskee, Hughes, Pittsburg, Latimer, LeFlore, Haskell and Sequoyah. Vacant.

District No. 7. Pawnee, Osage, Washington, Tulsa, Creek, Nowata and Rogers. N. W. Mayginnis, Tulsa.

District No. 8. Craig, Ottawa, Delaware, Mayes, Wagoner, Cherokee, Adair, Okmulgee, Muskogee and McIntosh. J. H. White, Muskogee.

STATE BOARD OF MEDICAL EXAMINERS.

Melvin Gray, M. D., Durant, President; B. L. Denison, M. D., Garvin, Vice-President; J. J. Williams, M. D., Weatherford, Secretary; O. R. Gregg, M. D., Waynoka, Treasurer; E. B. Dunlap, M. D., Lawton; Ralph V. Smith, M. D., Tulsa; W. LeRoy Bonnell, M. D., Chickasha; Wm. T. Ray, M. D., Gould; W. E. Sanderson, M. D., Altus; H. C. Montague, D. O., Muskogee.

Reciprocity with Georgia, Kentucky, Mississippi, Nevada, North Carolina, Wisconsin, Kansas, Arkansas, Virginia, West Virginia, Nebraska, New Mexico, Tennessee, Iowa, Ohio, California, Colorado, Indiana, Missouri, New Jersey, Vermont, Texas, Michigan.

Meetings held second Tuesday of January, April, July and October, Oklahoma City.

Address all communications to the Secretary, Dr. J. J. Williams, Weatherford.

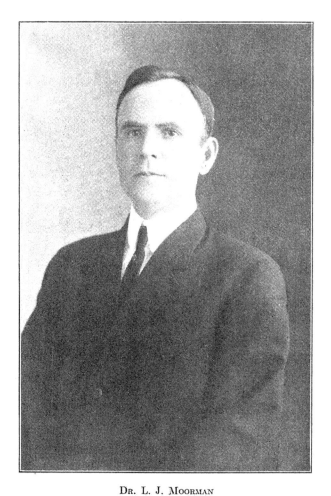

Dr. L. J. Moorman

OKLAHOMA CITY, OKLAHOMA

President Oklahoma State Medical Association, 1919-1920.

Dr. Moorman is a native of Leitchfield, Kentucky. He took his B. S. degree at Georgetown College in 1898, and M. D. at University of Louisville in 1901. He practiced medicine at Jet, Oklahoma, from 1901 to 1905, and at Nashville, Oklahoma, from 1905 to 1906, locating in Oklahoma City in in 1907.

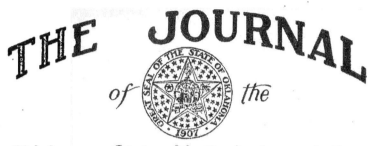

THE JOURNAL

of the

Oklahoma State Medical Association

| VOLUME XII | MUSKOGEE, OKLA., JUNE, 1919 | NUMBER 6 |

PRESIDENT'S ADDRESS.*

27TH ANNUAL MEETING, OKLAHOMA STATE MEDICAL ASSOCIATION.

L. S. WILLOUR, M. D.

MC ALESTER, OKLAHOMA

Members of the Oklahoma State Medical Association, and Guests:

It is indeed a very happy surprise to be with you at this Twenty-seventh Annual Meeting of the Association.

April 19th, I was still in France, and knowing so well the many delays in embarkation and demobilization, it seemed impossible for me to reach Muskogee by this date. However, I have been fortunate, and can be here with my friends who have honored me with the Presidency of this organization.

During the past two years I have met many of you, some here at home, and others in France, and I have always been proud to recall the fact that I am President of an organization which has given such undivided support to our Government during the Great War in which the country has put forth every effort to bring a successful culmination.

It is almost impossible for me to address you on any subject other than one pertaining to the War. I will not, however, discuss any scientific question, but rather try in a brief way to tell some of the experiences our Oklahoma Doctors have had in doing the tasks they have been called upon to perform.

First, I wish to mention the men who were refused commissions, and worked on the various boards here in the States. These men were true American citizens, and when Uniformed Military Service was denied them, they gave the only service for which they seemed to be fitted; their work was of a most important nature and was almost universally faithfully done.

Many of our men, some of whom were early in the service, never went overseas, but were assigned to various positions here at home. Their work was the making of our Great Army—work of a constructive nature—and in many instances not at all pleasant, but never-the-less most important. In some cases, the physical condition of the officer was such that he could not stand the strain of hard campaign and long hours on duty; in other instances, he seemed so perfectly fitted for his position as advisor, examiner, or at a training camp, that his services seemed of greatest value in such capacity.

Some of our best men have given their lives while serving here at home, and are due the same tribute as the men who fell on "The Field of Honor". Let us

---

*Read before the 27th Annual Meeting, Muskogee, May, 1919.

not forget them and their families, and the supreme sacrifice they made during the dark hours of the great War.

The men who went over-seas have had a great experience, in many cases not of a professional nature, but those who went to the Front saw our men in action, while those at the Base Hospitals or attached to the various organizations in the Service of Supplies, saw the vast work of supplying an army, and the immediate results of modern warfare.

The ones in the back areas had to work hard and endure much, at times their bed was one of mud and three or four blankets. The so-called rest camps which all officers so well remember, were very poorly equipped, and men not accustomed to hard living found these places very trying. The marches to these camps were long and usually wet, the ever-present mud of France was there, and the food and sleeping accommodations left much to be hoped for, but it was a part of practically every doctor's trip to his station in France, and accepted by him as a part of his duty to our country.

Later, many of these camps were very much improved, and on my return I visited both Pontenazen and Kerhuon camps at Brest, and found them with very good accommodations for both officers and men.

The work with organizations in the Service of Supplies and in the Base Hospitals, while not accompanied with danger, was at times very hard, twenty hours overseeing operating teams without rest was not unusual, and in the advanced section where our Evacuation Hospitals were stationed, the operative and dressing work, during a push was enormous. This work was done in both Evacuation and Base Hospitals by many of our own members, and to their skill and untiring efforts, many a noble American soldier owes his life.

These men worked without rest for long hours, and in most instances the wounded received not only the professional care his individual case demanded, but a silent prayer was breathed by the operator and entire staff that they might be able to save a life or limb, and return the wounded man to his friends at home, for a life of usefulness.

Some two thousand American Medical Officers served with the British, both with troops and in hospitals. I am informed (not authentically, however) that the casualty rate among these officers was 12 1-2 per cent. These men had no service with our own army, but rendered valiant service to our noble allies.

Convoy surgeons on troop ships and hospital trains have all had their part to play, and have done well the work assigned them.

The Boche put forth a constant effort to destroy our lines of communication, both on land and sea, they made as dangerous as possible the transportation of both our combat troops and sick and wounded, and it was under such circumstances that these Medical Officers carried on their work.

Now we come to our brave members who served with troops at the Front in Field Hospitals and Ambulance Companies. It was theirs to face the real dangers of War, and some of our members now lie beneath the "Poppies of Flander's Fields". These men often suffered from exposure to the elements, long marches, and hard campaigning. It took young men with physical training to stand these hardships. They were obliged to work rapidly, and under the most adverse circumstances. When the troops to which they were attached were in action, it meant not only hard work of a professional nature, but they were constantly under fire, and their lives in imminent danger. A temporary dressing or immobilization splint was quickly applied at the First Aid Station, and the wounded man rushed to a place of comparative safety, where a more thorough exploration and dressing of his wounds could be accomplished.

These men were called upon not only to witness the suffering of our boys immediately after injury, but to watch many pass to the Great Beyond, there to join others of our Great American Army.

My return from Europe was made on the Leviathan, with Headquarters of the 42nd Division, and much praise was given the Oklahoma Ambulance Company that formed a part of this Unit. It was theirs to witness the very hardest campaigning, and they participated in most of the hard fighting of the American Army. We may well be proud of Ambulance Company Number 167, which is distinctly an Oklahoma Unit.

The Medical personnel of the 36th Division was made up largely of Oklahoma and Texas Doctors. This Division never fought with the American Army, but was attached to the 4th French Army. These men saw some activity, and in a personal interview with a French officer, I was informed that their service was of a high order and merited the praise they received from their French associates.

Let us know that our Medical Officers at the Front were brave and true, it was their lot to face shot and shell, but unwavering they stood at their post of duty, and gave relief to our wounded men. Not all of these Medical Officers can return to us, the shell of the Boche has forever closed their eyes in the sleep of death. May we never forget their valiant service, and crown them with the same laurel wreath of bravery that will adorn the brow of every fallen patriot in this great cataclysm.

. Oklahoma has had in the Service 500 doctors, and we are proud of every one of them. The deaths of men in the Service from this number are 12, of these 2 died in Foreign Service, and 10 in this Country.

I feel as a State we have done our full duty, and now as we who are returning to civil life taking up our work at home, may we feel that we have given to our country only that which she deserves. Let us live through the coming years with an eye single to the good of humanity, as we have done during our Military Service, and may we all work to accomplish much in forwarding the aims of medicine and surgery.

Let me not stop until I voice an expressoin of appreciation, and a word of tribute to the noble women of our State who have joined the Army Nursing Corps, and stood side by side with the Doctors in the care of our sick and wounded. They have accomplished a great work, and their tender ministrations to the sick and wounded soldier has been of inestimable value. May God bless every woman of this organization, and may she know that her work is thoroughly appreciated.

I wish now to thank the members of the Oklahoma State Medical Association for the honor conferred upon me in electing me your President. I have rendered the organization no service, as during the entire year my time has been occupied with military duties, and I am very sorry that circumstances have been such that I could not keep in closer touch with matters pertaining to the work of the association.

I shall always remember with pride the fact that I have been your President, and will continue to work to help accomplish the things which will improve organized medicine in Oklahoma.

PERIRENAL HEMATOMA

K. A. Meyer, Chicago (*Journal A. M. A.*, May 17, 1919), reports two cases of rupture of the kidney, a rare condition of which only thirty cases have been previously reported. One case was fatal; in the other a good recovery was recorded. There was a history of pneumonia in the fatal case, with systolic murmur at the heart apex, which might indicate that the lesion was originally a hemorrhagic infarct. Severe pain in the kidney region and the presence of a variably sized tumor-like mass, with evidence of internal bleeding, are the important symptoms. The pain is variable in character, radiating usually downward, but sometimes from the shoulder, sometimes closely simulating renal colic. The presence of blood in the urine is important. In only one case has the diagnosis been made before operation.

SOME STUDIES IN PYELOGRAPHY*

Jas. H. Hays, M. D.

ENID, OKLAHOMA

Fellow Members:

I assure you that it is with pleasure I assume the duties of chairman of this section. While the work of our section is comparatively new, it is exceedingly important.

Five years ago there were only a few men in the larger centers of population devoting their time and attention to urology or radiology; now practically every town of five to ten thousand population has two or three or more men who are devoting a majority of their time to one or the other.

The dermatologist has been known for a much longer period; but in the years gone by, he has given considerable of his tine to some other line of work. There are, indeed, few physicians today that are capable of making a correct diagnosis or prognosis of a skin lesion. The general knowledge among physicians today of the various skin lesions is less than that of any other organ of the human body. I hope that in the future meetings of this section that we may have more papers on dermatological subjects.

The participation of our country in the recent war has demonstrated the importance of the urologist and the genito-urinary surgeon. Our Government during the past two years has probably educated and trained more physicians in this line of work than have all our colleges in the past ten years. The Government has found out that syphilis and gonorrhoea has rendered more men unfit for service than practically all other diseases combined. Our Government also discovered that the radiologist is one of the importamt aids in the proper diagnosis of many pathological conditions, so she early in the war began training many physicians in this line of work. The difficulty has been that we have not always known when we had a good radiograph, or how to properly interpert it. There are many men doing radiographic work who are not able to read their radiographs. In my judgment, radiography is only beginning to enter its field of usefulness.

I believe it would be a valuable plan, if the various sections of the Oklahoma State Medical Society could so arrange their program that not more than two of the sections would be in session at the same time, each section to have a definite time for its sessions, beginning and closing promptly on time. This will give the men, especially the general practitioner, an opportunity to attend at least two of the sections.

Pyelography is a comparatively new study in diseases of the kidney. By the pyelograph we get an outline of the pelvis of the kidney. Braasch and Dr. Bransford Lewis, and others, discovered that most all diseases of the kidney produced some irregularity or distortion of the kidney pelvis. About four years ago, Braasch published a book on pyelography with many cuts illustrating the appearance of the kidney pelvis in many of these diseases. This book stimulated many cystoscopists to get pyelographs of diseased kidneys, which has proven to be a great aid in the diagnosis, treatment, and prognosis of the diseased kidney. Unfortunately, I have not a plate of the pelvis of a pair of normal kidneys. In private practice it is difficult to secure an individual who will submit to the preparation and examination necessary to secure the pyelograph.

In preparing these few slides for our study, the pelvis of the kidney was filled with a fifteen per cent. solution of thorium nitrate, the catheter left in situ and a radiograph taken. In preparing the patient, it has been my custom to have him drink large quantities of water previous to the examination. About 30 minutes before hand I have him given, hyperodmically, one-fourth grain of morphin. After the patient is placed on the cystoscopic table, one grain of

*Chairman's Address, read in Section on Genito-Urinary and Skin Diseases, Annual Meeting, Muskogee, May, 1919.

cocain in tablet form is placed in the urethra. In the male, one-half grain in the prostatic urethra and one-half grain just inside the external meatus, cystoscope is carefully and gently passed into the bladder, and the bladder thoroughly irrigated with a sterile boric-acid solution. The ureteral catheter is then passed up into the pelvis of the kidney. I prefer a soft pliable catheter; with such a catheter the operator can do no harm and will usually pass more readily than a stiff one. Before filling the pelvis of the kidney with the thorium solution it is a good plan to draw off through the catheter whatever urine there is in the pelvis of the kidney and save a specimen of it for microscopic examination. The majority of these cases have been operated, the kidney removed and carefully examined which greatly aided me in the proper interpretation of these plates.

Plate No. 1 is a pyelograph of the left kidney of a woman 47 years old who had been suffering with pain in the left side for the past 7 years. This patient had been going from hospital to hospital, cystoscoped and radiographed several times, and twice prepared for operation, but operation deferred. The pelvis of this kidney required 36 c.c. thorium solution to fill. I wish to call your attention to the lower part of the pelvis of this kidney. It has the appearance of a large dilation of the ureter and so far as position is concerned is thoroughly drained. This ureter was patulous and a No. 10 catheter was readily passed. The urine from this kidney contained much pus and many pathogenic organisms, principally, staphylococci and colon bacilli. You will notice the irregularity of the cavity of the pelvis in its extension into both poles of the kidney. This patient had irregular attacks of pain in the left kidney region, varying from a day to three months apart: not the sharp cutting pain but a dull aching pain. She was sallow and toxic in appearance and had become addicted to the use of opiates. This kidney was removed April 2, 1919, the kidney was adherent to all the surrounding tissues and had to be decapsulated to be removed. It was about two-thirds of the normal size, firmly fixed in place by adhesions. The lining of the pelvis was thick and tough; a small stone was found in the upper pole about half the size of a pea. The major part of the secreting portion of the kidney was gone. There were areas of scar tissue all through the cortex. This is a demonstration of a chronic pyelo-nephritis; the beginning may have been due to a calculus, if so the stone had been passed before coming under my observation.

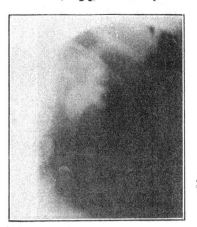

PLATE No. 1

Plate No. 2 is a pyelograph of the right kidney of a man 52 years of age, that was brought to my office on a stretcher in January, 1919. This man was suffering with terrible pain in the right kidney region which radiated downward to the end of the penis, had frequent and scanty urination, nausea, and vomiting. His physician stated that he had been in this condition for three days. Pain could be relieved only by large doses of opiate frequently repeated. Catheter was passed into the bladder and about 20 ounces of urine was drawn which contained considerable pus. Patient was taken to hospital and prepared for radiograph.

Cystoscope was passed into the bladder, ureteral catheter was readily passed up under left ureter but unable to pass it more than one inch up the right. Patient

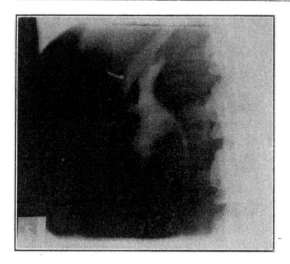

PLATE No. 2

was then anesthetized and again attempted to pass the catheter up the right ureter but failed. Two days later patient was again prepared for radiograph, a half grain morphin given, hypernatically, patient again cystoscoped and attempted again to pass the catheter up this same right ureteralopeningbut would only pass as before, about one inch. By careful examination along the right side of the trigone, down near the neck of the bladder, I noticed another ureteral opening; I passed a catheter into this opening about two inches and could not pass it any farther. I withdrew this catheter, and passed up this same opening a small No. 4. very soft and pliable catheter. It passed up about the same distance and would go no farther. I manipulated it for some time, and all at once it apparently passed the obstruction. I passed the catheter in about two inches farther, and I noticed the end of it coming out of the other right ureteral opening. I undertook to withdraw the catheter and it required as much time and patience to remove it as it did to get it inserted. I then inserted a No. 8, olive tipped, ureteral catheter, into the second opening up to the point of obstruction, injected olive oil into the catheter, until I could see it returning around the catheter and by manipulation passed the obstruction and the catheter passed readily into the pelvis of the kidney, drew off about 3 ounces of urine, which contained a great deal of pus, passed 60 c.c. of thorium solution into the pelvis of this kidney and

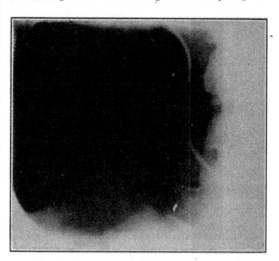

PLATE No. 3

got this remarkable picture. The urine from this kidney contained pus and colon bacilli. Thorium solution was withdrawn from the pelvis, the catheter removed and the patient was greatly relieved.

Only once after this examination did the patient require opiates for the relief of pain. Four days later I again passed a No. 8 catheter, drew off all the urine, filled the pelvis of the kidney with one-half per cent. silver nitrate solution, and left it there for 30 minutes. About two hours later the patient had a mild chill, temperature 101 degrees. This procedure was repeated four times at intervals of four days each, without any more reactions. Patient was completely relieved. This is a case of hydronephrosis produced by a stricture of the ureter at the point of bifurcation. The hydronephrosis had become infected with colon bacillus. There are reports of many cases of double ureter openings on one side of the bladder; most of them end in a blind pouch, from one to six inches in length. There are a few reported with two complete ureters for one kidney.

I regret that I had not left the first catheter that came out of the second ureteral opening in place, filled it with thorium solution and had it radiographed, because I was never again able to repeat the trick, nor was I able to pass a catheter up the first ureteral opening into the kidney, although opening must have been patulous.

Plate No. 4 is of the right kidney of a young man 18 years old, brought to me by his physician in January, 1917. This patient complained of painful and frequent urination, loss of flesh, some "night sweats", inability to sleep because of pain in the bladder. The bloody urine was loaded with pus, some blood, contained colon bacilli and staphylococci. Patient was prepared and anesthetized, and it was with some difficulty that the bladder was cleansed through the cystoscope. The mucous membrane all around the right ureteral opening was eroded and very angry in appearance. Catheters were passed up both ureters, urine of the left kidney was normal, urine of the right kidney contained some pus and many tubercle bacilli. You will note that there is no definite outline of the pelvis of this kidney. It has the appearance that thorium permeated irregularly all through the kidney. This kidney, with as much as possible of its fatty capsule and about four inches of the ureter, were removed. Patient made a good recovery, the wound healing in about four

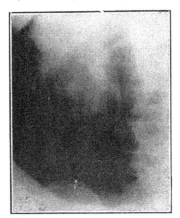

PLATE No. 4

months time. Six months ago all the complaint the patient had was some frequency of urination, but no pains. Dissection of this kidney from pole to pole showed that the kidney was practically broken down, caseated, and no definite pelvis.

Plate No. 5 is a pyelograph of the right kidney of a woman 32 years of age, that was referred to me in August, 1918, as a floating kidney. This kidney could be easily palpated and could be pushed downward to the brim of the pelvis. This patient complained of loss of flesh, constipation, some frequency of urination. She had an evening temperature of 100 to 101 degrees. You will notice that the pelvis of this kidney is rather dimly outlined, and small opaque areas apparently outside of the pelvis. The urine from this kidney contained only a small amount of pus, no pathogenic organism found. After the second lavage with one-half per cent. silver nitrate and rest in bed, the temperature did not rise above normal, and we decided to do a fixation of this kidney. Opening down on to the kidney, and removing a portion of the capsule along the outer border, discovered a focus of pus. On close examination, found a number of these foci in the cortex. The kidney was removed, and on dissection many foci of pus were found all through the body of the kidney.

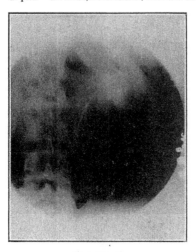

Unfortunately, this kidney was mislaid, and no microscopic examination was made, but I am inclined to believe that it was tubercular because of the thick caseous condition of the pus, and there was no infection of the wound. Patient made a rapid recovery. She was in my office a few days ago, with a temperature of 100 1-2. Urine was negative. She was referred to the internist for a diagnosis and he later reports to me that the patient is tubercular.

Plate No. 6 is a pyelograph of the left kidney of a woman 32 years of age sent to me by her family physician February, 1918. When this patient came to me she had a temperature of 101 degrees, pulse 100, stating that she had been bedfast for six weeks, having had chills, fever, and sweats. Her family physician informed me that she had lost weight, had attacks of pain that required opiates to relieve her. Center of pain was in the region of the bladder, and seemed to radiate all over the abdomen.

PLATE No. 5

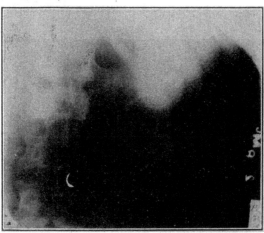

PLATE No. 6

She had been previously operated for appendicitis but was not relieved. A catheterized specimen of her urine contained red blood cells, pus and colon bacilli. She at times had frequent urination, and always during these periods there would come these severe attacks of pain. Cystoscopic examination of the bladder showed the left ureteral opening to be red, swollen, pouting and angry in appearance. The right ureteral opening was normal. Catheter passed up the right ureter readily, but was unable to pass the catheter up the left ureter more than an inch. The obstruction felt hard; injected olive oil through the catheter for ten or fifteen minutes, got by the obstruction three or four inches, when I could neither pass the catheter farther nor draw it back. I gave the catheter a good, hard jerk and it gave way, catheter came back and blood flowed freely from the ureteral opening. Washing away the blood, I could see a little stone in the mouth of the ureter, which I removed with a pair of forceps.

Three days later, I again cystoscoped this patient and the catheter readily passed up the left ureter and drew off one and one-half ounce of urine which contained pus and colon bacilli. Filled the pelvis with thorium and secured this pyelograph. Lavaged the kidney four times with one-half per cent. silver nitrate solution at four-day intervals, and sent her home. She was home about two weeks, and had chills with fever and sweats but no pain. She was bed-fast for about two weeks with a daily temperature of from 100 to 102. She returned and I dilated the ureter with a No. 10 catheter and lavaged the pelvis again with the same solution of silver nitrate three times, each time using the large catheter. I saw her six months later. She was in excellent health and stated that she had not felt so well in years.

You will notice the large size of the ureter as well as the large and rather indefinite outline of the pelvis of the kidney. This is a case of partial obstruction of the ureter with a small renal calculus, down near the bladder, which had produced a dilation of the ureter above the obstruction as well as of the pelvis of the kidney.

Plate No. 7 is a pyelograph of the left kidney of a man 38 years old, who had been having attacks of pain in the left kidney region for five years—at irregular intervals of from one to six months apart. He first consulted me about a year before this radiograph was taken, stating that he had a stone in the left kidney, but I declined to advise or treat him till he would consent to a cystoscopic or radiograhpic examination. In January, 1918, he submitted. Catheter readily passed up to the pelvis of the kidney and I drew three ounces of urine, which did not contain any pus, but did contain many epithelia. I then passed a No. 8 catheter and filled that pelvis of the kidney with thorium. This is a poor plate, taken from a good radiograph. You will notice the similarity of this plate to No. 6. These plates were taken within three weeks of each other. Their descriptions of their attacks of pain were very similar, but this patient had no temperature

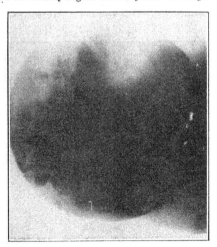

PLATE No. 7

though he said that he had lost considerable flesh. In this case there was no difficulty in passing the ureteral catheter. After his examination the patient was so relieved that he would not consent to an operation, and he was free from attacks of pain till November, 1918, when he had a rather mild attack of pain. I again cystoscoped him, passed a No. 10 catheter into the pelvis of the kidney and drew nearly three ounces of urine, which was still negative except that it was of low specific gravity, 1006. This is a case of hydronephrosis of the left kidney; the cause of which I do not know. The kidney cannot be palpated, and there is no obstruction in the ureter. The patient does not give any history of having passed a stone. .

Plate No. 8 is a poor pyelograph of a right kidney of a rather interesting case—a physician's wife—28 years old. This patient was brought to me by her husband, was six months pregnant, and complained of a dull heavy pain in the right side of the back with frequent and painful urination. The bladder urine

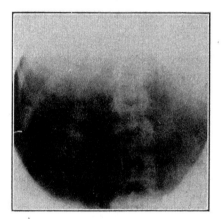

PLATE No. 8

contained a great deal of pus and colon bacilli. She was cystoscoped. Catheter passed into the pelvis of the right kidney and 8 ounces of urine was drawn from this kidney which contained pus and colon bacilli. Kidney was lavaged with one-half per cent. silver nitrate solution. She returned at intervals of two weeks for similar treatments till she was confined. This pyelograph was taken about four weeks ago, soon after her confinement. Kidney pelvis at this time contained about 4 ounces of urine.

You will notice that this kidney lies far below the normal position and it is with difficulty pressed upward. It can be readily palpated. It is twice the size of a normal kidney. Since confinement this woman has been free of pain and appears in excellent health. This is an extreme case of hydronephrosis of the right kidney of a woman of child-bearing age. Hydronephrosis of the right kidney is very common in women. The right kidney in women is often moveable and the motion downward produces a kinking of the ureter, thereby obstructing the free outflow of urine from the kidney. The downward and inward swing of the kidney behind the ascending colon, pressing forward on the colon, increases constipation. The second symptom so common in this class of cases. It is this class of cases that is so often mistaken and operated for chronic appendicitis. I believe that simple pyelitis and hydronephrosis of the right kidney in women are mis-diagnosed more frequently than any other kidney lesion, and yet they are the most common.

CONTROL OF VENEREAL DISEASE*

F. W. EWING, M. D.

MUSKOGEE, OKLAHOMA

With the creation of the Interdepartmental Social Hygiene Board and the establishment of the Division of Venereal Diseases in the United States Public Health Service, one of the most important movements ever undertaken in connection with the prevention of disease was launched.

The United States Government has recognized that venereal diseases are enemies to the public health, and are to be fought just as yellow fever, malaria, tuberculosis and hookworm have been fought.

The whole problem of venereal disease control is being approached from every angle: and the era of pessimistic beliefs and sporadic attempts at control has been replaced by an era of rational study, unbiased experiment and determined action.

A great number of contributing factors are recognized: not one of them must be neglected if we are to attack this problem in the same sound scientific spirit in which we have attacked other disease problems. Into it enter such other well defined problems as those of general school education, recreation, economic readjustments, national customs, national psychology and morals.

When the Division of Venereal Diseases was created, two great needs were especially evident, the need for an effective organization for venereal disease control as an integral part of every State board of health, and the need for educating the general public on the venereal disease problem as rapidly as possible. The first need was met by each state board of health being invited to organize a bureau for the control of venereal diseases in charge of a man of their own selection. These men were appointed as acting assistant surgeons of the Public Health Service in order to give them further authority and to conform to the regulations making available the funds for venereal disease control in the various states.

Almost every state has adopted measures and accepted the co-operation of the Public Health Service by placing an officer of that service in charge of the work.

In the states which have passed adequate regulations, appointed a man and received federal appropriation, the work for the control of venereal diseases is being organized along four chief lines:

1. Establishment of venereal disease clinics in towns sufficiently large to support them.

2. Education of the public on the nature of venereal diseases and the means required for their control.

3. Law enforcement measures for the repression of prostitution.

4. Establishment of detention homes and other institutions for the proper quarantine of cases dangerous to the public health and for the rehabilitation of persons of previously immoral life.

Clinics are established in the various sections of the states, particularly in the towns that reach a large outlying community, as well as in the large cities. Each clinic is placed in charge of local doctors of suitable training and ability and whose staff should include a female nurse, a female social worker and a male attendant.

Skillful medical treatment, education and the rehabilitation and replacement in society of those who for a time have been anti-social in their habits are the principal functions of the clinic.

---

*Chairman's Address, read in Section on General Medicine, Mental and Nervous Diseases, Annual Meeting, Muskogee, May, 1919.

The problem of education is being met in part through the state boards of health and their clinics. In part, however, this matter demands a nation-wide campaign and this is being successfully carried on by the Division of Venereal Diseases of the Public Health Service. The objects of this campaign are to combat and correct ancient misunderstandings and misconceptions; to provide accurate information inoffensively presented; to arouse interest and active co-operation, and to make possible the teaching of sex hygiene.

It should be stated here that the teaching of sex hygiene, as now understood, does not contemplate the delivery of a few formal lectures on the subject, dissociated from all other instructions, and to be listened to with bated breath and emotional discomfort. It means first the education of parents, so that they will know how to answer the questions of growing children and to be able to inspire them with a reverent attitude towards sex. It includes also the study of biology in the schools, so that children will learn the essential facts regarding the development of life without having the subject made unduly prominent in their minds. In fact, they will learn what they need to know about sex without at all realizing that they are receiving sex instructions. Contrary to making the subject prominent, it will become merely one small part of the instruction in the care of their bodies and in right attitude towards life.

The generel results of the government's campaign against venereal diseases during the past two years have been very interesting, and in some respects contrary to what many persons expected. It has often been said that nothing could be done to stem the tide of venereal diseases, because the problem was bound up with unchangeable human nature. The results, however, as seen in the medical departments of the army and navy, have shown that a great deal can be done with good effect.

It has been said that the people were not ready to support such a campaign as this. Quite to the contrary, it has everywhere been found that the people are intensely interested in this problem; that they are astounded at the facts shown by the draft as to the prevalence of venereal diseases in the civilian communities; that they are indignant that things have been allowed to progress so far before a radical remedy was devised and applied, and that they are now determined that the venereal diseases shall be checked and their great prevalence reduced so far as possible. The support of the people in this work is absolutely assured, and for this we are indebted and should always be grateful for the epoch-making work of the surgeon-generals of the army, navy and the public health service and their medical officers.

DELIVERING THE PLACENTA

A procedure for delivering the placenta is proposed by J. L. Baer, Chicago (*Journal A. M. A.*, May 24, 1919), which does away, he thinks, with some of the possible dangers. It utilizes, he claims, the natural powers of the woman without danger of too much traumatism causing metritis or rupture of a pus tube. In most cases the inability to accomplish expulsion spontaneously is due to the loss of tone of the abdominal wall, so long overstretched. His method is as follows: "After the usual period of waiting, averaging half an hour, and when the uterus is at the height of a contraction, as evidenced by both feeling it and by the pain the woman is experiencing, I grasp the abdominal wall crosswise above the fundus and pull the rectus muscles together, thus taking up all the slack. I then encourage the woman to bear down, and in practically every case in which expression on the fundus would have succeeded, this procedure has succeeded. If, then, there should be adherent membranes, they are treated in exactly the same fashion as following any other method of expression." The advantage claimed is the avoidance of handling the uterus, which he considers always advisable.

SYPHILIS AND ITS RELATION TO THE DISEASES OF THE EYE.*

R. O. EARLY, M. D.

ARDMORE, OKLAHOMA

This paper must of necessity be brief, for to go into the pathological changes of each structure of the eye caused by a disease so widespread as syphilis would in itself entail a length of time that I have no desire to occupy. When one stops to think that in some of the diseases of the eye, namely, iritis, that syphilis is found to be the cause in from 30 to 60 per cent of the cases, this disease becomes one all ophthalomogists are always vitally interested in. I will endeavor to take up briefly the different ocular tissue, as none are immune, but more especially do I wish to speak of this disease in relation to the uveal tract.

Syphilis of the Cornea: Most important of the specific corneal affections is parenchymatous keratitis, the etiology being divided into two forms: (1) Inherited parenchymatous keratitis and (2nd) the acquired form. It is stated by most authorities on this subject that 60 per cent. of the cases depend on inherited syphilis, with the disease most frequent between the ages of 5 and 15 and more common among girls than boys.

The symptoms are quite characteristic, namely, after a few days of ciliary congestion, spots of haziness appear in the cornea which, with oblique illumination, will be seen to be in the parenchyma of the cornea. In a couple of weeks, the whole cornea will have become involved, giving a ground glass appearance; this, together with the formation of new blood vessels, gives the cornea the so-called "Salomon patch" appearance. The above symptoms are always complicated by iritis and iridocyclitis with often a rise in tension.

These symptoms, together with the general manifestation of the disease-dwarfed stature-sunken nasal bridge, malformed teeth, etc., generally make the diagnosis easy. The routine use of making a Wassermann test in these cases has simplified the diagnosis where any doubt has remained. You are all familiar with the long and tedious time consumed in the treatment of these cases, of the almost certainty of the involvement of the second eye, all of which the patient should be warned.

Two to ten per cent. of the cases of this type are due to acquired syphilis and appear usually in the late secondary or tertiary period of the constitutional diseases. Its cause is more rapid and, unlike the inherited form, usually is unilateral and appears between the 20th and 50th years of life.

Syphilis of the Iris: As stated before, it has been found that from 30 to 60 percent. of all cases of iritis are due to syphilis. The beginning of the ocular affection may be from six weeks to 18 months after the initial lesion, rarely it arises during the late tertiary manifestations. Clinically we may divide this type of iritis into three varieties:

(1) Acute syphilitic iritis. In this form are found the usual signs of iritis, with no lesions that would of themselves justify the diagnosis of syphilis, we having to depend on the history and Wassermann reaction.

(2) True, syphilitic iritis, sometimes called iritis papulosa. In this form there appears in the inflamed iris one or more yellowish or reddish brown nodules which vary in size from a small seed to a small pea; as a rule these papules are situated at the pupillary border of the iris; the usual signs of iritis—pericorneal injection, synechia, etc., are of course present.

(3) Gummatous iritis is really a manifestation of gumma, almost always found at the ciliary border as a yellowish white growth. It is an uncommon manifestation and belongs to the late stages of syphilis.

---

*Chairman's Address, read in Section on Eye, Ear, Nose and Throat, Annual Meeting, Muskogee, May, 1919.

Syphilis of Choroid, diffuse or disseminated, is in a large percentage of cases due to this disease.

In the first mentioned, after a period of diffuse grayish exudation, the ophthalmoscope shows large areas of exposed sclera, separated from each other by apparently normal choroid with irregular pigment fringing their borders.

In the disseminated form, after a period of grayish exudation, numerous irregular spots are formed, surrounded either completely or partly by black margins with often spots of pigment in the center of the white area.

A certain number of syphilitics acquire after a year or two a form of retinitis which is subject to relapses. Treatment in these cases is often unsatisfactory, owing to atrophy of the optic nerve and extensive choroiditis. With the advent of salvarsan and neosalvarsan the treatment of syphilis, especially as regards diseases of the uveal tract, has been much more satisfactory. I believe that it is worth every man's time to go thoroughly into every case of doubtful iritis, have a Wassermann made as a routine practice and if positive, get the patient on proper anti-syphilitic treatment at the earliest possible moment.

GENITO-URINARY SURGERY

A. R. Stevens, New York (*Journal A. M. A.*, May 31, 1919), remarks on the infrequency of wounds of the urinary tract, at least in the hospital admissions, and their high mortality. This is perhaps explained by the obvious possibility of frequent fatal hemorrhage from wounds in this region. Various statistics show that the kidney was involved in from 4 to 9 per cent. of abdominal wounds, and in from 4 to 7 per cent. of wounds of the bladder. While he has no reliable figures himself, he says that few of these cases reach the hospital, and his experience is the same as that of other surgeons. Two cases of some interest are reported, and also his one record of kidney wound discovered before nephrectomy. A recent French publication, giving collective statistics, states that uncomplicated bladder wounds give a mortality of 56 per cent., and out of fifteen cases with co-existing intestinal wounds, all except one resulted fatally. His own records of eleven patients with wounds of the bladder or vicinity show six fatal cases, and in four patients wounded through the perineum, there was only one recovery. As regards supra-pubic wounds, Stevens thinks it advisable, as a rule, to close the bladder wound occurring on the peritoneal surface but to drain an extraperitoneal opening. Two cases showing a deviation from the latter part of this rule, impairing the patient's prospects, are reported. Importance of removing all loose bits of bone in complicated fractures of the pelvis is pointed out. Penetrating buttock wounds are notoriously grave, and the possibility of bladder or ureteral injury is to be considered. He has seen no case of fistula involving both intestinal and urinary tract, though simple fecal fistulas are not so rare. The bladder complications of spinal gunshot wounds are of special interest. The symptoms vary greatly in different cases, but there is usually some retention before incontinence sets in, and different methods have been employed to meet the conditions. Some English surgeons have strongly advised against attempts to relieve the retention. This plan is not, in Steven's opinion, a good universal rule, but it is probably best when it can be borne. Any harm done by a large amount of residual urine in the bladder is probably less risky than the danger of infection from frequent catheterization. Hematuria in soldiers was of interest and many cases were studied with the cystoscope. It was surprising that 90 per cent. of them represented what has been rather loosely termed "war nephritis," a condition which is not discussed in this paper.

JOURNAL OF THE OKLAHOMA STATE MEDICAL ASSOCIATION

VOLUME XII   MUSKOGEE, OKLA., JUNE, 1919   NUMBER 6

PUBLISHED MONTHLY AT MUSKOGEE. OKLA., UNDER DIRECTION OF THE COUNCIL

DR. CLAUDE A. THOMPSON. EDITOR-IN-CHIEF
308 SURETY BUILDING, MUSKOGEE

DR. CHAS. W. HEITZMAN, ASSISTANT EDITOR
BARNES BUILDING, MUSKOGEE

ENTERED AT THE POST OFFICE AT MUSKOGEE, OKLAHOMA, AS SECOND CLASS MAIL MATTER, JULY 28, 1912

THIS IS THE OFFICIAL JOURNAL OF THE OKLAHOMA STATE MEDICAL ASSOCIATION. ALL COMMUNICATIONS SHOULD BE ADDRESSED TO THE JOURNAL OF THE OKLAHOMA STATE MEDICAL ASSSOCIATION. 308 SURETY BUILDING, MUSKOGEE, OKLAHOMA.

The editorial department is not re-ponsible for the opinions expressed in the original articles of contributors.

Reprints of original articles will be supplied at actual cost, provided request for them is attached to manuscript or made in sufficient time before publication.

Articles sent this Journal for publication and all those read at the annual meetings of the State Association are the sole property of this Journal. The Journal relies on each individual contributor's strict adherence to this well-known rule of medical journalism In the event an article sent this Journal fo publication is published before appearance in the Journal, the manuscript will be returned to the writer

Failure to receive the Journal should call for immediate notification of the editor, 307-8 Surety Building, Muskogee, Okla

Local news of possible interest to the medical profession, notes on removals, changes in address, deaths and weddings will be gratefully received.

Advertising of articles, drugs or compounds unapproved by the Council on Pharmacy of the A. M. A. will not be accepted.

Advertising rates will be supplied on application. It is suggested that wherever possible members of the State Associa tion should patronize our advertisers in preference to others as a matter of fair reciprocity.

EDITORIAL

PROCEEDINGS, OKLAHOMA STATE MEDICAL ASSOCIATION, MUSKOGEE, MAY 20-22, 1919.

HOUSE OF DELEGATES:

Called to order by the President, Dr. L. S. Willour, McAlester.

The minutes of the last meeting, May, 1918, as published in the Journal of June, 1918, were adopted.

The following committees were appointed:

Credentials—Drs. B. H. Brown, Muskogee; R. H. Harper. Afton; R. T. Edwards, Oklahoma City.

Special Necrology Committee—Drs. C. W. Heitzman, Muskogee; J. E. Davis, McAlester; B. J. Vance, Checotah.

Resolutions Committee—Drs. S. DeZell Hawley, Tulsa; W. O. Rice, Alderson; R. F. Terrell, Stigler.

It was stated that the auditing committee of the Council—Drs. Heitzman, Muskogee; Ellis Lamb, Clinton; L. C. Kuyrkendall, McAlester—would render report after study of the books of the Secretary-Treasurer-Editor, to the Delegates.

The report of the Secretary-Treasurer-Editor was received. (See page 163).

The House adjourned on call of the President.

HOUSE OF DELEGATES, MAY 22, 1919, 9:00 A. M.

Called to order by the President.

The Credentials Committee reported present 33 delegates including officers.

Election of officers resulted as follows: President-elect, Dr. John W. Duke, Guthrie; 1st Vice-President, Jackson Broshears, Lawton; 2nd Vice President, Dr. G. Pinnell, Miami; 3rd Vice President, Dr. J. A. Hatchett, El Reno; Delegate to A. M. A., 1920-21, Dr. L. S. Willour, McAlester.

Councillors: District 1—Dr. G. A. Boyle, Enid, to succeed himself. District 3—Dr. M. E. Stout, Oklahoma City. District 5—J. L. Austin, Durant.

Meeting place for 1920, Oklahoma City.

The President appointed Dr. LeRoy Long to escort the President-elect, Dr. J. W. Duke, to the chair. On introduction to the House, Dr. Duke made a short address in appreciation of his election, assuring the members he would continue his efforts for the advancement of the highest ideals of the medical profession.

The Auditing Committee of the Council reported that the books of the Secretary-Treasurer-Editor had been audited and found correct and in accordance with the printed report submitted to the House. (See report page 163).

May 21, 1919.

To the Officers and Members of the Oklahoma State Medical Association:

The undersigned members of auditing committee desire to report: That after an examination of the books of your Secretary-Treasurer, we find the same in accordance with the report submitted by him.

Respectfully,

Charles W. Heitzman, Chairman.
L. C. Kuyrkendall.

The Council report was adopted.

The Special Necrology Committee reported as follows:

Mr. President and Fellow Members of the Oklahoma State Medical Association:

Let us stand and pay tribute to those of our membership, who since our last gathering have passed to that "Beautiful Island of Somewhere". And as we stand here there must appear to us the memories personified of those we knew and loved. The recollections of their lives is disseminated around us like the clear sunshine of this beautiful May-day: as we gaze about us at nature arrayed in her bounteous verdure, the blooming flowers and the animal life each in their way bearing testimony to a fullness of animation, we cannot realize that our friends and companions are gone. And then we think had we the power not to be born we certainly would not have accepted existence upon conditions that are such a mockery. But we still have power to die, though the days we give back are numbered. It is no great power, it is no great munity.

DEATHS

This year has scored heavily upon us in deaths among our members. As nearly as is ascertainable we have lost since our last report the following members:

Deaths, May 1, 1918, to April 30, 1919.

Henry Blender, Okeene	Blaine County
P. E. A. Fling, Hugo	Choctaw County
T. F. Laidig, Drumright	Creek County
N. P. H. White, Clinton	Custer County
W. E. Hagood, Bison	Garfield County
H. B. McKenzie, Enid	Garfield County
R. J. Gordon, Ninnekah	Grady County
Thos. J. Horsley, Mangum	Greer County
A. B. Callaway, Stigler	Haskell County
T. B. McClure, McCurtain	Haskell County
S. P. Rawls, Altus	Jackson County
D. E. Wilson, Elmer	Jackson County

C. C. Northrup, Braman_____Kay County
J. R. Dale, Hobart_____Kiowa County
A. L. Wagoner, Hobart_____Kiowa County
C. L. Kerfoot, Prague_____Lincoln County
G. M. Wilkinson, Nowata_____Nowata County
R. L. Hull, Oklahoma City_____Oklahoma County
F. B. Sorgatz, Oklahoma City_____Oklahoma County
A. H. Herr, Okmulgee_____Okmulgee County
Harry Walker, Pawhuska_____Osage County
G. H. Rutledge, Afton_____Ottawa County
J. Paul Gay, McAlester_____Pittsburg County
T. G. Palmer, A. E. F._____Pittsburg County
C. S. Wilkerson, Roff_____Pontotoc County
J. P. Bartley, Bartlesville_____Washington County
T. B. Dickson, Ramona_____Washington County

While they are gone from our midst yet their having once lived still acts as an inspiration for us to become better physicians and thereby attain to that greater inherent nobility of character within us: so that when our final summons comes, we go not to our death like quarry slaves scourged to their dungeons; but with that nobler better faith that will enable us to meet "Our Pilot face to face when we shall cross the bar."

Respectfully submitted,

Charles W. Heitzman, Chairman.
John W. Duke.
L. C. Kuyrkendall.

It was suggested that a copy of the Journal containing the report of the Necrology Committee be sent to the surviving members of the deceased physicians, if practicable. The Secretary stated that such had been the custom heretofore where the address of such survivors was obtainable.

Motion carried to make the Necrology Committee a permanent committee.

The Resolutions Committee reported that they would later submit their report. It was ordered that the report be printed when received.

Dr. G. A. Boyle, Enid, moved that the Governor be commended by resolution for vetoing a certain special bill passed by the Legislature which sought to direct that a physician not able to qualify to the usual and customary rules of the State Board of Medical Examiners in order to be examined, be legislated into such status, that the Board be directed to examine him without applying the rules applied to other applicants. The motion was opposed by Dr. C. W. Heitzman, Muskogee, who stated that it was not the province of the State Medical Association to take action commending the Governor for doing his proper duty, that too much suggestion from the profession had already been made to lawmakers whose sworn duty it was to enact proper and sensible laws for the people. He cited the recent refusal of the Legislative Committee of the Ohio Medical Association to appear before a legislative committee and give their opinions on certain legislation pending, which ordinarily is opposed by all state medical associations, and the consequent overwhelming defeat of the bill by the body. He advanced the opinion that allowing the lawmakers free hand for a time would be more effective than sending representatives to plead with them to do what was their obvious duty.

Other speakers in favor of the adoption spoke on the question.

The motion was adopted, and the Secretary directed to prepare and forward suitable resolutions covering the matter.

The Southern Medical Association telegraphed its best wishes and greetings and extended an invitation to Oklahoma physicians to attend their meeting at Asheville, N. C., November, 1919.

A motion was made by Dr. Ross Grosshart, Tulsa, and carried, that a committee from the House be appointed to aid the Legislative Committee, to draft a law and ask the Legislators to enact the same providing Counties in Oklahoma power to vote bonds for the erection and maintenance of County Hospitals,—for the treatment for the sick and handling all. quarantine cases, that said law should prescribe the management of such Hospitals be kept out of poiltics, so that the poor sick should receive the proper treatment and care from the best scientific men in the County, regardless of their political faith.

The motion was carried.

The President appointed: Drs. Ross Grosshart, Tulsa: A. B. Leeds, Chickasha; Jackson Broshears, Lawton.

The House adjourned.

Resolution Committee's Report was as follows:

Be it resolved: That the Oklahoma State Medical Association thoroughly appreciate the entertainment and facilities furnished for our meeting by the Muskogee County Medical Society and the Physicians of Muskogee.

Be it further resolved: That we thank the ladies of Muskogee who so generously entertained the visiting ladies at the luncheon and automobile drive.

Be it also resolved: That we appreciate the patriotism of our members who gave up their practice and went forth to do their bit in the Great World War which is just finished and we especially want to extend to them the greatest compliments for the noble sacrifice which they made.

We further appreciate the efforts. of our officials who have worked so faithfully for a united and harmonious profession. For it is only through meetings of this kind that we aid the Physicians of this state to keep abreast of the times and to keep in touch with the rapid developments in medicine and surgery.

Respectfully submitted,

S. De Zell Hawley.
W. O. Rice.
R. F. Terrell.

COUNCIL, MUSKOGEE, MAY 20, 1919, 11:00 A. M.

Present: President, L. S. Willour; Drs. G. A. Boyle, L. C. Kuyrkendall, Ellis Lamb, N. W. Mayginnis, C. W. Heitzman, Secretary-Treasurer-Editor, C. A. Thompson.

The following committee was appointed: Auditing—Drs. Heitzman, Lamb and Kuyrkendall. Report of Secretary-Treasurer-Editor for the fiscal year, May 1, 1918, to April 30, 1919, with all books, vouchers, duplicate deposit sheets and papers pertaining to the office were received by the committee.

A motion was adopted that a recommendation be made to the House of Delegates that a Councillor committee, with power to act, be appointed to study the present plan of collection of dues and inaugurate such changes as might be deemed necessary to improve and simplify the work of collection. The committee consisted of Drs. Mayginnis, Lamb and the President and Secretary, ex-officio.

A spirited discussion on the duties of councillors was indulged in, after which it was unanimously declared the policy of the Council that each county society be visited during the year, that a list of members and non-members eligible to membership be prepared by the Secretary's office and forwarded to the councillor concerned as soon as practicable, on which concerted effort was to be made to increase membership wherever expedient. Adjourned.

COUNCIL, MAY 22, 1919.

Report of committee on collection of dues was referred, the committee to continue investigation and make report by mail of findings through the Secretary's office, to the Council who would vote such changes as necessary.

A motion by Dr. Willour was adopted after lengthy discussion, that Dr. C. W. Heitzman, Muskogee, be appointed as Assistant Editor of the Journal and to act as representative of the Council in Muskogee in such matters as were delegated to him from time to time.

A motion by Dr. Kuyrkendall to increase the salary of the Secretary-Treasurer-Editor to $100.00 monthly was adopted.

A motion was made and carried authorizing the Secretary to submit to the Council by mail any matter he deemed of urgency or of such nature that might be acted upon by the councillors by mail, or deemed not of sufficient importance to warrant calling a meeting for the action of the Council.

It was ordered that such bills of expense properly incurred and rendered by members of the council be paid by the Secretary-Treasurer. Adjourned.

ANNUAL REPORT OF THE SECRETARY-TREASURER-EDITOR.

(For Fiscal Year May 1, 1918, to April 30, 1919.)

To the House of Delegates, Council and Members, Oklahoma State Medical Association.

Gentlemen:—

I herewith submit my report of affairs of my office for the time indicated.

Membership: The membership for 1918 reached the highest point in our history, running to 1540 at the close of the year.

Members in good standing April 30, 1918, 1386.

Members in good standing April 30, 1919, 1434.

As is well known to the initiated, the prosperity of a county society as indicated by regular meetings, be the membership ever so small; and a membership in proportion to the number of physicians of the county, is almost solely dependent, with rare exceptions, on the activity, energy and tact of one physician—the County Secretary. It is not the province of your secretary to suggest an innovation looking to improvement in certain sections of the State, but it is not out of place to suggest to you that the Council or House of Delegates appoint a committee to closely calculate the number of physicians in each society, and if it is believed proper to suggest to the members of certain societies that they elect some one of their number secretary, who has the energy to look after their affairs in proper form. The justification of this lies in the fact that many good physicians lapse their membership from careless, or no attention on the part of the secretary. Every ethical man in the State should join us and cooperate in our problems. Non-membership on their part is our loss as well as theirs.

Membership carries with it implied obligations from the member to the entire membership. Insofar as medical defense is concerned, a careless statement on the part of a physician may cause a suit, utterly baseless, against some fellow physician. Students of these matters are of the opinion that in nearly every case they are due to some intentional or unintentiomal statement, deliberate malice, or to a "Golden Silence", more dishonest and damaging than active criticism, when their fellow physician is under discussion. Your defense attorneys have just successfully concluded two cases, the first we were called on to defend without the defendants being required to even state or present their defense. The cost of this defense is quite an important item, but the most puzzling feature of all in the matter is that the county society membership has dwindled to three members for 1919.

In one county where we are called to defend a difficult and expensive case, the most insistent urging and repeated notices of pending lapses and correspondence was necessary to keep it from having, proportionately, the largest loss in membership. This was due solely to carelessness on the part of a poorly selected secretary.

To cure this neglect is difficult, but the suggestion that a member who is lapsed after a certain date and proper notice be required to pay an additional sum for reinstatement seems worthy of trial. Certainly the general and majority body of members who are prompt and of least trouble should not be required to expend their money in carrying the negligent. Each year the two or three hundred who wait to the last moment cost the membership more in labor and correspondence than all others combined.

MEMBERS IN MILITARY SERVICE.

Most county societies carried their absent members but there are some marked exceptions, and some notably in counties which are under unusual obligations to the State Association. This office is under the impression that these cases or lapses, however, are more due to lack of permanent organization, lack of attention on the part of the county secretary or those remaining at home while the secretary is absent in war service and in some instances a misunderstanding that the State Society would carry members in the Military Service, when that duty obviously fell upon the county society. By an unprecedented amount of correspondence to the officers of county societies or physicians remaining in the county, most of such absentees have been provided for. Many deserving members, however, have been cut from membership lists while still absent in Military Service, due to the failure of their fellow members to provide for them.

DEATHS.

(See report of Special Necrology Committee on another page.)

MEDICAL DEFENSE.

The legal rights of those of our members who have been sued and who were entitled to defense have been unusually well cared for. In every case satisfaction has been expressed, so far as is known. In this connection, however, some unwarrantedly irritating circumstances arose in the administration of the Fund according to the rules laid down. In spite of repeated publication of the rules, wide dissemination of them, physicians sued insisted on its protection when the facts clearly showed them not entitled to defense. Once again attention of members is called to the rules. Your cooperation is asked to make this phase of our work the success it now seems assuredly it will be if the fund is administered justly and sensibly to all alike. And habit of deviation from strict rule in handling these cases exactly as a business matter will result in failure eventually.

FINANCIAL STATEMENT.

For information of the Council and House of Delegates there is appended herewith a condensed statement of receipts and expenditures for the Fiscal year ending April 30, 1919, including all balances as shown by report of April 30, 1918.

All cash books, duplicate deposit sheets, checks and stubs of checks have been audited and submitted to the Council for their information. The business interests of the Association have grown to such respectable proportions that it is no longer feasible or practical to render a detailed or printed statement of them, so all the books are submitted to the Council and its auditing committee for their inspection and report. The condensed report of their findings will be published as usual in the June Journal.

Receipts.

Balance April 30, 1918	$	2,076.39
Advertising		3,373.26
Time Deposit Surrendered		1,000.00
Interest on Time Deposit		20.00
Interest on Liberty Bond		20.00
County Secretaries		4,727.50
		$ 11,217.15

Expenditures.

Printing Journal, etc.	$	3,476.17
Reporting Meetings		265.82
Councilors and Delegates Expense		279.82
Attorneys Fees and Legal Expense		300.50
Secretary's Salary		900.00
Stenographic and Clerical Work		562.35
Office Rent		130.00
Guests Expense		103.15
Refunds		97.50
Treasurer's Bond		10.00
Auditing Books		10.00
Telephone, Telegraph and Express		43.87
Office Supplies		34.48
Postage		169.50
Press Clippings		35.25
Transfer to Medical Defense Fund		1,400.00
		$ 7,818.41
May 1, 1919, Balance Cash on hand		3,398.74
		$ 11,217.15

Balance on Hand in Bank	$	3,398.74
Liberty Bond		500.00
Total	$	3,898.74

Medical Defense Fund.

Receipts.

May 1, 1918, Balance on Hand	$	577.55
May 28, 1918, Surrender on Time Deposit		168.00
April 26, 1919, Oklahoma State Medical Association		1,400.00
April 30, 1919, Interest on Time Deposit		80.00
		$ 2,225.55

Expenditures.

Attorneys' Fees	$	437.20
Time Deposit, (Commercial National Bank)		1,000.00
		$. 1,437.20
May 1, 1919, Balance on Hand		788.35
		$ 2,225.55

Balance on Hand in Bank_____$ 788.35
Time Deposit_____ 3,000.00
War Savings Stamps_____ 832.00

Total_____$ 4,620.35

Respectfully submitted,

C. A. THOMPSON,

Secretary-Treasurer-Editor.

CURRENT MEDICAL LITERATURE
Conducted by
DR. CHAS. W. HEITZMAN, Barnes Building, Muskogee

Contributions and observations of Oklahoma physicians collected by them in the course of study of American and foreign medical literature, deemed to be of sufficient interest and value to the profession, are especially invited to this department. Such contributions should bear the name of the sender, which will be appended to the abstract or omitted, as desired.

TREATMENT OF BURNS.
By A. L. McDonald, Duluth, Minn.
(Annals of Surgery, March, 1919)

McDonald discusses his experiences with severely burned patients, following the forest fires around Duluth. He states that when over one-half of the body was burned they all died. Several died with lung complications and a few from late toxemia.

His treatment is as follows: He states in the first aid care of extensive burns, the dressing with gauze soaked in 10 per cent. or stronger bicarbonate of soda, and kept moist, is the simplest, and gives greatest comfort. This is preferable to attempts at a more complicated technic. Morphine should be used to give rest but must be administered with care since there is often severe reaction and depression and the drug may do harm. Treatment of shock with posture, heat, hot drinks, and stimulants may be necessary.

Paraffin is much preferable to gause with oily dressings, and should be substituted as soon as possible, at least within thirty-six hours. With the use of the air pump and atomizer the method can be simplified, and rendered quite painless, dressings on gauze should be abandoned.

Dichloramine-T in oil is painful and of slight value. If there is extensive slough, wet dressings or antiseptic powders are preferable.

The use of adhesive strapping over the raw surface is highly satisfactory, and simplifies the treatment since dressings may be extended to two or three days.

The general conditions of the patient must be carefully followed and built up by stimulants, tonics or transfusions.

Skin grafting is rarely necessary, nor does it offer much advantage to the healing with paraffin or adhesive.   C. von Wedel, M. D.

ON SOME LESIONS OBSERVED IN OPERATIONS FOR OLD INJURIES TO THE SPINAL CORD, WITH REMARKS AS TO TREATMENT.
By Charles A. Elsberg, New York.
(Annals of Surgery, March 1919)

Elsberg goes into considerable detail as to the appearance of the cord and dura following old injuries; some he states show marked congestion, some the scars of adhesions, and some bands of firm tissue.

As to treatment, he aptly says that all opinions are still at great variance. The question what symptoms and signs justify operative interference is the all important one. Repeated examination and good x-ray pictures are necessary. First, surgical relief is impossible in complete transverse lesions. Second, there is no hope of relieving patients with symptoms and signs of incomplete cord lesions who have large bed sores, or are much emaciated. Third, individuals who have after spinal trauma improved considerably for a period of months, but in whom improvement has stopped before useful function of the limbs has been regained, should be operated upon either if a marked angulation of the cord has remained or the x-ray shows a narrowing of the spinal canal by dislocated or new formed bone, unless the examination shows there is a dissociated disturbance of superficial sensation. Four, if there has been a considerable return of power in the lower limbs, and the condition has become stationary, and if locomotion is interfered with by the spasticity, a laminectomy and division of the appropriate posterior nerve roots is often followed by satisfactory results. Five, severe root pains at or near the upper level of the lesion, if they cannot be relieved by immobilization of the spine, may demand operative interference—namely, wide decompressive laminectomy. Sixth, can we benefit a patient who has vesical incontinence left after an old spinal injury? This question is a most important one. Theoretically, the regeneration of the anterior nerve roots should be possible, but practically, up to present time, experiences in man have been inconclusive.   C. von Wedel, M. D.

FLY TIME.

Prof. R. I. Smith, entomologist at the North Carolina State Agricultural station, says:

"Formalin is a very successful poison for flies in spite of many reports to the contrary. I have recently used it extensively with excellent results. The method which I have found most successful is the use of formalin in milk with the following proportions:

"One ounce (two tablespoonfuls) of formalin:

"Sixteen ounces (one pint) of equal parts milk and water.

"In this proportion the mixture seems to attract flies much better than when used in scwetened water. The mixture should be exposed in shallow plates. A piece of bread in the middle of the plate furnishes more space for the flies to alight and in this way serves to attract a greater number of them."

PERSONAL AND GENERAL NEWS

Dr. C. L. Hill, Haskell, is moving to Muskogee.

Dr. L. W. Cotton, Enid, is visiting New York for special work.

Dr. C. H. Lockwood, Medford, is doing special work in Chicago.

Dr. J. J. Fraley, Hominy, is the new president of the city council.

Dr. Z. J. Clark, Cherokee, is attending the clinics of New York City.

Dr. G. M. Clifton, Norman, has been appointed health officer of Cleveland County.

Dr. W. R. Leverton, Hobart, has been discharged from army service and resumed his old location.

Dr. W. G. Brymer, located at Dewar for many years, is preparing to locate in San Antonio, Texas.

Dr. C. J. Brunson, Adamson, who recently returned from overseas service is preparing to locate at McAlester.

Dr. J. N. Shaunty, Eufaula, has returned from overseas service and awaits discharge at Camp Zachary Taylor.

Dr. M. K. Thompson, Muskogee, was elected by an overwhelming majority to the school board, after a bitter fight.

Dr. Ross D. Long, Oklahoma City, has been discharged from the army and is doing special work in New York City.

Dr. J. J. Dial, Muskogee, is returning to his old location in Texas, Sulhpur Springs. Dr. Dial has resided in Muskogee for several years.

Dr. H. M. Stricklen, Tonkawa, has received his discharge from the army, and returned to his old location. He has just been appointed health officer of Kay County.

Dr. Walton H. McKinzie, Enid, has been appointed health officer of Garfield County, a position he formerly held. His many friends over the state are gratified at his appointment.

Dr. L. B. Oldham, Muskogee, visited Alabama in May to attend graduation exercises of his daughters. He says interstate "Hard Surfaced Roads" appeal to him. He used an automobile for the trip.

Dr. D. Armstrong, Durant, has been appointed health officer of Bryan County. Dr. Armstrong is one of the good men of southern Oklahoma, and one of our best secretaries. Bryan county will not suffer in its health administration.

McAlester is to have a health survey. On the suggestion of the Lion's Club the Pittsburg County Medical Society selected Drs. R. K. Pemberton, J. A. Smith and W. C. Graves to investigate all matters affecting public health affairs.

Major W. P. Lipscomb, M. C., U. S. A., who is in France with the 36th Division, writes the Journal he expects soon to be discharged, after which he will spend a year in New York in eye, ear, nose and throat work and then return to his home in Oklahoma City

The Victor Electric Company emerged with flying colors and complete exoneration after an extended hearing before the Federal Trade Commission, which handed down its decision in Washington March 10th. It was charged that in purchasing certain businesses necessary to the proper conduct of the Victor Company a violation of the law, more technical than practical, had been made. A thorough investigation by the United States authorities refutes the charge which was dismissed to the credit of the company.

WILLIAM C. HIGH.

Dr. William C. High of Maysville died in Temple, Texas, May 5, 1919, after an illness of many months superinduced by the excessive demands made upon him as a consequence of the epidemic of 1918 which he attempted to make, eventually paying the penalty of death. A resident of Oklahoma for years prior to statehood in that part of Indian Territory now known as Carter County, he moved to Maysville in 1903.

Dr. High was born in Canton, Texas, March 19, 1870, obtained medical education at Memphis, Dallas and Ft. Worth, later doing special work in New Orleans. He has been a member of our Association since organization. He is survived by a wife at Ardmore and two sons. Interment was made at Ardmore under Masonic auspices.

Dr. T. F. Harrison, Wewoka, has been appointed health officer of Seminole County, vice Dr. M. M. Turlington. Dr. Turlington, it will be remembered, is the physician once elected to the Legislature who never appeared or qualified as a lawmaker, stating that the needy sick of his county needed him more than the law making body.

Dr. W. L. Kendall, Enid, former superintendent of the State School for Feeble Minded Children, was awarded a verdict of twelve thousand five hundred dollars against the Oklahoma Publishing Company, Oklahoma City. The suit grew out of articles appearing in certain Oklahoma City papers during the last legislature, in which charges of various mismanagement, etc., were alleged against Dr. Kendall.

Medical Men of War Organized. Under suggestions from the American Medical Association and Dr. Hubert Work, President of the House of Delegates of that body, who served in Washington throughout the war on the Staff of the Provost Marshal-General, Oklahoma physicians eligible to membership perfected a tempory organization at the Muskogee meeting. Dr. L. S. Willour, McAlester, Major, M. C., U. S. A., was selected President. Dr. S. J. Fryer, Muskogee, Captain, M. C., U. S. A., selected secretary. Dr. Rex Bolend, Oklahoma City, Captain, M. C., U. S. A., was selected Treasurer. A very respectable number of former medical officers of the Army and Navy, members of local and advisory boards, applied for membership to the body. A permanent organization will be further perfected at the annual meeting of the A. M. A. at Atlantic City, June 9-13.

DISCHARGES FROM THE ARMY.

Rex Bolend, Oklahoma City	R. D. Long, Oklahoma City
J. H. Sanford, Muskogee	R. V. Smith, Tulsa.
J. M. Bonham, Hobart	A. N. Lerskov, Claremore
W. G. Lemmon, Tulsa	Carl Puckett, Pryor

STATE HOSPITAL ORGANIZATION.

A State hospital organization was organized at the Muskogee meeting under the auspices of the State Committee on Hospitals, Drs. F. S. Clinton, Tulsa; M. Smith, Oklahoma City, and C. A. Thompson, Muskogee, ex-officio member. A banquet was tendered the body by Dr. Clinton at which the following subjects were presented: Object of the Meeting, F. S. Clinton, Oklahoma Hospital; Hospital Standardization, F. K. Camp, Wesley Hospital; Minimum Requirements of Case Records, LeRoy Long, Oklahoma University Hospital; Hospitals as Health Centers, J. A. Hatchett, El Reno Sanitarium; The Doctors' Part, V. Berry, Okmulgee Hospital; The Hospital's Part, A. S. Risser, Blackwell Hospital; Laboratory Requirements of a General Hospital, Equipment and Management, M. Smith, St. Anthony's Hospital; Let's Go, Sessler Hoss, P. and S. Hospital, Muskogee.

Officers elected were: President, F. S. Clinton, Tulsa; 1st vice president, J. A. Hatchett, El Reno; second vice-president, A. S. Risser, Blackwell; Executive secretary, Paul Fessler, Oklahoma City; Treasurer, Sessler Hoss, Muskogee. Mr. Fessler was selected to attend the American Hospital Association as delegate. The object of the organization is to standardize Oklahoma Hospitals in every respect.

MISCELLANEOUS

MALARIA.

C. C. Bass, New Orleans (*Journal A. M. A.*, April 26, 1919), describes the treatment of malaria-infected persons, adopted in Bolivar and Sunflower counties, Miss., after three years' observation in an attempt to learn the most effectual and practical method, as follows: "The treatment for adults is 10 grains of quinin sulphate every night before retiring for a period of eight weeks. For children the dose that gives the same results as 10 grains in adults is: under 1 year, 1-2 grain; 1 year, 1 grain;

2 years, 2 grains; 3 and 4 years, 3 grains; 5, 6, and 7 years, 4 grains; 8, 9, and 10 years, 6 grains; 11, 12, 13 and 14 years, 8 grains; 15 years or older, 10 grains. The 6, 8 and 10 grain doses are best administered in the form of two tablets (or if preferred, capsules), containing 3, 4 or 5 grains each. The smaller doses are best administered in aromatic syrup of yerba santa (syrupus eriodictyi aromaticus, N. F.), so prepared that one teaspoonful contains the required dose." The patient should be advised to omit no doses, as the treatment must be continuous for the full term of eight weeks. Those with acute attacks of malaria should be given one dose of 10 grains, or a proportionate dose for children, three times a day for three or four days, which relieves the acute symptoms, and then the eight weeks' treatment will eliminate the infection. The treatment described will disinfect 90 per cent. of the cases. To disinfect the whole would require three months or over. Some persons require much longer treatment than others. If there are indications that the carrier is of that type, the eight weeks' treatment should be extended without waiting for a relapse. A malaria carrier is liable to relapse at any time, and with the varying methods used by different physicians few victims are actually and thoroughly disinfected. Quinin and its other similar alkaloids are the only remedy for malaria, and the sulphate is as good as any. The administration by mouth is the only method to be considered. Bass advises those who give it hypodermically to take a few doses themselves, which will quiet their enthusiasm for that method. The daily continuous administration is much better than the intermittent treatment for a few days each week, though some hold the contrary opinion.

T. A. B.

Typhoid fever, which has a record of disabling ten per cent of the personnel of armies in cam-. paigns, is no longer a disease which needs to be reckoned with by our military authorities. By the simple expedient of three hypodermic injections into the arm of each soldier the menace of this disease has been entirely eliminated. It is obvious that if every person outside the army could be induced to submit to the same treatment the disease would just as quickly disappear from civil life.

There is just one measure—and that an extremely simple one—by which the menace of typhoid fever may be entirely removed, and that is prophylactic vaccination.

It was in 1912, after careful study of the subject, that the Mulford laboratories first advocated the use of the Triple Typhoid Bacterin or Vaccine (Typhoid, Paratyphoid "A" and Paratyphoid "B") now commonly known as TAB. The use of Triple Typhoid Vaccine in the armies has since become universal.

The Mulford Laboratories have also made available "sensitized" vaccine or "serobacterin," in which the suspended bacilli have been acted upon by their own immune serum. The chief advantage of the sensitized vaccines or serobacterins lies in the fact that they bring about the immune state more rapidly than do the plain or unsensitized bacterins—and this is an extremely important point in civil communities in the midst of epidemics—and, as a rule, the local and general reactions following their use are milder than those following the use of unsensitized bacterins. When serobacterins are used it is therefore possible to administer twice the number of killed bacteria used in the unsensitized bacterins.

EMPYEMA.

Empyema as observed at Camp Mills, L. I., is discussed by H. B. Phillips, A. G. Langman, and C. L. Mix, Camp Mills, Garden City, L. I. (*Journal A. M. A.*, May 3, 1919). The successful treatment of empyema depends on a recognition of the basic pathology of the condition. Unlike pus collections elsewhere in the body, adequate drainage is not the only essential. The indications for the most successful treatment are the establishment of adequate drainage together with the recognition and exclusion of atmospheric pressure. They give a summary of a previous preliminary report by Philips on the efficacy of adequate and continuous drainage, and describe the special apparatus, the cannula, bottle, negative-pressure manometer, and connecting rubber tubing. The cannula is of a special construction to be used as a trocar cannula for the thoracotomy, and to be also nonobstructible, remaining in the chest wall until the empyema sac has been obliterated by firm adhesions. The advantages are numerous, the control over the negative pressure assures against primary collapse of the lung. There was no respiratory impairment. The lung could be kept expanded, and the original dressing was the only one; also the duration of treatment was much reduced. They refer to the original article in describing the methods used in fifty cases of empyema. The Philips apparatus was not available at the beginning of the treatment, and they had to make repeated aspirations with aseptic technic in the earlier cases, striving to keep atmospheric air from the pleural sac during the puncture and resorting in the cases to either intracostal drainage or the rib-resection operation. The cases are divided into four groups: first, those treated by simply repeated aspirations, which method is not favorably spoken of. The contraindications are thus deducted: "1. The character of the exudate such that it obstructs the cannula or needle. 2. Absence of improvement following this treatment. 3. The appearance of a complication pneumothorax, following aspirations. 4. Severe toxemia of the patient." The second group, treated by intercostal drainage, consisted of ten cases, with a mortality of 30 per cent., none of the cases being complicated with actual pneumonia. These cases all showed the disadvantages of open pneumothorax in addition to those of inadequate drainage. There were twelve cases treated by rib resection. The impressions given by this group indicate that the postponement of the operation makes it easier for the patient and the operation less risky. This advantage, however, seems to be paid for in convalescence time, the adhesions forming in the partially collapsed lung and enhancing the chronicity. Sixteen cases were treated with the Philips apparatus. Seven of them had coincident complicating pneumonia, of whom five died, through the treatment seemed to prolong their lives. At this time the majority of cases have been too short a time under this treatment to speak of their final termination. In none of the cases has there been any open pneumothorax observed, nor any signs of shock or respiratory embarrassment after the application of the apparatus. Leakage occurred in but two of these cases, due to the patients' delirium; but this did not occur until after a five days' continuous expansion of the lung in one case, and eight days' expansion in the other. The most prominent facts noted with the apparatus are summarized as follows: "1. Complete expansion of the lung was secured in an average of three days after application of the apparatus. 2. The mortality of the straightforward cases of empyema has been *nil.* 3. A large pneumothorax is exceedingly improbable (not encountered in our experience); and the open pneumothorax and all its dangers, so thoroughly and carefully considered and cautioned against by Graham and Bell, is impossible after the apparatus has been applied only a few days, for by this time the lung has been considerably expanded and a good part of it has become adherent to the chest wall in its expanded condition. 4. The duration of empyema, as such, is very materially shortened." The advantages of the apparatus are enumerated in detail, all the improvements observed being mentioned. Atmospheric pressure is excluded and the necessity for operation is done away with. Secondary infection is also excluded. The duration of treatment is shortened, and a functionating lung is obtained from the start, while a clean, sanitary, pleasing, economical and simple method gets rid of the pus. Repeated aspiration as a curative procedure is in most cases not feasible, and as a palliative measure usually permits pneumothorax to occur. Intercostal drainage is impossible without this complication, according to their experience, and rib resection is the preferable operation when the apparatus is not available. Too much must not be expected of the apparatus, but it is valuable if it only lessens mortality. It cannot prevent the formation of a pneumothorax from within if there is a leak from a bronchial tube, which, however, is not a frequent cause. Neither can it prevent the intoxication of the patient by absorption. Some cases of *Streptococcus hemolyticus* infection rapidly become extremely septic and fatal before drainage can help. It is a mistake to think that all cases can be cured by immediate and continuous drainage, but with the above-mentioned limitations the usefulness of the Philips apparatus has been amply demonstrated.

"PROCAINE", A NEW FREE BOOKLET WHICH MAY BE HAD FOR THE ASKING.

"Procaine for Local Anesthesia in Surgery, the Specialties, and Operative Dentistry" is the title of a new booklet by Dr. F. H. McMechan, Editor of the American Yearbook of Anesthesia and Analgesia. It is an editorial abstract of a series of articles on local anesthesia prepared by Doctor McMechan, and presents in simple, boiled down, yet detailed style the advantages of Procaine over other local anesthetics; the various solutions and combinations used and how to prepare them from marketed products; indications and contraindications; and the technic for its use in spinal, sacral, venous, ophthalmic, rhinolaryngologic, and dental anesthesia. A number of excellent illustrations add to its value.

This booklet may be had *free* by any physician, hospital superintendent, surgeon or dentist sending his request to The Abbott Laboratories, 4757 Ravenswood Avenue, Chicago, Ill. Everyone who secures it will find it distinctly worth while.

The Abbott Laboratories are making Procaine under license from the Federal Trade Commission and supplying it in standard market packages under the well-known guarantee of purity and accuracy.

PNEUMOTHORAX

B. P. Stivelman and Joseph Rosenblatt, Bedford Hills, N. Y. (*Journal A. M. A.*, May 17, 1919), report two cases of pneumothorax showing a characteristic protrusion of the distended pleural sac into the untreated side. The observation was confirmed by roentgenoscopy as well as by physical signs. The cause of such protrusion in pneumothorax is explained by the meeting of the two pleurae opposite the second and third ribs, anteriorly, in the median line. The degree of displacement of the mediastinum was rather marked in both of these cases. The most important factors, the authors say, that facilitate mediastinal displacement are absence of pleural and pleuropericardial adhesions, and the distensibility of the ligaments that hold it in place. Both patients were young adults, and these factors are more liable to exist in such than in older persons. The article is illustrated.

ROSTER OF MEMBERS OF COUNTY SOCIETIES, 1919.

ADAIR COUNTY

Beard, D. A._____Westville
Beard, J. H._____Watts
Berry, F. O._____Westville
Chambers, D. P._____Stilwell
Collins, B. F._____Nowata
Evans, S. R._____Stilwell
Goldberg, B. C._____Watts
Medearis, P. H._____Tahlequah
Patton, J. A._____Stilwell
Robinson, J. A._____Westville
Sands, A. J._____Oklahoma City
Sellers, R. L._____Westville
Williams, T. S._____Stilwell

ALFALFA COUNTY

Ames, H. B._____Burlington
Clark, A. J._____Cherokee
Evans, M. T._____Aline
Frasier, E. A._____Jet
Hibbard, J. S._____Cherokee
Lile, H. A._____Aline
Ludlum, E. C._____Carmen
Rhodes, T. A._____Cherokee
Tucker, J. M._____Carmen

ATOKA COUNTY

Briggs, T. H._____Atoka
Fulton, J. S._____Atoka
Gardner, C. C._____Atoka

BECKHAM COUNTY

Edmonds, R. L._____Foss
Lee, I. A._____Erick
McComas, J. M._____Elk City
Palmer, T. D._____Elk City
M. Shadid_____Carter
Speed, H. K._____Sayre
Standifer, J. E._____Elk City
Steel, J. M._____Berlin
Tisdal, V. C._____Elk City
Warford, J. D._____Erick
Windle, O. N._____Sayre
Yarbrough, J. E._____Erick

BLAINE COUNTY

Barnett, J. S._____Hithcock
Browning, J. W._____Geary
Buchanan, M. W._____Watonga
Buchanan, F. R._____Canton
Doty, H. W._____Watonga
Green, G. T._____Drumright
Griffin, W. F._____Greenfield
Hamble, V. R._____Homestead
Krebs, H. M._____Eagle City
Leisure, J. B._____Watonga
Milligan, E. F._____Geary
Murdoch, L. H._____Okeene
Norris, J. A._____Okeene
Padberg, A. F._____Canton
Stough, D. F._____Geary

BRYAN COUNTY

Allen, J. R._____Caddo
Armstrong, D._____Durant
Austin, J. L._____Durant
Bates, J. A._____Coalgate
Bates, C. W._____Atoka

Durham, J. H._____Durant
Fuston, H. B._____Bokchito
Gray, M._____Durant
Green, J. C._____Durant
Griffith, J. K._____Kemp
Haynie, J. A._____Durant
Jackman, F. M._____Mead
Kay, J. H._____Durant
Keller, J. R._____Calera
McCarley, W. H._____Colbert
McCalib, D. C._____Utica
McKinney, H. B._____Durant
Mullenix, C. S._____Roberta
Rains, W. S._____Platter
Rappolee, H. E._____Caddo
Reynolds, J. L._____Durant
Richardson, W. F._____Colbert
Sawyer, R. F._____Durant
Shuler, Jas. L._____Durant
Wells, A. J._____Calera
Yeats, H. W._____Durant
Yeiser, C. C._____Colbert

CADDO COUNTY

Anderson, P. H._____Anadarko
Blair, S._____Apache
Bird, Jesse_____Cement
Brown, B. D._____Apache
Bryan, J. R._____Cogar
Campbell, S. T._____Anadarko
Cannon, R. S._____Hydro
Cantrell, J. H._____Carnegie
Chambers, Claude S._____Anadarko
Coker, Geo. B._____Cyril
Dinkler, F._____Ft. Cobb
Downs, E. W._____Hinton
Edens, M. H._____Anadarko
Hawn, W. T._____Binger
Henke, J. J._____Hydro
Hobbo, A. F._____Hinton
Hume, Chas. R._____Anadarko
Johnston, R. E._____Bridgeport
Kerley, W. W._____Anadarko
Lane, C. W._____Okanogon, Wash.
McClure, P. L._____Ft. Cobb
McMillan, Chas. B._____Gracemont
Myers, P. B._____Apache
Padberg, J. W._____Carnegie
Putnam, Claude E._____Eakly
Putnam, W. B._____Carnegie
Rector, R. D._____Anadarko
Rogers, W. F._____Carnegie
Sanders, P. I._____Bremerton, Wash.
Smith, C. A._____Hinton
Smith, R. Earle_____Gracemont
Taylor, A. H._____Anadarko
Wheeler, J. W._____Gracemont
Willard, A. J._____Cyril
Williams, S. E._____Hydro
Williams, R. W._____Anadarko

CANADIAN COUNTY

Aderhold, T. M._____El Reno
Arnold, C. D._____El Reno
Brown, H. C._____Okarche
Catto, W. B._____El Reno
Clark, F. H._____El Reno

CANADIAN COUNTY (Continued)

Dever, H. A._____El Reno
Hatchett, J. A._____El Reno
Herod, Phil. F._____El Reno
Lane, Thos._____El Reno
Lynde, L. W._____Okarche
Miller, W. R._____Ponca City
Muzzy, W. J._____El Reno
Richardson, D. P._____Union City
Riley, Jas. T._____El Reno
Ruhl, N. E._____Piedmont
Runkle, R. E._____El Reno
Sanger, S. S._____Yukon
Taylor, G. W._____El Reno
Wolff, L. G._____Okarche

CARTER COUNTY

Alexander, M. S._____Healdton
Amerson, Geo. W._____Milo
Barker, E. R._____Healdton
Barnwell, J. T._____Graham
Best, Jesse C._____Ardmore
Boadway, F. W._____Ardmore
Booth, T. S._____Ardmore
Cameron, J. H._____Healdton
Cantrell, D. E._____Healdton
Cox, J. L._____Ardmore
Cowles, A. G._____Ardmore
Denham, T. W._____Ardmore
Dowdy, Thomas W._____New Wilson
Early, R. O._____Ardmore
Fox, U. R._____Ardmore
Gillespie, L. D._____Berwyn
Goodwin, G. E._____Ardmore
Gregory, David A._____Ardmore
Hardy, Walter_____Ardmore
Hathaway, W. G._____Pooleville
Henry, Robt. H._____Ardmore
Higgins, H. A._____Springer
von Keller, F. P.____Ardmore
Martin, J. A._____Ranger, Texas
McRae, J. P._____Coalgate
McNees, J. C._____Ardmore
Shelton, J. W._____Ardmore
Smith, J. H._____Healdton
Sullivan, C. F._____Ardmore
Taylor, Dow_____Woodford
Ware, T. H._____Okmulgee
Willard, Robt. S.____Ardmore

CHOCTAW COUNTY

Askew, E. R._____Hugo
Chambliss, T. L._____Soper
Clark, J. L._____Hugo
Gee, R. L._____Hugo
Fling, P. E. A. (deceased)____Hugo
Hampton, K. P._____Soper
Hale, C. H._____Boswell
John, W. N._____Hugo
Marsh, G. O._____Ft. Towson
McPherson, V. L._____Boswell
Miller, J. S._____Hugo
Moore, J. D._____Hugo
Oliver, W. M._____Boswell
Shull, R. J._____Hugo
Swearingen, C. H.____Hugo
White, H. H._____Hugo
Wolf, Reed._____Hugo
Yeargan, W. M._____Soper

CLEVELAND COUNTY

Bobo, C. S._____Norman
Boyd, T. M._____Norman
Clifton, G. M._____Norman
Day, J. L._____Norman
Ellison, Gayfree____Norman
Gable, J. J._____Norman
Grady, C. W._____Norman
Graham, S. H._____Norman
Griffin, D. W._____Norman
Hargrove, R. M.____Norman
Lambert, J. B._____Lexington
Lowther, R. D._____Norman
McLaughlin, J. R.__Norman
McClure, J. B._____Norman
Melton, J. W._____Shamrock
Northcutt, C. E.____Lexington
Thacker, R. E._____Lexington
Thurlow, A. A._____Norman
Torrey, J. P._____Norman
Williams, J. M.____Norman

CHEROKEE COUNTY

Allison, T. P._____Sand Springs
Allison, J. S._____Tahlequah
Baird, A. A._____Park Hill
Blake, W. G._____Tahlequah
Duckett, B. J._____Hulbert
Duckworth, J. F.____Tahlequah
Hill, Israel_____Gideon
McCurry, L. E._____Tahlequah
Morrow, B. L._____Salina
Thompson, Jos. M.__Tahlequah

CUSTER COUNTY

Boyd, T. A._____Weatherford
Clohessy, T. T.____Clinton
Comer, M. C._____Clinton
Davis, S. C._____Oklahoma City
Gordon, J. Matt.__Weatherford
Gore, Victor M.____Clinton
Gossam, K. D._____Custer
Jeter, A. J._____Clinton
Lamb, Ellis_____Clinton
McBurney, C. H.____Clinton
McCullah, Robert__Arapaho
Murray, P. G._____Thomas
Parker, O. H._____Custer City
Parker, W. W._____Thomas
Omer, William J.__Thomas
Rogers, McLain____Clinton
Williams, J. J.____Weatherford

COMANCHE COUNTY

Angus, H. A._____Lawton
Baird, Chas. W.____Lawton
Barber, Geo. S.____Lawton
Broshear, Jackson__Lawton
Dunlap, P. G._____Lawton
Dunlap, E. B._____Lawton
Gamble, J. F._____Fletcher
Gooch, L. T._____Lawton
Gooch, E. S._____Lawton
Hammond, F. W.____Lawton
Harned, W. B._____Chattanooga
Hood, J. R._____Indiahoma
Hues, J. T._____Lawton
Joyce, Chas. W.____Fletcher
Janney, J. G._____A. E. F.
Kerr, G. E._____Chattanooga
Knee, Loren C.____Lawton
Malcolm, John W.__Lawton

COMANCHE COUNTY (Continued)

Martin, Chas. M._____Elgin
Mason, W. J._____Lawton
Mead, W. B._____Lawton
Milne, L. A._____Lawton
Mitchell, E. Brent_____Lawton
Myers, D. A._____Lawton
Perisho, J. Allen_____Cache
Rosenherger, F. E._____Lawton
Shoemaker, Ferdinand_____Lawton
Stewart, A. H._____Lawton

COAL COUNTY

Bates, Frank_____Coalgate
Blount, W. G._____Tupelo
Brown, W. E._____Lehigh
Cates, Albert_____Tupelo
Clark, J. B._____Coalgate
Conner, L. A._____Coalgate
Cody, R. D._____Centrahoma
Goben, H. G._____Lehigh
Hill, R. M. C._____Coalgate
Hipes, J. J._____Phillips
Logan, W. A._____Lehigh
Nelson, J. A._____Centrahoma
Rushing, F. E._____Coalgate
Rutherford, H. P._____Clarita
Sadler, F. E._____Coalgate
Wallace, W. B._____Coalgate

COTTON COUNTY

Dice, R. J._____Randlett
Holsted, A. B._____Temple
House, C. F._____Hastings

CRAIG COUNTY

Adams, F. M._____Vinita
Bagby, Louis_____Vinita
Bell, C. P._____Welch
Bradshaw, J. O._____Welch
Campbell, W. M._____Vinita
Cornwell, N. L._____Bluejacket
Craig, J. W._____Vinita
Hays, P. L._____Vinita
Herron, A. W._____Vinita
Hughson, F. L._____Vinita
Jackson, W. W._____Vinita
Johnson, H. Lee_____Vinita
Marks, W. R._____Vinita
Mitchell, R. L._____Vinita
Morgan, E. A._____Vinita
Neer, C. S._____Vinita
O'Leary, D. W._____Welch
Pickens, F. A._____Grove
Staples, J. H. L._____Bluejacket
Stough, D. B._____Vinita
Walker, Chas. F._____Grove

CREEK COUNTY

Avery, Amos_____Sapulpa
Bone, Wade J._____Sapulpa
Conger, D. W._____Mounds
Coppedge, O. C._____Bristow
Coppedge, O. S._____Depew
Croston, G. C._____Sapulpa
Fry, Melvin_____Drumright
Garland, H. S._____Sapulpa
Haas, H. R._____Sapulpa
Harris, Ben C._____Sapulpa
Hoover, J. W._____Sapulpa
Izgur, Leon_____Drumright
King, E. W._____Bristow

Longmire, W. P._____Sapulpa
Neal, Wm. J._____Drumright
Newman, M. H._____Oklahoma City
Mattenlee, J. M._____Sapulpa
Reese, C. B._____Sapulpa
Reynolds, E. W._____Bristow
Reynolds, S. W._____Drumright
Schrader, Chas. T._____Bristow
Schwab, B. C._____Sapulpa
Smith, L. L._____Sapulpa
Stafford, G. S._____Kiefer
Sweeney, R. M._____Sapulpa
Taylor, Z. G._____Mounds
Wells, J. M._____Bristow
Wheeler, F. R._____Mannford

DEWEY COUNTY

Allen, F. W._____Leedy
Saba, W. E._____Leedy

GARFIELD COUNTY

Aitken, W. A._____Enid
Baker, J. W._____Enid
Barnes, J. H._____Enid
Bishop, H. P._____Carrier
Bitting, B. T._____Enid
Boyle, Geo. A._____Enid
Bunker, L. L._____Enid
Cotton, Lee W._____Enid
Davis, Frank P.____Enid
Field, Julian_____Enid
Francisco, Glenn____Enid
Francisco, J. W.___Enid
Freisen, Julius____Enid
Gill, W. W._____Ringwood
Hays, Jas. H.____Enid
Harris, D. S.____Drummond
Hinson, T. B.___Enid
Huddleson, J. W.__Enid
Hudson, F. A.____Enid
Kelso, M. A._____Enid
Kendall, W. L.___Enid
Lamerton, W. E.__Enid
Looper, S. A.____Enid
Mahoney, J. E.___Enid
Mayberry, S. N.__Enid
McKee, E. N.____Enid
McInnis, A. L.___Enid
McMahon, A. M.__Hilldale
Newell, W. B.___Hunter
Piper, A. S.____Enid
Rhodes, Wm. H.__Enid
Smithe, P. A.___Enid
Stone, Roy D.___Covington
Swank, J. R.___Enid
Thompson, C. E.__Enid
Vandiver, H. F.__Lahoma
Wilkins, A. E.__Covington
Wolff, E. J.___Waukomis

GARVIN COUNTY

Branum, T. C._____Pauls Valley
Callaway, J. R._____Pauls Valley
Callaway, J. R._____Marfa, Texas
Erwin, J. O._____Ashland
Gaddy, Lewis_____Stratford
*High, W. C._____Maysville
Hoover, A. J._____Paoli
Johnson, G. L._____Pauls Valley
Keever, A. P._____Lindsay
Lain, E. H._____Paoli
Lindsay, J. K._____Elmore City
*Deceased

GARVIN COUNTY (Continued)

Lindsay, N. H._____Pauls Valley
Matheney, J. C._____Lindsay
Markham, H. P._____Pauls Valley
McDaniel, W. B._____Maysville
Mitchell, C. P._____Lindsay
Morgan, J. B._____Foster
Norvell, E. E._____Wynnewood
Polk, W. T._____Maysville
Pratt, C. M._____Pauls Valley
Ralston, B. W._____Lindsay
Robinson, A. J._____Pauls Valley
Robberson, M. E._____Brady
Settles, W. E._____Wynnewood
Shannon, J. B._____Pauls Valley
Spangler, A. S._____Pauls Valley
Sullivan, C. L._____Elmore City
Sullivan, E._____Oklahoma City
Tucker, J. W._____Purdy
Webster, M. M._____Stratford
Wilson, H. P._____Wynnewood
Wilson, S. W._____Lindsay
Young, J. A._____Maysville

GRADY COUNTY

Antle, H. C._____Chickasha
Ambrister, J. C._____Chickasha
Baze, R. J._____Chickasha
Baze, W. J._____Chickasha
Barry, W. R._____Bradley
Bonnell, Wm. L._____Chickasha
Boone, U. C._____Chickasha
Bledsoe, Martha_____Chickasha
Cook, W. H._____Chickasha
Cox, C. P._____Ninnekah
Dawson, E. L._____Chickasha
Downey, D. S._____Chickasha
Emanuel, L. E._____Chickasha
Fuller, T._____Amber
Ganes, Frank M._____Verden
Gerard, G. R._____Ninnekah
Hampton, P. J._____Rush Springs
Hume, R. R._____Minco
Leeds, A. B._____Chickasha
Little, J. S._____Minco
Livermore, W. H._____Chickasha
Marrs, S. O._____Chickasha
Masters, H. C._____Minco
Renegar, J. F._____Minco
Shaw, R. M._____Alex
Stinson, J. E._____Chickasha
White, A. C._____Chickasha
Winborn, L. H._____Tuttle

GRANT COUNTY

Hardy, I. V._____Medford
Lockwood, C. H._____Medford
Martin, J. T._____Deer Creek
Saffold, B. W._____Gibbon

GREER COUNTY

Austin, C. W._____Brinkman
Border, G. F._____Mangum
Bray, G. T._____Reed
Cherry, G. P._____Mangum
Dawson, W. D._____Henryetta
Dodson, W. O._____Willow
Jeter, O. R._____Brinkman
Lansden, J. B._____Granite
Mabry, E. W._____Mangum
McGregor, Frank H._____Mangum
Merridith, J. S._____Duke

Neel, Ney_____Mangum
Nunnery, T. J._____Granite
Pierson, L. E._____Camp Pike, Ark
Poer, E. M._____Jester
Wiley, G. W._____Granite
Willis, T. L._____Granite

HARMON COUNTY

Collins, C. E._____Gould
Jones, J. E._____Hollis
Patrick, J. B._____Vinson
Pendergraft, W. C._____Hollis
Pendergraft, R. L._____Hollis
Ray, W. T._____Gould

HASKELL COUNTY

Billington, J. E._____Enterprise
Davis, John_____Stigler
Gilliam, W. C._____Spiro
Hill, A. K._____Stigler
Johnson, Emmett_____Kinta
Van Matre, M._____Keota
Mayfield, T. B._____Britton
Mitchell, S. E._____Stigler
McDonald, J. W._____Brooken
Terrell, R. F._____Stigler
Thomas, Ernest_____Quinton
Turner, T. B._____Stigler
Waltrip, J. R._____Kinta

HUGHES COUNTY

Felix, T. B._____Holdenville
Hicks, C. A._____Wetumka
Hicks, Fred B._____Wetumka
Mitchell, P. E._____Wetumka
McCary, D. Y._____Holdenville
Scott, Hugh_____Holdenville

JACKSON COUNTY

Abernethy, E. A._____Altus
Brown, R. F._____Headrick
Buck, D. C._____Eldorado
Clarkson, William H._____Blair
Crow, E. S._____Olustee
Hardin, T. H._____Elmer
Hix, J. B._____Altus
Hyde, R. H._____Eldorado
Lowe, J. T._____Blair
McCray, J. W._____Martha
McConnell, L. H._____Altus
Miles, E. P._____Hobart
Rudell, W. P._____Altus
Rutland, W. H._____Altus
Sanderson, W. E._____Altus
Spears, C. G._____Altus
Strother, S. P._____Holdenville
Stults, J. S._____Olustee
Taylor, H. R._____Eldorado

JEFFERSON COUNTY

Ashinhurst, T. E._____Waurika
Browning, W. M._____Waurika
Collins, D. B._____Sugden
Cranfill, A. C._____Grady
Derr, J. I._____Waurika
Edwards, F. M._____Ringling
Lewis, A. R._____Oklahoma City
Maupin, C. M._____Waurika
Shankle, H. D._____Hartshorne
Stephens, J. M._____Hastings
Sutherland, L. B._____Ringling
Wade, L. I._____Ryan
Wilton, G. C._____Ryan

JOHNSTON COUNTY

Cottrell, W. P.------------------------Milburn
Booth, J. E.--------------------------Mill Creek
Clark, Guy.---------------------------Milburn
Crocker, A. S.------------------------Tishomingo
Ellis, J. M.--------------Mt. Pleasant, Texas
Kniseley, H. B.-----------------------Tishomingo
Looney, J. T.------------------------Tishomingo
Stobaugh, F. B.----------------------Mannsville
White, F. A.--------------------------Wapanuka

KAY COUNTY

Barker, C. J.------------------------Kaw City
Bishop, H. H.-----------------------Dilworth
Gearheart, A. P.---------------------Blackwell
Gowey, H. O.------------------------Newkirk
Havens, A. R.-----------------------Blackwell
Hawkins, J. C.----------------------Blackwell
Johnson, W. M.---------------------Peckham
Jones, J. A.-------------------------Tonkawa
Lively, M. M.-----------------------Blackwell
Lowery, Allen-----------------------Blackwell
Martin, W. M.----------------------Blackwell
McCullough, S. S.------------------Braman
Miller, D. W.-----------------------Blackwell
Newlon, B. F.----------------------Ponca City
Nieman, G. H.----------------------Ponca City
Nuckols, A. S.----------------------Ponca City
Orvis, E. J.------------------------Blackwell
Risser, A. S.------------------------Blackwell
Robertson, W. A. T.---------------Ponca City
Waggoner, E. E.--------------------Tonkawa
Walker, I. D.-----------------------Blackwell
Woll, J. C.-------------------------Tonkawa

KINGFISHER COUNTY

Cavett, E. R.-----------------------Loyal
Dixon, A.---------------------------Hennessey
Fisk, C. W.-------------------------Kingfisher
Gose, C. O.-------------------------Hennessey
Meredith, A. O.--------------------Kingfisher
Overstreet, J. A.-------------------Kingfisher
Pendleton, J. W.-------------------Kingfisher
Rector, Newton--------------------Hennessey
Scott, Frank.-----------------------Kingfisher
Share, A. L.------------------------Kingfisher
Wagner, C. E.----------------------Hennessey

KIOWA COUNTY

Barkley, A.-------------------------Hobart
Bonham, J. M.----------------------Hobart
Bryce, J. R.------------------------Snyder
Dobson, A. T.----------------------Hobart
Hamilton, J. T.---------------------Snyder
Hathaway, A.-----------------------Mt. View
Land, J. A.-------------------------Lone Wolf
Leverton, W. R.-------------------Hobart
Martin, F. F.-----------------------Roosevelt
McIlwain, W.----------------------Lone Wolf
Miller, W. W.----------------------Gotebo
Muller, J. A.-----------------------Snyder
Stewart, G. W.---------------------Hobart
Watkins, B. H.---------------------Gotebo
Weeden, A. J.----------------------Mt. View

LATIMER COUNTY

Dalby, H. L.-----------------------Wilburton
Evins, E. L.------------------------Wilburton
Henry, T. L.------------------------Wilburton
Kilpatrick, G. A.-------------------Wilburton

Morrison, C. R.---------------------Wilburton
McArthur, J. F.---------------------Wilburton
Munn, J. A.------------------------Wilburton
Rich, R. L.--------------------------Red Oak
Talley, I. C.------------------------Red Oak

LE FLORE COUNTY

Billingsley, C. B.-------------------Cowlington
Booth, G. R.------------------------LeFlore
Campbell, E. A.--------------------Heavener
Collins, E. L.-----------------------Panama
Dean, S. C.-------------------------Howe
Doler, Calhoun---------------------Bokoshe
Duff, W. M.------------------------Braden
Fair, E. N.--------------------------Hodgens
Fowler, J. D.-----------------------Heavener
Harbour, J. T.----------------------Cowlington
Hardy, Harrell---------------------Poteau
Hardy, J. J.-------------------------Poteau
Hartshorne, W. O.-----------------Spiro
Mahar, C. H.-----------------------Spiro
McClaine, W. Z.-------------------Heavener
Minor, R. W.-----------------------Williams
Mixon, A. M.-----------------------Spiro
Morrison, C. A.---------------------Poteau
Plumlee, John L.-------------------Poteau
Shaw, C. C.-------------------------Poteau
Shepard, R. M.---------------------Talihina
Shippey, E. E.----------------------Wister
Wear, J. B.-------------------------Poteau
Winter, John D.--------------------Poteau
Woodson, B. D.--------------------Poteau

LINCOLN COUNTY

Adams, J. W.-----------------------Chandler
Erwin, P. F.------------------------Wellston
Erwin, F. B.------------------------Wellston
Glenn, J. O.------------------------Stroud
Hannah, R. H.----------------------Prague
Marshall, A. M.--------------------Chandler
Morgan, C. M.---------------------Chandler
Norwood, F. H.--------------------Prague
Pendergraft, W. A.----------------Carney
Williams, H. M.--------------------Wellston
Wyman, F. W.---------------------Stroud

LOGAN COUNTY

Barnes, F. M.----------------------Marshall
Barker, Pauline--------------------Guthrie
Barker, C. B.-----------------------Guthrie
Barker, E. O.-----------------------Guthrie
Berry, Leo A.----------------------Navina
Cotteral, C. F.---------------------Guthrie
Duke, J. W.-------------------------Guthrie
Hahn, L. A.-------------------------Guthrie
Houseworth, J. I.------------------Guthrie
Melvin, J. L.-----------------------Guthrie
Lovelady, Benton------------------Guthrie
Petty, C. S.------------------------Guthrie
Richmond, H. T. C.----------------
Ritzhaupt, L. H.-------------------Guthrie
Rucks, W. W.----------------------Oklahoma City
Stevens, David---------------------Guthrie
Trigg, F. E.-------------------------Lovel
West, A. A.-------------------------Guthrie

LOVE COUNTY

Autry, D.---------------------------Marietta
Batson, W. B.----------------------Marietta
Jackson, T. J.----------------------Marsden

MAYES COUNTY

Adams, J. L.----------------------------Pryor
Branson, C. S.------------------Locust Grove
Bryant, W. C.----------------------------Choteau
Hollingsworth, J. E.------------------Strang
Leonard, J. D.------------------------Strang
Mitchell, J. L.----------------------------Pryor
Pierce, E. L.------------------Locust Grove
Puckett, Carl----------------------------Pryor
Rogers, Ivadell------------------------Pryor
Smith, F. W.----------------------------Pryor
Whitaker, J. W.------------------------Pryor
White, L. C.----------------------------Adair

MAJOR COUNTY

Anderson, J. V.--------------------Fairview
Johnson, B. F.--------------------Fairview
McCall, P. C.------------------------Okeene
Specht, Elsie L.--------------------Fairview

MARSHALL COUNTY

Crume, F. M.----------------------------Lark
Ballard, A. E.------------------------Madill
Baker, J. F.------------------------Woodville
Belt, M. D.------------------------Woodville
Blaylock, T. A.------------------------Madill
Ballard, C. B.------------------------Kingston
Davis, W. L.------------------------Kingston
Ford, W. H.------------------------Kingston
Gaston, J. I.------------------------Madill
Gordon, T. M.------------------------Kingston
Haynie, W. D.------------------------Powell
Holland, J. I.------------------------Madill
Lewis, E. F.------------------------Kingston
Logan, J. H.------------------------Lebanon
Reid, J. E.------------------------Madill
Robinson, P. F.------------------------Madill
Rutledge, J. A.------------------------Woodville
Ussery, W. H.------------------------Lebanon
Welborn, O. E.------------------------Kingston
Winston, S. P.------------------------McMillan

McCLAIN COUNTY

Cochran, J. E.----------------------------Byars
Dawson, O. O.------------------------Wayne
Kolb, I. N.------------------------Dibble
McCurdy, W. C.------------------------Purcell
Smith, C. B.------------------------Washington
West, J. W.------------------------Purcell

McCURTAIN COUNTY

Baird, W. T.------------------Broken Bow
Chastain, J. B.------------------Broken Bow
Clarkson, A. W.------------------------Valliant
Graydon, A. S.------------------------Idabel
Hammond, O. O.------------------Broken Bow
Hooper, Z. A.------------------------Idabel
Huckabay, C. R.------------------------Valliant
McBrayer, W. H.------------------Haworth
McCaskill, W. Burns------------------Idabel
McDonald, C. T.------------------Broken Bow
Miller, W. A.------------------Liberty, Mo.
Moreland, B. F.------------------------Shultz
Moreland, J. T.------------------------Idabel
Moreland, W. A.------------------------Idabel
Oliver, R. B.------------------------Bokohoma
Sherrill, R. H.------------------Broken Bow
Taylor, W. D.------------------------Haworth
Weaver, R. E.------------------------Idabel
Williams, R. D.------------------------Idabel

Wisdom, W. E.--------------------Bismark
Woods, N. B.--------------------Millerton

McINTOSH COUNTY

Bennett, Dyton--------------------Texanna
Graves, G. W.--------------------Hitchita
Jacobs, L. L.--------------------Vivian
Lee, N. P.--------------------Checotah
Little, D. E.--------------------Eufaula
McColloch, J. H.--------------------Checotah
Monor, S. W.--------------------Hitchita
Montgomery, A. B.--------------------Checotah
Pope, A. J.--------------------Hanna
Rice, J. F.--------------------Eufaula
Rushing, B. F.--------------------Hanna
Shaunty, J. N.--------------------Eufaula
Snelson, A. J.--------------------Checotah
Smith, F. L.--------------------Fame
Tolleson, W. A.--------------------Eufaula
Vance, B. J.--------------------Checotah
Watkins, J. C.--------------------Checotah
West, G. W.--------------------Eufaula
Womack, W. F.--------------------Checotah

MURRAY COUNTY

Adams, J. A.--------------------Sulphur
Bailey, H. C.--------------------Sulphur
Baldwin, W. S.--------------------Cotter, Ark.
Brown, I. N.--------------------Davis
Brown, A. P.--------------------Davis
Dunn, R.--------------------Davis
Luster, J. C.--------------------Davis
Powell, W. H.--------------------Sulphur
Ponder, A. V.--------------------Sulphur
Salter, J. M.--------------------Sulphur
Simmons, J. H.--------------------Sulphur
Slover, G. W.--------------------Sulphur
Slover, J. T.--------------------Sulphur
Tucker, W. M.--------------------Del Rio, Texas

MUSKOGEE COUNTY

Ballantine, H. T.--------------------Muskogee
Berry, W. D.--------------------Muskogee
Blakemore, J. L.--------------------Muskogee
Buchanan, Jas. E.--------------------Haskell
Brown, Benj. H.--------------------Muskogee
De Groot, C. E.--------------------Muskogee
Dill, E.--------------------Boynton
Dial, J. J.--------------------Muskogee
Donnell, R. N.--------------------Muskogee
Dwight, K. M.--------------------Muskogee
Earnest, A. N.--------------------Muskogee
Ewing, F. W.--------------------Muskogee
Farris, R. C.--------------------Porum
Fite, Wm. P.--------------------Muskogee
Fite, F. B.--------------------Muskogee
Floyd, W. E.--------------------Muskogee
Fullenwider, C. M.--------------------Muskogee
Graves, J. R.--------------------Council Hill
Fryer, S. J.--------------------Muskogee
Harris, J. G.--------------------Muskogee
Harris, A. W.--------------------Muskogee
Heitzman, C. W.--------------------Muskogee
Hill, C. L.--------------------Haskell
Hoss, Sessler--------------------Muskogee
Hollingsworth, J. I.--------------------Muskogee
Joblin, W. R.--------------------Porter
Jones, R. E.--------------------Braggs
Keith, Emma Starr--------------------Muskogee

MUSKOGEE COUNTY (Continued)

King, F. S._____Muskogee
Klass, O. C._____Muskogee
Lee, John E._____Haskell
Lovell, A. J._____Dalhart, Texas
Morrow, Milton_____Muskogee
Nesbitt, P. P._____Muskogee
Nichols, J. T._____Muskogee
Noble, J. G._____Muskogee
Oldham, I. B._____Muskogee
Plunkett, J. H._____Porum
Rafter, J. G._____Muskogee
Reynolds, John_____Muskogee
Rice, C. V._____Muskogee
Rogers, H. C._____Muskogee
Sanford, J. Hoy _____Muskogee
Scott, H. A._____Muskogee
Stocks, A. L._____Muskogee
Stolper, J. H._____Muskogee
Tilly, W. T._____Muskogee
Thompson, C. A._____Muskogee
Thompson, M. K._____Muskogee
Vittum, J. S._____Muskogee
Walton, F. S._____Muskogee
Warmack, J. C._____Muskogee
Warterfield, F. E._____Muskogee
White, J. H._____Muskogee
Wilkiemyer, F. J._____Muskogee

NOBLE COUNTY

Brafford, S. F._____Billings
Cavett, Robt. A._____Morrison
Coldiron, D. F._____Perry
Dorough, John L._____Perry
Kuntz, R. L._____Perry
Mavity, Ralph P._____Billings
Owen, B. A._____Perry
Stewart, L. D._____Perry

NOWATA COUNTY

Allen, R. I._____Nowata
Brookshire, J. E._____Nowata
Collins, J. R._____Nowata
Collins, E. F._____Nowata
Lawson, D. M._____Nowata
Nairn, W. M._____Nowata
Roberts, S. P._____Alluwee
Scott, M. B._____Delaware
Strother, L. T._____Nowata
Sudderth, J. P._____Nowata
Thomas, J. G._____Alluwee
Waters, Geo. A._____Lenapah
Wilkinson, J. T._____Delaware

OKFUSKEE COUNTY

Bloss, C. M._____Okemah
Bombarger, C. C._____Paden
Carroll, W. B._____Okemah
Davis, W. M._____Castle
Griffith, W. C._____Weleetka
Hilsmeyer, F. E._____Weleetka
Jenkins, W. P._____Bearden
Keyes, R._____Okemah
Kennedy, J. A._____Okemah
Lucas, C. A._____Castle
May, H. A._____Okemah
Nye, L. A._____Okemah
Pemberton, J. M._____Okemah
Preston, J. A._____Weleetka
Rollins, J. S._____Guthrie
Stephenson, A. J._____Okemah
Watts, B._____Okemah

OKLAHOMA COUNTY

Alford, J. M._____Oklahoma City
Allen, E. P._____Oklahoma City
Andrews, Leila E._____Oklahoma City

Bailey, F. M._____Oklahoma City
Baird, A. B._____Oklahoma City
Barker, C. E._____Oklahoma City
Bee, Archie._____Oklahoma City
Blesh, A. L._____Oklahoma City
Bolend, Rex._____Oklahoma City
Buchanan, T. A._____Oklahoma City
Burus, T. C._____Oklahoma City
Buxton, L. Haynes_____Oklahoma City

Camp, F. K._____ ___Oklahoma City
Chase, A. B._____Oklahoma City
Christian, O. C._____Oklahoma City
Chumbley, C. P._____Oklahoma City
Clement, W. R._____Tulsa
Clymer, C. E._____Oklahoma City
Coley, A. J._____Oklahoma City
Crawford, Paul H._____Oklahoma City
Cummings, W. C._____Oklahoma City
Cunningham, S. R._____Oklahoma City

Davenport, A. E._____Oklahoma City
Davis, Edward F._____Oklahoma City
Day, C. R._____Oklahoma City
De Mand, F. R._____Oklahoma City
Dixon, W. E._____Oklahoma City

Earnheart, E. G._____Oklahoma City
Edward, J. T._____Oklahoma City
Edwards, R. T._____Oklahoma City

Ferguson, E. S._____Oklahoma City
Fishman, C. J._____Oklahoma City
Flesher, T. H._____Edmond
Fowler, W. A._____Oklahoma City
Fulton, Fred._____Oklahoma City
Fulton, Geo. _____Oklahoma City

Gay, Ruth._____Oklahoma City
Gibson, R. B._____Oklahoma City
Gipson, H. H._____Oklahoma City
Guthrie, A. L._____Oklahoma City

Haas, Karl._____Harrah
Hall, Jas. F._____Oklahoma City
Harbison, J. E._____Oklahoma City
Hartford, J. S._____Oklahoma City
Henry, J. W._____Oklahoma City
Hinchee, G. W._____Oklahoma City
Hirshfield, A. C._____Oklahoma City
Holliday, J. R._____Oklahoma City
Howard, R. M._____Oklahoma City
Hubbard, J. C. _____Ft. Amador, Canal Zone
Hunter, G. M._____Oklahoma City
Hunter, S. M._____Oklahoma City
Inman, L. E._____Oklahoma City
Jolly, W. J._____Oklahoma City
Kelly, J. F._____Oklahoma City
Kuhn, J. F._____Oklahoma City
Lain, E. S._____Oklahoma City
LaMotte, Geo. A._____Oklahoma City
Langsford, Wm._____Oklahoma City
Langston, Wann_____Oklahoma City
Lauderdale, T. L._____Oklahoma City
Lawson, N. E._____Oklahoma City
Lee, C. F._____Oklahoma City
Lipscomb, W. P._____Oklahoma City
Long, Le Roy_____Oklahoma City
Long, R. D._____Oklahoma City
Longmire, T. R._____Oklahoma City
Looney, R. E._____Oklahoma City

OKLAHOMA COUNTY (Continued)

Mahr, J. C.....................Oklahoma City
Martin, J. T.................Oklahoma City
Maxwell, J. H...............Oklahoma City
McHenry, D. D..............Oklahoma City
McLean, G. D...............Oklahoma City
McNair, O. P...............Oklahlma City
Messenbaugh, J. F..........Oklahoma City
Moorman, L. J..............Oklahoma City
Morgan, S. L...............Oklahoma City
Mraz, J. S.................Oklahoma City
Newton, L. A...............Oklahoma City
Nowlin, N. R...............Oklahoma City
Phelps, C. R...............Oklahoma City
Pine, J. S.................Oklahoma City
Postelle, J. M.............Oklahoma City
Reck, J. A.................Oklahoma City
Reed, Horace...............Oklahoma City
Riely, L. A................Oklahoma City
Riley, J. W................Oklahoma City
Roland, M. M...............Oklahoma City
Rolater, J. B..............Oklahoma City
Sackett, L. M..............Oklahoma City
Salmon, W. T...............Oklahoma City
Sanger, F. M...............Oklahoma City
Sanger, Winnie M...........Oklahoma City
Smith, M...................Oklahoma City
Stevens, J. W..............Oklahoma City
Stout, M. E................Oklahoma City
Sullivan, E. S.............Oklahoma City
Taylor, C. B...............Oklahoma City
Taylor, W. M...............Oklahoma City
Todd, H. C.................Oklahoma City
Townsend, C. W.............Oklahoma City
Underwood, E. L............Oklahoma City
Vincent, D. W..............Oklahoma City
von Wedel, Curt............Oklahoma City
Wallace, W. J..............Oklahoma City
Walker, A. J...............Oklahoma City
Weir, M. M.................Oklahoma City
Wells, Eva.................Oklahoma City
Wells, W. W................Oklahoma City
West, A. K.................Oklahoma City
West, W. K.................Oklahoma City
Westfall, L. M.............Oklahoma City
White, A. W................Oklahoma City
Will, A. A.................Oklahoma City
Wilson, Kenneth................Spencer
Wood, Ira J.......................Jones
Wynne, H. H................Oklahoma City
Young, A. D................Oklahoma City
Young, A. M................Oklahoma City

OKMULGEE COUNTY

Adams, A. C........................Kusa
Alexander, R. M..................Bryant
Ferguson, Jas. B...............Okmulgee
Alexander, L...................Okmulgee
Bercaw, J. E...................Okmulgee
Berry, V.......................Okmulgee
Bollinger, I. W...............Henryetta
Boswell, H. D.................Henryetta
Breese, H. W..................Henryetta
Bryan, E. C...................Okmulgee
Brymer, W. G.....................Dewar
Burrows, O. S..................Wetumpka
Carnell, M. D.................Okmulgee
Coleman, A. W....................Dewar

Cott, W. M....................Okmulgee
Crawford, T. O...................Dewey
Culp, A. H.......................Beggs
Edwards, J. G.................Henryetta
Hole, B. W....................Okmulgee
Holmes, A. R..................Henryetta
Hollingsworth, F. H..............Beggs
Horine, Wm. M.................Henryetta
Larrabee, W. S...........El Paso, Texas
McKinney, G. Y................Henryetta
Mitchner, W. C................Okmulgee
Mooney, R.....................Henryetta
Milroy, J. A..................Okmulgee
Myers, E. C...................Okmulgee
Nagle, Wm.....................Muskogee
Nelson, J. P...................Coalton
Pigg, W. B....................Okmulgee
Randel, H. O..................Okmulgee
Randel, D. M..................Okmulgee
Randel, B. W..................Okmulgee
Riley, J. Lee.................Henryetta
Robertson, I. W...............Henryetta
Robinson, J. C................Henryetta
Sanderson, W. C...............Henryetta
Simpson, N. N.................Henryetta
Stephenson, W. L..............Henryetta
Thompson, Wm. A...................Kusa
Torrence, L. B................Okmulgee
Vernon, Wm. C.................Okmulgee
Wallace, V. M....................Morris

OTTAWA COUNTY

Allen, J. B.....................Quapaw
Barham, J. B..................Tar River
Bewley, J. D.....................Miami
Bowman, W. R.....................Quapaw
Braselton, B. F..................Miami
Brewer, T. W.....................Miami
Cannon, R. F.....................Miami
Cooter, A. M.....................Miami
Cunningham, J. B.............Hockerville
Dawson, J. R......................Afton
Deal, Fred.......................Miami
DeTar, Geo.......................Miami
DeArman, M. M....................Miami
Dodson, T. J....................Picher
Garrison, Geo. I.................Quapaw
Hampton, J. B.................Commerce
Harper, R. H......................Afton
Jacobs, J. C.....................Miami
James, E. D..................Joplin, Mo.
Leisure, E. A..................Fairland
Lewis, E. M.....................Douthat
Lightfoot, Earl C......West Mineral, Kansas
Lightfoot, J. B..................Miami
Lively, C. O..................Tar River
Mason, B. B.....................Picher
McNaughton, G. P.................Miami
McCullum, Charles...............Quapaw
McLelland, C. A..................Miami
Miller, H. K...................Fairland
Mitchell, W. C................Commerce
Phillips, I.....................Picher
Pinnell, G.......................Miami
Points, Blair....................Miami
Rowley, W. T.....................Miami
Sibley, W. A..................Tar River
Smith, Ira....................Commerce
Smith, W. B....................Fairland
Squibb, H. W....................Quapaw
Troutt, L. W......................Afton

OTTAWA COUNTY (Continued)

Webb, G. O._____Tar River
Whorton, J. T._____Picher
Willis, M. P._____Commerce
Williams, J. Clay_____Miami
Wilks, F. M._____Bernice
Woodcock, J. H._____Miami
Wormington, Frank_____Miami

OSAGE COUNTY

Aaron, W. H._____Pawhuska
Berry, T. M._____Hominy
Chase, W. W._____Bigheart
Colley, K. L._____Bigheart
Colley, T. J._____Hominy
Goss, C. W._____Pawhuska
Hall, R. L._____Pawhuska
Herron, W. F._____Houston, Mo.
Jones, F. F._____Pawhuska
Mullins, Ira_____Hominy
Neal, Q. B._____Pawhuska
Shoun, D. A._____Fairfax
Shoun, J. G._____Fairfax
Skinner, Benj._____Pawhuska
Smith, A. J._____Pawhuska
Summers, H. L._____Osage
Walker, Roscoe_____Pawhuska
Wortin, D._____Pawhuska

PAWNEE COUNTY

Arnold, W. E._____Jennings
Ballaine, C. W._____Cleveland
Barber, L. C._____Ralston
Beitman, C. E._____Skedee
Gayman, M. W._____Ralston
Fleming, J. R._____Keystone
Herrington, D. J._____Terlton
Phillips, G. H._____Pawnee
Roberts, J. A._____Cleveland
Robinson, E. T._____Cleveland
Thompson, E. M._____Cleveland

PAYNE COUNTY

Beach, C. H._____Glencoe
Cash, J. B._____Glencoe
Cleverdon, L. A._____Stillwater
Davis, Benj._____Cushing
Harris, E. M._____Cushing
Holbroke, R. M._____Perkins
Hudson, W. B._____Yale
Hughes, Eli_____Stillwater
Janeway, D. F._____Stillwater
Manning, H. C._____Cushing
McQuoin, H._____Red Rock
Morris, I. C._____Antlers
Murphy, J. B._____Stillwater
Sexton, C. E._____Stillwater
Simmons, C. D._____Stillwater

PITTSBURG COUNTY

Allen, E. N._____McAlester
Barton, V. H._____McAlester
Baum, F. J._____Savannah
Bevill, S. D._____McAlester
Browning, R. L._____Haileyville
Brunson, C. J._____Adamson
Carlock, A. E._____Hartshorne
Chapman, T. S._____McAlester
Davis, J. E._____McAlester
Echols, J. W._____McAlester

Foster, M. H._____Alderson
Graves, W. C._____McAlester
Gray, J. W._____Quinton
Griffith, A._____McAlester
Grubbs, J. O._____North McAlester
Hailey, W. P._____Haileyville
Harris, Chas. T._____Kiowa
Harris, A. J._____McAlester
Hudson, W. R._____Gowen
Johnson, C. A._____Kiowa
Johnston, J. C._____McAlester
Kilpatrick, G. A._____McAlester
Kuyrkendall, L. C._____McAlester
Lewallen, W. P._____Canadian
McCarley, T. H._____McAlester
Munn, R. A._____Kiowa,
Norris, T. T._____Crowder
Pemberton, R. K._____McAlester
Rice, O. W._____Alderson
Sames, W. W._____Hartshorne
Turner, G. S._____Krebs
Smith, J. A._____McAlester
Street, Graham_____McAlester
Troy, E. H._____McAlester
Wait, W. C._____McAlester
Watson, F. L._____McAlester
Williams, C. O._____McAlester
Willour, L. S._____McAlester
Wilson, McClellan,_____McAlester

PONTOTOC COUNTY

Akers, Wm. W. D._____Ada
Breckinridge, N. B.___Merida, Yucatan, Mexico
Breco, J. G._____Ada
Burns, S. L._____Maxwell
Castleberry, R. T._____Ada
Craig, J. R._____Ada
Cummings, I. L._____Ada
Dawson, B. B._____Ada
Deen, J. A._____Ada
Faust, W. D._____Ada
Harrison, Edith_____Stonewall
Harrison, Fred_____Stonewall
Hill, T. A._____Roff
Jeffress, J. I._____Roff
Lewis, M. L._____Ada
McNew, M. C._____Ada
Meredith, H. D._____Ada
Orr, C. L._____Ada
Overton, L. M._____Fitzhugh
Richey, S. M._____Francis
Ross, S. P._____Ada
Sullivan, B. F._____Ada
Threlkeld, C._____Ada
Weeden, H. J._____Sasakwa
Sturdevant, S._____Vanoss

POTTOWATAMIE COUNTY

Anderson, R. M._____Shawnee
Applewhite, G. H._____Shawnee
Ball, W. A._____Wanette
Baker, M. A._____Shawnee
Baxter, G. S._____Shawnee
Bradford, W. C._____Shawnee
Brown, R. A._____Prague
Butler, W. R._____Maud
Byrum, J. M._____Shawnee
Calhoun, Z. T._____McComb
Campbell, H. G._____Asher

(POTTAWOTAMIE COUNTY (Continued)

Carson, F. L. ....Shawnee
Colvert, Geo. W. ....Tecumseh
Connally, G. A. ....Romulus
Cordell, U. S. ....Romulus
Culbertson, R. R. ....Maud
Culbertson, J. ....Maud
Cullum, J. E. ....Tecumseh
Fortson, J. L. ....Tecumseh
Gallaher, W. M. ....Shawnee
George, L. G. ....Stuart
Goodrich, E. E. ....Tecumseh
Gray, E. J. ....Tecumseh
Hughes, J. W. ....Shawnee
Kaylor, R. C. ....McLoud
McFarling, A. C. ....Shawnee
McGee, W. N. ....McAllen, Texas
Owen, A. H. ....Meeker
Phillips, W. D. ....Maud
Rawls, W. E. ....Asher
Rowland, T. D. ....Shawnee
Royster, J. H. ....Wanette
Reeder, H. M. ....Shawnee
Rice, E. E. ....Shawnee
Sanborn, G. H. ....Shawnee
Sanders, T. C. ....Shawnee
Scott, J. H. ....Shawnee
Stooksbury, J. M. ....Shawnee
Turner, Jas. H. ....Shawnee
Wagner, H. A. ....Shawnee
Walker, J. A. ....Shawnee
Walker, J. E. ....Earlsboro
Wilson, H. H. ....Shawnee

PUSHMATAHA COUNTY

Acheson, F. I. ....Antlers
Bills, R. C. ....Moyer
Burnett, J. A. ....Crum Creek
Guinn, Edw. ....Antlers
Henderson, Thomas ....Ft. Towson
Huckabay, B. M. ....Tuskahoma
Johnson, H. C. ....Antlers
Lawson, J. S. ....Clayton
Patterson, E. S. ....Antlers
Robinett, Geo. ....Albion
Walker, E. B. ....Belzoni
Wright, P. E. ....Antlers

ROGERS COUNTY

Anderson, F. A. ....Claremore
Arnold, A. M. ....Claremore
Bassman, Caroline ....Claremore
Busheyhead, J. C. ....Claremore
Elliott, C. V. ....Inola
Ewell, J. E. ....Catoosa
Haley, J. H. ....Chelsea
Hays, W. F. ....Claremore
Howard, W. A. ....Chelsea
Lerskov, A. N. ....Claremore
Means, J. F. ....Claremore
Mills, W. P. ....Claremore
Rutherford, S. C. ....Inola
Smith, J. C. ....Catoosa
Smith, W. E. ....Collinsville
Stemmons, J. M. ....Oolagah
Strickland, Geo. ....Claremore
Taylor, J. C. ....Chelsea
Waldrep, J. G. ....Claremore
Young, B. O. ....Talala

ROGERS MILLS

Ballenger, B. M. ....Strong City
Cary, W. S. ....Rankin
Dorrah, Lee ....Hammon
Wallace, Geo. H. ....Cheyenne

SEMINOLE COUNTY

Black, W. R. ....Seminole
Harber, J. N. ....Seminole
Harrison, T. F. ....Wewoka
Huddleston, W. T. ....Konowa
Kiles, H. A. ....Konowa
Knight, W. L. ....Wewoka
Long, W. J. ....Konowa
McAlister, E. R. ....Seminole
Perkins, J. H. ....Wewoka
Van Sandt, Guy B. ....Wewoka
Turlington, M. M. ....Seminole
Warhurst, M. A. ....Sylvian

SEQUOYAH COUNTY

Breedlove, J. C. ....Muldrow
Cheek, J. A. ....Sallisaw
Coffman, J. S. ....Sallisaw
Collins, T. W. ....Muldrow
Green, E. P. ....Sallisaw
Holcomb, J. L. ....Marble City
Hudson, V. W. ....Sallisaw
Hunter, W. M. ....Vian
Jones, S. B. ....Sallisaw
Loftin, W. T. ....Sallisaw
McKeel, Sam A. ....Sallisaw
Morrow, J. A. ....Sallisaw
Pinner, L. J. ....Gans
Sandling, J. T. ....Vian
Taylor, R. Z. ....Vian
Wood, T. F. ....Sallisaw

STEPHENS COUNTY

Bartley, J. P. ....Duncan
Conger, H. A. ....Duncan
Cowman, John P. ....Comanche
De Meglio, Edw. ....Oklahoma City
Dicker, M. F. ....Comanche
Frie, H. C. ....Duncan
Garrett, S. S. ....Dixie
Haraway, P. M. ....Marlow
Harrison, C. M. ....Comanche
Ivy, W. S. ....Marlow
Long, D. ....Duncan
Mavity, A. R. ....Marlow
Montgomery, D. M. ....Marlow
Montgomery, R. L. ....Marlow
Mullins, J. A. ....Marlow
Neiweg, J. W. ....Duncan
Rice, S. A. ....Alma
Spears, W. S. ....Velma
Taylor, J. I. ....Loco
Thomason, E. B. ....Velma
Wharton, J. O. ....Duncan
Williamson, S. H. ....Duncan

TEXAS COUNTY

Hayes, R. B. ....Guymon
Langston, Wm. H. ....Guymon
McMillen, Jas. ....Goodwell
Risen, Wm. J. ....Hooker

TULSA COUNTY

Allison, Ira	Tulsa
Ament, C. M.	Sapulpa
Atherton, Lytle	Tulsa
Atkins, P. N.	Tulsa
Ball, C. H.	Tulsa
Beesley, W. W.	Tulsa
Beyer, W. J.	Tulsa
Bland, J. C. W.	Tulsa
Boso, F. M.	Tulsa
Boutros, A.	Tulsa
Brodie, W. W.	Tulsa
Brown, Paul R.	Tulsa
Burdick, J. R.	Tulsa
Butcher, J. P.	Tulsa
Calhoun, C. E.	Sand Springs
Capps, J. A.	Tulsa
Carlton, L. H.	Tulsa
Case, W. H.	Tulsa
Childs, H. C.	Tulsa
Childs, J. W.	Tulsa
Clinton, Fred S.	Tulsa
Clulow, Geo. H.	Tulsa
Cohenour, E. L.	Tulsa
Cook, W. A.	Tulsa
Coulter, T. B.	Tulsa
Cronk, Fred Y.	Tulsa
Davis, G. M.	Bixby
Dillon, C. A.	Tulsa
Douglas, R. A.	Tulsa
Dunlap, R. W.	Tulsa
Dutton, W. F.	Tulsa
Emerson, A. V.	Tulsa
Felt, R. A.	Tulsa
Flanigan, O. A.	Tulsa
Ford, H. W.	Tulsa
Franklin, Onis	Tulsa
Geissler, P. C.	Tulsa
Gessler, Henry	Tulsa
Gilbert, J. B.	Tulsa
Glass, Fred A.	Tulsa
Gorrell, J. F.	Tulsa
Grosshart, Ross	Tulsa
Gunn, Howell	Tulsa
Gwin, H. B.	Tulsa
Halm, C. T.	Sand Springs
Harris, Bunn	Jenks
Haskins, Thos. M.	Tulsa
Hawley, S. DeZell	Tulsa
Hayden, E. F.	Tulsa
Hendershot, C. L.	Tulsa
Henderson, F. W.	Tulsa
Hillie, H. L.	Collinsville
Hooper, J. S.	Tulsa
Houser, M. A.	Tulsa
Johnson, Chas. B.	Tulsa
Irvan, H. D.	Tulsa
Kimball, M. C.	Tulsa
Lareau, H. G.	Tulsa
Latham, L. D.	Tulsa
Laws, J. H.	Broken Arrow
Lemmon, W. G.	Tulsa
Linn, C. P.	Broken Arrow
Lynn, R. S.	Broken Arrow
Mangan, P. A.	Broken Arrow
Margolin, Bertha	Tulsa
Mayginnis, N. W.	Broken Arrow
Mayginnis, P. H.	Tulsa
McCarty, Chas.	Tulsa
McLean, B. W.	Jenks
Mohrman, S. S.	Tulsa
Morgan, J. H.	Tulsa
Mullens, Robt. B.	Broken Arrow
Murdock, H. D.	Tulsa
Murray, S.	Tulsa
Newlin, W. B.	Tulsa
Oden, B. N.	Tulsa
O'Hern, C. D. F.	Tulsa
Perry, M. L.	Tulsa
Pigford, A. W.	Tulsa
Pleas, E.	Collinsville
Price, H. P.	Tulsa
Price, Horace T.	Tulsa
Reeder, C. L.	Tulsa
Rhodes, R. E. L.	Tulsa
Rogers, J. W.	Tulsa
Rogers, W. H.	Tulsa
Roth, A. W.	Tulsa
Roy, Emill	Tulsa
Smith, R. V.	Tulsa
Smith, R. R.	Tulsa
Springer, M. P.	Tulsa
Stallings, T. W.	Tulsa
Stevens, J. C.	Drumright
Stroud, E. F.	Tulsa
Trainer, W. J.	Tulsa
Wagner, R. S.	Tulsa
Wall, G. A.	Tulsa
Wallace, J. W.	Tulsa
Ward, H. P.	Leonard
Watkins, Frank L.	Tulsa
Webb, J. E.	Tusla
White, Daniel	Tulsa
White, P. C.	Tulsa
Wiley, Ray	Tulsa
Wiley, C. Z.	Tulsa
Woods, Charles J.	Tulsa
Woody, W. W.	Tulsa
Wright, John W.	Collinsville

TILLMAN COUNTY

Arrington, J. E.	Frederick
Briggs, I. A.	Stillwater
Fuqua, W. A.	Grandfield
Gillis, J. A.	Frederick
Hays, A. J.	Frederick
Howell, C. A.	Oklahoma City
Mitchell, I. A.	Frederick
Spurgeon, T. F.	Frederick
Wilson, R. E.	Davidson
Wright, Harper	Grandfield

WAGONER COUNTY

Bates, S. R.	Wagoner
Brewer, A. J.	Coweta
Carder, A. E.	Coweta
Cobb, Isabella	Wagoner
Gordon, G. R.	Wagoner
Hayward, C. E.	Wagoner
Jobe, G. W.	Wagoner
Martin, C. E.	Wagoner
McCourt, E. T.	Wagoner
Shinn, T. J.	Wagoner

WASHINGTON COUNTY

Athey, J. V.	Bartlesville
Bradfield, S. J.	Bartlesville
Chamberlain, D. E.	Bartlesville
Crawford, H. G.	Dewey

WASHINGTON COUNTY (Continued)

Dunn, J. C._____Bartlesville
Green, O. I._____Bartlesville
Hudson, J. O._____Copan
Hudson, L. D._____Dewey
Kingman, W. H._____Bartlesville
Kiser, J. D._____Bartlesville
Koppenbrink, Walter_____Higginsville, Mo.
North, A._____Bartlesville
Parks, S. M._____Olathe, Kansas
Rammel, W. E._____Bartlesville
Shipman, W. H._____Bartlesville
Sommerville, O. S._____Bartlesville
Smith, J. G._____Bartlesville
Staver, B. F._____Bartlesville
Sykes, W. M._____Ramona
Terrill, R. J._____Vera
Weber, H. C._____Bartlesville
Woodring, G. F._____Bartlesville
Wyatt, M. C._____Bartlesville
Yazel, H. E._____Bartlesville

WASHITA COUNTY

Baker, B. W._____Cloudchief
Bennett, D. W._____Sentinel
Bungardt, A. H._____Cordell
Dillon, G. A._____Dill City
Farber, J. E._____Cordell
Freeman, I. S._____Butler
Harms, J. H._____Cordell
Kerley, J. W._____Cordell
Neal, A. S._____Cordell
Sherburne, A. M._____Cordell
Stephens, E. F._____Foss
Stoll, A. S._____Foss
Tidball, Wm._____Sentinel
Tracy, C. M._____Sentinel
Weaver, E. S._____Dill City
Weber, A. A._____Bessie
Witt, J. W._____Colony

WOODS COUNTY

Bowling, J. A._____Alva
Clapper, E. P._____Waynoka
Fewkes, John W._____Alva
Grantham, Ei._____Alva
Munsell, L. S._____Beaver
Welsh, S. H._____Dacoma
White, C. T._____Alva

WOODWARD COUNTY

Amos, C. L._____May
Bamber, W. J._____Arnett
Brace, A. J._____Sharon
Davis, C. E._____Woodward
Duncan, J. A._____Forgan
Cockerill, H. S._____Mooreland
Eiler, P. G._____Quinlan
Forney, C. J._____Woodward
Goddard, R. K._____Supply
Hill, C. B._____Supply
Messersmith, J. W._____Floris
Miller, E. M._____Buffalo
Newman, O. C._____Shattuck
Patterson, J. L._____Woodward
Patterson, Fred_____Woodward
Pierson, O. A._____Woodward
Racer, F. L._____Woodward
Rollo, J. W._____Shattuck
Rose, W. L._____Woodward
Stecher, H. E._____Supply
Slusher, W. M._____Brownwood, Texas
Triplett, T. B._____Mooreland
Tedrowe, C. W._____Woodward
Workman, J. M._____Woodward
Workman, R. A._____Woodward
Steele, J. M._____Sayre
Walker, H._____Rosston
Westfall, G. A._____Harper, Kansas

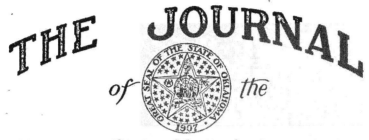

THE JOURNAL of the

Oklahoma State Medical Association

| VOLUME XII | MUSKOGEE, OKLA., JULY, 1919 | NUMBER 7 |

CANCER OF THE CERVIX; A PLEA FOR ITS EARLY DIAGNOSIS.

GREGORY A. WALL, M. D.

TULSA, OKLAHOMA

According to Prof. Wilson of Birmingham (I), among individuals of the age of 35 and upwards one male in every twelve, and one female in every eight, dies of cancer. In the female the uterus is the site in nearly 30 per cent. of the total number of cancers; so that among women living at the age of thirty-five and upward, one in twenty-seven, or nearly four per cent., will eventually die of cancer. Cancer of the various organs of the human occurs in all continents and among all races, no matter what their condition of servitude may be. It is no respecter of persons, and the rich and poor alike are subject to it; it occurs as often in the negro as it does in the caucasian; neither does it slight the young.

Cancer of the cervix appears most commonly between the ages of forty and fifty. In a series of cases (6071) reported by Koblanck 33.7 per cent. occurred between the ages of thirty and forty and 24 per cent. occurred between thirty and sixty. Occasionally cases are seen later than sixty and earlier than thirty. Graves saw one at twenty-five years and Cragin reports one at the age of eighteen. Cancer of the cervix has a very constant and definite etiology, in that it occurs almost exclusively in the cervices that have some inflammatory or traumatic lesion, usually the result of childbirth. It is estimated that 95 to 98 per cent. of women with cancer of the cervix have had children and the greater majority have been multiparous: and those cases—(I) New System of Gynecology, Lockyer and Eden: Vol. II, p. 421—which show an ectropion of the cervical membrane, or an erosion of the lips, have a special predisposition for cancer. The most commonly accepted cause for this condition is a lacerated cervix uteri. Why cancer is rare in procidentia, is answered by supposition that the epidermis becomes so thickened and hypertrophied in this condition that it acts as a protection.

The symptoms of cancer of the cervix in its incipiency are so treacherous and come on with such slight evidences that it behooves us to be more on the lookout for it than we are. In the early stages of cancer of the cervix there are no definite symptoms to arouse our suspicion and consequently the disease is often far advanced before any alarming signs occur. The three cardinal symptoms of cancer of the cervix are: (1) leukorrhea, (2) bleeding, and (3) pain, in the order named. In the early stages the vaginal secretion does not differ from one due to hyperemia except as to quantity, but later on the discharge assumes a watery consistency, which is quite characteristic of cancer and is one of the chief clinical signs and should arouse suspicion, and call for a very thorough examination at once. In the later stages still, when necrosis and infection take place, the discharge becomes exceedingly foul and the odor nauseatingly characteristic. Bleeding is the next most prominent clinical symptom and from the fact that it is usually venous, is no particular menace to life. An important sign is the very free bleeding upon the slightest manipulation, and does not exist in the same degree in any other condition. Pain, the third symptom, is of no diagnostic value in the early stages, since it is only the announcement that the disease has ceased to be limited to the cervix and has passed into the parametrical tissues and adjacent lymphatics.

Far too many physicians place too much stress upon the "change of life" and attribute symptomatology to it which does not belong there. How often women come to the family physician with the suggestion that they are having "change of life" and they want something done for excessive bleeding which is dragging them down. An examination shows to our amazement a large bleeding fungous mass, bathed in a foul-smelling, nauseating, purulent discharge. One glance at the condition tells us that we have a cancer of the cervix, far advanced and usually beyond hope of cure, and all because this woman was not advised properly by her doctor, or if she was it was not stressed enough. Perhaps she had been told by some physician that she was merely having the "change of life"—and she was having a change of life, for she was very rapidly changing from the mortal to the spiritual one, all because of false advice. Had she been forcibly reminded by her medical advisor of the probable dangers to her from cancer, at every opportunity, she might have been saved, in all probability she would have been. Since it is now generally accepted as a fact that cancer in its early stages is a local disease, primarily confined to the tissues affected, if it be removed or destroyed while still confined to these tissues, it should be, in fact it will be cured. Knowing this to be a fact, can there be any excuse for any physician in this day of enlightenment to neglect to examine his patients and make the diagnosis while the disease is yet a local one, and amenable to surgical procedure? We know that the complete excision of the most virulent form of cancer, while it is yet a local condition, will in all probability be a stop against its recurrence. The question comes to the writer, How long does cancer remain a local disease? No one in the world can answer that question, as the time is a variable one, depending on the malignancy and the variety of the cancer, as well as on the resisting power of the individual. Recent observations have shown that some varieties of cancer have a very short period of localization, and that all forms are shorter in duration than we formerly supposed. No one can say anything about the resisting power of the individual; one's resisting power may be good this day and the very next it may be very low, in fact it may change from hour to hour. We do know that certain bodies have a good resisting power against disease while others have a poor one, but up to now no scientist has been able to tell us a way of measuring that power.

The life destroying power of cancer is measured by its ability to extend into the lymphatics and blood vessels, and adjoining structures, thus progressing from a local to systemic disease. For this reason, if for none other, it should be our bounden duty to prevent this condition taking place, for no systemic cancer ever got well or was cured by operation. Knowing as we do, that instead of years or months before the disease breaks down the protecting barriers and becomes systemic, it may be only weeks or even days or hours, are we not guilty of the grossest negligence if we do not strive to so make ourselves better and more careful diagnosticians, so that we may be able to give the proper advice at the proper time, and thereby save a life that may be very necessary to the welfare of a large family. I am of the opinion that the profession as a whole is learning the value of an early diagnosis in this condition, and that fewer cancers are coming to the surgeon, where the parametrium is involved. Still, there is plenty of room for improvement along the line of early diagnosis, and many men are still permitting their patients to walk in the valley of the shadow of death, by failure to give them a careful examination on every occasion, when there may be the slightest chance that they have incipient cancer. There are not enough vaginal examinations made by the family physician on his child-bearing patients and not enough advice about the dangers of cancer. Too many physicians do not keep records enough and do not get thorough histories from their clients. They look at the tongue, feel the pulse, look wise and then proceed to write a prescription for H. V. C. or liquor sedans and forget about the case until it comes back again with all the signs of a fully developed cancer, beyond the only known cure, viz: surgery. Had this patient received the proper examination at the time of the first visit, the condition would in all probability have been found and the proper advice given, and another victim of carelessness or ignorance would not have gone to an early grave.

It always was a wonder to the writer why so much commotion was caused in a neighborhood when the doctor failed to diagnose an obscure incipient contagious disease, and how little was said if he failed to diagnose an early cancer of the uterus. Just let some doctor make a mistake in the diagnosis of smallpox in its early stage and see what a howl is set up, and yet cancer of the uterus kills more women than does smallpox, and the early diagnosis is easier than that of early smallpox.

The writer is convinced that we do not take the people into our confidence enough, and this brings us to the realization that this must be done as forcibly as we know how, by constantly telling every one, at every chance, of the dangers of cancers in the child-bearing woman. Make it so forcible that they will take it home to ponder over. Cancer of the womb robs more homes of useful wives and mothers, at their most active and useful period of life, than does tuberculosis, so do you not think that the family physician who is in a way the custodian of these lives, should realize his responsibility and trust more fully than he does? Only an ignoramus does not know at the present time all that is necessary to know about cancer of the womb in order to have his suspicions aroused and, then if he fails to do his duty, he is meriting the contempt of every modern physician. The medical profession has a bounden duty to perform and that is, face the question fairly and squarely, and meet it with a determination to stamp out inoperable cervical cancer. The man who calls himself a specialist in diseases of women, and there are many incapable ones, should be able to give a resume of all the facts about cancer. He should emphasize the fact that cancer of the uterus is inevitably fatal without early recognition and proper treatment, and that proper treatment is complete removal before the disease becomes systemic, for the mortality of systemic cancer is 100 per cent.

In every case before metastases has taken place, the mortality is but 25 per cent., and in the very early cases the death rate will be about nil. In many cases the failure to diagnose the case early lies directly with the woman herself, who delays examination or declines to permit one being made when urged to do so, but this does not relieve the doctor entirely from responsibility, for had he frequently impressed her with the dangers of the various cervical laccrations and leukorrheal discharges, she might have possibly been brought to a realization of the possibility of cancer taking place.

If the people are ever going to know the facts about cancer of the womb, these facts must come from the physician, and the family advisor is the proper one. The commoner symptoms of the disease must be taught the woman, and these should be impressed on her mind at every occasion. Next in importance to teaching them that there is a way at their command to definitely determine in nearly every instance whether they have cancer or not, is to teach the public more about it. If it is cancer, the woman should be told so, without equivocation or faltering, not to scare the life out of her, but to scare life into her. The doctor who advises his patient who has one single sign of cancer, "to wait awhile and see," is criminally inefficient. There should be nothing but contempt for the doctor who sends his patient away without making a vaginal examination, giving her a vaginal douche, and a snapshot diagnosis of "change of life" or some other equally absurd diagnosis.

Still, the Cancer Commission of the great State of Pennsylvania for the year 1912 shows that of the developed cases of cancer of the womb that consulted physicians, 10 per cent. of them never had a physical examination made, and 20 per cent. of those had been given worse than useless advice. If this can happen in this highly enlightened and populous state, where the glare of the sun of twentieth century knowledge shines brightest, what would be the results of an investigation in less favored communities? Let us therefore resolve that in the future we will more faithfully and more carefully take up the burden of cancer of the womb and give it more thought, more study, more talk, so that in the end we may save lives now so ruthlessly lost. To that end only shall we have done our duty to our patients, to our profession and to the people.

Conclusions.

Since cancer of the womb is curable in the period of localization, and this being the time when the symptoms are so insidious, we should endeavor to place in the woman's hands some literature which would assist her in coming to the conclusion that there is something wrong, and she should consult her physician and tell him her troubles at once.

To this end the writer would suggest that the State Society, through a committee, issue a small pamphlet on this condition which should be elementary in character, so that it could be placed in every home and could be read and understood by the laity.

GONORRHEAL EPIDIDYMITIS

A. B. James, Toronto, Canada (*Journal A. M. A.*, May 24, 1919), says that the war has given a special opportunity for observing cases of gonorrheal epididymitis in army practice. The incidence is given by various writers as from 10 to 25 per cent., and was 15 per cent. the last year at the Canadian Special Military Hospital at Etchinghill, England. The cases show a longer stay in the hospital than other complications of gonorrhea. He has observed two distinct types: first, the subacute, coming on slowly with slight pain or constitutional symptoms, slight enlargement of the epididymis and little redness and edema of the scrotum. Such cases rarely develop into the second or acute type, in which the symptoms are much more severe. The infection may travel by direct extension from the urethra, as held by most observers; through the lymphatics, which James considers most frequent, or by way of the blood, which is least likely. The pathology of the condition is described, and James finds the globus minor most frequently involved. The advantages of surgical procedure in all types are numerous, and the author considers the operation justifiable, though it is only for the relief of pain. He reviews the objections to epididymotomy, but he says it is simple and should take only a few moments. He notices the opinions of other authors on the subject, and says nearly every contributor agrees that the operation tends to minimize the chances of sterility. In his series of 115 cases of epididymotomy, twelve were bilateral, six of which showed living spermatozoa, and he believes that, with longer observation, this number would have been increased. He describes his operative technic. In advanced cases he advises general anesthesia, on account of the dense adhesions that have formed. His conclusions are as follows: "1. Early operation is advised to prevent destruction or occlusion of the tubules. 2. The pain is relieved almost immediately by surgical interference. 3. The process is considerably shortened. 4. No accurate conclusions as to sterility may be made except in bilateral cases, but present evidence favors epididymotomy as a means of preventing sterility. 5. There is less liability of a relapse of the urethritis. 6. The operation should be more generally employed."

THE PREVENTION OF CANCER.

WALTON FOREST DUTTON, M. D.

TULSA, OKLAHOMA

A great deal has been written about the etiology, pathology, and treatment of cancer, but not a great deal about prevention. There is no field in medicine where the correlation of facts is of more importance than in the study of cancer. The collection of statistics, relative etiology, pathological findings, and treatment should receive more painstaking effort.

Cancer is one of the most dreaded diseases that effect the human family. It does not make any great progress toward spontaneous recovery, and little can be done for the disease when far advanced. Cancer is often cured in the incipient stage by proper treatment. This, however, is, unfortunately, true only in a small percentage of cases. Owing to a lack of diagnostic ability, the great number of cases go on to the incurable stage. Hence, it is useless to attempt radical operation in these late cases.

It is extremely difficult to draw correct conclusions concerning the distribution of cancer, owing to the unreliable manner in which vital statistics are secured. The greater accuracy in the compilation of the causes of death show a higher mortality. This will account, in a measure, for the belief that cancer is so prevalent among uncivilized peoples.

A fairly accurate compilation of statistics has been made so that one can estimate conditions as follows:

In the United States approximately 5 per cent. of the deaths after the age of thirty are due to cancer.

England, out of a total of 141,241 deaths of males over 35 years of age, in 1907, shows that 12,695 died of cancer, and out of 140,607 deaths of females over 35 years of age, 17,671 died of cancer.

Switzerland has a more accurate way of obtaining the death rate. There the death rate from cancer is estimated at 0.129 per cent.

Holland attributes 0.101 per cent of the death rate to cancer.

The figures in Spain, Hungary and Latin-American countries are unreliable.

The yearly increase in the mortality from cancer has an important bearing upon the question of the public health and the economic welfare in all civilized countries. W. Roger Williams ("Natural History of Cancer," 1909) states that there has been a yearly increase in the cancer death rate from three to five per cent during the past twenty years.

The statistical evidence obtained from the autopsy table presented by various authorities, in every country, lays at rest any doubt as to the increase of cancer. It is maintained that cancer increase is limited to certain organs, while other organs have not shown any perceptible increase.

Bashford has shown for England that cancer of the uterus is decreasing while cancer of the gastro-intestinal tract has slightly increased. The accuracy of reports of various authorities in England, United States, Switzerland, France, and Italy is of considerable importance from a statistical view point.

It is a self-evident fact that cancer is a disease of decadence, and should be attacked as early as feasible. Cancer is a disease that rarely attacks before the age of thirty, and in the majority of cases occurs between fifty and sixty years of age.

In the study and prevention of cancer, the etiological factors must of necessity be kept uppermost in mind.

A paper on "The Relative Etiology and Pathology of Cancer" (Journal Oklahoma State Medical Association, July, 1918) offers in its conclusions a graphic guide to both physician and surgeon. It unfolds step by step the etiological and pathological factors in cancer. A thorough study of this paper will enable the physician to grasp an idea of the logical procedure in the prophylactic treatment of cancer.

Diet and hygiene are factors not to be overlooked in the prophylactic treatment of the disease.

Heredity influences should be attacked by keeping the individual in the best physical and mental condition. This often may be accomplished by removing some chronic focus which has proved fatal to the progenitors of the individual. Decadence must be warded off by clean living and proper care of the physical being. Especial attention should be given those organs most frequently subject to continuous irritation. Acute local conditions should never be allowed to become chronic. Cancer is non-inoculable and non-communicable, but that does not obiviate the fact that certain acute local conditions if allowed to become chronic will eventually become cancerous.

The logical sequence of this fact establishes the necessity of removing all ulcers of the stomach; all precancerous growths in the breasts; all lacerations and chronic ulcerations of the uterus; and all chronic ulcerations of the rectum. Gallstones if not removed most always cause cancer. Any precancerous condition of the mouth, tongue, and throat should be removed at the earliest possible moment. All moles, warts, and other growths of like nature upon the body should be removed. Any condition in any part of the body suspected of being precancerous should be removed, provided it does not shorten the life of the patient. Any practice, creed, or sect that teaches other than the radical treatment of cancer should be prevented from exercising their practice or teaching by due process of law.

Persons suspecting a cancerous or precancerous condition should consult a competent physician every three months.

Cancer hospitals should be established by and in every state and territory.

STREPTOCOCCIC INFECTIONS

W. B. Blanton, C. W. Burhans and O. W. Hunter, Camp Custer, Battle Creek, Mich. (*Journal A. M. A.*, May 24, 1919), report on the streptococcic infections observed at Camp Custer, since its establishment. Sixty-five per cent of the acute infections coming to necropsy have been due to these. Excluding the month of October, 1918, when influenza was epidemic, 75 per cent of the fatal acute infections were from this cause. The camp was several months old when they first appeared, chiefly as secondary infections. Two methods of invasion are to be considered; first, such as occurs after a sudden, severe antecedent disease has lowered the patient's resistance, and, second, such as occurs when the virulence of the streptococcus is the principal determiung factor. The authors give in detail the conditions and incidence of these infections and summarize as follows: "1. Streptococci as observed at Camp Custer have manifested themselves almost uniformly as secondary invaders. 2. It is impossible to divorce a discussion of streptococcic infection from such antecedent diseases as influenza, measles and the acute upper respiratory inflammations. 3. Important factors in the incidence of streptococcic infections and their outcome are disclosed after investigating the effects of length of service, rural and city life, and bodily fatigue and exhaustion. 4. Streptococci have been responsible for a variety of lesions, but their predilection for the respiratory system far exceeds all other localizations."

SOME SUGGESTIONS ON THE CAUSE OF CANCER.

Arthur W. White, A. M., M. D.

OKLAHOMA CITY, OKLAHOMA

Quite recently as a result of some of the continous studies on the cause of malignancy, some new conclusions seem to have developed.

In going over the literature on cancer for the past few months this phase of the question appealed to me a little more than any other at this time, except, possibly, the question of metastasis, about which seemingly nothing had been written for some considerable time.

What is contained in this paper is drawn principally from conclusions reached by Leo Loeb, Doctor Spain, Fibiger and Bulkley, from observation on tissue and tumor growth.

Tissue growth is started by external factors, which bring about similar or identical results in the tissue, even though the causes themselves differ. These are considered primary causes and are referred to by most of these men as "formative stimuli" in order to distinguish them from functional stimuli.   It may be that both the formative and functional stimuli are the same, acting in a similar manner; the difference in result depending on the difference in strength and time and in the systems on which they act.

The primary causes may be either physical or chemical. The physical are either mechanical or electrical, the rays of which are held by the tissues. The chemical causes are produced somewhere in the organism itself. Even in the case of parasitic organisms the change is partly through chemical agencies which they produce, there may be also a mechanical effect.

Loeb has shown that chemical stimulus brings about changes in the effected tissue. These changes are partly chemical as is shown by increased oxidation and partly physical as shown by increased water content in the cells.

Doctor Spain demonstrated that small quantities of various rays produce stimulation on various tissues, while large quantities cause destruction.

If a strong stimulus be applied to tissues, which are under any otherwise unfavorable condition, an abnormal response takes place with the formation of giant cells, and syncytia. If the conditions of nourishment to these tissues become still more unfavorable, necrosis results.

It seems that these conditions apply both to normal tissues under abnormal conditions and to tumors, but are much more evident in malignant tumor. Further that these same physical factors when acting over a long period, on normal tissue, produce tumors or cancer. Fibiger has found it possible to produce cancer experimentally by the application of physical and physico-chemical factors, as already referred to. Apparently from his report the transformation from normal tissue to cancer was a slow one, passing through several intermediate steps.

The formative stimuli act the same upon tumors and cancers as upon the normal tissues, which makes it seem to me in a measure explain why the cancer mortality under surgical management increased from 63 to 100,000 in 1900 to 81.8 in 1919, or over 28 per cent.

Loeb was able by cuts, incomplete extirpation, transplantation of tumors, etc., to excite new growths in tumors, both benign and malignant; which teaches us that a tumor probably should not be sectioned for examination, unless that tumor be removed quite soon thereafter, also it may explain why following the disturbance, incident in operation, of a small cyst or other tumor we have later developing a malignancy.

Chemical formative stimuli undoubtly play a considerable part in the natural growth and development of normal tissue.

The difference in the growth of certain organs in the young and the old, and in different races of people, and in the different climates, seems to suggest the difference not only in the chemical substances circulating in the blood which affect the growth not only in normal tissues, under normal conditions, but also the tissues, under abnormal conditions, that is with reference to nourishment, oxidation, etc., but also that there is a varying resistance on the part of the tissues in certain systems against the effect of these chemical formative stimuli. Analagous substances seem to favor growth or delay of tumors in several types of animal life. The amphibia for example. We see from Loeb's reports some indications that during pregnancy tumors may assume large proportion in the rat, while in the mouse, pregnancy seems to exert a very unfavorable influence on the growth or development of transplanted tumors so that it may be in the future that original and secondary, or primary and metastatic, tumors will be considered as separate and distinct things.

The corpus luteum bears a specific relation to the uterine wall and the mammary gland in the normal course of metabolism, also artificially given it has a definite effect upon the ovary in its essential function, that of ovulation. So that this probably comes under the second class, that of metastatic conditions. A Japanese investigator recently in some experiments with corpus luteum on the hen demonstrated beyond question that it has a positive inhibitory action on ovulation. It has been proven experimentally in the case of cancer of the mammary gland in mice that there can be no doubt that these special substances play an important part in changing normal into cancerous tissue. By extirpation of the ovaries at maturity, the spontaneous development of cancer of the breast, so common in certain strains of mice, can be almost altogether prevented.

There is another class of substances which prevent growth, as for example iodine, which according to Marine prevents compensatory hypertrophy of the thyroid, likewise according to Pearl calcium seems to counteract certain effects of the corpus luteum substances, as well as having a tendency to somewhat inhibit the growth of inoculated tumors. Again, certain of these formative stimuli established in the etiology of tumor growth may bring about a converse condition, as for example assuming that heredity forms a part, along this line, the development of stimulus may reach the point where it prevents the growth of tumor for one or two generations, when having lost its power or met new conditions in succeeding generations again acts as a productive factor.

In considering then a fully established cancer, it might be concluded that cancer is tissue growth in which a chemical stimulus probably not very differemt from that necessary to normal development is constantly at work producing changes which accompany all growths. So that internal secretions may be responsible for the production of cancer. It has been an accepted fact for some time that long continued stimulation may produce cancer; whether the chemical stimulus must be transmitted to the cells by an outside agency or whether long continued stimulation of tissue ultimately leads to such a change in the cell that the cell itself is unable to produce continuously the substance, which propagates the growth, is probably the thing yet to be decided.

Of the attempts to unite the various facts into consistent theory of tumor and tissue immunity and growths, only two recent ones seem to have attracted any particular attention, one by E. E. Tyzzer explains the immunity as due to a local anaphylactic reaction, that is, some substance is given off by the tumor cells which combines with the body fluid. The other by Loeb has to do with the mutual chemical incompatibility of the body fluids of one individual with the tissues of the other, which form abnormal products which are induced to produce dense fibrous tissue.

Williams remarks "a mass of evidence could be adduced to show that cancer is a disease of hypernutrition;" this may mean when taken with the findings of others that normal nutrition can be overdone, or that the complex of modern civilization with all its temptations and errors in regard to eating and drinking, together with the nervous strain and the absence of physical exercise does produce such a disturbance of the normal internal stimuli as to produce new growths.

At any rate the fact remains that while cancer is very infrequent among primitive people and among animals living in the state of nature, it is on the increase in morbidity and mortality with the increase of civilization. There can, therefore, be hardly any other conclusion than that this dire disease depends largely upon the conditions developed by or associated with our artificial existence, to which is given the name "modern civilization".

MALIGNANT DISEASE OF THE LARGE INTESTINE*

LeRoy Long, M. D., F. A. C. S.

OKLAHOMA CITY, OKLA.

In the development of malignant disease of the intestinal tract there are certain areas of predilection. Notwithstanding the close embryological relationship, the small bowel is not often involved. According to Bland-Sutton, 2 per cent of cancers of the alimentary tract are in the small intestine, while 25 per cent. involve the large intestine. In other words, the relative frequency of cancer of the small intestine to cancer of the large intestine is as two is to twenty-five.

Several theories have been presented in an effort to explain the frequency of development in the large intestine. One of the most familiar is that which takes into consideration the supposed etiological relationship of mechanical irritation. It is pointed out that the contents of the small intestine are in a relatively liquid state, while in the large intestine the contents have been dried out, and as a result, the mucosa receives injuries on account of the constant contact with such material. In support of this theory, it is pointed out that cancer of the stomach is relatively frequent, and that it may be explained in the same way— that is, that the gastric mucosa is repeatedly injured by the coarse mass of alimentary substances before the mass has been changed to a more liquid state by the process of digestion.

Ochsner is of the opinion that the chemistry of the alimentary tract has a good deal to do with the development of cancer. He calls attention to the fact that cancer is found much more frequently where the contents have an acid reaction. On the stomach side of the pylorus the contents are acid, and cancer is frequent. On the duodenal side the contents are alkaline and cancer in that locality is extremely rare. On the proximal side of the ileo-cecal valve the contents are alkaline, while there is an acid reaction on the distal side. In the first locality cancer rarely occurs, while it is relatively frequent in the second. He remarks that every farmer knows that noxious weeds grow in an acid soil, while clover and the useful plants grow best in an alkaline soil.

In the large bowel the places of predilection in the development of cancer are the cecum, the hepatic and splenic flexures, and especially the sigmoid and the pelvic colon. This fact would seem to support the mechanical irritation theory.

Carcinoma is by far the most frequent malignant disease of the large bowel, the sarcomata and the lymphosarcomata being extremely rare.

According to the schematic division by Ribbert, the epithelial tumors—that is to say, the carcinomata—of the large bowel may be divided into three general classes, all of them being composed of cylindrical epithelium: First, carcinoma cylindrocellulare adenomatosum, which is subdivided into (a) solidum, (b) polymorphum; second, carcinoma cylindrocellulare scirrhosum; third, carcinoma cylindrocellulare gelatinosum. Of these three the most frequent in the large bowel, according to Bastianelli, are carcinoma cylindrocellulare adenomatosum and carcinoma cylindrocellulare scirrhosum. The first may be carc. aden. simplex, hav-

*Read in Surgical Section, Annual State Meeting, Muskogee, May 21, 1919.

ing a connective stroma not quite scirrhous, and a non-medullary parenchyma, or it may be carc. aden. medullare, in which case it may form an enormous tumor with ulceration in the center. The lumen of the bowel may not be encroached upon; it may even be made larger by ulceration. Generally, however, there are fungating masses on the inside, and these serve to make the opening irregular and interfere with the fecal current. There is, too, infiltration about the walls which are stiffened and immobile.

In carcinoma scirrhosum there is a small, hard tumor of slow growth. The lumen may be encroached upon to the point of obliteration.

In carcinoma gelatinosum there is a large infiltrating hard growth with a deep ulcerating center, but without fungating masses.

It is pointed out that the insidious character of scirrhous carcinoma makes of it a hopeless condition for the reason that it is already an old standing one when it makes itself manifest, and disastrous metastases have already taken place. The gelatinous form is considered extremely malignant.

Practically, then, with our present knowledge, but little hope is had in any of these conditions save in connection with the adenomatous type, but in this type many patients may be relieved if operated early after symptoms have developed.

In the opinion of Bastianelli, the main questions to be considered, from a clinical point of view, are: (a) The extension of the parietal involvement; (b) visceral metastases; (c) glandular metastases; (d) peritoneal dissemination or grafting.

To ocular examination the parietal involvement may seem to stop abruptly, but Handley has pointed out that the microscope will show cancer cells far beyond the apparent boundary between the normal and the diseased areas.

It is impossible to determine the beginning or the extent of metastasis, for metastasis takes place often as soon as the connective spaces are penetrated. Attention is called to the fact, however, that the largest glands are not always the most dangerous, for the reason that they may be the seat of an inflammatory process, only. The condition of hardness and deformity of glands is much more significant.

To amplify a statement already made, three particular areas may be considered in connection with the matter of location of the cancer. Beginning at the origin of the large bowel, the first area is the cecum and the ascending colon. The second takes in the hepatic flexure, the transverse colon and the splenic flexure. The third area takes in the remainder of the colon down to the rectum, that is to say, the descending colon and the sigmoid, it being understood that the sigmoid embraces the pelvic colon, a term which is now in rather common use, and rightly so. By far the greater number of cancers occur in this third area— that is, the descending colon and sigmoid.

In the cecal region the neoplasm may grow from the ileo-cecal valve, the cecum proper or the ascending colon. They are mostly of the adenomatous type, either simplex or medullary. They are frequently large and often movable. The frequency in this region is second to that in the third region.

Bastianelli groups the principal symptoms as being the expression of two conditions, which he designates mechanical and septic. The mechanical element may be responsible for constipation, chronic obstruction with crises, acute obstruction and invagination. It would seem, however, that obstructive symptoms are not nearly so common in cecal cancers as they are in those of the terminal colon. Desmerest reports 220 cases with chronic obstruction in 20 and acute obstruction in 6, and the reports of other investigators practically agree.

Invagination is reported in about the same percentage of cases, the most frequent cause being the growth of the tumor on a limited portion of the valve or the cecum, and being pushed onwards by contractions of the ileum.

Septic complications may be expressed as fever, anemia, loss of weight, or they may be more direct, as abscess, perforation, peritonitis.

In the second area, malignant neoplasms have a special significance. Notwithstanding the fact that growths of the transverse colon may be found by physical examination much more readily than in any other portion of the large bowel, W. J. Mayo has found that the mortality is very high, probably because the lymph nodes about the head of the pancreas are involved very early.

Cancers of the third area involve the descending colon and the sigmoid, and for all practical purposes, our attention may be directed to the sigmoid exclusively, for it is in this location that the large majority of the left side tumors occur.

Quenu and Duval divide the sigmoid into three zones. First zone, from the descending colon to the brim of the pelvis—the ileo pelvic zone. Second, the pelvic portion of the sigmoid. Third, the zone at the junction of the pelvic colon with rectum, tumors at this point being called recto-sigmoidal tumors.

Van Hook and Kanaval, in an effort to systematize the symptomatology, group the manifestations of malignant processes in the large intestines under four heads:

1. Symptoms due to the progress of the neoplasm in the tissue of the affected organ.
2. Symptoms due to obstruction of the lumen of the intestine.
3. Symptoms due to metastases.
4. Symptoms due to adhesion and ingrowth to neighboring structures.

These authors say that, as a rule, the first symptoms of value are due to ulceration, and are diarrhea, fetid discharge, hemorrhage.

Taking into consideration the fact that cancer of the hidden organs is one of our most formidable problems, it would seem that we ought not to wait for these rather significant symptoms before directing our attention to an investigation with the view of clearing up, if possible, the existence or non-existence of a malignant process.

In studying the histories of these cases, clinicians call attention to several manifestations of importance.

1. Irregularity of the bowels—now constipated, now loose.
2. Soon there develops uneasiness and discomfort of the abdomen.
3. A little later there is pain and tenderness—sometimes colicky pains. Bastianelli emphasizes the importance of repeated attacks occurring somewhat like appendicitis, except as to location of pain.
4. Loss of flesh and strength greatly out of proportion to the pain.
5. If there is ulceration, the appearance of blood stained mucous, shreds, broken down tissue and pus in the stools.
6. The development of anemia as the result of absorption, and the underfeeding on account of poor appetite.
7. Obstinate constipation in those cases in which the cancer is causing a narrowing of the lumen.

As the process advances there are more postive symptoms:

1. Partial obstruction, which, especially if the carcinoma is in lower sigmoid, results in narrow or pencil like stools.
2. Visible peristalsis, which may indicate an almost complete, or a complete obstruction.
3. Complete obstruction, the signs of which will depend upon the location. Anschutz has called attention to the very marked distention of the cecum when the obstruction is low. Even when it is in the lower sigmoid the distention of the cecum may be so great that it is distinctly palpable and may lead one to believe that the pathology is in the cecal region. This has been called *local meteorism* by Anschutz.

Obstruction is more and more frequent the lower the seat of the tumor. In some cases a scirrhous of the pelvic colon may constrict the bowel as if a string was tied about it—*cancer en ficelle.*

In certain cases of great narrowing there may be sudden obstruction on account of the lodgment of a foreign body. A case is recalled in which the patient died as the result of an obstruction that was not operated. Autopsy showed a *cancer en ficelle*. There was enormous distention on the proximal side, and the distended area was packed full of bran, which the patient had been eating to relieve his obstinate constipation, the bran being packed into the tiny opening at the site of the cancer.

In an involvement of the lower sigmoid the sigmoidoscope should be used after the technique of Hanes of Louisville. In this way the lower part of the sigmoid may be examined. The x-ray is invaluable, particularly if there is narrowing.

Attention is called to the fact that benign tumors are rarely found in connection with the intestinal tract. Any evidence, then, pointing to tumor formation should lead one to suspect malignant disease.. However, benign or mixed types are occasionally found. Grossly considered, a differential diagnosis may be impossible.

A brief history in the case of a patient recently operated for a neoplasm of the terminal pelvic colon may be of interest.

Mr. C. L. W. White, age 52, dealer in automobiles, consulted me February 21, 1919, his principal complaint being frequent desire to defecate, the desire being preceded by pains in the lower abdomen.

The patient declared that he had always been well, with the exception of piles for which he had some kind of an operation seven or eight years ago, without complete relief, and an attack of pyorrhea for which he was treated about a year ago.

About four or five weeks before the consultation his mouth became sore. Having had pyorrhea he thought that was the trouble, and he, on his own responsibility, took some kind of ipecac tablets and a patent cathartic medicine, and other cathartics. He insisted that he was not constipated, the cathartics being taken under the impression that they would be of service in curing the sore mouth.

About the same time he began this treatment he noticed pains about the hips, but more pronounced about the left hip. He consulted a physician who told him that he had "rheumatism".

A few days after first noticing the pains about the hips there developed a frequent desire to defecate. At first the desire was not associated with pain, but gradually the desire became more frequent, and accompanied by sharp pains in the lower abdomen and in the rectum, the latter symptom being dwelt upon by the patient, obviously for the reason that he had had piles seven or eight years before.

At the time of the examination he complained of "continual aching" in the lower abdomen, and of a desire for the bowels to move ten or twelve times a day, there being but little discharge, and sometimes no discharge at all.

The patient had a good appetite, but he said that the taking of food was followed in five or ten minutes by a desire for the bowels to move.

The patient stated that he had not observed blood in the stools, that he had not passed black stools, but that he had had a few evacuations that looked like "undigested watermelon".

Apparently his general condition was good. He had not lost weight. The blood pressure was 124-80. The reflexes, the pupils, the station were normal. The teeth and gums were fair. The head, neck, chest, extremities, negative. The back, the kidney areas, the sacro-iliac joints were negative. Aside from a little tenderness over the right external ring and extending to a point to the inner side of the crest of the right ilium, the abdomen was negative to physical examination. No enlargements could be felt; no tympany could be made out. An examination of the rectum for six inches was negative. There were several small piles of neglible importance about the anal margin.

At the time of the first examination it was suspected that the patient might be developing a malignant tumor along the course of the intestinal tract, but the diagnosis was not clear.

The patient was sent home with the suggestion to his physician to have him return in a week or ten days, if the symptoms were not relieved. He did not return until April 5th when the picture was an entirely different one. He related that he began to-pass blood soon after the former examination; that his diarrhea had been worse; that he was losing weight and that he felt very bad.

A physical examination showed that he had a little stiffness of all the abdominal muscles, and there was a little tenderness in the lower part of the abdomen, more particularly on the right side. His pulse rate was 80, blood pressure 114-75. He was sent to the hospital and a consultant was asked to see him. At first the consultant felt very strongly that the patient might have an amebic dysentery, but a careful examination of the stools was negative. The stools, in fact, were practically normal. Although examined several times, there was no occult blood found. The gastric examination was negative. The examination of the urine was practically negative. The blood examination showed 80 per cent. hemoglobin, R. B. C. 4,200,000, W. B. C. 12,200, polynuclear 63, lymphocytes 34, eosinophiles 1. A Wassermann was negative.

Another consultant was asked to make a proctoscopic examination. He reported the findings negative.

Finally some x-ray plates were made, first with the injection into the rectum. The plate showed that the injected material ballooned the rectum and extended but a short distance into the pelvic colon. Another plate made twelve hours after the ingestion of a chemical meal showed a distinct narrowing at exactly the same point indicated by the rectal injection. It may be remarked that the various laboratory examinations were negative with the exception of the x-ray, which gave very positive and very important information, for upon the x-ray findings a diagnosis of a neoplasm in the pelvic colon was made.

Operation disclosed a large tumor at the extreme lower extremity of the pelvic colon and involving the bowel for a distance of about six inches. Grossly, it was an adenomatous carcinoma. What seemed strange at the time was that there were no enlarged glands found in the neighborhood, but there were many small papillomata scattered over the adjacent peritoneal surfaces. The tumor was adherent to the bladder and to the coils of the small intestine which had fallen down about it. There was also a rather broad attachment to the omentum. The pathologist reported that the tumor was a myxadenoma.

References

1. Malignant Disease of the Large Intestine, by Bastinelli, reported in the proceedings of the International Congress of Medicine, London, 1913.

2. Principles and Practice of Surgery, by A. P. C. Ashhurst.

3. Section on Malignant Disease of the Intestinal Tract, by J. Garland Sherrill, Louisville, Ky., in reference Handbook of the Medical Sciences, 1914.

Discussion

Dr. A. L. Blesh, Oklahoma City: The discussion of Dr. Long's paper was an honor thrust upon me. I did not have the pleasure of seeing the paper before coming here, and have just now heard it read. To my mind the great lesson here is that of early diagnosis. Under the relations at present existing between the medical staff of the hospital, its laboratory, the full power of the latter is not available as an aid in clinical diagnosis for the simple reason that the average patient is financially unable to meet the expense. This radiograph most beautifully emphasizes the lesson that it should have been made earlier. It is to be said for our Government, that it not only equipped its hospitals liberally, but insisted—yes, ordered—that the equipment be used. No doubt a radiograph taken when this patient first consulted the essayist would have located the seat and nature of the trouble at a time when the surgery of it would have been much simpler, and the results correspondingly better. Every neoplasm of the sigmoid colon should be looked upon with a strong suspicion of malignancy. A closer relationship must be established between the laboratory and the staff, in the patients interest.

Dr. Long, closing: I thank you very much for your kind references to the paper in general, but since the criticism has seemed to develop about the case operated:—When this man presented himself you will remember he was in good general condition. He had frequent bowel movements, but there was nothing about him particularly that would indicate at that time, very strongly, that he had a neoplasm. With the exception of this disturbance, he seemed to be in good general condition. A consultant thought it was a case of dysentery, which seemed to have a good basis, and I thought ought to be investigated very carefully. When he came back to the hospital he had taken bismuth and it was sometime before we had his stools in condition so examination of the stools would be conclusive. When he came back to the hospital the second time—or was sent to the hospital at that time—he had lost some weight, but was not anemic. He had not been eating much, because when he would eat it would make him feel bad and his bowels would act pretty soon. Finally, investigation developed he had a neoplasm.

Answering another question that was raised by one of the gentlemen kind enough to discuss the paper, I think that the statement that was made in the paper was that among the different manifestations of malignant diseases of the intestinal tract would be manifestations due to extensions in the organ involved, due to visceral and glandular metastases and so on. One ought not expect these things in the early cases. It was simply mentioned that these things happen later. It is possible they may happen where they are not very apparent. It is usually too late to do anything for the patient when they exist, and it was not mentioned as a matter upon which we should base a diagnosis in the early case, because these things occur late, and when they occur it is usually too late to do anything particularly for the patient.

NOTE.—The patient referred to above returned to hospital June 16, 1919, with symptoms of intestinal obstruction. A large, somewhat nodular mass was made out by palpation. It seemed to practically fill the abdomen. Abdominal section disclosed an enormous neoplasm involving omentum and intestinal coils. Numerous papillamata were scattered over the peritoneal surfaces. The clinical diagnosis of carcinoma seemed to be only too clearly supported.

A cecostomy performed with difficulty, on account of the extensive involvement limiting mobilization, gave temporary relief. The patient died today (July 3, 1919). An autopsy was done, but the report of the pathologist is not yet in my hands.—Author.

ABDOMINAL SPONGE

Accidents will happen, and out of 27,250 abdominal operations at the Mayo Clinic during the last five years, thirteen were for the removal of sponges left in the abdomen. In most of the cases the patients were from rural districts, and had probably been operated on for acute conditions by general practitioners with very mediocre assistants. This is the statement of J. C. Masson, Rochester, Minn. (*Journal A. M. A.*, May 31, 1919), who remarks that the only wonder is that there are not more such accidents under such circumstances. The patient usually recovers after a stormy convalescence, but has a persistent sinus left, and while he has to thank the original operator for saving his life he will seldom hesitate to sue for unlimited damages, if he learns the facts. Masson, therefore, has the sponges made with a silver ring placed around the base of the tape and firmly sewed to both sponge and tape with strong thread. If a sponge is reported missing, its whereabouts will be indicated by the metal band, as show by roentgen ray. In hospitals this procedure should be especially applicable.

THE DIAGNOSIS OF CANCER.

A Plea for Greater Care in Examination.

BENJAMIN H. BROWN, A. B., M. D.

MUSKOGEE, OKLAHOMA

Statistics quoted by Ewing in his *Neoplastic Diseases* show a remarkable increase in the recorded deaths from cancer during the last fifty years. In England in 1840, one of every 129 deaths reported was from cancer, while in 1905 the ratio had risen to 1 in 17. Ewing believes, from an analysis of the data, that there has been little if any increase in the actual incidence of cancer, and that the apparent increase is due to improved methods of diagnosis and to the longer tenure of life dependent upon the rapid strides of preventive medicine, improvement in hygiene, and more efficient methods of treating disease. In the more progressive countries during the same fifty year period the increase in the average expectation of life ranges from ten to twenty-five years. This is equivalent to saying that the majority of mankind, instead of dying before middle age, as was the case a generation ago, now attain to the years when cancer is more prevalent. Riechelman states that in Berlin hospitals in 1902 there was room, through improved diagnostic methods, for a 20 per cent. increase in cancer deaths.

Although there may be doubts as to whether there is an increase in the incidence of cancer at a given age as compared with former years, there can be none that cancer is one of the leading factors in the mortality tables, indeed crowding close to the top of the list in middle life and old age. It is also clear that in the past the diagnosis of cancer has been grossly unsatisfactory, and that even now there is abundant room for improvement along this line.

Aside from prophylaxis directed against predisposing and irritating factors, the only way in the present state of our knowledge of the subject in which we can improve the statistics is by the complete eradication of the diseased tissue, which depends upon treatment while the disease is still localized, which depends upon early diagnosis. It behooves us, then, as physicians to do our duty in the premises by making every effort of which we are capable to take this first and essential step.

Leaving out of consideration those forms of internal cancer which are obscure and difficult of diagnosis, the physician too often fails to recognize those which are begging for a diagnosis, and in which a little care and attention to detail would prevent the scarring of professional reputations and perhaps result in the saving of life. It is not genius that is required to obviate the more common blunders, but thorough history taking, painstaking examination, and prompt action where findings justify. In order to minimize the most frequent sources of diagnostic failure, careful consideration should be given to the following points:

(1). In general, malignancy should be excluded, regardless of age, in all patients with stomach and other abdominal symptoms, in all who have lost weight or are anemic.

(2). Every lump and every obscure pain in a woman's breast should make us think of cancer, even though in a majority of cases the suspicion may be without foundation.

(3). In every abdominal condition which might be cancer a rectal examination should be made. The finding of metastases sometimes clears the diagnosis. The same procedure should be adopted with every patient complaining of sciataca or abnormal sensations in the lower back or legs. Not only have neoplasms been often discovered in this way, but other conditions as well, such as a tuberculous abscess pointing in the pelvis. A local examination should be made whenever there is complaint of hemorrhoids, hemorrhage, pain or other rectal symptoms.

(4). Metrorrhagia is a mandatory indication for a careful examination by palpation and inspection, especially if the patient is near or past the menopause.

(5). We should not lose sight of the fact that hematuria is one of the symptoms, frequently the first, of tumor of the kidney, bladder or prostate.

The observations made above are not intended to be complete, but are suggestive and directed against the most common oversights. In addition they are elementary and obvious. However, no apology is offered for presenting them. The important is often obvious and the obvious is often overlooked. It is only by constantly keeping before us their importance that we can avoid the mistake of neglecting the simple means of diagnosis which are ready at hand, as well as that of failure to resort to the more complicated methods of laboratory and examining room.

CLINICAL REPORT OF OPERATION ON UNDESCENDED TESTES.

FRED S. CLINTON, M. D., F. A. C. S.
PREIDENT AND CHIEF SURGEON OKLAHOMA HOSPITAL
TULSA, OKLAHOMA

A few weeks ago there was presented for the care of the writer a fourteen year old boy with double undescended testes, and after a careful survey of the literature it was found that one of the most responsible and satisfactory descriptions of the development of successful operation was in the December (1918) number of *Surgical Clinics of Chicago* by Dr. Arthur Dean Bevan. Inasmuch as his experience and operative technic is based upon the study of over 400 cases, his teaching was followed in the case presented.

The parents, in presenting the boy for examination, requested a written opinion as to whether he should be operated upon and I therefore advised that:

(a) At this age, 14 years, he has the best chance of getting good results.

(b) There can be no doubt that the individual is better off with organs in a normal position than if they are in the abdominal cavity or in the inguinal canal or in the external rings.

(c) If in an abnormal position such as the inguinal canal, they are more subject to injury and more dangerous to the balance of the body if diseased than if in a normal position.

(d) The present deformity is invariably associated with great risk of hernia or rupture.

(e) There is some evidence to show that undescended testes are more apt to be the site of malignant disease than those in normal position.

(f) There is associated with these cases particularly, as in all malformations, a certain psychic element which must be considered.

Our effort to correct the deformity of course would be in principle as follows:

(a) Endeavor to restore the testes to their normal position.

(b) To correct the tendency to hernia.

(c) Diminish the danger of trauma or injury to the testes.

(d) Relieve the patient from mental worry associated with this deformity.

(e) Lessen the element of risk of malignant degeneration.

The technic of the operation together with the illustrations are best understood by the study of the original report above indicated.

This, the same as any other successful reconstructive plastic surgery, must be free from: (a) sepsis, (b) hemorrhage, (c) tension, (d) with adequate blood supply.

The results in lengthening the cord some five inches, as described by Dr. Bevan, and placing the testes in their new beds, was so satisfactory that I felt it was desirable to call the attention of some other members of the profession who may have needs for this particular information.

REPORT OF MEETING OF THE CLINICAL SOCIETY OF ST. ANTHONY HOSPITAL.

Dr. J. W. Riley, Chairman.   Dr. Lelia Andrews, Secretary.

Section 1.—Report of Deaths in Hospital for Previous Month.

Dr. M. Smith: There have been many cases in which the cause of death has been very interesting to me and probably to some of the rest of us. The health department, I think, very wisely, too, are demanding diagnoses as to the cause of death. You have to give the exact cause of death. Now in cases in which the patient has sustained an injury and dies immediately it can be reported as such, but if he lives a few days this diagnosis is no longer acceptable as the exciting cause of death.

The patient I am reporting on tonight is a railroad engineer, Mr. C. V., who while attempting to jump from his engine as engine left the track was so caught under the engine as to suffer severe crushing injuries, the exact extent of which could not be determined. In addition patient received a simple fracture of the right tibia and fibula and was severly scalded. On entering hospital patient was found to be in a semi-conscious condition but complained of pain over epigastrium. Four hours later patient was catheterized and a small amount of urine obtained. Physical examination demonstrated nothing but what has been mentioned above. Cause of death, internal injury, the exact nature of which was not determined as no post-mortem was allowed.

Dr. J. F. Kuhn: The case I am reporting was treated by Dr. Lea Riley and myself. Patient, Miss D. S., age two years Personal and present illness: Patient's birth was affected by employment of high forceps. Since birth, has not progressed normally in a mental way and some impairment of proper use of feet has always been present. On the night of March 2, 1919, patient ate a small portion of banana. Following morning parents noticed nothing unusual concerning baby until noon when baby suddenly lost consciousness. A physician was called at once and the temperature found to be 107. Physical examination made a few minutes later in the hospital revealed nothing other than a failure in reaction of pupils to light and the presence of nystagmus, and marked distention of abdomen of gaseous nature. The laboratory reported albumin in urine along with diacetic, many W. B. C. and hyaline and granular casts. The blood count showed 18500 W. B. C. with 68 Poly. count; R. B. C. normal. Treatment consisted of immersing body in tepid water until temperature was under control and the administration of sodium bicarbonate, whiskey, and bromides as indicated. Intake of proper amount of water was maintained with stomach pump. On night of arrival a lumbar puncture was done and 30 c.c. withdrawn under marked pressure, clear in appearance. Laboratory reported spinal fluid negative. On night of March 6, 1919, patient died without having regained consciousness and with the marked elevation of temperature still persisting. Diagnosis: acute toxic enteritis.

Dr. J. W. Riley: I have a case to report, a Mr. R. V., age 19 years. This case belongs to the medical men but I was asked to do a lumbar puncture. The history in brief, which was obtained through an interperter, consisted of vertigo and tinnitus aurium which began one year ago and which became so severe during the last eight months as to render it necessary for the patient to remain in bed. About three weeks ago patient noticed a dimness of vision which increased in severity rapidly and resulted in total blindness in seven days. About three months ago patient noticed an impairment of use of left arm with development of ataxic gait. Two years ago had an initial lesion on genitals which was followed in a few weeks by a rash over body.

Physical examination showed a total amblyopia and absence of pupillary reaction. Epitrochlears not enlarged. Impaired gait present.

The laboratory reported the routine examination of blood and urine negative. The Wassermann and Hecht-Gradwohl negative, with the blood. Negative results were also reported with the spinal fluid.

On February 28, 1919, I was asked to do the lumbar puncture which we did, turning him on his left side. There was no trouble in getting the fluid and I took an ordinary test tube, half full, which was probably six or seven c.c. I asked the interperter a few questions and he told me of these headaches, vertigo, etc. This was done about 10:00 o'clock and about 1:00 o'clock I learned that the man was not breathing well and in a few minutes he died. The autopsy showed that he had a tumor of the right hemisphere, which was elongated, of firm consistency and which encroached upon the ventricle. This tumor was perhaps as large as a good sized walnut. It cut firmly on section, and appeared brown externally and white internally. The Wassermann was negative and the cell count about normal, I understand. The tumor was turned over to the pathological laboratory and will now be reported by the pathologist.

Dr. L. A. Turley: I took a section and run it through in the usual manner; on placing it under the microscope, found it was a mass of connective tissue, not infiltrated, so the diagnosis was gumma of the brain.

Dr. J. W. Riley: Dr. Lea Riley has a death to report.

Dr. Lea Riely: This man gave the following history: Two weeks ago he had chills, fever, and aching over the entire body, followed with a cough. I was asked by the firm employing him to see him in connection with the physician looking after him. I went to see him and found that he had a broncho-pneumonia at base of left lung as far as the third vertebrae. I saw him a couple of days and his breathing was very rapid, respiration high and tongue dry. After the second day the dullness was succeeded with flatness and the breath sound was further away and not so distinct in lower portion of lungs. I inserted a needle between the sixth and seventh ribs, and had him removed to the hospital here. On arriving here we removed about 500 c.c. of purulent material from pleural cavity in which the laboratory reported pneumococcus and staphylococcus, both by smear and culture. The next morning, after removing this pus, his breathing became much better and his heart beats were stronger. This continued for 24 hours followed with a return of the symptoms. I now put in a spinal puncture needle between the fourth and fifth lumbar vertebrae and drew off about 67 c.c. of fluid. This fluid was clear but had been cloudy on previous punctures. No bacteria found in fluid. Following the puncture the patient revived and regained his senses and was much better for another twelve hours. Next morning his condition was alarming and in about three hours he died.

This brings up a point to me in connection with this case, that I do not feel exactly satisfied with, and one which I have been studying a great deal. This epidemic of influenza has been particularly selective to the cerebro-spinal type. I believe it was a case of potential meningitis, because this fellow was always much better after relieving the pressure. It became more active after lumbar puncture, and there are two theories whether or not the release of pressure allows the germs to enter the spinal fluid or whether the lumbar puncture produces inflammation of the meninges.

Some experiments have been brought out along this line of injecting animals with toxic bacteria. Two animals are used, one a control animal on which the lumbar puncture is not done and one in which this procedure is carried out. The latter animal develops meningitis, showing that this came into the meninges and produced meningitis. The question is whether this puncture hastens the meningitis or not. For instance, two men in Philadelphia who treat cerebro-spinal lues, give an injection of 606 and then do a lumbar puncture and get the effect from this. We did not take a blood culture from this man but I am sure he had pneumonoccic bacteria. Cause of death, pneumonic meningitis.

SECTION 2.—PRESENTATION OF CLINIC BY DR. A. A. WILL.

GUNSHOT WOUNDS OF LEFT CHEST, TWO BULLETS ENTERING BELOW COSTAL BORDER
AND BOTH PERFORATING CHEST WALL POSTERIORLY IN EXIT.

Dr. A. A. Will: This particular man entered the marines last October and while stationed in Virginia had this accident, which was a gun shot wound of left chest. Now the question comes up, this man had contracted lues about three years ago which he did not mention in history. Has lost weight since injury but thinks that this was not due to the resulting empyema but to the fact that he ate very little food. Since that time patient has been running a very irregular course of fever and has lost about thirty pounds in weight. I saw him the day he arrived here, his temperarure was 101. The next day I did not see him. The following day his temperature was 105 1-2. Still the drainage was not very profuse from his side. During the examination the right lung was apparently clear. The left side was flat. On the ninth day I sent him to the hospital. The second day here the temperature dropped to 104. At that examination I discovered pneumonia in the right lower lobe. His temperature continued runing high and on the seventh day his temperature was still 105 and on the eighth day 104 1-2. Then he had a crisis and it went to 96 3-5, and from that time on he ran more or less temperature until a week ago when it became normal, and remained so ever since.

This boy is interesting from several points. The first is we have never known whether the bullet pierced the diaphragm or not; when he arrived here the tubes were not in the abscess cavity. Upon removal of the tube, the tube was found absolutely closed. There was a small opening near the tip of the tube. Evidently when his chest became fully filled it would drain through this small opening. This tube had been in there for five weeks; when it was full it would overflow at the end of the tube or result in the patient having a coughing spell.

Four weeks following the injury he had a rib resection done. He was unconscious during this time and was simply put to bed and kept quiet. I have some X-ray pictures that will be of interest, I want to demonstrate the empyema of the lung. This tube was low down. The abscess, as we have mapped it out, was down lower. Each time it would flow in here it came out through the tube. After we removed this tube we put in one of our tubes. This is our air space. These pictures were taken as the pneumonia had more or less cleared up, in right lung. We stethoscoped this man several times and did so this morning and every time he had a pneumothorax. The question arose in our minds whether this space was above or below the diaphragm. This man is better and is on his way to recovery. In fact he has been up and around several days. We treated this the same way as the empyema (drainage tubes with irrigations of Dakin's solution). The pathological reports are coming along very nicely.

The third thing that is interesting is what I have contended all the time, that it is poor surgery not to do a resection of the ribs when you have thick pus, but it has been demonstrated to me that you can remove the pus and get good results without it. (This was accomplished in this case with irrigation with Dakin solution through drainage tube). Now, Dr. Moorman I wish you would demonstrate this X-ray which I am not able to do.

Dr. L. J. Moorman: I was asked to see this boy soon after he came into the hospital and might state that we found at that time in connection with these photos, compression of the lung, which I think the x-ray shows. There is an air space that you can see, a tube going into that space. Evidently with this perforating wound we had considerable collapse of the lung. There is a good deal of mottling of the lung; the boy going through what he did before he came here resulted in conditions that would account for that. I think that the boy is very lucky to have lived at all. Now in the first place the bullets entered below the costal line, and I do not see how they came out without perforating the diaphragm. It seems to me, regardless of the pathological report and the outcome of this case, that the bullets must have perforated the diaphragm in order to have traversed from the abdomen to the region of the scapula, and we are quite sure that these bullets perforated the lung and left pneumothorax. This illustrates very clearly the value of laboratory procedure and the danger of incompetent interpretation. We guessed that this air space, apparently below the diaphragm, was gas in the stomach. There was little movement of the diaphgram. We had him under the fluoroscope and it was suggested that we give him some bismuth to see if the pocket of gas really represented the stomach. To our surprise the bismuth passed on down and located the stomach far below the normal position.

It seems to me that this boy would have gotten along much better if the wounds had been properly cleaned and sealed at the time. I believe it is the practice of the surgeons at the Front to take that chance on these cases.

Dr. LeRoy Long: Anything further Dr. Will? Gentlemen, you have heard this interesting report. It is now open for discussion.

Dr. Riley: There are certain things about this case that appear to me to be interesting. In the first place you have a pneumothorax here, the diaphragm does not show quite so plain on the affected side and I think there is pus in here and it is a sub-diaphragmatic abscess.

Dr. M. Smith: Is the pus thick?

Dr. Will: It was at first but the Dakin solution cleared it up.

Dr. Smith: I have watched a lot of these cases that the war men had and I like to watch the improvement. Recently I have seen some brilliant and succesful work with nine radical operations. I think that a large number of those cases where you get thick pus, if you use Dakin solution it will completely melt it down. Now there must be something in it and we will all be using it more in the future than we in the past.

Dr. Lea Riely: Dr. Will spoke of the pus being negative. I wonder if a smear would show any of the germs. It seems after the Dakin solution the germs are dead, but the smear will sometimes show them. They are in the smear, Dr. Will, are they not?

Dr. Will: Yes, they are still in the smear.

Query: There was a differential count of 70 when he first came in, was there not?

Dr. Will: When he first came in the white count was 10,400. The differential 78 and 22. His temperature now runs about 99 in the afternoons.

Dr. Long: I am not sure whether it is understood from his remarks that it is the accepted way to heal wounds of the chest as long as we have any debris in the chest. Wounds may be closed when we have a clean wound, not only a clean wound but a wound full of vitality. It has been carried on to this point, that practically any wound, especially large wounds, but on any wounds where it is possible to vitalize the tissue then it may be sewed up right away, and if I understand it, that was the practice. But understand, that does not mean to sew up or close up hermetically any wound if devitalized tissue is present or to sew it up on the assumption that there will be no trouble. The physicians point out that it may be about thirty hours before there will be any trouble. If the wound has been cleaned and we have only sound tissue, then let it alone. If it shows staphylococcus, then let it alone but watch it. If it shows streptococcus, then you are in trouble. I do not believe that it was ever intended, especially in wounds of the lungs, to seal them up hermetically as long as we have devitalized tissues. You should put on clean gauze after it has been cleansed, but do not stop up hermetically, because it is understood that there will be more or less drainage. A few times we may have pus develop from wounds of the chest. I agree with those gentlemen that this bullet went through the diaphragm.

Dr. Moorman: I heard Devaul, the Italian, and two English surgeons on surgery of the chest. They state that they would take a chance with trouble within with devitalized tissue removed. They always prepared for a second opening if necessary but would close these wounds in this way. If they had a serious wound, they would deliver the lung from the pleural cavity and free it from foreign matter and put it back and still close it completely. The Italian used artificial pneumothorax in case of hemorrhage. This is where I got my authority for this statement.

Dr. Long: I remember that statement made by these men. I was impressed that Devaul operated without removing the lung but the lung was just brought out, the chest cleaned up and lung replaced and sewed up, but that was after devitalized tissue had been removed. I do not think that just running gauze through it would be right. Just exactly opposite is Dr. Barton Ellis' procedure. I think that is the outstanding thing we have learned in connection with the war, that when devitalized tissue is removed we can sew it up or do anything we want to do with it.

Dr. W. K. West: I had a course in Bellevue a year and a half ago. There instead of resecting a rib, a lateral intercostal incision was made and tractors applied, separating the ribs so that the lung was delivered.

Dr. Will (closing): It makes you appreciate how much you get from these clinics. I think Dr. Moorman will tell you that we have fooled with this case for several weeks and we are not sure of the diagnosis. We were sure but are not now. We thought we had a sub-diaphragmatic abscess. It is worth a great deal to us for you men to declare it is a sub-diaphragmatic abscess. This boy, instead of having a torn wound or any wound you would get from a schrapnel, had a clean wound and I do not suppose very much lacerated tissue. The Sister (in charge of dressings) has said many times that she believed there was a drainage from that cavity, as one day she would get practically no pus and other days large amounts.

SECTION 3.—DEATH REPORTS FOR MARCH, 1919.

Dr. George La Mott:—Empyema. Baby D., age two and one-half years. Influenza followed by pneumonia six months ago. She developed marked dullness on the right side, which was diagnosed empyema. There was some dyspnea and orthopnea at times but patient had never been subject to spasms or convulsions prior to this attack. The condition was so acute that I did not operate her the day she came into the hospital, but the increasing sepsis made it impossible to delay it over one day.

On the second day after the child came in, I used 30 cc. of 0.2 per cent solution of cocaine and introduced a needle into the ninth interspace posteriorly. I withdrew about one-half ounce of tenacious ropy pus, then injected one-half ounce Dakin solution and again withdrew a small amount of pus. At this time patient suddenly became rigid and the needle was withdrawn. After a brief spasm the child succumbed. Heat and stimulation were of no avail. The pulse remained good until immediately before death. Slight cyanosis of the lips, but finger nails remained pink. I was unable to get an autopsy.

Now gentlemen, what was the cause of death? I feel like it was due to embolism, yet the element of pleural shock must be considered. I would be very glad to hear some discussion on the case.

Discussion.

Dr. D. D. McHenry. This is a very interesting case to me since death might have been from any one of several causes. A child of this age and general condition would be very susceptible to the cocaine anesthetic, but the entire amount injected was no more than one-sixth grain.

Dr. L. J. Moorman. I have read a great deal about pleural shock, but have never seen a case. I am frank to say I don't exactly understand the condition but it seems to me that if the anesthetic was carried through the parietal pleura it might lessen the danger of pleural shock.

Dr. Le Roy Long. The older writers classify the cause of death under three heads: 1. Failure of the heart itself. 2. Changes in the lungs. 3. Death through the central nervous system.

I think we can eliminate the first cause because there was no previous cardiac disturbance and the pulse remained good up to the time of·death.

The second cause may be eliminated since there was only slight cyanosis, the finger nails remained pink.

I think, then, we can say death was through the nervous system. The most probable cause being cerebral embolism.

Dr. M. Smith:—Osteo-sarcoma. Mr. E. A. J., age 60, traveling man. The trouble began as small nodule on left scapula. This was removed several years ago, but recurred. He was subjected to repeated operations.

About eight months ago he again came into the hospital. At this time he had a sloughing ulcer on his back extending from the scapular region down to the lumbar region extending almost the entire length of his back, the toxins of which were enough to produce death. The large sloughing ulcer was the result of a "cancer paste" which was applied at one of the so-called "cancer hospitals." The damage done by the caustic was far more grave than the·malignancy. He was given a general anesthetic and I removed all the necrotic tissue, even to a portion of the left scapula, which had been necrosed by the paste. Cautery was applied to the bleeding vessels and later skin grafts were done.

The patient came back to the hospital a few weeks ago, very weak and emaciated. There was evidence of general metastasis and the pain was intense. He succumbed from toxemia.

Dr. L. J. Moorman:—Broncho pneumonia complicating influenza. Mrs. M. W., age 45, the mother of nine living children. The youngest child was two weeks old when the mother died and seven of the children were brought to the hospital with the mother on account of influenza. The patient entered the hospital forty-eight hours after the onset of the illness in a state of extreme prostration, dyspneic and cyanotic with signs of meningeal irritation. The physical examination revealed evidence of extensive broncho-pneumonia involving both lungs. The white count was 4,500. Patient died twelve hours after entering hospital. Autopsy was not secured.

Dr. L. J. Moorman:—Empyema following influenza. John M. C. N., age 45. Patient gave history of several attacks of malaria, otherwise history negative. Contracted influenza November, 1918, from which he never recovered. He entered the hospital March 15 in a delirious state, apparently suffering from some overwhelming toxemia.

Diagnosis. (1). Extensive empyema of the right chest. The liver was displaced downward and the mediastinal structures pushed far to the left. (2). Mitral insufficiency. (3). Pulmonary tuberculosis (dullness and moisture in upper lobe of the left lung). The latter condition probably explains the so-called attacks of malaria which preceded the influenza. Patient died in less than twenty-four hours after entering hospital.

The history and clinical findings with autopsy report, which appears below, cause one to wonder how the case could have gone on so long without recognition and treatment.

Autopsy Report. Right lung completely collapsed from apex to base. Numerous white areas, one to ten mm. in diameter in the lower lobe. Pleura covered with corrugated thickenings. One gallon and a half of greenish fluid escaped from the pleural cavity. The left lung adherent to the chest wall in places, contained many white areas over the surface. Caseous tuberculosis in both lungs. Complete atelectasis in right lung. Pyothorax in right side. Mild acute nephritis beginning. Arterio-sclerosis of the aortic ring and mitral valve.

Case Report—Aortic Aneurism.

Dr. J. T. Martin, Oklahoma City. Mr. A. G. B., age 58, contractor. History of penile sore, twenty years ago.

I reported this case before the society six years ago. At that time he complained of rheumatism, asthma and a pain in the chest with a brassy cough. The diagnosis of aneurism was easy. He had a marked polyuria, passing from fourteen to twenty quarts of light colored urine per day, and an excessive thirst. No edema. Chest negative, one knee jerk absent. Romberg sign negative. Members of the society estimated his life at six to eight months. He was put on mercury and potassium iodide treatment and advised to lead a quiet life on account of his aneurism.

I present the case again tonight with a smaller aneurism than he had six years ago. This shows that we can never know what may happen. The pulsating tumor in his chest is smaller and the pains are less severe. His tabetic signs and symptoms, however, are more prominent. He now has the Argyll-Robinson pupil and shows some ataxic gait. He has some arterio-sclerosis but no heart lesion. There is no appreciable difference in the two radial pulsations.

I have presented this case because it showed the unusual termination of aneurism in a man of this age.

OSTEITIS FIBROSA

J. L. DeCourcy, Cincinnati (*Journal A. M. A.*, May 31, 1919), reports a case of osteitis fibrosa in the upper portion of the humerus in a boy of twelve. A cyst, about 2 1-2 inches in length, filled with bloody matter, was dissected out with some healthy bone, and a strip from the tibia was transplanted into its place. A few isolated giant cells were demonstrated in sections from the cyst, and, with its gross appearance, justified a diagnosis of osteitis fibrosa. He holds that such tumors should be considered malignant, and curettage, therefore, is contraindicated. A bone graft is a proper treatment, provided one can exclude infection after full resection of the cyst or tumor.

JOURNAL OF THE OKLAHOMA STATE MEDICAL ASSOCIATION

VOLUME XII   MUSKOGEE, OKLA., JULY, 1919   NUMBER 7

PUBLISHED MONTHLY AT MUSKOGEE, OKLA., UNDER DIRECTION OF THE COUNCIL

DR. CLAUDE A. THOMPSON, EDITOR-IN-CHIEF
308 SURETY BUILDING, MUSKOGEE

DR. CHAS. W. HEITZMAN, ASSISTANT EDITOR
BARNES BUILDING, MUSKOGEE

ENTERED AT THE POST OFFICE AT MUSKOGEE, OKLAHOMA, AS SECOND CLASS MAIL MATTER, JULY 28, 1912

THIS IS THE OFFICIAL JOURNAL OF THE OKLAHOMA STATE MEDICAL ASSOCIATION. ALL COMMUNICATIONS SHOULD BE ADDRESSED TO THE JOURNAL OF THE OKLAHOMA STATE MEDICAL ASSSOCIATION, 308 SURETY BUILDING, MUSKOGEE, OKLAHOMA.

The editorial department is not responsible for the opinions expressed in the original articles of contributors.

Reprints of original articles will be supplied at actual cost, provided request for them is attached to manuscript or made in sufficient time before publication.

Articles sent this Journal for publication and all those read at the annual meetings of the State Association are the sole property of this Journal. The Journal relies on each individual contributor's strict adherence to this well-known rule of medical journalism. In the event an article sent this Journal fo publication is published before appearance in the Journal, the manuscript will be returned to the writer

Failure to receive the Journal should call for immediate notification of the editor, 307-8 Surety Building, Muskogee, Okla

Local news of possible interest to the medical profession, notes on removals, changes in address, deaths and weddings will be gratefully received.

Advertising of articles, drugs or compounds unapproved by the Council on Pharmacy of the A. M. A. will not be accepted.

Advertising rates will be supplied on application. It is suggested that wherever possible members of the Sta`e Associa tion should patronize our advertisers in preference to others as a matter of fair reciprocity.

EDITORIAL

CANCER PREVENTION.

Observers long ago noted that those diseases most difficult of cure or classed as incurable were invariably accompanied in materia medica, surgical manoeuvers and therapeutic literature by suggestions for control in ratio to the difficulty of cure or treatment.

Cancer stands unchallenged as the leader in this class. No system or department of medicine offers the sufferer, even average hope of permanent cure or arrest. Brushing aside the claims of the criminal exploiter of the cancer sufferer; the recurrent absurd claims of the charlatan in our own ranks, often with some pretensions of ability and plausability; and the occasional very highly-rated physician, who becomes paranoically wedded to his pet theory; the medical profession has had brought home to it forcibly, the following tenatively accepted ideas of etiology and management:

The cause is certainly not known or proved, but from the mass of experience the predominant possible factors seem to be.

Departure from cell type, due to nearly any trivial cause, but especially traceable to some form of constant irritation. Among the commoner being, neglected tears of the cervix. "Harmless" lumps in the female breast, "dyspepsia", indigestion, the various gastric disturbances, the very common growth about the face; and, other causes of lesser occurrence.

Whether these are to be accepted as causes is not so much our concern, but the safe and easy eradication of most of them, if recognized in time, is universally admitted by everyone. It follows that the responsibility of discovery and warning lies with, not the expert surgeon, but with the family physician, the man brought daily into contact with potential cancer. This conclusion has become absolute logic to observers, who accept with reservations, the ideas of cause and prevention.

If there is now any practical prevention it lies in acceptance of the rules suggested, and with the man who sees the case first and recognizes its dangers. It is his duty to advise his patient of the possibilities and the relative ease of correction. Any other course is unwarranted when the ease of early correction is compared with the tragic possibilities of non-recognition, pitiably useless and dangerous makeshifts so often noted when the case is beyond hope of relief. In many fatalities due to cancer the severe indictment of almost unbelieveable neglect on the part of a trusted family physician may be justly and properly lodged.

In the light of our present lack of information and divergence as to etiology, hair-splitting argument is well enough, indeed most useful in keeping the subject alive, but the only course the physician may follow with the maximum of benefit, is that of sane watchfulness, emphatic statement of the dangers of neglect and prompt removal of all abnormalities reasonably assignable as factors in production of cancer.

SYNTHETIC, VERSUS NATURAL SODIUM SALICYLATES.

Pernicious, financed and systematic activity of the ubiquitous "Detail" man, invariably biased and pregnant with inaccurate conclusions based on unauthenticated alleged research work; as a rule backed up with statements from some physicians equally biased and wholly unfitted to present opinions on technical, chemical, clinical or laboratory investigations, render it imperative that the attention of the hard worked physician, with no time to devote to investigation, be called again to the subject. The fact that Oklahoma has recently been most thoroughly "worked" by detail men, glibly misleading the busy doctor as to the merits of "Natural", over Synthetic Sodium Salicylates, warrants a statement of the findings in the matter.

In the first place the indisputable findings are not new to the informed, but the average physician has neither time or inclination to read the mass of matter, good and bad, coming to his desk. He is especially prone to ignore the weekly reports of his personal, uninspired—except to ascertain the truth,—scientific corps of investigators, the Council on Pharmacy and Chemistry of the American Medical Association. He has never reflected that, almost without variation, whatever the Council has assailed as unworthy in the years of its work, has come to oblivion and discredit. Among the investigations the Salicylate question was made and settled long ago. The conclusions are:

There is no difference between the toxicity of natural and synthetic sodium salicylate.

Clinical reports of differences are unsatisfactory and inconclusive as based on most inaccurate and questionable trial.

No significant chemical impurities are discoverable in the synthetic product.

Hilpert in 1913 investigated for the Council eleven specimens ranging from the cheapest commercial bulk sodium salicylate at 0.45 cents per pound to the highest-priced "Sodium Salicylate from True Natural Oil of Wintergreen" at $14.00 per pound. His conclusions were that there was no difference as to properties and composition.

A. W. Hewlitt the same year (*Journal A. M. A.*, August 2, 1913, page 319) published a compilation of the most thorough investigations of a corps of investigators. These were supplied with every conceivable specimen of salicylates, but without the slightest information of identity as to whether they were synthetic or natural. The clinical investigation was conclusive. Not one of them was able to distinguish between the two classes of products.

These findings have been substantiated so often that citations are useless.

We call attention to the matter now in order that physicians may be able to reject the active "Educator" calling on him for the purpose of disseminating misinformation on a matter which he often pays little or no attention to.

CURRENT MEDICAL LITERATURE
Conducted by
DR. CHAS. W. HEITZMAN, Barnes Building, Muskogee

Contributions and observations of Oklahoma physicians collected by them in the course of study of American and foreign medical literature, deemed to be of sufficient interest and value to the profession, are especially invited to this department. Such contributions should bear the name of the sender, which will be appended to the abstract or omitted, as desired.

LE PALUDISME A BORD DE "LA MARSEILLAISE" SUR LA COTE OCCIDENTALE DE L'AFRIQU

(Malaria on board the La Marseillaise on the west coast of Africa).

By Dr. G. Goett, medecin de 1re classe de la marne. Arch de Med. et Pharmacie Navales, No. 2, August, 1918, p. 118.

The very interesting, instructive and, in many respects, dramatic story of the author of the ravages made by malaria on board the Marseillaise is so typical of the havoc this disease can create on board a cruiser that the reviewer considers himself justified in presenting it to the readers of Military Surgeon in the author's own words as nearly as this can be done:

"La Marseillaise, coming from Brazil, arrived at Dakar on September 23, 1917. The sanitary conditions on board were excellent; the ship was ordered to go into drydock for some repairs to her bottom, and then to continue on her voyage to Agadir.

"It was the season during which the colony was the most insalubrious, and we learned on our arrival that there was a great deal of malaria on shore and that the first cases of blackwater fever had already made their appearance. Everybody on board was immediately put on preventive doses of quinine.

"Between September 23 to 28 we were at anchor in the roadstead, and saw but few mosquitoes. But, soon after having gotten into dock, September 28, the ship was invaded by anophelines. In one single night the ship was filled with them, and this for two cogent reasons: in the first place, the dock was extremely dirty, and even during normal times a veritable nest for mosquitoes; and, in the second place, the wind blew from the direction of a swampy plain, known to be full of fever and mosquitoes. Sufficient protection by mosquito netting or the closing of all the open places by wire screens not being available, we resorted to the use of an ointment consisting of equal parts of camphor and salol and with which we anointed the bodies of the men, with the view of keeping off the mosquitoes and of relieving the pain from their bites. On October 4 (six days since getting into dock) we left Dakar, having on board but four cases of malaria, but a steady increase in the number of cases could be noted from day to day, and on the 7th, when we arrived at Port-Etienne, we had 125 cases in beds; we departed on the 8th with 145 sick. On the 11th we had a maximum of 289 cases.

"The recurrent seizures were all alike, sudden, with violent headaches, intense lumbar pain and stiffness, face red and swollen, eyes brilliant, temperature rising without chilly rigors, no bilious vomiting in the beginning.

"Many of the recurring seizures became bilious, with nausea and vomiting, whenever the temperature began to rise. The attacks continued for six to eight days, some lasting for twelve days. There were cases of syncope occurring in men who were on their way from hammock to closet; some were delirious for several hours, the delirium disappearing with the fever, leaving but a light mental confusion. On the 18th day of October, the day of our arrival at Agadir, we still had 144 sick in bed, but the daily admissions decreased, and with the decrease in atmospheric temperature the number of mosquitoes declined.

"On October 27, the day of our return to Dakar, we had but few new cases a day, while the relapses became numerous and occurred without showing any regularity as to time; all, without exception, were tertians.

"The attacks occurred always during the morning, the patients reporting at the sick-bay after the 11 o'clock meal with voilent chilly rigors, the temperature rising. The fever lasted from six to eight hours and terminated in an intense perspiration. Quinine had a more marked action in these tertian forms than in the preceding remittent cases; they were made to disappear after the third day.

"Out of a complement of 598 men, 440 were attacked; 307 suffered a second tertian invasion, furnishing 532 relapses. Out of these 307 tertian cases 154 had one relapse, 101 had two, 32 had three, 20 had four.

"Observed complications.—On our arrival at Agadir, one of the mechanics had an attack of Raynaud's disease (local asphyxia of the extremities of the blue form). This was followed by gangrene of the toes and even of the feet, where blackish sloughs began to form: he was sent to the hospital at Casablanca. One of the sharpshooters, after an attack of remittent fever, presented a keratitis, followed by an ulcer of the cornea. Edemata were observed frequently. One case even showed general anasarca, heart and kidneys being absolutely normal. Aside from this case, the edemata were partial, attacking the malleoli and the scrotum, painless, white, causing but slight formications during their being absorbed. Amenesias and deliria, followed by mental confusion and disappearing with defervescence, were observed.

"One breveted sharpshooter, for the period of a week, was the victim of a dreamy delirium, seeking to find one of his relatives in every part of the ship and to wash his garments. A second master gunner was temporarily delirious, jabbering unintelligible phrases, afterwards remembering nothing that had occurred during the period. Another master gunner, with neurasthenic tendencies, panphobic and suspicious, suffering from insomnia, lived a life of sadness and solitude, speaking to no one, answering hardly any questions, except complaining of severe 'migraines.' Several cases of an urticaria-like eruption, during the febrile period, were observed.

"A steward presented a beautiful case of intermittent torticollis that lasted several days. Convalescents complained of diverse forms of neuralgia; intercostal, lumbar, scapular, crural, etc., all of which disappeared on a few grams of quinine. Tremors, 'a grandes oscillations,' increasing during intentional movements and persisting for a long time, were observed; one of the quartermasters had them even during his sleep for more than a month.

"*Pernicious attacks.*—Three of these were very striking. On our arrival at Agadir, 'second-maitre' I., for three days down with bilious remittent and showing nothing but slight agitation, so that he could scarcely be kept in his hammock, his temperature going down on the fourth day, when, suddenly, during the evening, he had an algid attack; the pulse became small and intermittent, extremities grew cold; dark circles appeared around the eyes. In a few hours, in spite of injections of ether-quinine, his head, shoulders and arms were covered with cold perspiration, while other parts of the body remained hot. Temperature 37 degrees. He did not feel cold. His temperature went down to an alarming degree, his features became drawn more and more, his eyes retreated and his lips became cyanosed, while he remained perfectly conscious and answered all the questions. He died at the very moment when the temperature went up to 40 degrees C.

"On our arrival at Fort-de-France, quartermaster D., after coaling all day the previous day, was taken suddenly, at morning quarters, with a pernicious epileptic seizure. After a serious of slight crises, frequent to overlapping, these crises terminated in a furious delirium; he remained delirious all day at the hospital into which he was transferred, developing new crises, nessitating the straitjacket; he saw himself pursued by his comrades wanting to strike or kill him; gradually recovering, regaining consciousness without the slightest recollection of what had occurred. Prodromata, in the form of 'migraines' and tremors, had been noted by his comrades, he having become vindictive and irritable.

"Another case of the delirious form, presenting similar symptoms as the preceding, occurred in the person of 'matelot timonnier' Le G.

"Finally, choleric and dysenteric forms occurred, the stools being frequent and sanguinolent, or simply serous and copious.

"There were on board the *Marseillaise* a certain number of parrots, parochites, a striped monkey and a baboon. Many of these died on our trips between Dakar, Agadir and Fort-de-France, without the cause of death having been determined; but the striped monkey and the baboon, having presented chills, followed by somnolence and bilious vomiting, may be assumed to have died from malaria."

Such is the pathetic story of malaria on the *Marseillaise*, which will surely interest those of all our naval colleagues who, like the reviewer, could tell similar, if not identical, tales from experience.

H. G. BEYER.

(From *Military Surgeon*, March, 1919).

PERSONAL AND GENERAL NEWS

Dr. W. B. Pigg, Okmulgee, visited St. Louis clinics in June.

Dr. J. L. Adams, Pryor, attended the Rochester clinics in June.

Dr. H. T. Ballantine, Muskogee, has returned from army service overseas.

Dr. T. H. Briggs, Atoka, has been appointed health officer for Atoka county.

Dr. N. H. Lindsay, Pauls Valley, is visiting the Rochester and Chicago clinics.

Dr. J. W. Graves, McAlester, has been appointed health officer for Pittsburg County.

Dr. C. M. Bloss, Okemah, has been reappointed superintendent of health for Okfuskee county.

Dr. E. L. Bagby, Vinita, has been appointed superintendent of the State Hospital at Supply.

Tulsa County Medical Society adjourned for the summer after the meeting of June 23rd.

Drs. L. J. Moorman, Oklahoma City; Chas. R. Hume, Anadarko, and C. W. Heitzman, Muskogee, represented the State Medical Association at the Atlantic City meeting.

Dr. G. R. Booth, LeFlore, has returned from New Orleans where he has been doing special work.

Dr. W. J. Wallace, Oklahoma City, visited New York and the Atlantic City meeting in June and July.

Dr. J. N. Shaunty, Eufaula, has been discharged from the army and returned to his home, after overseas service.

Dr. C. A. Dillon, Tulsa, is attending Dr. Richard Cabot's course at Harvard University during the month of July.

Dr. J. A. Deen, Ada, has been appointed health officer for Pontotoc county. He succeeds Dr. Catherine Threlkeld, the only woman health officer in the state.

Dr. F. W. Ewing, Muskogee, has been appointed county superintendent of public health. Dr. Ewing held the office during the absence of Dr. Claude Thompson who was in military service from November, 1917, to January, 1919.

Dr. G. A. Wall, Tulsa, had as his guests Drs. S. S. Glasscock, Kansas City, Kansas, and A. R. Lewis, State Commissioner of Health, Oklahoma City, when they attended the meeting of the Tulsa County Medical Society June 23. Dr. Wall tendered a dinner to several guests on the occasion.

Ottawa County Physicians held a joint meeting with physicians from Cherokee County, Kansas, and Jasper County, Missouri, June 19. It goes without saying the meeting was held on the "Missouri" side and in characteristic Missouri style and vein. The organization rightly denominated the "Society of Good Fellowship", was made permanent and will be continued. Nearly one hundred physicians attended, enjoying the lunch and other refreshments. Dr. F. L. Wormington, Miami, was elected President and Dr. Loudermilk, Galena, Kansas, Secretary.

Lieutenant Commander R. B. H. Gradwohl, Medical Corps, U. S. N. R. F., has returned from the Service and resumed his work as director of the Gradwohl Biological Laboratories and Pasteur Institute of St Loius. Owing to the efficient organization of the Gradwohl Laboratories, they were not closed during the war period, and now that Dr. Gradwohl has returned, the profession is assured that renewed efforts will be made to assist all those who are in need of laboratory aid.

Dr. C. E. Putnam, Lieutenant, M. R. C., Eakley, sends his regards to the *Journal* from Berlin, Germany. Dr. Putnam is one of the few fortunate enough to reach the much desired goal and assures us he likes Oklahoma better and will be with us soon.

Oklahoma Baptist Hospital, Muskogee, announce the opening of their new institution. The board of trustees inviting the public to inspect the new building July 2 and 3.

Dr. J. A. Mullens, Marlow, is visiting the Denver Clinics. He is accompanied by his wife and daughter who will take a cottage in Colorado Springs for the summer.

Dr. H. T. Ballantine, Muskogee, has been reappointed health officer for the City of Muskogee, Dr. Sessler Hoss, who held the place in his absence, resigning.

Dr. F. B. Fite, Muskogee, is in New York to meet his son, Captain William P. Fite, M. C., U. S. A., who has been over seas with the 36th division.

Dr. J. C. Mahr, in charge of the Federal and State Venereal Work, is directing the seizure of many patent medicines heretofore sold and lauded as cures.

Tulsa physicians are protesting against discrimination toward their profession by office building owners who, they claim, refuse to rent offices to them.

Dr. T. A. Hartgraves, Lieutenant M. C., U. S. A., Soper, has received his discharge from the army. He did laboratory work in France.

Captain J. Hutchins White, M. C. U. S. A., Muskogee, who has been overseas for more than a year, is on his way home.

Dr. L. A. Hahn, Guthrie, who served as a captain in the army, has been discharged and returned to his home.

Dr. C. J. Brunson, Adamson, who has been in the army for some time, has located in McAlester.

MISCELLANEOUS

DOCTOR JEAN-PAUL GAY.

This is sacred Memorial day,
    When we visit the city of the dead.
We pay respect to their memory,
    Thinking of things we might have said.

The little things we did not do,
    Words of cheer we left unsaid,
All come home with sad regret
    When we visit graves of sacred dead.

We visit the grave of lamented Paul,
    Co-worker and friend of a few short years,
And read the name —Jean-Paul Gay—
    With mingled sorrow, pride and tears.

Did you know our friend Jean–Paul?
Did you know Doctor Gay?
If not, you can never understand
Our loss when he was taken away.

Did you know Gay? the sacrifice he made
When his country called him to go?
See him smile in the face of adversity,
When others were scampering so.

The adverse side of Jean–Paul's life,
Which critics would all parade,
Was dotted with deeds of charity work,
For which no credits were made.

Too modest to mention his deeds of love,
His aid to thousands that came,
For his services whether gratis or not,
Given with a smile just the same.

A born physician, a heart of love,
The soul of honor and of right.
If you have not known him thus to be,
You have not known him as you might.

Peace to Thy ashes, friend o'mine,
And, until the judgment day,
Sleep ye, peacefully, comrade;
Rest ye, my friend—Jean–Paul Gay.

—J. W. Echols, M. D.

COUNCIL ON PHARMACY AND CHEMISTRY
AMERICAN MEDICAL ASSOCIATION

This report is limited according to the ideas and opinions as to its usefulness and practicability to Oklahoma physicians. A complete report is obtainable upon request from the Council, 535 North Dearborn St., Chicago.

ARTICLES ACCEPTED.

Abbott Laboratories: Liquor Hypophysis, U. S. P., Abbott.   Procaine Hypodermic Tablets, 3-4 grain.   Procaine-Adrenalin Hypodermic Tablets—Abbott.

E. R. Squibb and Sons: Protargentum—Squibb.

NEW AND NONOFFICIAL REMEDIES.

Barbital–Abbott Tablets, 5 grains: Each tablet contains 5 grains of barbital–Abbott (see New and Nonofficial Remedies, 1919, p. 82).   The Abbott Laboratories, Chicago.

Procaine Hypodermic Tablets, 3-4 grain: Each tablet contains 3-4 grain of procaine–Abbott (see New and Nonofficial Remedies, 1919, p. 30).   The Abbott Laboratories, Chicago.

Procaine–Adrenalin Hypodermic Tablets: Each tablet contains procaine–Abbott 1-3 grain and adrenalin 1-2500 grain (see New and Nonofficial Remedies, 1919, p. 30).   The Abbott Laboratories, Chicago (*Journal A. M. A.*, May 17, 1919, p. 1463).

Protargentum–Squibb: A compound of gelatin and silver containing approximately 8 per cent. of silver in organic combination.   It has the actions and uses of silver preparations of the protargol type (see New and Nonofficial Remedies, 1919, p. 307).   Protargentum–Squibb is used in 0.25 to 5 per cent. aqueous solutions, prepared freshly as required.   E. R. Squibb and Sons, New York (*Journal A. M. A.*, May 24, 1919, p. 1543).

PROPAGANDA FOR REFORM.

Phosphorus Metabolism: The more recent investigations on digestion and absorption all point to the probability that phosphorus from the digestive tract reaches the general circulation only in the form of inorganic phosphates and that all organic phosphorus compounds are synthesized in the body cells.   This is in support of the conclusion of the Council on Pharmacy and Chemistry in forming an estimate of the therapeutic potency ascribed to preparations of organically bound phosphorus, such as lecithin, glycerophosphates, phytin, nucleic acid and phosphoproteins.   All the newer researches give indication that the body is dependent on a ready made supply of phosphatid (phosphorized fat) in the diet to maintain normal nutrition (*Journal A. M. A.*, May 3, 1919, p. 1294).

Iodex: Iodex is a black ointment marketed by Menley and James with the claim that it is a preparation of free or elementary iodin minus the objectionable features that go with free iodin. As a result of an investigation of Iodex made in the A. M. A. Chemical Laboratory, the Council on Pharmacy and Chemistry reported in 1915: 1. The composition is incorrectly stated; the actual iodin content is only about half of that claimed. 2. The action of Iodex is not essentially that of free iodin, although that is the impression made by the advertising. 3. The assertion that iodin may be found in the urine shortly after Iodex has been rubbed on the skin has been experimentally disproved. As the manufacturers of Iodex still persist in their claim that the product contains free iodin, the A. M. A. Chemical Laboratory has again examined Iodex. It reports that Iodex gives no test for free iodin, or, at most, but mere traces (*Journal A. M. A.*, May 3, 1919, p. 1315).

Two Misbranded Nostrums: Bull's Herbs and Iron Compound was a weak alcoholic solution containing iron, phosphates, sugar and vegetable derivatives, among which were quinin, red pepper, gentian and podophyllum. It was falsely and fraudulently represented as a remedy for weak nerves, ailments peculiar to women, scrofula, rickets, liver, kidney and bladder diseases, etc. Efferescente Granulare consisted of over 13 per cent. sodium bicarbonate, 61 per cent. of sugar, 3 per cent. of borax, and 17 per cent. potassium bitartrate. Though invoiced as "Eff. Magnesia" it contained no magnesia. Both were declared misbranded (*Journal A. M. A.*, May 3, 1919, p. 1316).

Collosol Manganese: Stephens, Yorke, Blacklock, Macfie, Cooper and Carter reporting in the *Annals of Tropical Medicine and Parasitology* the results of their investigation for the English government of Collosol Manganese, conclude that Collosol Manganese in the doses used is of no value in the treatment of simple tertian malaria (*Journal A. M. A.*, May 3, 1919, p. 1318).

Helpful Hints for Busy Doctors: A comparatively recent issue of the *International Journal of Surgery* has an editorial on "The Questionable Etiology of the Present Epidemic," signed "G. H. Sherman, M. D." It was to the effect that one can best immunize against influenza by using "a combined vaccine containing the influenza bacillus, pneumococci, streptococci, the *Micrococcus catarrhalis* and staphylococci." In the advertising pages of the same issue was an advertisement of "Influenza Vaccine No. 38," which "will abort Colds, Grippe, Influenza and Pneumonia," and which was made by "G. H. Sherman, M. D." The vaccine contained the various bacilli and cocci mentioned in the G. H. Sherman editorial. One wonders if in the succeeding issues of the *International Journal of Surgery* one may look for editorials by the proprietors of Bellans, Phenalgin and other products advertised in the publication (*Journal A. M. A.*, May 10, 1919, p. 1372).

Administration of Arsphenamine: The U. S. Public Health Service has issued a circular concerning the dilution and the rate of administration of arsphenamine solutions. A study as to the cause of the disagreeable results following the use of the various preparations of arsphenamine has indicated that most disagreeable results are not inherent in the preparations but are produced through faulty steps in the administration of the remedy, chiefly from the use of a too concentrated solution and by too rapid administration (*Journal A. M. A.*, May 10, 1919, p. 1372).

Tyree's Antiseptic Powder: An advertising leaflet for Tyree's Antiseptic Powder recently received by a physician is devoted largely to a report of a bacteriologic examination of the Tyree's preparation. The physicians who receive this advertising material might easily overlook the fact that the reported bacteriologic tests were made in 1889 and that the investigation of the Council on Pharmacy and Chemistry in 1906 brought out that the examination applied to a product differing radically in composition from that of the preparation now marketed. The Council found that although the Tyree preparation was advertised as a mixture of borax and alum, it was essentially a mixture of zinc sulphate and boric acid. Here then we have a manufacturer publishing in 1919, in behalf of a certain product, tests that were made in 1889 with a product of different composition although of the same name (*Journal A. M. A.*, May 17, 1919, p. 1482).

Peptenzyme: Peptenzyme was reported on by the Council on Pharmacy and Chemistry along with a number of other products of Reed and Carnrick in 1907. The report "Reed and Carnrick's Methods" announced that none of the products examined were eligible for New and Nonofficial Remedies. The following is an abstract of the report on Peptenzyme: Peptenzyme elixir and powder are said to contain "the enzymes and ferments of all the glands which bear any relation to digestion;" therefore, the peptic glands, pancreas, salivary glands, spleen and intestinal glands. The preparations are said to be "not chemical extracts, but pure physiologic products." Apparently Peptenzyme powder consists of the glands dried and powdered, while elixir is an extract. It is stated that these preparations digest proteids, starch and fat, and in addition stimulate and nourish the digestive glands, and that the ferments in these preparations do not interfere with or digest one another. Examination by the Council showed that these preparations were practically devoid of any power to digest proteids or fat when tested by the U. S. P. method. The claim that the product contained ferments which would not show this activity in the test tube, but become active in the alimentary canal, is contrary to known facts and could not be substantiated by the manufacturer. The claims made for Peptenzyme powder and elixir were held to be unwarranted (*Journal A. M. A.*, May 17, 1919, p. 1484).

Kline's Nerve Remedy: This epilepsy nostrum was analyzed by the A. M. A. Chemical Laboratory and found to be a bromid preparation and practically identical with Waterman's tonic restorative.

Nuxated Iron: The analysis in the A. M. A. Chemical Laboratory indicated that Nuxated Iron Tablets contained only 1-25 grain of iron, while the amount of nux vomica was practically negligible. Nuxated Iron has been advertised by an extensive campaign of misrepresentation and exaggeration (*Journal A. M. A.*, May 24, 1919, p. 1560).

The Williams Treatment: According to the Dr. D. A. Williams Company, which sells it on the mail order plan, the Williams Treatment "conquers kidney and bladder diseases, rheumatism and all other ailments when due to excessive uric acid." The Williams Treatment was analyzed in the A. M. A. Chemical Laboratory and from the results of the examination it was concluded that it is essentially a mixture containing in 100 cc. 48 gm. potassium acetate in solution and in about 7 gm. potassium bicarbonate, the latter being largely undissolved. The mixture is colored with caramel and flavored with oil of wintergreen or methyl salicylate (*Journal A. M. A.*, May 31, 1919, p. 1632).

Investigation Based on False Premises. One sometimes reads in supposedly "Original Articles" in medical journals statements that seem puzzlingly familiar. If one is sufficiently inquisitive and possessed of a germ of Sherlock Holmesism, the familiar statement may be traced to the "literature" for some proprietary medicine with which the author's article deals. The unwisdom of authors accepting the unconfirmed statements of the promoters of proprietary remedies is well illustrated in a recent report of the Council on Pharmacy and Chemistry on "Collosol Cocaine", a preparation claimed to contain 1 per cent. of cocain in colloidal and relatively nontoxic form. The report brings out that men of good standing had reported "Collosol Cocaine" to be much less toxic than cocain. These men, however, did not verify the statement of its composition, and subsequent investigation by others brought out the fact that "Collosol Cocaine 1 per cent." contained but 0.26 per cent. cocain, and that its toxicity was in accord with the amount of cocain found. Those who investigated the action of drugs must recognize more fully than has often neen done in the past, that a study of a medicament is of no scientific value whenever the identity of the substance is not established (*Journal Indiana State Medical Association*, May 1919, p. 134).

Therapeutic Evidence: Has the medical profession learned to distinguish between real therapeutic evidence and chance observation? If so, the profession will not be impressed by certain testimonials for a widely advertised ointment. The wise physician who reads the testimonials will ask: Was it the "baking" or the proprietary ointment which produced the "remarkable results" in "rheumatic affections and ankylosis"? Was the "contracting arm chronic" benefited by time and friction or by the proprietary? How did the physician know that "anointing the nostrils" prevents attacks of influenza? Those who are inclined to give credit to drugs for naturally occurring events may be interested in the statement of a prominent chemist that he has been free from his periodical colds since he arranged for an inoculation with a "cold" vaccine but was prevented from keeping the appointment. (*Penn. Medical Journal*, May 1919, p. 524).

Dichloramine–T and Petrolatum Dressing for Burns: Torald Sollmann reports that solution of dichloramine–T in chlorcosane do not protect the large open surfaces of burns against mechanical irritation and access of air. On the contrary, the solution is absorbed by the dressing, which is then glued by the wound secretions and causes pain and injury when the dressing is changed. As a result of a study of the decomposition of dichloramine–T by different solvents, Sollmann proposes the use of an ointment of three parts of surgical paraffin and seven parts of liquid petrolatum as a protective dressing on wounds (burns) treated with dichloramine-T-chlorcosane solution. It may even be used as a basis for a dichloramine–T ointment (*Journal A. M. A.*, April 5, 1919, p. 992).

Stevens' Comsumption Cure: C. H. Stevens, a discredited London quack, has been attempting to exploit Canadian veterans at the Mountain Sanatorium for the treatment of pulmonary tuberculosis at Hamilton, Ont. The nostrum was claimed to contain "Umckaloabo root" and "Chijitse," but the analysis made for the British Medical Association showed it to contain no active drugs except alcohol and glycerine. The following is a brief history of this "cure": In 1904 Stevens was selling "Sacco" in Capetown, South Africa, but got into the courts and found it expedient to leave Capetown. In 1906, Stevens was in Johannesburg trading as the "South African Institute of Medicine" and selling his stuff as "Lungsava"; was twice convicted of violating the law and left for England. In 1907, Stevens was in London selling his "cure" and in 1910 was declared by the courts to be guilty of intentional fraud and his "cure" pronounced a quack remedy. In 1915 Stevens' "cure " appeared in the United States under the name of "U. C. Extract" exploited by the Umckaloabo Chemical Company of New York City. Today, Stevens is attempting to exploit tuberculous Canadian soldiers who have acquired the disease in the service of their country (*Journal A. M. A.*, April 5, 1919, p. 1018).

Surgical Solution of Chlorinated Soda (Dakin's Solution): According to New and Nonofficial Remedies, 1919, Surgical solution of chlorinated soda may be prepared: 1. By the electrolysis of a sodium chlorid solution. 2. By the action of chlorin on sodium carbonate. 3. By the interaction of chlorinated lime and sodium carbonate solutions with subsequent treatment with either boric acid or sodium bicarbonate to reduce the alkalinity (*Journal A. M. A.*, April 5, 1919, p. 1021).

Procain Anesthesia: There is no evidence of latent injury to the dental nerves from repeated injections of procain to control supersensitiveness of the teeth. If an isotonic solution is used and this solution made sterile by boiling, it is not probable that it will be injurious (*Journal A. M. A.*, April 8, p. 1022).

Iodex: According to Pharmacal Advance, a house organ extolling the products exploited by Menley and James, Iodex has all the virtues of free iodin without its drawbacks. The claim that a given proprietary represents all the desirable therapeutic properties of a drug but not its drawbacks has been so often proved unwarranted that the claims made for Iodex should receive scant consideration. The report of the A. M. A. Council on Pharmacy and Chemistry on Iodex included a report from the A. M. A. Chemical Laboratory which showed that Iodex, despite the advertising claims, contains no free iodin;—to be exact, when a test for free iodin was made on five specimens, four yielded only minute traces of iodin, while the fifth yielded none (*Journal Mo. State Medical Association*, April, 1919, p. 127).

Buttermilk Therapy: For reliable information with regard to new therapeutic measures and reliable brands of drugs proposed for them, New and Nonofficial Remedies should be consulted. This book contains a chapter which discusses the probable value of the Metchnikoff sour milk therapy. The book also describes those brands of preparations which the Council on Pharmacy and Chemistry found to be reliable and exploited recently (*Journal A. M. A.*, April 12, 1919, p. 1099).

The Advertising of Sal Hepatica: There are two ways of advertising a "patent medicine"— by direct advertisement to the public and by means of propaganda which will lead the medical profession to acquaint the public with it. Sal Hepatica is advertised by the indirect method (*Journal A. M. A.*, April 12, 1919, p. 1079).

Collosol Cocaine Not Admitted To N. N. R. Collosol Cocaine (Anglo-French Drug Co. Ldt., New York) is claimed to be a preparation containing 1 per cent, of cocain in colloidal form and is alleged to possess a remarkably low toxicity. However, the A. M. A. Chemical Laboratory found that a specimen contained not more than 0.4 per cent. of alkaloid; hence it does not have the composition claimed and is in effect misbranded. Further, in England it was conceded that the preparation was not an "absolute colloid" and that the declaration with regard to the percentage of cocain was incorrect (Barger, Dale and Durham reported that a specimen was found to contain but 0.25 per cent. of cocain). Without considering other objections, the Council on Pharmacy and Chemisrty declared Collosol Cocaine inadmissible to New and Nonofficial Remedies because its composition was not correctly declared (*Journal A. M. A.*, April 12, 1919, p. 1094).

Goldenrod and Hay Fever: In spring hay fever is caused chiefly by the pollens of grasses. The fall hay fever in the Northern, Eastern and Southern states is for the most part attributed to the pollens of ragweeds. In the Pacific and Rocky Mountain states they are replaced by the wormwoods. Schepperell has concluded that goldenrod does not cause hay fever (*Journal A. M. A.*, April 19, 1919, p. 1162).

Germany and The American Chemical Industry: The Alien Property Custodian has issued a report which, in part, is devoted to a discussion of the influence which Germany has had on the chemical industry of the United States. It outlines how the German government obtained a practical monopoly in the United States in dyes, fine chemicals and synthetic drugs. The report explains how by-products of the dye works were converted into explosives—trinitrotoluene, for instance—and the advantage which the production of these explosives gave to Germany as a military power. The report explains that in medicinal chemicals very little real manufacture existed in the United States. The report discusses the ramifications of the "Big Six"—the German concerns which controlled the dye industry—in American industrial life and describes how their American branches were shown to be enemy owned and therefore taken over by the custodian. The "Big Six" were: Badische Anilin and Soda Fabril, Farbenfabriken vorm. Friedr. Bayer and Co., Actien-Gesellschaft fur Anilin-Fabrikation, Farbwerke vorm. Meister Lucius and Bruning, Leopold Cassella, G. m. b. H., and Kalle and Co. Aktien-Gesellschaft. The Americarn firms were: Badische Co. of New York, Bauer Chemical Company, Bayer and Co. (Inc.) Berlin Aniline Works, Casella Co., Farbwerke Hoechst Co., Heyden Chemical Works, Kalle and Company, Merck and Co., Roessler and Hasslacher Chemical Company and Synthetic Patents Co. (Inc.). The report closes with a description of a corporation to be known as the Chemical Foundation, Inc., which is to acquire by purchase the German patents which in the past have formed a colossal obstacle to the American dyestuff industry. The Alien Property Custodian has sold to this company for the sum of $250,000 approximately 4,500 patents (*Journal A. M. A.*, April 19, 1919, p. 1176).

·Anthelmintics: The earth worm reacts with symptoms of toxicity to all clinical anthelmintics just as do the parasitic intestinal worms. This fact has enabled Torald Sollmann to reinvestigate the claims long made for certain drugs. Spigelia was found to have rather feeble toxicity, but fresh pumpkin seed and squash seed were quite highly efficient (*Journal A. M. A.*, April 26, 1919, p. 1228).

Annual Meeting of the Council on Pharmacy and Chemistry: Among the subjects considered at the recent meeting were: The Council decided to publish at an early date a report on unscientific and commercial propangada for nonspecific protein therapy. The Council appointed a committee to study the problems of serum and vaccine therapy with a view of publishing the evidence obtainable regarding both the value of, and also the dangers incident tó, the use of serums and vaccines. A special committee was appointed to report on the present status of pollen extracts on the prophylaxic and treatment of hay fever. The Council adopted a resolution urging legislation which shall require the Public Health Service to extend its control of serums, vaccines, toxins and antitoxins to cover other potent remedies that are used hyperdomically or intravenously. The Council passed a resolution that the control of arsphenamine by the Public Health Service shall be continued and the price controlled by the government. The Council decided to describe in a separate section of New and Nonofficial Remedies proprietary preparations of therapeutic value which are so exploited as to be inadmissible to New and Nonficial Remedies. A · committee was appointed to establish fuller cooperation between teachers of therapeutics and pharmacology in medical schools and the Council. A committee was appointed to determine the present status of radium water therapy (*Journal A. M. A.*, April 26, 1919, p. 1243).

Veracolate Tablets: The Council on Pharmacy and Chemistry examined Veracolate (Marcy Co.) in 1915 and found it to be semisecret in composition, unscientific in combination and exploited under unwarranted claims (*Journal A. M. A.*, April 26, 1919, p. 1245).

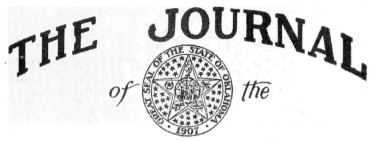

THE JOURNAL of the

Oklahoma State Medical Association

VOLUME XII   MUSKOGEE, OKLA, AUGUST, 1919   ·   NUMBER 8

PREPARATION AND USE OF THE CARREL-DAKIN ANTISEPTIC SOLUTION*

MILLINGTON SMITH, M. D.

OKLAHOMA CITY, OKLAHOMA

During the past few months much has been written concerning the Carrel-Dakin antiseptic solution which is being used so extensively in wound sterilization in the war zone. Remarkable results have been obtained. The surgeons of our own country find that this solution is of equal value in open wounds encountered in civic life and in the industries. We have been using the preparation in our local hospitals for the last eight months and have obtained some remarkable results.

In the numerous articles that have appeared in our journals on this subject great stress has been laid on the methods of application. Dr. Carrel says that 40 per cent. of its value depends on the care that is used in its application. Not so much has been written concerning the technique of its preparation, which· is of no less importance. Very briefly I wish to mention the formula and points which must be observed in order to obtain a solution of greatest value.

This antiseptic is an aqueous solution of sodium hypochlorite of a concentration not less than 0.45 per cent., no more than 0.5 per cent. Clinical experience proves that under 0.45 per cent. its bactericidal effect is not the best, and over that it is irritating. The formula that laboratories have found to give a solution nearest correct is the following:

Chlorinated lime_____200 gms.
Sodium carbonate_____ 80 gms
Sodium bicarbonate (dry)_____100 gms.

Our laboratories have found that the majority of brands of commercial chlorinated lime contain not 33 per cent. of available chlorin, as is official, but from 24 to 25 per cent. Of course, if the lime has a higher percentage of available chlorin than 25 per cent., a smaller amount of lime must be used.

Put into a twelve liter flask the 200 gm. of chloride of lime and five liters of ordinary water; shake vigorously for a few minutes and leave to macerate for five or six hours.

At the same time dissolve in five liters of cold water the carbonate and bicarbonate of soda. After the maceration of the lime mix the soda solution with it and shake thoroughly. Leave stand until the calcium carbonate which is pre-

---

*Read in Surgical Section, Annual State Meeting Muskogee, May 21, 1919.

cipitated is settled out. Siphon off the supernated liquid and filter. This liquid is the finished product.

On account of the variation of commercial products, it is best to standardize the finished product. This procedure is one that any druggist of technical training can do. Our laboratories have checked up products prepared by our local druggists and have found them very satisfactory. For an explanation of the technique of the standardization, I shall refer you to the December number of the *Southern Medical Journal*, 1916, or the December 2nd number of the *American Medical Journal*

Action of the Solution: How does this solution act as an antiseptic? How strong a bactericidal agent is it? Why is it a better antiseptic than Labarraque's solution, which many of you used so extensively a few years ago? How does its action differ from alcohol, bicloride of mercury, peroxid of hydrogen and other antiseptics, are questions which are interesting to all of us.

We are frank to say that we are not definitely able to state wherein its bactericidal power lies. It has been proven to the satisfaction of many chemists and bacteriologists that its action is due to two substances. Sodium hypochlorite is a very unstable compound. When it comes in contact with the carbonic acid of the necrotic tissue nascent chlorin is liberated which in turn reacts with the water of the tissues, liberating nascent oxygen, which is a very active oxidizing agent, destroying the bacteria by the simple process of oxidation.

Some of the salt is not broken down until it has well penetrated the pus and necrotic tissue, as it must come in contact with carbonic acid before the nascent oxygen is liberated. This preparation acts as a bactericidal agent just as the chlorinated lime acts which you use in the sewer. It is an antiseptic of high bactericidal activity and of little toxic and irritating quality. It has marked pyocytohemolytic power, being able to dissolve pus, blood-clots and necrotic tissue. The living tissue is not affected by the solution.

It differs in its action from hydrogen peroxid inasmuch as hydrogen peroxid is so unstable that its oxygen is liberated before the solution penetrates very deeply.

It differs from Labarraque's solution inasmuch as the latter is alkaline in reaction, which neutralizes the carbonic acid, thus preventing the liberation of the nascent oxygen.

Its action differs materially from alcohol and mercuric bichlorid, as the action of the latter two is that of destroying the bacteria by coagulation. At the same time the pus and tissue debris is coagulated, interfering with drainage. Part of the antiseptic power of this solution lies in the fact that hypochlorite coming in contact with protein material forms complex compounds known as chloramins, which have marked antiseptic properties. It is upon this principle that Dr. Dakin has prepared his so-called chlorazene antiseptic tablets, which can be bought on the market at the present time. These tablets are stable and from them the antiseptic solution can be made. However, for hospitals the solution made up from the chemicals as has been described is much more satisfactory, as it is much cheaper. The actual cost of the material used in the solution is about twenty-eight cents for five gallons. Where a laboratory is accessible the time spent in the preparation of the solution is not very much.

Application: Concerning the technique of the application of this solution, as carried out by Dr. Carrel, you have no doubt read the extensive articles that have appeared in the *American Medical Journal, Journal of Surgery, Gynecology and Obstetrics, Southern Medical Journal* and others. The preparation has not been used in this country very much, but where used it has proven that the technique is just as applicable to the treatment of wounds encountered in civic life as in war.

Dr. Noland, the chief surgeon of the Tennessee Coal and Iron Railroad

Company, says that in his service the use of mercuric chlorid, iodin, iodin and benzin, alcohol and similar antiseptics for the early and late treatment of wounds has been entirely abandoned and all classes of open wounds are treated with Dakin's solution.

Fresh wounds are cleansed with gauze soaked in the solution and all minor wounds are put up in wet dressings of the same. This dressing is thoroughly moistened every two hours, by the patient if he is treated in his home, or by the nurse if he is treated in a hospital. One precaution which must be taken is to see that the skin surrounding the wound is protected with vaseline, as the antiseptic is irritating to the skin. Burns of all degrees are treated in exactly similar manner. More serious and deep wounds, especially those involving bone and joint, are treated by the instillation method.

We have found in our experience with the solution for the past eight months that infected wounds, even where deep-seated cavities are involved, are quickly sterilized if the technic is carefully observed, i. e., if the tubes are so arranged that every portion of the wound is reached at two-hour intervals. We have had several cases of hands that have been severely torn and lacerated and severely infected, which under the treatment have healed with wonderful rapidity and with a small amount of scar formation.

From my experience with the solution and from the experience of some of my colleagues I have been convinced that we have obtained results which we never have been able to secure with other antiseptics.

Discussion.

Dr. A. A. Will, Oklahoma City: Gentlemen, I believe that one of the reasons why the Carrel-Dakin solution has not become more popular with the surgeons over the United States is the fact that it was really a chemist who brought this solution to our notice, and we have a great many skeptics at present who continue to question its value. I believe they are skeptical because—not because they don't know the technique or don't know that the solution is perfect—but because they have not given the solution a trial in the selective cases.

I heard Doctor Bevan last year, or saw him present a number of cases of badly infected limbs. At the time, I believed that Dakin's solution, as an antiseptic, would never become very popular. The cases he showed were infections and contused wounds of the limbs, using the drainage tubes, hot bags of salt solution, bichlorid, the active use of iodin; and in some of the cases they used the Dakin solution. At that time, if you will remember, Dakin's apparatus consisted of a container with a large tube running down and several small tubes going into the wound, the wound closed. Now, the trouble with that apparatus is that we don't know how to use it. These small tubes lead down deep into the infected wounds and there is no way for the solution to return—it simply remains in there and dissolves the pus and there is no way for the solution to pass out. Major Davis, who was in the First British Unit and had control of the base hospital, from Chicago, told me a year ago that he did not believe Dakin's solution would prove of great value in the war zone, for the simple reason that the technique was too complicated, and he used a large bottle—not a Dakin solution, but practically the same thing—I haven't the formula, I have forgotten it. This bottle could be used in the evacuation hospital at the front. The soldier was given this bottle with two tubes, one ingress and one leading out—every hour, every half hour, every two hours, if necessary. This syringe that was given them was placed in the mouth of this large bottle which contained the solution—simply take the clamp off of the end of the tube entering the wound and inject three or four ounces of that solutoin—simply passes through and passes out the other tube. Now, that was the procedure carried out by the wounded men coming from France to England, or from the evacuation hospital to the base hospital at that time. Since that time I understand Major Davis has been more or less convinced that the same procedure can be carried out with Dakin's solution and better results obtained.

The use of Dakin's solution in the chest conditions as we have used it at home, and I suppose that that was taken from the war service, a simple tube is put into the chest proper; the Dakin solution is put into the cavity under pressure; your solution is allowed to remain there a few minutes; no matter how thick that material may be the first time, you aspirate the chest. You may get very little material, but after two or three injections of the Dakin solution your material passes out easily. Now, then, to do this with a degree of ease they simply have this vacuum pump, and each time the Dakin solution is put in it is allowed to remain a few minutes and withdrawn. Every day a bacteriological count is made and kept. The few cases I have treated at the hospitals have done remarkably well. Now, then, if we could say the Dakin solution does nothing more than have a certain effect on these patients whereby they do much better and that it does away with a lot of the odor, which the saline will not do—you remember how disagreeable it became to the patient and everyone surrounding him—it has served a useful purpose. That is one thing Dakin's solution does do—it clears up that odor. In using that solution a method of treatment is carried out every two hours and it is gradually lengthened out as the bacterial count grows better. When it gets down to where the bacterial count is practically nil, you simply close that cavity. We use following the Dakin solution, or where we are sure the cavity is practically, a form of formalin and glycerin solution and fill the cavity remaining and close the wound. I don't know what the experience has been in the war zone of the complete healing of these cases, but we do know some of them come back and have to be reopened and cleared up, and we do know the use of the glycerine solution following this, and using the straight chlorin solution to simply finish up the job, has certainly simplified the treatment of empyema of the chest.

I have had a small experience in treating, and I suppose all of us have treated tubular stricture of the rectum, which is one of the conditions we all side-step; and the great trouble has been, and will continue to be, that following dilation more scar tissue forms. I used all the other antiseptics and stimulation solutions, but in the very few cases I have tried Dakin's solution in, it does heal that stricture—heals that lining membrane—with less scar tissue than you have ordinarily, so that we are getting some results in the treatment of these cases, and it clears up the pus. I use a return catheter for the solution and it works out very nicely.

Just another reason why Dakin's solution has not been more popular. That is the fact, as Doctor Smith has said, that the proportions have to be exact. Now an apparatus has been made whereby a doctor, in his private practice, can use it by making up his solution. This apparatus I think will be inexpensive and the solution is certainly much cheaper than anything else we can use. I really believe it lessens the amount of scar tissue; it apparently does in large surface wounds. All in all, I am like Doctor Smith—I believe I am thoroughly convinced, and that is only in the past year, that Dakin's solution is going to prove of considerable value to us in the treatment of all suppurating wounds.

Dr. A. Ray Wiley, Tulsa: My personal opinion of this Carrel-Dakin solution reminds me very much of a star shell. It goes up, flares, throws out a little light, settles down in its own niche and stays there. It was my good pleasure to work in the Rockefeller Demonstration Hospital at Rockefeller Institute during the winter of nineteen seventeen and spring of nineteen eighteen with Major Stewart and Lieutenant Sullivan, and those of you who have been there will know these men. I worked at the right-hand of Carrel and had every opportunity to observe the way the solution was made and the results they got—and I will say that they did get some results—but, it is a most tedious and laborious thing—most tedious and laborious technique and very expensive in any ordinary institution. Rockefeller can afford it, but the ordinary institution cannot afford it—not in the manner of making your solution, not in the manner of making your medicine, but in the number of nurses and assistants it takes to handle the technique and in the number of persons it takes to make the changes in changing the dressings. For instance, the ordinary technique: That the injection has to be made every two hours. If the patient is capable of making that injection himself, all well and good, but a majority of them are not and it takes the nurse, or whoever the assistant is—it requires them to be on the job every two hours, day and night, and it takes lots of assistants in making the change every twenty-four hours. We had there about six nurses to each surgeon, only making the change in the dressing. One of them handled this and one of them handled that, and somebody else something else. They got in your way most of the time, but nevertheless, that was the instructions.

The great virtue I found in the use of the Dakin solution is very similar to what Doctor Will said here. I have treated four cases of empyema with Carrel-Dakin technique in my private practice. I used it with two of them as the Doctor has utilized it, and that was in those chronic empyemas. One of three years standing, and the other of eight months standing. Those two were treated with ordinary Dakin solution. The one of three years standing was healed up in three months and the one of eight months standing was healed up in one month. The other two cases I used the chlorazene and got good healing in both cases.

Doctor M. Smith says regarding the manufacture of the solution, that all limes do not contain the same amount of chlorin; that it is easy for a person who has not had a laboratory to make up that solution. How are you going to determine how much chlorin you have in your lime solution if you don't have a laboratory to analyze your lime?

Another thing, Dakin's solution is subject to rapid deterioration and changing, so it should be analyzed at least every twenty-four hours if you are going to get good results.

Another thing, it has a certain applied place. You cannot try anything and everything with Carrel-Dakin, nor Dakin never expected that. It has been unjustly criticized because the men who have taken it out have tried to treat everything with it and, naturally, did not get the results they expected. That is their fault and not the fault of Carrel or Dakin.

It must be used in proper technique and according to the men who have had experience with it, and if you don't use it according to their technique you will not get the result they get. But, for practical purposes, I will say that it can only be used in a large institution with a corps of workers and assistants who do know the technique and who keep it in proper condition every day and know what they are doing. It cannot be used in the ordinary hospitals in smaller communities.

Dr. J. S. Hartford, Oklahoma City: We always have the man who is conservative to check the man who is over-enthusiastic, and that goes as a safeguard in our lines of treatment that are new and possibly not well settled. In the clinic at the University of Oklahoma we have quite a large number of pus tubes. Sometimes it is a question whether or not we drain. Most cases we do not. Quite a number of those cases have been followed by infection. We have had some nice results by Carrel-Dakin solution in the treatment of those cases, but the question of a few cases is not the thing. The question of a hundred cases or the question of a thousand cases is not the thing. We must put alongside the positive thousand cases another thousand cases that have been treated by some other method, and then we must compare those two. A report of two thousand cases is not right unless you put another two thousand cases alongside, operated by some other method and compare them. I heard Vaughan, at the Congress of Clinical Surgeons, in summing up the treatment of wounds. Vaughan went on to say that the Carrel-Dakin solution was impractical in warfare; then he took a series of cases that had been treated by Carrel-Dakin and a series treated by other methods and he compared them, and he wound up in such a beautiful way—I presume he did this because of the fact that a representative of the Surgeon General of the French Army was present at this meeting. He wound this paper up in such a beautiful manner that it appealed to me. He said, "In our experience the best results have been obtained in the cases in which it might not have been used".

Dr. Ralph Smith, Tulsa: It so happens that I have been situated for the past nine or ten months where I have seen some cases treated by the Carrel-Dakin method. Like all other remedies, if used properly and in the proper class of cases, it is of value. There are those who would have us believe that it is the most excellent treatment for all classes of wounds. I want to sound warning right here. You are standing on a false bottom. I have seen many cases treated by the Dakin method. My first training in the use of the Dakin method was in France, where I was located in what is perhaps the best equipped American hospital in France, and surgeons are sent there for instruction in the use of the Carrel-Dakin method and the practice of war surgery. They used the Dakin method almost exclusively in that hospital. The technique was beyond criticism. However, the best results in the treatment of these wounds are following the Dakin method in connection with the De Page and Chantreau method, which is mechanically cleansing. When you stop to consider that the Dakin solution is only effective for two minutes or less after it comes in contact with the wound, you will readily understand that two hours is too great an interval. Carrel statistics were taken from a series of cases in what is considered a very small hospital, possibly enough to receive seventy-five or eighty at the best. He had a corps of trained assistants and nurses and had expert laboratory men to use in the preparation of the solution, so that he did get excellent results. The point of the essay hinges upon one sentence. That is, that the solution must come in contact with all parts of the wound, which is practically an impossibility. The wound is an open cavity, in a vast number of these war cases, which perhaps represents five inches in diameter and capable of holding a pint of solution, or more, and yet with walls collapsed it would have in it a few tubes and thought to have been Dakinized, and I have taken them out and found a little channel following these tubes, and the solution is following the tube right out to the surface. Now there is one practical way you might get the solution to all parts of this wound, and that is by packing the wound wide open with gauze. Now, what are these half dozen tubes going to do with this large wound with collapsed walls? Simply pack that wound and put your Dakin tubes around the outside of all your packing and you may get your solution in nearly all parts of this wound, but not all. Take compound fracture cases, eight, ten or twelve weeks standing, and they are still sticking Dakin tubes in there, and imagine their getting results. Where is the source of the pus? Maybe five inches from the end of the tube. And then, when you do your secondary operation and remove these sequestra, then you can Dakinize again with hope for success. It is a good treatment if properly carried out, but it is almost an impossibility. I believe it is a delusion. I remember one occassion in particular. We had two quite similar cases. One had the tubes in and had plenty of gauze packing, and the other had a wound and no tubes in his wound—his wound being packed wide open and never had had Dakin's. I have seen those wounds clear up and ready for secondary closure in six, eight and ten days. I have seen them without a Dakin tube in them and have seen the man next to him with the Dakin tube, so you cannot figure it all from the Dakin solution. It is good, but it is hard to apply, and its technique must be absolutely perfect. The minute that piece of shrapnel goes through the clothing and into the flesh you have an infected wound. After the first dressing is applied the next, perhaps, will not be for three or four days and you will have some pus present.

I expect to use the Dakin solution, but it must be especially prepared. It is irritating, even in the weaker solution. Carrel says the vaseline is unnecessary, but it is necessary. It should be protected and I have seen some very serious results because they didn't begin using the gauze early enough. At Fort Des Moines I have seen the Dakin method carried out in the most minute form, and that was by a surgeon trained in the Rockefeller Institute and the army hospital at Washington. We, over here, have no conception of what real infection means. It is a foolish idea to think you can clean all wounds with Dakin solution.

Dr. A. L. Blesh, Oklahoma City: Let us go back to first principles. It was not very long ago that we thought a wound could not get well unless it was dressed every few hours—meddlesome surgery. However, it wasn't long until we found out that meddlesome surgery was just as bad as meddlesome midwifery. Every time a wound is dressed, it is immaterial what antiseptic is used, a risk of infection is incurred. Mechanical sterilization is the greatest of all antiseptics—the load the tissues have to carry is thereby reduced.

Secondary hemorrhage in the use of the Carrel-Dakin solution is not uncommon. The chlorin has the power of decomposing animal ligatures, thus necessitating the use of non-absorbable material for ligatures. This in turn predisposes to the maintenance of the already existing infection.

I am not opposed to the Carrel-Dakin solution where the facilities and the trained personnel are at hand for its proper use; but maintain that with the average man, in the average little hospital, in the way it is ordinarily used, it is worse than a failure, because the surgeon in relying upon it is leaning upon a broken reed. It will not take the place of good surgery, and where good surgery is practiced it is seldom needed. Of course, it is understood that its use in any hands necessitates frequent meddling with the wound which as a principle is bad. Meddlesome surgery is fully as bad as meddlesome midwifery. It takes an expert to be able to meddle with wounds frequently, and keep out of trouble. Believing myself, that I am not expert enough to do it, I haven't the hardihood to meddle much with the wounds under my care.

Dr. M. Smith, closing: I have never read a paper in my life that gave me such supreme gratification as this one has. We all very well know that when a paper is read and everyone present agrees with the paper, that it does not amount to much. The different ideas expressed in this discussion are beneficial to me, especially from men who have had, I might say, unlimited experience in the use of the "Dakin solution", which enables you to parallel your various experiences, keeping me out of the enthusiastic rut that we so often fall into. However, in regard to Dr. Blesh's discussion, I think we are aboslutely in hearty accord with the one subject—namely: dressing of wounds every few hours. I know, and Dr. Blesh and every surgeon in this house knows, that the less you disturb a wound the better it is. This is prima-facia evidence and needs no argument. When you have a clean wound, and make a septic wound out of it, you are responsible for the results. In this instance in the Carrel-Dakin solution, you have something that will come to your rescue and help you out, which it will do if you use it judiciously.

This paper was not intended for anything but dirty, septic, infected wounds or cavities in any part of the body, and not for fresh wounds, unless we have reason to believe they are septic.

I have foot-notes as to what the leading surgeons on the war front have to say after a number of years experience as to the efficacy of this solution. We all know that clean surgery is good surgery. Dr. Blesh mentioned in his discussion the effect that this solution has on various kinds of ligatures, causing them to be dissolved or macerated, and very conducive to secondary hemorrhage. This, in a measure, is quite true no doubt, but I might say that under those conditions it may have possibly been due to the slough and not altogether to the bad effect of the solution on the ligatures.

I read with a great deal of interest in the *American Medical Journal*, eight or ten months ago, an article by Mr. Monyhan, giving in detail his experience with the "Dakin solution", and he sums it up by saying "that they probably would have done just as well without the use of it"—instead advocating the various other so-called antiseptic solutions. This, I think, was a matter of personal experience, and not a general denial.

I was also very much interested in Doctor LeRoy Long's discussion, and fully agree with him that it is necessary in all lacerated wounds to remove all of the tissue that has been devitalized and established drainage, thereby endeavoring to lessen the probabilities of infection by doing clean surgery. My experience with Dakin's solution in fresh wounds has been limited, but very satisfactory, preventing, as I believe, infection of various kinds by keeping the wound aseptic. However, it is hard for us to know just how much tissue to remove in badly lacerated or crushed wounds, knowing the shock of the tissues may extend far beyond what we may consider healthy tissue, lowering its resistance and especially conducive to infection.

I was also interested in Dr. Ralph Smith's discussion. In this paper I am going to pay special attention to it. I am not an army surgeon, and the one regret of my life is that I could not be. Certain things come up in our lives that we cannot help, even though we may want to do them. I tendered my services to my country and the saddest time of my life was that the line of demarkation had been established and the "die was cast", consequently I could not go. I would not send my boy or your boy any place I would not go myself. It makes little difference what becomes of me, but our boys must be cared for.

I will now read you a paragraph from Hughes and Banks War Surgery, page 302, as follows:

"During a rush it is impossible for a surgical specialist at a casualty clearing station to excise and deal with every wound, and of necessity he has to evacuate to the base hospital cases which in quieter times he would certainly retain. Of the rushes on this front we can give the valuable information that in *every case, however grave, in which the Carrel-Dakin treatment, very imperfect as it was in some cases, had been started at the casualty clearing station, not a limb or life was sacrificed: but in many cases which appeared at the casualty clearing station to be of minor importance, and were therefore evacuated without the Carrel-Dakin treatment, gas gangerene had supervened by the time the base hospital was reached, and both limbs and lives were lost.*"

Now, in your personal experience can you work out a treatment more satisfactory than that? I do not claim it a panacea for all wounds—there are cases that it will not benefit. There are cases that diphtheria anti-toxin does not do any good.

I want to say a few words in regard to the method of use; it must be used judiciously and systematically. Have your drainage tubes so arranged that the solution will come in contact with every recess of your wound, and in from twelve to thirty-six hours after its use, even though you have experienced sloughing and a very offensive odor emanating from the wound, or cavity, you will have the pleasure when you enter the room of your patient of being relieved from unpleasant odors of decomposition, to that of a mild chlorin inhalation. Now, can you do this with drainage, salt solution, boracic acid solution, bichlorid solution, or in fact any other of the various solutions you may choose? I answer emphatically, No.

Question by Dr. Ralph Smith: How about several thousand cases treated with dry gauze?

Reply: I am glad you asked that. When you do clean surgery that is a different proposition. I did not read this paper on fresh wounds—it was not the intention, but you got off on it, and consequently I must answer it. Clean surgery, with normal resistance power of your patient, does not need any solution, and the several thousand you mention, seems to come under this head.

I can hardly close this paper without calling your attention again to Hughes and Banks War Surgery, page 322, as follows:

"We would like once again to emphasize the important observation, taken now over 2,000 consecutive cases of severe wounds, *that in all cases, however gross and severe, especially compound comminuted fractures of the femur and the like, where Carrel's treatment had been commenced early at the casualty clearing station, limbs and lives were saved: But in all cases where rush of work prevented the Carrel-Dakin treatment from being carried out, such limbs were gangrenous by the time the base hospital was reached, and had to be sacrificed, and in a considerable number of cases lives were lost.*"

"We cannot overestimate the immense importance of a system of continuity in treatment; for today, when we see extensive compound comminuted fractures of the femur, which a year ago would have been submitted to amputation, united and healed and the man up on crutches at the end of six weeks; cases of severe compound comminuted fracture of the humerus with union and good function at the end of five weeks, etc., it gives much ground for reflection. By the regularly organized standard method of wound treatment where continuity can be kept up, we are not only saving life and limb, a very important point in the economy of any army, but we are also saving much subsequent expense to the State."

During the recent epidemic of influenza there has been a number of cases of empyema treated by simple trocar puncture, drainage tube inserted, and Dakin solution injected into the cavity with a 20 c.c. glass syringe, and immediately syphoned out by a suction apparatus the nose and throat men use for taking up the mucous and blood in the throat during operation. This is repeated every two to four hours during the day, and in every instance marked improvement has been quite apparent in two or three days.

Instead of resecting a rib or ribs, as we used to do, we now under local anthesia, insert a tube as above described, with much more satisfactory results, it being very exceptional now that we think it necessary to subject our patient to the rib resection.

Dr. Hartford spoke very nicely regarding its use in gynecological work with offensive leukorrhea discharge, for which I thank him.

Now in conclusion, we will ask again, What is the ideal antiseptic? It must possess the following properties:

(1) It must be a highly potent bactericide.

(2) It must be innocuous to sound tissue, but must rapidly remove dead tissue and sloughs.

(3) It must be non-poisonous to the individual when applied in large quantities to an extensive wound.

(4) It must be innocuous to leukocytes and not delay their functions.

(5) It must act in the presence of serum or wound exudate.

(6) It must not delay, but rather hasten, tissue repair.

(7) It must be an antiseptic which will help the patient for the first few days following his injury, and not rely upon the patient helping himself.

(8) It should be cheap and must be easily prepared.

Again thanking you for the discussion and assuring you of my most sincere appreciation of same.

OVARIAN FUNCTION*

John S. Hartford, M. D,, F. A. C. S.

PROFESSOR OF GYNECOLOGY, SCHOOL OF MEDICINE, UNIVERSITY OF OKLAHOMA,
OKLAHOMA CITY, OKLAHOMA

The history of the study of the ovary has been one of the most interesting in medical and surgical research. This study has been greatly stimulated in the last decade, since the dire results of ovarian castration became well established. In the earlier days we thought of the ovary only as it referred to menstruation and the propagation of the specie. Through the study and the experimental research of Loeb, Fraenkle, Ancel, Bouin, Marshall, Robert Myer, Shroeder, Martin and others, we know now that the ovary has a dual function, and that the function of life is possibly not as great as the glandular element that influences the entire physical, nervous and psychical make-up of women, and it is the latter function we wish to emhasize in this paper.

The sexual and child-bearing function of the ovary has been well established for a long time. We know that following the rupture of the graafian follicle carrying the ovum, that the phenomena of menstruation follows, caused by some chemical substance not well known. It has also been fairly well established, that preceding, during and immediately following menstruation, pregnancy is most likely to take place. Removal of the ovaries will stop menstruation, followed by sterility.

Recently, some very interesting studies have been made, showing that the height of sexual desire in women, precedes, accompanies and immediately follows menstruation, with a secondary curve midway between the period. Thus we see that the greatest period of sexual desire is synonymous with and immediately following the rupture of the graafian follicle. The dual functions of the ovary are not well separated, and we see them closely related in many instances, namely, we know that the pregnancy will not develop unless there is a corpus luteum. The corpus luteum extract of the market is usually selected and made from animals that were pregnant when slaughtered; the corpus luteum from sows and cows giving one of the most reliable preparations.

The portion of the ovary containing the glandular secretion has not been entirely classified, but is presumed to come from the interstitial portion. But for us the consideration of the elements is sufficient, which consists of the graafian follicles and their contained ovum; the corpora lutae originating from degenerated graafian follicles.

It appears that the harmones of the graafian follicles are not alone the origin of the secretion, as there appears to be sufficient secretion in the child to cause growth and development of the genitals, up to the time of puberty, when the ripening of the graafian follices stimulates menstruation and sexual life, and at this period the breasts begin to develop. If the ovaries are removed before puberty there is lack of development of the genitals and probably mal-development of the body with absence of the sexual nature. Steinbauch, in his experiments with animals, has proven that the interstitial portion of the ovaries is responsible for the genital development, and that when ovaries were transplanted, the genitals continue to develop and the sex instincts were present.

Ovarian secretion has some relation to the other secretory glands. Castration of young animals causes slight enlargement of the thymus and hypophysis and decreases of weight of the adrenals.

Oophorectomy causes certain metabolic changes in the body, osteomalacia is favorably influenced by removal of the ovaries, and usually there is an increase in the weight of the body. Loewy Richer reports that the removal of ovaries in dogs caused a marked decrease in the consumption of oxygen. After a few

*Read in Surgical Section, Annual State Meeting, Muskogee, May 21, 1919.

weeks, ovarian extracts fed to these dogs caused them to assume, not only normal oxygen intake, but caused them to use an increased amount of oxygen. The above experiments and observations point to a specific influence in the body metabolism.

There are a chain of general symptoms which gynecologists report in their patients after the removal of the ovaries, and which are many times associated with the natural menopause. These symptoms have not been regularly classified, but in a recent article by Richardson of Baltimore upon "The Effect of Hysterectomy Upon Ovarian Secretion", he has outlined a tentative classification, which he divides into two divisions:

First: Symptoms from the domain of autonomous nervous system:

1. Vasomotor—Hot flushes; headaches; dizziness; vertigo; fainting; dermatographia; urticaria; erythemata; cold hands and feet.

2. Cardiac—Palpitation; tachycardia; (mild, with normal heart).

3. Gastro-intestinal (motor and secretory)—Digestive disturbances with flatulence; eructation, nausea and occasional vomiting; stasis; meteorism; constipation; diarrhea.

4. Urinary—Irritable bladder; polyuria.

5. Endocrine—Thyroid; hyper- and hypo-function; pituitary, e. g. hypotension; gonads, e. g. voice; body conformation; countenance; facial hair; breasts; external genitalia.

6. Sweat glands, e. g. sudden sweating.

Second—Psycho-neurotic symptoms:

1. Psychic—Fatigability (mental and psychical); emotivity; hypersensitiveness; irritability; changed temperament; anxiety and apprehension; insomnia; excitability; hysteria; psychoses; depression; apathy and indifference; lack of energy; impaired memory; aphasia; indecision; self-condemnation; suicidal ideas.

2. Neurotic—Exaggerated reflexes; tremors and epigastric quivering; visual and auditory disturbances; lowered muscle tones; paraesthesia.

You will find from the above classification that you will be able to place most any case, and some cases will present the entire symptom complex. I wish to call especial attention to the skin manifestations coming from ovarian hormones. Dutoit has recently written a very interesting article showing the effect of ovarian secretion upon the skin. The effect upon the genitalia of ovarian castration is very marked upon young women or those in child bearing period. The labia majora and minora becomes rapidly thinned out and contracted. The opening of the vagina becomes atrophied and hard, many times resembling kraurosis.

I believe that with present knowledge of the functions of the ovaries, and the chain of symptoms that follow their removal, that they never should be removed, only for the soundest pathological reasons, either before or after the menopause, and if they are removed, their loss should be compensated for by the transplantation of sections of the ovary in the abdominal wall, broad ligaments, libia majora or some location where the blood supply is good, and the careful administration of corpus luteum extract over a long period.

Discussion.

Dr. M. Smith, Oklahoma City: This is quite a change from the heated discussion on the "Dakin solution", to the high altitude of the ovarian function. I was very much interested in the paper, and Doctor asked me to open the discussion.

I think there is a great deal in connection with the glandular system that we are now upon the verge of knowing something more about, but as yet, we are still to a great degree groping in the dark, and it is not only an interesting subject, but a very deep subject, and the more we study it the more bewildered we become.

When a female child is born, according to some of our best text books, there are three hundred and fifty thousand ovules in the ovaries; this may seem incomprehensible if you will stop to think about it. I have had occasion recently to look up some literature on this subject, and noticed one very striking to me where a male was castrated and their grafting a portion of the ovary into the sack, and that instead of the male going on and developing, as he would have naturally done, he developed the feminine characteristics instead of the rough characteristics of the male. Instead of the hair of the head and pubes assuming the coarse rough nature peculiar to the male, it had a soft, velvety feeling that naturally appeals to the instinct of any man.

I was very much interested in the effect of the irritated bladder. A number of years ago, probably twenty-five—I do not remember exactly—I had occasion to remove some ovaries for an irritated bladder. I tried everything under the sun to give relief, finally in desperation I advised abdominal section. On opening the abdomen, I found what we would not call a pathological ovary. I removed those ovaries, and in less than four weeks the woman who had recently been incapacitated for a number of years before the operation, was doing her own washing and ironing and working in the field with her husband every day. This is only one of the several experiences that I might recite. I think physiology teaches us that there is a secretion in the ovary that is absolutely necessary for the development of the child on up until puberty has been attained.

I have had some cases where they menstruate after I have removed the tubes and ovaries—this is not a true menstruation, being only nature's way to relieve the pent up nerve energy—the true menstruation only occurs with ovulation and rupture of the graafian follicle, etc.

Another important point made by the essayist was to consider removing the ovaries before puberty, or even after, unless the pathology was in a measure sufficient. To attempt to rob a woman of her true womanhood is taking from her the most sacred of all her inheritance.

In Philadelphia in 1918, I had the pleasure of attending a clinic of Prof. E. E. Montgomery, who is pronounced the greatest gynecologist in the world. I saw him transplant the ovary in an abdominal wound at several different clinics. Also Dr. Bland, whose ability is beyond question, gave a beautiful operation, removing the transplanted ovary from the abdominal wound for cystic degeneration that he had transplanted four years before. The moral of this transplantation was very apparent to the gynecologist.

Dr. Hartford, closing: I thank the gentleman for the discussion and there are a few points brought out in the discussion I think it is well to consider. One point is that menstruation does not follow after the ovaries have been removed. There has been a great deal of experimental work along this line. For instance, the fellows who have the idea about the value of the corpus luteum figure that if the corpus luteum is a good thing to stimulate the ovary it ought to produce menstruation. If it is responsible for the bringing about of menstruation, or the feeding of it, it ought to produce menstruation. There is only one record or instance of that that I have been able to find—one man that claims he has removed the tubes and that those tubes are now in the hospital as entire specimens, and that following the removal of these tubes and ovaries this woman was fed corpus luteum and menstruation was established, which was brought about over a period of time. Yet I still have a doubt and question that particular thing, because there may have been supernumerary ovaries. There may be a portion of ovary left in the ovarian ligament, where it was tied off at the time of other operations. This is always a point it is good to follow—the ovaries should be tied off as far as possible and not injure the ovarian circulation—that is sometimes responsible for the mal-secretion of the ovary and for the condition that follows. I feel that the skin manifestation is an important field.

The question of the corpus luteum extract as compared with the testicular extract, which was advocated some time ago, shows there is a difference in the two glands. That is, that the ovarian tissue does contain a glandular substance that is necessary in the make-up of the woman.

As regards the question of passion, where the ovaries have been removed, that has always been a question. When you suggest to a woman that you expect to remove the ovaries there is always a question in her mind whether she will be able to perform the family duties as she did previous to that time, and it is a true fact, as was brought out in the discussion, that a certain per cent. of these women will have an excessive sexual desire after the removal of the ovaries, which we have not been able to account for, but Richardson, in his discussion of the removal of the uterus and leaving in the ovaries has brought out the point that where a complete history in that type of cases was kept fewer women had normal desires along that line than did those where the ovaries were left. Now, we must understand and cannot forget that even in women who never have had any disturbances to the ovaries—never had any operative procedure whatever—that there is a vast difference in the sexual desire and sexual appetite, if you please, so that on that question we are not sure.

EXFOLIATIVE DERMATITIS.

A case of exfoliative dermatitis, terminating fatally, due to arsphenamin, is reported by J. R. Latham, Camp Jackson, Columbia, S. C., (*Journal A. M. A.*, July 5, 1919). The death followed the intravenous injection of 0.8 gm. of arsphenamin, and the case bears the stamp of arsenical poisoning. · The patient, in a routine examination, gave a positive Wassermann, but there was no other evidence of syphilis in the history or examination, and his physical condition was excellent. The first injections of 0.4 gm. arsphenamin caused so severe a reaction that he was sent to the hospital for a week, before he returned to duty. The symptoms began to appear, and a second injection was given, and ten days later he was admitted to the base hospital. Four days after admission his skin began to exfoliate, the blood pressure fell, while fever and pulse mounted and the urine output steadily declined. As the exfoliation became more extreme mental hebetude deepened, and coma appeared as he gradually failed. Death occurred thirth-eight days after the first dose of arsphenamin. The following is the author's summary: "1. A fatality followed a therapeutic dose of arsphenamin, the equivalent of less than 3 grains of metallic arsenic. 2. Diarrhea and vomiting were absent during all stages of the intoxication. 3. Nephritis was not a marked feature at any time, and only appeared at the end. 4. There was apparently a decided affinity of the poison for the skin or for the trophic nerves supplying it. From the first to the last all toxic symptoms may be logically ascribed to impairment of skin function. 5. Arsenic was persistently present in the urine. This was remarkable in the absence of accompanying renal inflammation. 6. There was a high leukocytosis and eosinophilia, the latter related closely to the patient's resistance. The height of the leukocytosis followed that of the fever. 7. Arsenic was found at necropsy in every tissue in which it was sought."

BLOOD TRANSFUSION*

F. L. Carson, M. D., F. A. C. S., and R. M. Anderson, M. D.
SHAWNEE, OKLAHOMA

From the earliest dawn of the history of medicine the dream of the transference of blood from animals to man or from man to man has been recorded. To stay the advent of senility or to restore youthful vigor seems to have been a favorite illusion with our ancestors.

Ore[1] claims to have found many references among the early Egyptians to the subject of transfusion. In the light of our knowledge the actual performance of the operation as we now know it was probably not accomplished, or if blood was actually transferred from one individual to another, it was in such small quantities as to be negligible. Even the oft-quoted case of Pope Innocent VIII in 1492, where three boys were sacrificed in a vain attempt to save the life of the prelate, is subject to question, as the actual details are entirely lacking—an oversight not usually found in descriptions of other operations of the same period.

The heterogeneous transfusion, which was repeatedly attempted, all ended disastrously; the reason, of course, is well understood now, but was clouded with mystery at the time.

It was after the appearance of Harvey's epoch-making paper, in 1628, when the circulation was really understood, that intelligent attempts at direct transfusion were made. Lower, a physiologist in the latter part of the seventeenth century, was probably the first to make such an effort, using segments of goose quills to interpose between the segments of vessels of the donor and recipient. Sporadic attempts seem to have occurred from that time, usually resulting disastrously; either due to the clotting, or to improper selection of donors, until the latter part of the last century and the first part of this when use was made of defibrinated blood and more generally of so-called physiological saline solution. But even during this period we get the impression that investigators were not satisfied. Matas[2] in 1891, expressed the situation by stating that while mechanically and physically saline solution rivaled blood, physiologically it could never take its place; he further made the statement "In speaking of blood as a medium for transfusion, we mean, of course, only pure, entire living blood and not the altered pathological material known as defibrinated blood. We also mean blood of the same species and not that derived from heterogeneous sources." Even at that early date he must have had an idea of the incompatability of blood of different species.

It was not until Carrel, who was undoubtedly stimulated by the work of Matas on the surgery of vascular systems, had, after infinite labor, worked out the details of direct anastamosis of vessels by suture, that transfusion began to assume its present place in surgery. The method used was, however, too complicated to come into general use, and too few operators had mechanical dexterity to master its intricate details. Then came the various mechanical devices to facilitate the arteriovenous anastamosis. Chief among these were the Crile's canula, Brewer's tube, Bernheim's methods, and a great many other ingenious devices. All these methods were good, and in the hands of the originators worked very well, but they were too complicated to be generally adopted.

The disadvantages of any direct method of transfusion were very soon evident to those who attempted it; besides the technical difficulties, which were considable with even the simplified operation, the fact that the actual amount of transferred blood could at best be only approximated, caused investigators to turn to less complicated methods. Among the first to render the operation less difficult were Kimpton and Brown's[3] paraffined glass cylinder method; somewhat later Lindeman devised his justly popular syringe method: this was probably

*Read in Surgical Section, Annual State Meeting, Muskogee, May 21, 1919.

the best that had been advocated until'that time and within a short time it became very popular. The disadvantages were the number of assistants necessary, the multiplicity of syringes used and the fact that one vein in each donor and recipient was destroyed by the operation. Unger's[4] ingenious two-way-stop-cock apparatus found considerable popularity, but this also was open to the same drawback as the others.

Lewisohn,[5] in a preliminary paper, showed the feasibility of using sodium citrate as an anti-coagulant, and in a more extensive paper[6] gave in detail the method which bids fair to stand the test of time. This sodium salt had long been known as an agent to retard the coagulation of blood, but had been considered too toxic to be available in transfusion. The trouble lay in the fact that in the laboratory a one per cent. solution had been used and this was known to be too large a dosage if used in any considerable amount of blood; but by working in a narrow margin Lewisohn demonstrated that two-tenths per cent. would serve its purpose, and at the same time could be used in 500 to 1000 c.c.'s of blood with absolute safety, provided the proper precautions were observed. It has been claimed that reaction (chills and fever) following the citrate methods are more frequent than after the direct, but this statement seems open to question. Hunt[7] believes the patient's general condition is an important factor in the percentage of post-transfusion reactions; thus he found that pernicious anemia cases had 8.5 per cent higher reactions than when the operation was performed for other conditions. It is well known that the intravenous injection of any foreign substance may be followed by a chill, and it is possible that lack of observation of proper technique in keeping the blood warm may account partially for the reaction following this method.

Hektoen[8] pointed out in 1908, that under special conditions transfusion might prove dangerous, owing to red cell agglutination within the vessels of the recipient, and suggested that this might be avoided by selecting a donor whose corpuscles were not agglutinated by serum of the patient. It remained for Moss[9] to work out the iso-agglutinins and iso-hemolysins in detail and later[10] to suggest a practical easy method of determining the fitness of donors in given cases, by grouping. He found that every human falls into one of four groups according to the following modification of Moss' technique, by Sanford.[11]

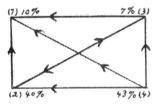

(7) 10%   7% (3)

(2) 40%   43% (4)

Moss agglutination groups (modified by Sanford); the corpuscles of the various groups are agglutinated by the serums of the groups from which the arrows lead.

Earlier investigators claimed that tests must be made before each transfusion,[12] but more recently it has been found that each individual remains permanently in his respective group.

It is better to have a donor in the same group as the recipient, but practically it has been found that if the serum of the donor does agglutinate the corpuscles of the recipient and the reverse is not true, no untoward effects will be noted—the serum of the donor being so rapidly diluted by the recipient's blood that agglutination does not occur. The reverse, however, must not occur, i. e. the serum of the recipient must not agglutinate the corpuscles of the donor.

So far nothing has been said about hemolysis, which is really the thing to be feared. Brem[13] pointed out that when hemolysis does occur it was always preceded or accompanied by agglutination. The reverse may not be true, i. e. there may be agglutination without subsequent hemolysis; but for practical purposes the agglutination test is utilized, owing to its simplicity.   Brem,[14] in the same article, modifies Moss' original technique, making it so simple that any but a novice in laboratory work may perform it.   It is as follows:

Let 11 represent a known blood belonging to group 2 and x a blood the group of which must be determined.   Five or six drops of 11 blood are collected in a small clean dry test tube or centrifuge tube, and one or two drops, according to the size of the drops, in another tube containing 1 c.c. of 1.5 per cent. sodium citrate in 0.9 per cent salt solution, which gives one approximately a five per cent. suspension of corpuscles.   The percentage does not have to be exact.   The x blood is collected in the same way in two similar tubes.   The bloods in the dry tubes are allowed to coagulate, the coagulum is loosened from the side of the tube with a platinum wire, and the tubes centrifugalized to separate the serum. Serum and corpuscles are now ready for the tests.   Platinum loopfuls of serum and corpuscles are placed on coverslips, which are inverted over an ordinary cell slide rimmed with petrolatum.   Two loopsful of serum are used and one of corpuscle suspension.   The slides are gently rolled from side to side to agitate the corpuscles in order to bring them into contact with each other.   Agglutination, if it occurs, takes place at room temperature within five minutes.   It can usually be detected with the naked eye, showing as brick red particles, but should be examined, also, with the low power objective of the microscope.   Rouleaux formation of red corpuscles must be differentiated from small clumps due to agglutination.

In emergency it is not necessary to group patients and the only test necessary is to see that the serum of the recipient does not agglutinate the cells of the donor.   Referring to the above table (Sanford's) we see that group four corpuscles are not agglutinated by the serum of any other group.   So anyone doing any considerable amount of surgery should have in readiness a few professional donors of this group for emergency purposes.   They can easily be secured for a consideration.   Of course one must be careful to prevent the transmission of syphilis by having frequent Wassermanns.

This technique may sound complicated but in reality it is very easy, especially if one has a known group of serum and corpuscles to start with.   We are prepared to furnish these to any one who desires.

The beneficial effects of transfusion in so many pathological states are so well understood that it would be superfluous to recount them.   It is sufficient to say that great good has been accomplished in our hands in secondary hemorrhages, shock, pellagra and pernicious anemia.   In the hemolysis that accompanied the recent influenza epidemic it seems to us that transfusion would have been of great benefit.   Unfortunately we only tried it on one case which was practically moribund.   She improved after the first transfusion but the second failed to revive her and the case ended fatally.   Should the occasion again occur, and the time permit, we shall again attempt the operation.

Cases with bleeding fibroids, where the hemoglobin is under forty per cent after one or two transfusions, are quickly changed from exceedingly poor operative risks to ones that stand surgical intervention well.

Of course, cures are not expected in cases of pernicious anemia, but nothing so rapidly causes amelioration of symptoms and a remission of disease as this agent.

As mentioned above, we have tried transfusion in pellagra, choosing only those desperately ill and in whom all other agents were unavailing.   The benefits are so prompt and apparently lasting that we feel great encouragement in this form of therapy.

It has been suggested that the causes for failure in skin and bone graft, where it is not autogenous, may be due to the difference in grouping.   We have not tested this but will in the near future.

References:
1. Ore: Etudes sur la transfusion do sang, 1868.
2. Matas: New Orleans Medical and Surgical Journal, 1891.
3. Kimpton & Brown: Journal American Medical Association, 1913.
4. Unger: Journal American Medical Association, 1915.
5. Lewisohn: Medical Record, 1915.
6. Lewisohn: Surgery, Gynecology and Obstetrics, 1915.
7. Hunt: Texas Journal of Medicine, 1918.
8. Hektoen: Journal American Medical Association, 1908.
9. Moss: Bulletin Johns Hopkins Hospital, 1910.
10. Ibid: Journal American Medical Association, 1917.
11. Sanford: Journal American Medical Association, 1918.
12. Lewisohn: Journal American Medical Association, 1917.
13. Brem: Journal American Medical Association, Vol. LXVII.
14. Ibid:

CLINICAL REPORT OF OPERATION ON FRACTURE OF PATELLA.

FRED S. CLINTON, M. D., F. A. C. S.

PRESIDENT AND CHIEF SURGEON OKLAHOMA HOSPITAL

TULSA, OKLAHOMA

On April 5, 1919, F. M. K., age 65, injured in an automobile accident, sustained numerous abrasions and contusions distributed over his entire body and a comminuted fracture of the left patella.

After the customary examination, including x-ray, emergency attention was given, immobilization on long posterior splint, bandage from the foot up, figure-of-eight about the knee, elevation of entire extremity, rest in bed, and application of ice cap. However, leg continued to swell about the knee joint on the following day accompained by much pain, and an operation was decided upon at once and was performed in the following manner, which has given very satisfactory results in other cases as well as this; however, it is not always desirable to operate on these patients at once although the tendency of the time would seem to suggest earlier operations than formerly.

(a) The leg and thigh having been thoroughly cleansed and made as nearly aseptic as possible, a horseshoe incision was made exposing the comminuted patella.

(b) Under the most rigid asepsis, and without hand contacting, blood clots were removed from the edges of the patella and from the cavity and all hemorrhage thoroughly controlled.

(c) The internal and external lateral ligaments were each united by two interrupted chromic catgut sutures. Fragments of patella were approximated by matress sutures of kangaroo tendon introduced as follows: drill was held obliquely so that it emerged on the fractured surface in front of the articular cartilage, not entering the cavity, and the capsule was closed by use of continuous chromic catgut.

(d) External wounds closed and an immobilizing posterior splint applied and patient returned to bed with extremity elevated.

Patient made an uninterrupted recovery and at the end of six weeks was able to get about with the aid of a cane and has at this time a functionally good leg.

Points of danger are: (a) Sepsis and subsequent stiffness, or (b) Possible loss of leg. (c) Possible loss of life.

These may be avoided as a rule by: (a) The enforcement of the most rigidly aseptic technic. (b) By avoiding all hand contacting of the wound. (c) By not traumatizing the tissues by rough or needless manipulation.

JOURNAL OF THE OKLAHOMA STATE MEDICAL ASSOCIATION

VOLUME XII   MUSKOGEE, OKLA., AUGUST, 1919   NUMBER 8

PUBLISHED MONTHLY AT MUSKOGEE. OKLA., UNDER DIRECTION OF THE COUNCIL

DR. CLAUDE A. THOMPSON, EDITOR-IN-CHIEF
308 SURETY BUILDING, MUSKOGEE

DR. CHAS. W. HEITZMAN, ASSISTANT EDITOR
BARNES BUILDING, MUSKOGEE

ENTERED AT THE POST OFFICE AT MUSKOGEE, OKLAHOMA, AS SECOND CLASS MAIL MATTER, JULY 26, 1912

THIS IS THE OFFICIAL JOURNAL OF THE OKLAHOMA STATE MEDICAL ASSOCIATION.   ALL COMMUNICATIONS SHOULD BE ADDRESSED TO THE JOURNAL OF THE OKLAHOMA STATE MEDICAL ASSSOCIATION, 308 SURETY BUILDING, MUSKOGEE, OKLAHOMA.

The editorial department is not responsible for the opinions expressed in the original articles of contributors.

Reprints of original articles will be supplied at actual cost, provided request for them is attached to manuscript or made in sufficient time before publication.

Articles sent this Journal for publication and all those read at the annual meetings of the State Association are the sole property of this Journal. The Journal relies on each individual contributor's strict adherence to this well-known rule of medical journalism. In the event an article sent this Journal for publication is published before appearance in the Journal, the manuscript will be returned to the writer.

Failure to receive the Journal should call for immediate notification of the editor, 307-8 Surety Building, Muskogee, Okla.

Local news of possible interest to the medical profession, notes on removals, changes in address, deaths and weddings will be gratefully received.

Advertising of articles, drugs or compounds unapproved by the Council on Pharmacy of the A. M. A. will not be accepted.

Advertising rates will be supplied on application. It is suggested that wherever possible members of the State Associa tion should patronize our advertisers in preference to others as a matter of fair reciprocity.

EDITORIAL

VACATION AND OUTING DANGERS.

Natural tendencies of mankind, attractively aided by alluring pictures and literature of transportation companies and resorts, cause a pardonable longing for the cool spots depicted to the restless reader. He is especially fond of the pictures showing a tent by a lake or stream, the camp fire and boat conveniently near and his companion landing trout or bass. Blithely he plans for weeks his trip to the woods, thoughtless of the very common dangers sure to confront him.

Camping out in Oklahoma, except in cold weather, is one of the most dangerous procedures we may undertake. Physicians easily recall from experience the trail of typhoid and malaria brought back home by the vacationists.

Physicians have the opportunity to safeguard their clientele, however, by insisting on very simple precautions of a preventive nature.

Tents can be made mosquito proof, often they are not, and they are not wholly protective against the ever-present anopheles along our streams, so the nightly harmless dose of quinine as a routine should be advised with fair assurance of protection from serious illness.

Foods of every class, cool well water, the farmer's milk and fruits are an ever-present danger to the country visitor. The amount of prevalent ignorance of the fundamental means of food protection, care and transportation in our rural districts is appalling. One only has to visit and observe the neglect of very well known means of protection to realize the danger. Against these dangers there are two means of protection. The first, vaccination, is practically a dead letter to most of our people despite the brilliant results shown by our army experience. The second, sterilization of all food supplies, is either unknown, ignored or so carelessly done as to increase the menace by the sense of false security.

Timely warning will obviate a great deal of malarial and typhoid infection if the simplest rules are followed. The difficulty lies in lack of interest of those concerned and their inability to receive advice. The whole matter is one of the problems of the hour to physicians and health officers.

CURRENT MEDICAL LITERATURE
Conducted by

DR. CHAS. W. HEITZMAN, Barnes Building, Muskogee

Contributions and observations of Oklahoma physicians collected by them in the course of study of American and foreign medical literature, deemed to be of sufficient interest and value to the profession, are especially invited to this department. Such contributions should bear the name of the sender, which will be appended to the abstract or omitted, as desired.

COMPULSORY HEALTH INSURANCE.

(Pennsylvani Medical Journal, June, 1919).

To deprive any citizen of the privilege of putting his life in the hands of a physician of his choice is un-American and it is equally un-American to compel a physician to attend a person in sickness when for a good reason he would like to be excused. If a man must submit his life to the dictates of a bureaucracy, such a man is robbed of his liberty and independence as it is related to that which is above all things sacred to him.

Where is the justice or equity of discriminating legislation that would advocate a bureaucracy to control and dominate the members of the medical profession to the extent that such beuraucracy shall determine the personnel of a physician's clientele and the fee he may charge regardless of the qualifications attained and the specially skillful service rendered? One cannot be in sympathy with such a contemptible statewide lodge practice. Why should the members of the medical profession who at present rank in qualifications with that of any other profession or calling, be commercialized at the instigation of comparatively few apparently self-appointed ultra enthusiasts who pose as deeply interested in the physical welfare of the people of our commonwealth and who do not see fit to apply the same principle in every other line of human endeavor? It is just as un-American for a bureaucracy to determine the clientele of a physician as it would be to determine the clientele of a butcher, a baker, or a candlestick maker. There is no difference in the application of the principle.

The physical welfare of our people was never so well taken care of as now. Preventive medicine has made tremendous progress and is the outgrowth of work accomplished by the organized medical profession. Nowhere in our country was it the result of the importation of any foreign scheme that has brought ruin to the profession wherever adopted. This whole propaganda appeals to one as artful sophistry, a species of Michiavelianism.   G. E. H.

BLOOD TRANSFUSION.

B. M. Bernheim, Baltimore (*Journal A. M. A.*, July 19, 1919), lays stress on the importance of actual blood transfusion which experience in the recent war has taught him. We have, he thinks, too often been told that it is the rarest thing for a patient to bleed to death, and that only a salt or gum infusion is necessary in urgent cases, and they will do all that blood can do. He says would that that were so: there would have been many fewer deaths among our soldiers in France, if it were. He questions the sustaining power of the rise in blood pressure from the gum solution, and while salt solution may be of tempory value it has no sustaining power. Blood on the other hand, has real sustaining power because of its oxygen-carrying properties and irs ability to remain intact as a circulating medium. He quotes striking cases of his own observation, illustrating the points he makes, both of the failure of the substances and of the value of actual blood. At his suggestion, he says, the sodium citrate method was adopted in the American Expeditionzary Forces, and also, at his further suggestion, all transfusion in France was turned over to the medical men; hence, it happens that many of them obtained a wide experience in this valuable line of practice.

PERSONAL AND GENERAL NEWS

Dr. J. H. Barnes, Enid, was seriously ill in July.

Dr. Ney Neel, Mangum, visited Texas points in July.

Dr. Roy Stone, Covington, visited Washington in July.

Dr. J. A. Jeter, Clinton, visited the Rochester clinics in July.

Dr. T. A. Buchanan, Oklahoma City, is visiting Colorado points.

Dr. C. A. Thompson, Muskogee, will take a vacation in Colorado in August.

Dr. A. V. Emerson, Tulsa, has returned from a visit to the Rochester clinics.

Dr. J. S. Hibbard, for many years at Cherokee, has moved to Witchia, Kansas.

Dr. R. A. Gardner, Marietta, has returned from postgraduate work in Chicago.

Dr. A. T. Dobson, Hobart, has been appointed health officer for Kiowa County.

Dr. Ralph Workman, Woodward, is taking his vacation in the mountains of Colorado.

Dr. A. R. Holmes, Henryetta, has returned from an automobile trip to Colorado points

Dr. G. N. Bilby, Alva, has been discharged from the army and assumed his old location.

Drs. E. E. Rice and J. M. Byrum, Shawnee, have returned from a visit to the Rochester clinics.

Dr. W. E. Simon, Alva, has returned from overseas service and is at work in his old location.

Dr. L. E. Pearson, Reed, has been discharged from the army and is back at his old location.

Dr. F. H. Hollingsworth and family, of Okmulgee, are driving to the Northwestern resorts and parks.

Dr. Wm. McIlwain, Lonewolf, visited the home folks in July on a short leave from military service.

Dr. A. W. Harris, Muskogee, has returned from overseas service and resumed his work at his old location.

Dr. C. L. McCallum, Sapulpa, has returned from overseas service, received his discharge and is back at work again.

Dr. J. J. Caviness, Altus, has received his discharge after protracted overseas service and will return to his old location.

Dr. Horace Reed, Oklahoma City, has returned from overseas service and is relocated at 611 State National Bank Building.

Dr. George Hunter, Oklahoma City, has returned to his work after overseas service. He was City Physician prior to his departure.

Dr. J. F. Messenbaugh, Oklahoma City, has returned from several weeks vacation in Missouri, the Rochester clinic and Colorado points.

Dr. C. B. Hill, formerly superintendent of the Supply State Hospital, has moved to Guthrie and is asssociated with Dr. John W. Duke.

Dr. Carroll A. Johnson, Kiowa, has returned from overseas service. Dr. Johnson was flight surgeon attached to the immediate unit of Captain Eddie Rickenbacker.

Dr. T. B. Triplett, Moreland, has been discharged from the army after overseas service and has returned to his home. He has formed a partnership with Dr. T. E. Dixon.

Dr. L. E. Emanuel, Chickasha, has returned from overseas service and assumed his former location. Dr. Emanuel returns a Major and while absent was reappointed health officer of Grady County.

Dr. T. A. Hartgraves, formerly of Soper but for many months attached to Base Hospital Laboratory work in the overseas army, has located in Muskogee and is connected with the Muskogee Clinical and Pathological Laboratory.

Oklahoma Pow-Wow, Oklahoma City, published monthly by the Oklahoma Tuberculosis Association, Edited by Jules Schevitz, Executive Secretary, is a bright little sheet now being issued in the fight against tuberculosis. The organization will mail it to any physician on request, and urgently invites the cooperation of all physicians to make the issues attractive.

Dr. Frank McGregor, Mangum, has returned from overseas service in the army. Dr. McGregor returns with the earned distinction of having received more decorations and honorable mentions for distinguished service than any other Oklahoma physician. He was decorated by the King of England for extraordinary service and valor under fire. He will resume his place and partnership as a general surgeon with Dr. Fowler Border, with whom he was associated before entering service.

DOCTOR G. C. WILTON.

Dr. G. C. Wilton, Ryan, died at his home after a month's illness, the cause of death said to have been cancer of the stomach. Interment was made at Ryan.

Dr. Wilton was born in Lamar County, Texas, March 1, 1859. He was educated in the common schools of Texas and graduated from the Ft. Worth University. He moved to the Indian Territory in 1889, locating at Grady, moving to Ryan nineteen years ago. He is survived by his wife and a son and daughter.

COUNCIL ON PHARMACY AND CHEMISTRY
AMERICAN MEDICAL ASSOCIATION

This report is limited according to the ideas and opinions as to its usefulness and practicability to Oklahoma physicians. A complete report is obtainable upon request from the Council, 535 North Dearborn St., Chicago.

PROPAGANDA FOR REFORM

Collosol Preparations. The Council on Pharmacy and Chemistry reports that Collosol Argentum, Collosol Arsenicum, Collosol Cocain, Collosol Cuprum, Collosol Ferrum, Collosol Hydrargyrum, Collosol Iodin, Collosol Manganese, Collosol Quinin and Collosol Sulphur are inadmissible to New and Nonofficial Remedies because their composition is uncertain. In the few cases in which the therapeutic claims for these preparations were examined, the claims were found so improbable and exaggerated as to have necessitated the rejection of these products on this account. The term "Collosol" appears to be a group designation for what are claimed to be permanent colloidal solutions, marketed by the Anglo-French Drug Company, Ltd., London and New York. Were this claim correct, the Collosols should contain their active constituent in the form of microscopic or ultramicroscopic suspensions. The Council was, however, obliged to question the colloidal character of the preparations. A number of samples submitted to the Council had separated and Collosol Hydrargyrum was not a colloidal solution at all; also the ampules of Collosol Ferrum contained a flocculent precipitate. If either of these two preparations were injected intravenously as directed, death might result (Jour. A. M. A., June 7, 1919, p. 1694).

Pulvoids Calcylates Compound. The Council on Pharmacy and Chemsitry publishes a report on Pulvoids Calcylates Compound (The Drug Products Co., Inc.), not so much because the preparation is of any great importance, but as a protest against the large number of similar irrational complex mixtures which are still offered to physicians. These "Pulvoids" are tablets, each of which is said to contain "Calcium and Strontium Disalicylate 5 grs., Resin Guaiac ½ gr., Digitalis ¼ gr., Colchium (Colchicum) Seed ¼ gr., Squill ¼ gr., Cascarin 1-16 gr. with aromatics." They were advertised among "Approved Remedies for La Grippe and 'Flu'" * * *. The Council admits that salicylates have a field in influenza in that they often afford relief from pain. There is no reason to suppose that a mixture of strontium and calcium salicylate—the calcium and strontium disalicylate of the "Pulvoids" is probably a mixture of strontium and calcium salicylates—has any greater salicylic effect than an equal amount of sodium salicylate. On the other hand it is worse than useless to give colchicum, squill and digitalis for the relief of such pain. No educated physician will give resin of guaiac and "cascarin" in fixed proportions with salicylates (Jour. A. M. A., June 14, 1919, p. 1784).

Antithyroid Preparations (Antithyroidin-Moebius and Thyreoidectin) Omitted from N. N. R. New and Nonofficial Remedies, 1918, contained a discussion of "antithyroid" preparations and described two of these: Antithyroidin-Moebius (E. Merck, Darmstadt, Germany) and Thyroidectin (Parke, Davis and Company, Detroit, Mich.). The "antithyroid" preparations have not realized the expectations of their promoters, and are viewed with skepticism by practicallly all critical clinicians. Consequently, notwithstanding the cautiously worded claims made for Thyreoidectin, the Council voted to omit this preparation from New and Nonofficial Remedies (Antithyroidin-Moebius had already been omitted because it was off the market) (Reports Council Pharm. and Chem., 1918, p. 50).

Borcherdt's Malt Extract With Alteratives. Each fluid-ounce of this was claimed to contain iodin 1-30 grain, calcium iodid 1 grain, potassium iodid 2 grains, calcium chlorid 8 grains. The preparation was declared inadmissible to New and Nonofficial Remedies: (1) because it did not contain free iodin as claimed; (2) because it was needlessly complex, and therefore irrational; (3) because the name of the preparation is not descriptive of its composition, but therapeutically suggestive (Reports Council on Pharm. and Chem., 1918, p. 51).

Cephaelin and Syrup Cephaelin-Lilly Omitted from N. N. R. and Syrup Emetic-Lilly not Accepted. New and Nonofficial Remedies, 1918, described cephaelin (an alkaloid obtained from ipecacuanha root) and listed Syrup Cephaelin-Lilly as a pharmaceutical preparation of it. In 1918 Lilly and Company advised that the name of its preparation had been changed to Syrup Emetic. The Council directed the omission of Syrup Cephaelin-Lilly and voted not to admit Syrup Emetic because the name does not indicate the potent ingredient of the simple pharmaceutical preparation and in that it is therapeutically suggestive. Emetics are powerful agents, and preparations containing them should not be sold under non-informing names. As the cephaelin syrup was the only preparation of cephaelin admitted to New and Nonofficial Remedies and as the alkaloid appears to have no important therapeutic field, the Council also omitted cephaelin from the book (Reports Council Pharm and Chem., 1918, p. 52).

Colalin Omitted From N. N. R. Colalin is a bile salt preparation claimed to consist essentially of hyoglyococholic and hyotaurocholic acids. It is manufactured by Rufus Crowell and Company, Somerville, Mass., and marketed by Schieffelin and Company. An examination of the current advertising for Colalin revealed that claims were made for it which were not in harmony with the known actions of bile preparations. As these claims were not substantiated by evidence nor revised in accordance with a request sent to the manufacturer and the agent, the Council directed the omission of Colalin from New and Nonofficial Remedies (Reports Council on Pharm. and Chem., 1918, p. 52).

Diphtheria Bacillus Vaccine Omitted From N.N.R.   The Council directed the omission of diphtheria bacillus vaccine from New and Nonofficial Remedies because the manufacturer of the only preparation of this vaccine advised that its sale had been discontinued (Reports Council Pharm. and Chem., 1918, p. 54).

Empyroform Omitted From N. N. R.   Empyroform is a condensation product of birch tar and formaldehyde.   The Council voted to omit the preparation from New and Nonofficial Remedies because its usefulness is doubtful and because the agents were not in a position to submit further evidence for its value (Reports Council Pharm. and Chem., 1918, p. 55).

Foral.   Foral is a depilatory preparation sold with special claims for its use for the removal of hair prior to surgical operation or the dressing of wounds.   The Council declared Foral inadmissible to New and Nonofficial Remedies: because it is an unessential and irrational modification of the well known depilatory composed of barium sulphid 2 drachms, zinc oxid 3 drachms and starch 3 drachms, and because it is marketed under a noninforming name and with unwarranted claims (Reports Council Pharm. and Chem., 1918, p. 55).

NEW BOOKS

Under this heading books received by the Journal will be acknowledged.   Publishers are advised that this shall constitute return for such publications as they may submit.   Obviously all publications sent us cannot be given space for review, but from time to time books received, of possible interest to Oklahoma physicians, will be reviewed.

The Surgical Clinics of Chicago.   Vo.ume III, Number 1 (February, 1919).   Octavo of 236 pages, 75 illustrations.   Philadelphia and London: W. B. Saunders Company, 1919.   Published Bi-Monthly.   Price per year: Paper $10.00, Cloth $14.00.

Reconstruction Therapy.   By William R. Dunton, Jr., M.D., Assistant Physician at Sheppard and Enoch Pratt Hospital, Towson, Md.; Instructor in Psychiatry, Johns Hopkins University.   12mo of 236 pages, 30 illustrations.   Philadelphia and London: W. B. Saunders Company, 1919.   Cloth, $1.50 net.

AN OUTLINE OF GENITO-URINARY SURGERY

By George Gilbert Smith, M.D., F.A.C.S., Genito-urinary Surgeon to Out-patients, Massachusetts General Hospital.   12mo of 301 pages with 71 illustrations.   Philadelphia and London: W. B. Saunders Company, 1919.   Cloth, $2.75 net.

This is a condensed but very practical work on Genito-Urinary Surgery, and is especially directed to the attention of the student and general practitioner.   The work is based on the practical experience of the author, the case histories entirely from his private work or his work at the Massachusetts General Hospital.   The illustrations are liberal and clear and from actual operations or specimens.

THE HEALTH OFFICER

By Frank Overton, M.D., D. P. H., Sanitary Supervisor, N. Y. State Dept. of Health, and Willard J. Denno, M. D., D. P. H., Medical Director of the Standard Oil Company.   Octavo of 512 pages with 51 illustrations.   Philadelphia and London: W. B. Saunders Company, 1919.   Cloth, $4.50 net.

This is a very readable work with unique and interesting features especially in the illustrations.   The author thought, and we hold with him, that the plainest primary fundamentals of disease dissemination may be "Greek" to some of our profession.   Experience in actual practice shows that an alarming percentage of doctors have either never learned the practical application of common knowledge of growth and spread of disease or ignore it and neglect it to the discredit of the medical profession.   With this idea in view he has inserted original drawings of accepted ideas on the subjects.   They show the diseases and their sources of growth directly or indirectly.

The problems and relations of the health officer in general are thoroughly considered in the text.   The work is so plainly written that it should be useful to everyone interested, whether physician, nurse or otherwise.

QUARTERLY MEDICAL CLINICS.

A Series of Consecutive Clinical Demonstrations and Lectures.   By Frank Smithies, M. D., Augustana Hospital, Chicago.   Volume 1, Number 1, January, 1919, Published by Medicine and Surgery Publishing Company, Metropolitan Building, St. Louis.   Annual Subscription, paper $5.00; cloth $8.00.   Single copies $1.50 in paper; Quarterly $2.50 in cloth.

This quarterly is a carefully edited report of the clinics and lectures given senior students of the School of Medicine of the University of Illinois at the Augustana Hospital.   Formerly stenographic reports were taken, mimeographed and given to the students. After repeated suggestion from visiting physicians that they be published and issued in consecutive order the work was undertaken and is now presented. The cases covering three months past. It is the aim to issue such a publication each quarter in the future.

The editor offers no excuse for the fact that some of the work is elementary, but advances the opinion that in teaching medical men very little must be taken for granted, that the simplest clinical and laboratory examination methods are often not clearly understood.

The subjects are those of every class presented for treatment at the hospital. Full histories, physical examination, special examination, x-ray examination, if any, discussion of the case, treatment, with any special suggestion as to technic and all other practical phases are given.

The work seems to be as valuable as were Murphy's Clinics to the student and practitioner. The illustrations are profuse and to the point.

DIET IN HEALTH AND DISEASE

By Julius Friedenwald, M.D., Professor of Gastro-Enterology in the University of Maryland School of Medicine and College of Physicians and Surgeons, Baltimore; and John Ruhrah, M.D., Professor of Diseases of Children in the University of Maryland and College of Physicians and Surgeons, Baltimore. Fifth edition, thoroughly revised and enlarged. Octavo of 919 pages. Philadelphia and London: W. B. Saunders Company, 1919. Cloth, $6.00.

This is a painstaking work covering closely every phase of diet affecting the organism. Elaborate tables, food values, diseases in which diet is a primary factor, diets adaptable to the healthy and the sick child, diseases caused by errors in diet, diet for the aged, in disease, in infections, in diseases of the stomach, liver, respiratory organs, circulatory system, genito-urinary system, nephritis, the nervous system, deficiency diseases, unclassified diseases, diseases of the skin, special diets as salt-free diets, etc., dietetic management of surgical cases, army and navy rations, prison and hospital dietaries and many other rare, but sometimes important conditions. Beverages, including lime water, milks, brandy and egg and allied mixtures of alcoholic content, fruit juices are noted. Cereals of every type, breads and vegetables have a place.

The work must be consulted to appreciate its thoroughness in every detail. Every physician should have the book near his desk for ready reference for the subjects embraced are those more often demanding attention than any other. It is a noticeable fact that works on diet and its many intricacies are those most often sought by physicians and intelligent patients from the library. The exacting details are too numerous to be remembered when needed, so it is necessary to constantly refresh the mind on them. This is the last word on the subjects.

SURGICAL TREATMENT

A Practical Treatise on the Therapy of Surgical Diseases for the Use of Practitioneers and Students of Surgery. By James Peter Warbasse, M. D., Formerly Attending Surgeon to the Methodist Episcopal Hospital, Brooklyn, New York. In three large octavo volumes, and separate Desk Index Volume. Volume III contains 861 pages with 864 illustrations. Philadelphia and London; W. B. Saunders Company, 1919. Per set (Three Volumes and the Index Volume): Cloth $30.00 per set.

This volume contains chapters on the Treatment of Hernia, their complications and forms; The Rectum and Anus; The Appendix, Liver and Gall-Bladder, the Genito-urinary organs, including the kidneys, uterus, suprarenal glands, bladder, prostate, penis, urethra and accessory organs; the testicles and scrotum, spermatic cord and testicles; vulva, vagina, uterus, ligaments, tubes, ovaries, etc. It also contains matter on the upper extremeties, not disregarding the too often lightly considered and unappreciated possibilities of felon, paronychia, cellulitis of the fingers, carbuncles, especially stressing the importance of proper treatment of the deep infections of the fingers, hands and arms. The lower extremeties are considered in like manner; their every conceivable abnormality being noted. Amputations in the light of the best end results are most thoroughly discussed. Plastic surgery and its incident indicated operations, electricity and radium, electric injuries are well noted. Many other fundamental conditions are noted.

"The Economics of Surgical Treatment" is a remarkably condensed statement of the practical problems confronting the profession. Under the head of "Surgical Practice Under Competition," "Surgical Practice Under the State," "Surgical Practice Under Group Experts" (The Mayo Clinic as an illustration), "Surgical Practice Under Co-operation" and "The Ultimate Needs and Destiny of Surgery"—a message full of import is written. The too long ignored fact, menace or inevitability of the injection of so-called socialistic methods, economic organizations of people, possibly some form of unionization applicable to medicine is recognized. But, in the statement that "Society will ever demand a special class who shall study the problems of human health . . ." is the barrier separating medicine, the most important of all sciences affecting modern life from the ordinary rules of organizations whose object is to demand the highest obtainable intrinsic reward for service rendered their fellows.

This volume completes the trio of works on surgery by Warbasse. It seems fair to say that the entire work is the most complete yet issued on the problems and work of the surgeon.

OFFICERS OF COUNTY SOCIETIES, 1919

County	President	Secretary
Adair	D. P. Chambers, Stilwell	J. A. Patton, Stilwell
Alfalfa	E. L. Frazier, Jet	J. M. Tucker, Carmen
Atoka-Coal	F. E. Sadler, Coalgate	W. T. Blount, Tupelo.
Beaver		
Beckham		J. E. Standifer, Elk City
Blaine	W F Griffin, Greenfield	J. A. Norris, Okeene
Bryan	H. B. Fuston, Bokchito	D. Armstrong, Durant
Caddo	P. H. Anderson, Anadarko	C. R. Hume, Anadarko
Canadian		W. J. Muzzy, El Reno
Carter	A G Cowles, Ardmore	Robert H Henry, Ardmore
Choctaw	C. H. Hale, Boswell	J. D. Moore, Hugo
Cleveland		D. W. Griffin, Norman.
Cherokee		
Comanche	A. H. Stewart, Lawton	E. B. Mitchell, Lawton
Coal-Atoka	F. E. Sadler, Coalgate	W. T. Blount, Tupelo
Cotton		
Craig	C. B. Bell, Welch	F. M. Adams, Vinita
Creek		H. S. Garland, Sapulpa.
Custer	K D Gossam, Custer	O H Parker, Custer
Dewey		
Ellis		
Garfield		L. W. Cotton, Enid.
Garvin		N. H. Lindsey, Pauls Valley.
Grady	Martha Bledsoe, Chickasha	J. C. Ambrister, Chickasha.
Grant		
Greer	Ney Neel, Mangum	Fowler Border, Mangum
Harmon		
Haskell	T B Turner, Stigler	R. F. Terrell, Stigler.
Hughes		Hugh Scott, Holdenville
Jackson	J. S. Stults, Olustee	J. B. Hix, Altus
Jefferson	D B Collins, Sugden	W M Browning, Waurika
Johnston		H. B. Kniseley, Tishomingo
Kay	G. H. Nieman, Ponca City	D Walker, Blackwell
Kingfisher	Frank Scott, Kingfisher	C. W. Fisk, Kingfisher.
Kiowa		A. T. Dobson, Hobart.
Latimer	E. L. Evins, Wilburton	C. R. Morrison, Wilburton
Le Flore	C. H. Mahar, Spiro	Harrell Hardy, Poteau
Lincoln		C. M. Morgan, Chandler
Logan		O. E. Barker, Guthrie.
Love		
Mayes	J. L. Adams, Pryor	L. C. White, Adair.
Major		
Marshall	J E Reed, Madill	J L Holland, Madill
McClain	J. W. West, Purcell	O. O. Dawson, Wayne
McCurtain	A W Clarkson, Valliant	W B McCaskill, Idabel
McIntosh	S. W. Minor, Hitchita	W. A. Tolleson, Eufaula
Murray	A P Brown, Davis	W. H. Powell, Sulphur.
Muskogee	J. L. Blakemore, Muskogee	H C. Rogers, Muskogee
Noble		B. A. Owen, Perry.
Nowata	J. E. Brookshire, Nowata	J. R. Collins, Nowata
Okfuskee	C. C. Bombarger, Paden	H. A. May, Okemah.
Oklahoma	W. J. Wallace, Oklahoma City	J. N. Alford, Oklahoma City
Okmulgee	Harry Breese, Henryetta	W. B. Pigg, Okmulgee
Ottawa	A. M. Cooter, Miami	G. Pinnell, Miami
Osage	A. J. Smith, Pawhuska	Benj. Skinner, Pawhuska
Pawnee		E. T. Robinson, Cleveland
Payne		J. B. Murphy, Stillwater
Pittsburg	L. C. Kuyrkeudall, McAlester	T. H. McCarley, McAlester.
Pottawatomie	E. E. Rice, Shawnee	G. S. Baxter, Shawnee.
Pontotoc	L. M. Overton, Fitzhugh	S. P. Ross, Ada
Pushmataha	H. C. Johnson, Antlers	Edw. Guinn, Antlers
Rogers	J H Haley, Chelsea	F A Anderson, Claremore
Roger Mills		
Seminole	W. T. Huddleston, Konawa	W. L. Knight, Wewoka.
Sequoyah	V W Hudson, Sallisaw	S A McKeel, Sallisaw
Stephens	J. W. Nieweg, Duncan	J. O. Wharton, Duncan.
Texas	W. H. Langston, Guymon	R. B. Hays, Guymon
Tulsa	G. A. Wall, Tulsa	A. W. Pigford, Tulsa
Tillman		J. E. Arrington, Frederick.
Wagoner	C E Haywood, Wagoner	C E Martin, Wagoner
Washita		A. S. Neal, Cordell.
Washington	O S Smerville, Bartlesville	J G Smith, Bartlesville
Woods		J. A. Bowling, Alva.
Woodward		

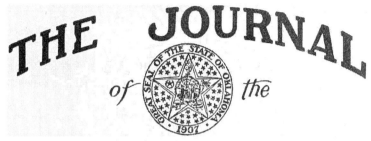

Oklahoma State Medical Association

VOLUME XII   MUSKOGEE, OKLA., SEPTEMBER, 1919   NUMBER 9

SYMPOSIUM ON SYPHILIS

The papers in this issue on the subject of Syphilis were read in the Section on Genito-Urinary Diseases, Skin and Radiology, at the Annual Meeting, Muskogee, May 21, 1919. Lack of space prohibits publication of all papers of the Symposium in one issue. The remainder with the discussion held by the section on all papers of the Symposium will be published later.

SYPHILIS

A Study of the Social Problem of Today

LIEUT. M. H. FOSTER, M. C., U. S..ARMY,

CHIEF OF THE GENITO-URINARY SERVICE,

FORT SILL, OKLAHOMA

As Bacon Saunders of Fort Worth preached the early operation for appendicitis some fifteen years ago and as Joe Bloodgood proclaimed the eradication of malignancy by removal of precancerous conditions about seven years later, we now venture an undertaking which is in keeping with the magnitude of the times, i.e., the control of syphilis in the present generation.

After extensive Wassermann surveys in 1915, Colonel Vedder found sixteen per cent of white and thirty-seven per cent of negro enlisted personnel to be syphilitic. He also found sixteen per cent of the recruits at that time suffering from an undetected syphilis.

In two series of routine Wassermanns done on pregnant women in Chicago in 1918, Cornell found that ten per cent of his charity cases at the lying-in hospital and three per cent of the cases selected from his private practice were syphilitic.

Pusey had previously estimated that the number of civilian syphilitics in America was 1,200,000, but Cornell, based on his three per cent findings, states that the number should be at least 4,320,000 and thinks that two or three times that number would be possibly nearer correct.

There is an enormous increase in venereal infections with all great movements of population. During the French Revolution this amounted to one man in four for the French army. In 1918 Thibierge estimated 200,000 syphilitics in the French fighting forces and on the same basis their number of infected soldiers during the present war must have far exceeded a quarter of a million.

Jolivet found that fifty-two per cent of his patients were infected by professional prostitutes and forty-eight per cent clandestinely by working girls, refugees, married women, etc.

The two striking factors about the increase of syphilis today, is first: the number of very young males—sixteen to eighteen year old boys. "Won't they soon be soldiers and must they not now prove their manhood?" Second: its augmentation among married women.

The hospital at Nancy, France, in 1914 admitted one woman in five patients syphilitic, but in 1918 this proportion rose to one syphilitic for each two admissions.

We come now to the two main considerations of this topic—

Diagnosis and Treatment

The achievement of an accurate diagnosis is our greatest obligation as well as our first service to the patient. Recently I saw a man diagnosed syphilis, but before treatment was begun further investigation disclosed the error and he was dismissed. At the same time another man had been circumcised on account of a troublesome balanitis. As further explanations seemed necessary to account for his tardy healing, a Wassermann was taken and reported positive two days later, but we did not need it then for the man had shown up a macular rash all over his body that morning at the sick call. These facts disclose that we cannot afford to be too happily optimistic when the diagnosis of syphilis is involved. Only last week a very intelligent soldier came to me with secondary syphilitic conditions acutely all over him. He had taken his primary sore to a doctor who said he merely had a herpetic blister and applied iodine. The sore dried up, hardened out, and healed over. But forty days later a papular rash broke out all over his body. This time he did not need a doctor to make a diagnosis for him, he knew what that was himself.

To be accurate, the diagnosis must be based on facts arrived at by an elaboration of the complete case history and enumeration of all manifestations, and a correlation of all clinical evidence with whatever laboratory investigations which may be relevant to the stage of the disease under consideration. Complete history and all manifestations should be written into the case record at the time of examinations. This will become valuable for reference when he begins to doubt that he ever had it.

Prior to 1910 certain of the older writers advocated withholding treatment until the secondary skin eruption would make the diagnosis certain. Then came the Wassermann reaction which was the greatest diagnostic aid of its time. Blumenthall (1912) found it positive in nine per cent of chancres up to three weeks old and in 68 per cent not more than seven weeks old. Klauder (1919) reports a positive Wassermann in 12 out of 33 chancres up to ten days old—or 36 per cent. But in 40 cases where the sore had been present 40 days or over, the same observer reports the Wassermann positive in 100 per cent. Let us inquire into this test, its variations, nature, and relation to the stage of the disease which it purports to indicate.

Kolmer concedes that the Wassermann serum test is readily subject to error in both a positive and negative way because it is not biologically specific for syphilis. Small traces of either acid or alkali added to a known negative will cause a falsely positive reaction according to Cummings, while a larger amount of either will produce a falsely negative reaction in a serum known to be positive. Thus a false reaction could be readily obtained at any time, the glassware and utensils used in the laboratory happening not to be chemically clean. Positive Wassermann reactions have at times been reported in almost every ill of man. I have obtained a positive Wassermann while the rash was present in two cases of dermatitis venenata. These cases were each negative two weeks after the rash disappeared on no treatment whatever. Kolmer believes that all errors should be reduced to one of two considerations: (a) unavoidable, and (b) avoidable. By unavoidable errors he means those positive reactions occurring in spirochetal diseases other than syphilis, i.e., frambesia. By avoidable errors he refers to inaccuracies due to biological reagent, careless technique, personal equation, etc., which we all agree should be largely eliminated by accurately standardized technique. After sending specimens of blood from each of 292 individuals to from four to ten laboratories, Uhle and McKinney of Philadelphia state "There is one chance in five that the tests will agree."

By nature the Wassermann test suggests to my mind a strikingly clinical correlary with the Widal test of typhoid. In typhoid we have the primary lesion occurring in the Peyer's patches to be followed after a fairly constant period of invasion by the notable secondary manifestations: rose colored spots on the skin and Widal serum reaction When this occurs we know that the condition has become firmly established throughout the entire system as a general constitutional malady.

Likewise the Wassermann reaction in syphilis follows a primary chancre after a more or less definite period of invasion, and its presence means that the infection has been carried throughout the system by the general circulation, and it must, therefore, be considered in the same stage of the disease with the skin lesions. It is, therefore, absent in early primaries, present with all variations of secondaries and unreliable in tertiaries; as it may either be present or absent. Then the Wassermann reaction is but a serological expression of the constitutional invasion of the entire system by syphilitic intoxication.

Serological immunization against syphilis is not here anticipated, but the diagnosis of syphilis in the early or pre-Wassermann stage is not only easier and more dependable than the Wassermann, but I think it is demanded by the present conditions if we are going to control the few million syphilitics in America before they become many millions more.

Should a case not present itself for examination before the second stage, then serological investigations become an important factor in diagnosis, but even then it is an aid rather than court of last resort. One of our patients admitted with a primary sore in October, 1918, gave a negative Wassermann which continued negative for five successive monthly tests. He was recently sent into the hospital with a macular rash over his body. Then the Wassermann became positive on the sixth test for the first time in this case history.

On several occasions, when symptoms and manifestations were absent, I have refused to diagnose syphilis even in the face of a positive Wassermann and have had this position verified by subsequent sera investigations; while on other occasions my clinical findings have determined a positive diagnosis for a patient giving a negative Wassermann.

In addition to being accurate, our syphilitic diagnosis must be early if it is hoped to effect complete cure in an appreciable number of the cases. It has been the routine custom in our hospital to send all venereal sores, and all suspected chancres in non-venereal locations, to the laboratory for scrapings and examinations by dark field, or of stained specimen for three successive days unless the spirocheta pallida is found on the first or second search. When the writer was placed in charge of the Genito-Urinary Service at Fort Sill, a review of our case records showed spirocheta found in about seven per cent of our cases. This represented some hundreds of examinations in sores of all ages, both treated and untreated. Other workers in this line from Camp Shelby, Mississippi, to Toronto General Hospital, were finding spirocheta in from from 60 per cent to 90 per cent of primary sores.

We determined to increase our percentage of findings, and considered the results obtained attributable to the two methods employed, first: a program of instruction among the regiments, and second: to careful search in the deeper portions of the sore for spirocheta.

When he sees that he is caught, a man naturally wants to believe that he only has a rub, a haircut, or local abrasion, and the prevailing manner of treatment according to the layman is to cauterize—the irresistible impule is to burn that sore. The men themselves sometimes treat their own sores with anything from hydrogen peroxide and metholatum to silver nitrate and nitric acid. One of our sergeants particularly proved his heroism. After becoming infected he cauterized the sore several times until multiple, or chancroidal eschars had developed and these in turn were followed by suppurating buboes. Now laying down the stick, he armed himself with a knife and split the buboes on both sides. In one side, however, drainage was not entirely according to his satisfaction, so he repeated the operation from a little different point of attack. Of course by this time a positive Wassermann relieved his mind of its few remaining misgivings.

Two cases had been treated at the dispensary, the surgeon believing that the cases presented merely simple abrasions. Bulletins were sent among the regiments and the men were told that we were here to treat them but that the first requisite for any treatment was the establishment of a diagnosis, and in the case of syphilis the diagnosis must be early if they hope for a cure to be effected. They were notified that whenever they doctored their own sores, even with talcum powder, that they usually made a pre-Wassermann diagnosis impossible, and thereby sacrificed their greatest hope of being completely cured.

Second: We began to make deep and diligent inquiries into the basal or induration portion of the lesions. The "exulceration" is often covered with a pellicle of excretion, and may contain most anything but spirochetes.

When the patient comes to us, thin pledgets of cotton wrung out of boiled water are at once applied to the sore and this dressing is frequently renewed until spirochetes are found or we have gotten negative reports for three successive days. In attempting a scraping, the sore may be first cleansed off and a drop or two of alchohol added to irritate and dilate local capillaries. This is flushed off with sterile water and the sore stroked with a dry gauze. The area may then be sucked out with an ordinary pipette or by means of a short Dakin tube. This is tied at one end, open at the other and tightly rolled up like a watch spring with the open end applied to the lesion. The tube is then allowed to slowly unroll. The best success has followed simply working down into the induration with platinum loop or instrument until sometimes a few red blood cells may show in the microscopic field.

Immediately our results were most gratifying. We got a bunch of new and untreated chancres. Two of these had appeared while the men were absent on furlough and they promptly returned before the expiration of their furlough for diagnosis and treatment. Spirochetes had been found in all but one of these new and untreated sores, or over ninety per cent, and their treatment begun before the Wassermann could become positive.

This then makes it possible to base a diagnosis on the three earliest manifestations. First, the primary sore with its history and characteristics; second, a local, or satellite adenopathy of Ravaut; third, spirochetes found in the lesion. This, besides being more definite and more direct than some six or eight later symptoms might be, has the real advantage of also being sufficiently early to base a hope of complete cure.

Treatment

For a decade the elemental treatment of syphilis has remained substantially the same. There have been variations in method and alterations in technique, but we have continued to deal during the past ten years with the same trinity—arsenic, mercury and iodine. With any specific disease it is desirable to standardize a rational basis of treatment for that infection, which at the same time possesses sufficient flexibility so that it may be readily adapted to the various requirements of the particular individual affected by the disease. It is not of as much importance to the patient whether he gets Vienna series, the familiar six and thirty of our army, or any other conventional establishment, as that each pateient gets the proper treatment, at the right time and on the interval which is best adapted to the stage and severity of his disease and to the toleration of his system.

While we endeavor to cure the syphilis, it is necessary that we do not kill the syphilitic. For this reason we have adopted a plan of management at Fort Sill which we believe offers the maximum safety and the minimum amount of danger. All patients for arsphenamin are admitted to the hospital in the morning and get a dose of salts first thing. The breakfast is practically liquid. They get nothing to eat at noon. At 1:00 p. m. every man lines up and presents his syphilitic register for review of treatment received and direction of further treatment necessary. An assistant gives every man a careful heart examination and a trained technician does the urinalysis. Water for mixing the drug has been distilled that day and is reboiled at noon. After sterilizing, the utensils are rinsed in distilled water and the mixing done, using 25 cc. of water for each milligram of arsphenamin or 150 cc. to the 0.6 gram dose. It is then neutralized, barely over, filtered and given in the vein by gravity at the rate of about one mgm. per thirty pounds of body weight, though the personal tolerance is often a better gauge of dosage than the body weight. They are kept quiet in bed for the rest of the afternoon and get some liquid refreshment six hours later. All duty patients are dismissed at noon next day, their register and notice which directs the regimental surgeon when they must be returned to the G. U. Service for further examination or treatment is sent out through channels and signed for.

It is amazing how rapidly and completely healing of primary lesion follows the use of arsphenamin. This is also true sometimes in less degree of certain active remissions of an earlier infection. In treating primaries with arsphenamin, there comes a time when the pronounced impression of the drug upon the infection no longer obtains as at the beginning, and we have come to doubt the wisdom of repeated injections of arsenic much beyond the point for the sake of giving the full number establishment for a series. This tolerance to arsenic on the part of the spirocheta is not surprising. I have seen paris-green slay caterpillars by armies, but if he webs up in a leaf, arsenic or no arsenic, there will be a butterfly soon. In like manner, when the spirocheta freezes up in an induration or mats down in scar tissue, he seemingly ridicules all efforts to get at him by continued repetition of arsenic.

Instead of the "sterilisatio magna," too previously announced by Ehrlich, we now have our attention called to the earlier onset of neuro-syphilis, or neurotropism of Ravaut. Since the advent of 606 meningeal and cranial nerve involvement is often a matter of months rather than a number of years after the primary infection. This seems due to the slaughter of spirochetes by the arsenic in such great numbers that the unhappily involved nerve tissues are grievously overcome by the proteid intoxication before it can possibly be eliminated. I have not seen this develop in any patient treated from a primary or spirochetal diagnosis, and I have been able to show, as claimed by Ravaut, that these nerve accidents may be modified in the patients treated from a secondary or Wassermann diagnosis, if the more rapid arsenic treatment be prefaced by the slower acting mecury. We must fight this war out by "attack and barrage" as the case may demand.

We have seen a number of vasomotor reactions manifested by blue-red flushing of face with edema of extremities and throat described by Milian of Paris, but have successfully treated all of them and no fatality has occurred on our service. These attacks have been warded off by giving the patient adrenalin and atrophin ten minutes before the next shot.

We have found neoarsphenamin less potent, and some patients claim about as much reaction from it as from arsphenamin. An Oklahoma soldier sent back from the front because of syphilis, got five shots of neoarsphenamin at Bordeaux. He then came to Fort Sill via New York, reaching us with secondary syphilis quite active. After getting one shot of arsphenamin, he told me that the one he got here had more kick to it than all the neo he got at Bordeaux.

We are without experience in the use of auto-salvarsan, but have tapped the spinal canal immediately after intravenous injection and have assumed that Williams of Toronto is correct when he claims that this gives equally good results.

Syphilis is notoriously prone to relapse and an insufficient amount of any kind of treatment will merely postpone and not prevent later manifestations. Sufficient treatment is a relative expression and cannot be made absolute. One case is recorded which produced a skin rash every six or eight weeks in spite of all treatment. The following case will illustrate what may be expected to occur after insufficient treatment. A non-commissioned officer brought a detail of men from Camp Kearney, Cal., to Fort Sill, in July, 1918, and went immediately into the hospital with secondary eruption over his body and a positive Wassermann. He got six shots of arsphenamin and thirty rubs of mercury, completing this series August 18, 1918. Then his register was lost and he got no further treatment. April 28, 1919, he was again admitted with macular rash over body, alopecia, mucous plaques in throat, marked general adenopathy, beaded tibial crests, and positive Wassermann.

Do we possess at this time satisfactory evidence that syphilis can be cured? Williams now announces that 82 per cent of cases treated on a primary diagnosis with symptoms and Wassermann absent after two years observation. The serum reaction is too unstable to rely upon either as a guide for determining the necessity for further treatment or as evidence of a cure having been affected. With symptoms remaining absent for years after completion of treament and the Wasserman being negative during life, Warthin of Ann Arbor demonstrated syphilitic lesions at autopsy from which he obtained spirochetes and he therefore concludes that cured syphilis is analogous to cured tuberculosis.

Present day methods of treatment have been employed for less than ten years and Warthin's tuberculosis analogy may be the most satisfaction afforded to us until we can observe the descendants of parents thus treated pass through the age of puberty.

Summary

1. This war has caused the large increase in venereal infections common to all great movements of population.

2. Existing conditions demand the early diagnosis of syphilis. Serum reactions belong to the secondary stage of syphilis. A pre-Wassermann diagnosis is most valuable.

3. Gravity of the situation requires that form of rational treatment which is best adapted to the needs of the patient. Treatment should be continued for a sufficient length of time, the stage of the disease being considered.

Conclusion

We have spent ten millions of dollars during the war, treating syphilis in the army. Now with the system of education, treatment and control bieng carried out by the National Public Health and the State, County and Municipal organizations, it will be possible to reduce the great increase in all venereal infections and to eliminate the carriers of syphilis if every doctor is continually alert in diagnosis and faithful with the treatment of these diseases. A certain number of primary sores will occur with time, but advanced lesions should usually be prevented. In this day of great conceptions and collosal achievements when typhoid is seldom seen and smallpox does not exist except when due to willful negligence or woeful ignorance, it is not too much to hope that the great social plague will be similarly controlled or eliminated.

THE PRIMARY SORE

J. Franklin Gorrell, M. D.

TULSA, OKLAHOMA

Gentlemen:

As I have been informed that this section expects to have a symposium on Syphilis, I will not use up our time in going into the history of the primary sore, as you'all know that it dates back to the earliest days of our history, and I believe also into Biblical days.

The primary sore is the first clinical manifestation of syphilis that we have, so it behooves the whole medical profession to make themselves familiar with the clinical methods of diagnosis of early syphilis, and to see that the future generation is thoroughly taught such methods.

The chancre may occur on any part of the body, but for the sake of convenience, it may be divided into genital and extra-genital sores. While we in this country generally think of it as a genital sore, it is claimed that in certain sections of Southeastern Europe, that the ratio between extra-genital and genital sores may be as high as twenty to one.

Gentlemen, in diagnosing a primary sore, four main points are usually sought for: first, the sore must be single; second, it must be indurated; third, it must not appear from four to six weeks after intercourse, and the lymphatic glands must be enlarged and hard.

Now let us take each of these points and see how far they are of value in helping us in making an early diagnosis of syphilis. McDonagh says, that in about 30 per cent of cases of syphilis there is more than one primary sore, when the infection is a genital one. When extra-genital, the sore is nearly always single.

Induration, when present, may be valuable proof of syphilis, but its absence by no means negatives syphilis. Induration, is in part, a process of healing, and a sore becomes most indurated when it is about to disappear, so if we withhold our diagnosis until that stage is reached, the chances are greatly in favor of the generalization stage having already started. Many sores, I believe, heal and vanish without ever becoming indurated.

The sore must not appear from four to six weeks after intercourse. Gentlemen, the history of the period of incubation may mislead you, that is, the sore may develop from eight to sixty days, and in the second place many men have intercourse weekly and they will often blame the woman with whom they last had intercourse.

The lymphatic glands in the groin must be enlarged and hard. It is claimed that in about five per cent of cases no palpable changes in the lymphatic glands can be ascertained. Then it is often hard to distinguish an enlargement due to syphilis from an enlargement caused by any other venereal disease, as in about 90 per cent of all cases of acute gonorrhea the lymphatic glands are enlarged. Hardness, if present, is characteristic of syphilis. But gentlemen, again, that tells us that it has reached the generalization stage, which we hope in this day to be able to make our diagnosis early so as to be able to avoid that stage if it is possible.

If there is any doubt, we must resort to the bacteriological examination, if the spirocheta pallida is found, it is proof that the sore is syphilitic, but gentlemen, if it is not found, we are not justified in telling our patients at once that it is not syphilitic. Make repeated examinations to try and find the organisms and in the meantime do not use spirocheticidal drugs before you are positive of your diagnosis. Dr. Klauder reports that in 33 cases examined ten days after their appearance, 31, or 93.9 per cent, showed the spirocheta pallida.

Although the primary sore may appear in a variety of forms, the majority of cases present certain characteristic features, enabling them to be considered under a few headings, so in order of their relative frequency they may be classed as: first, chancreous erosions; second, chancreous ulcerations; third, indurated papules.

Erosive chancres are the most common and are very frequently multiple, and McDonagh says the chancres are 90 to 1 that they are syphilitic. They may encircle the corones and when they encircle the glans, they are most difficult sores to diagnose. When they are on the glans-penis they are multiple, beautifully circumscribed and circular; however close the sores may be to one another there is no tendency to coalesce. And it is the chancre from which the spirocheta is the most easily obtained.

Chancrous Ulcerations: This form of chancre exhibits a deeper ulceration than the erosion, and is comparatively rare. There is formed a deep ulcer with sloping edges, moderate sero-sanguineous discharge and typical extensive induration into which the ulcer seems to have eaten.

The Indurated Papule: This is the primary lesion which differs from the erosion in the fact that the skin is not broken. It is hard, raised, dusky-red tubercle, sharply defined from the surrounding tissues. It may be large or so small as to escape notice of the patient. Gentlemen, there are many subdivisions of these three forms, but since our time is limited I will not attempt to classify them.

Extra-Genital Chancres

They may occur anywhere and are generally very easy to diagnose. The sore is nearly always single, but occasionally erosive chancres of the lip and anus are multiple, in which case the sores are contiguous, but as a rule these sores have been present for sometime before the patient seeks advice; thence an enlargement of the lymphatic glands draining the infected site is practically never missed. However big the sore may be, the amount of surrounding inflammation is always minimal and this at once excludes a pyogenic lesion.

A common extra-genital sore is the digital, and as a rule it is situated on the margin between the nail and the skin. There is nearly always a swelling of the epitrochlear gland which often suppurates. So it should always raise the suspicion of a digital chancre, and not a cellulitis, especially so if it develops in the region of the inner side of the elbow.

In the differential diagnosis of a chancre, it may be confounded with a soft sore or chancroids. The incubation period of the chancroid is a few days. It is an ulcer almost always from the start, at first quite superficial and later deep. The circumference is irregular, although sharply circumscribed because one pole of the ulcer tends to heal, while the other pole is spreading. The edges are often undermined. Ducrey's bacilli is the one most often found. Soft sores are very chronic and they may become pseudo-indurated, but they nevertheless retain the characteristics described above.

Herpes Genitalis: It is primarily a vesicular eruption of nervous origin and apt to recur. The lesions are grouped. They may become craterform ulcers and if treated with caustics, pseudo-induration is sure to follow. As a rule, herpes is only confounded with syphilis when under energetic treatment; the lesions get worse instead of better. It is generally due to irritation, therefore it follows, the longer the irritation is kept up the more chronic the lesions become.

SKIN MANIFESTATIONS OF SYPHILIS

Curtis R. Day, M. D.

OKLAHOMA CITY, OKLAHOMA

An understanding of the skin lesions of syphilis is had only by the knowledge of the anatomy and physiology of the skin and the character and progress of the development of the spirocheta pallidum.

The organism of syphilis enters the system through an abrasion of the skin or mucus membrane where it lives and thrives for a time in the lymphatic spaces of the outer skin. It is to be remembered that there are no lymphatic vessels in this part of the skin. This fact prevents the rapid spreading of the infection to other parts of the body.

During this stage of the disease it is purely a local affair. This is the chancre or primary lesion, which is a punched-out ulcer with a ring-like indurated border. The darkfield or staining method of examination of the secretion from these ulcers will demonstrate the presence of the spirocheta pallidum and thereby confirm the clinical diagnosis.

Just at this time allow me to emphasize the importance of a correct diagnosis. If the diagnosis of syphilis is made on a person not suffering from the disease, untold injury is done to this individual. On the other hand, the failure to properly diagnose a case of syphilis is endangering society equally as much.

The physician who makes the diagnosis of syphilis from the viewpoint of the fee to be obtained from the treatment is the worst form of criminal.

After sufficient destruction of the tissues has occurred, the lymphatic vessels are exposed and the organism enters them, and through this source enters the blood stream.

Prior to this time the syphilis is a local disease and frequently the primary lesions heal without treatment, only to re-appear wherein the infection has progressed far enough to produce general skin symptoms or the secondary lesions.

The secondary lesions assume all forms known in skin disease. The secondary lesions will also disappear without treatment. Because the chancre heals and the secondary lesions disappear without treatment, many cases of latent syphilis are discovered and it requires considerable effort on the part of the diagnostician to get the patient to recall the time when the infection occurred.

The third stage is when the organism enters the cells of the body and produces new growth or gumma. This is the destructive stage and the skin as well as other tissues of the body becomes involved.

It is this stage of the disease when the malignant lesions first appear. The most important observation to be made from a diagnostic viewpoint is that all lesions are annular or crescentic in formation and arrangement. This is true of the chancre, the secondary lesions and the gumma formations.

A careful consideration of these facts together with our present methods of laboratory diagnosis, i. e., the darkfield examinations of the secretion from the chancre, and the Wassermann tests of the blood and the spinal fluid, causes us to take a very different view of the treatment from that taken by Didy and other investigators who wrote authoritatively nearly a century ago. It was the belief of these writers that no treatment should be instituted during the primary stage because it only retarded the appearance of the secondary lesions.

They also stated that any radical treatment during the secondary stage only postponed the manifestations of the tertiary stage. They therefore advised no treatment until after the disappearance of the secondary symptoms, believing that all other treatment only prolonged the disease.

It has been but a few years since we were taught to withhold all treatment until the secondary skin lesions appear in order that we might be more positive of our diagnosis. Today we believe a treatment of a rigid type should be instituted and carefully followed before the appearance of any secondary lesions.

We should make our diagnosis from the scrapings of the chancre with the dark-field or staining method and begin treatment at once. If the physician sees the case in time he can thus avoid the manifestations of any further symptoms of the disease.

The theory of watchful waiting method of diagnosis and the deferred methods of treatment alike belong to the discard of yesterday, and they are both alike, a discredit to the medical profession.

When we learn, and when we instill into the minds of the laity that the diagnosis of syphilis can best be made at the very first appearance of the chancre, while it is yet a local affair, then we will be able to properly handle the various lesions of syphilis, for by so doing we will have to deal only with the primary lesions, for no other will exist.

In this day when the world has awakened to the awfulness of syphilis, let the medical profession come to the front and not only do reconstructive work but do constructive work and banish from our text books any description of any lesions of syphilis except the chancre.

SYPHILIS AND MENTAL PSYCHOSIS.

D. W. GRIFFIN, M. D.
NORMAN, OKLAHOMA

I suppose there is not a question before the medical world today more widely discussed and talked about than the subject of syphilis, and its relation to mental and nervous diseases, and thanks to the press which is at last waking up to the importance of laying bare before the people the truth. For many years these matters when mentioned by the press were in such a camouflaged manner the average person did not understand what was being talked about, but the great war brought about a change of conditions. When our boys began to arrive at camp and the alarming condition of so many thousand of them diseased with this, perhaps the worst of all social diseases, the people began to awaken. Our government immediately found itself confronted with a great enemy at our own door.

We had to first fight this social enemy before we could go across the great sea to drive home the truths of democracy and world's freedom to the enemy on the other side. So before our fighting men went across it was seen to that only those who were clean were permitted to go, and you know the result, when these pure, clean men struck the enemy, he went down. Are we going to soon forget this great lesson? I think not; already the campaign has extended far into our school system where it should have gone long ago. This great enemy of mankind destroying our young manhood and nobody taking a hand has got to stop. Ere long our high school boys and girls will know the meaning of the word syphilis and when they are properly warned they will know how to protect themselves. This is the day of preparedness, and if we do not do our duty, not only as physicians but as fathers and mothers, teachers, and preachers, we will be withholding from our children a sacred truth that will live to curse us. The truth concerning this social evil must be our light by day and pillar of fire by night.

Now to get back home; you do not have to go more than a hundred miles from this very hall to see some of the damaging effects of syphilis. For a few moments take a little mental excursion with me down to your own State hospital at Norman; there I will show you row upon row, not yet beneath the beautiful poppies, but a thousand times better off if they were. Out of a thousand inmates I can show you 10 per cent. of this thousand diseased with paresis, a disease directly traceable to syphilis. These are mostly young men, men of middle life. They are not the defective type of individuals you think of when you think of insane people, but usually men of affairs, active business men. I could show you men who have been worth thousands of dollars, whose lives have been wrecked by this disease. Not only does it wreck the individual but in nearly every instance does it wreck the home financially, socially, and otherwise. In many instances little diseased children are left to share the awful disease of the father, a disease many times worse than death. This is the disease that fills our homes for the feebleminded, and houses of correction. Its limitations are boundless.

You will recall that I have said at least 10 per cent. of our patients are paretics, which is syphilis. I feel that on the account of our limited facilities for examination I am too conservative. In New York where they have made a very extended study of this disease they report 12½ per cent.

Let us look at this thing from an economic standpoint, and see just what it is costing us per year for the care of those who have been driven insane by its action on the nervous system. Take 10 per cent. of our 2500 insane, and you have 250 paretics, directly traceable to syphilis, and to care for these 250 insane at $200 per capita, you have the grand total of $50,000 per year. These figures are almost to a cent what this thing is costing us each year for the care of insanity caused by this disease. What would you say of taking this $50,000 and appropriate it to the prevention? To do so for even five years would practically drive it from our borders.

I wish it were possible to take every high school boy and girl in this State and show them through our State hospitals for the insane and explain to them insanity produced by syphilis. Oh, but some poor ignorant mother would cry out, "Don't do that, I would not have my innocent minded boy or girl see and know those horrid things for any thing in the world"; but in such case I would suggest that you say to such person, "Preparedness is the great protector."

Why should not these boys and girls know the function of the pelvic organs? They should know, as they perhaps do, that these organs in the normal state are reproductive, that is, when the boy or girl grows up and properly marries under the laws of society, these laws come into play for the purpose of reproducing, and if they go out of this regular prescribed course of society, there is danger ahead. Nature has provided an army of germs for good as well as for evil, and when a boy goes out and takes the evil course there lies in his path germs of danger, viz, syphilis and gonorrhea. This is nature's army of protection. These germs do what they can to destroy the normal germ of life. God did not intend we should reproduce out of the regular prescribed course. When God made man he gave him a pure, clean woman. Why? To have children, of course. The greatest gift to man is the power of reproduction and every child coming into the world has a right to be born clean. We have a law which protects the child against being injured, wrongfully by accident or malice. Then why should it not have the same right of protection from a diseased syphilitic father or mother which is a thousand times worse than being deformed by some railroad or other accident?

When either a man or woman in middle life, without having shown some previous psychosis, breaks down mentally or nervously, you can be on your guard for syphilis. It is in middle life we look for the beginning of this trouble, usually between thirty and forty-five years of age, right at the very time in life when the earning power of the individual should be at its highest. Now when your patient begins to show mental or nervous symptoms about this period of life, you look for some other cause rather than overwork, family troubles, worry, failure in business, and so on—these things alone do not produce insanity.

No doubt your patient will make all kinds of foolish deals; very frequently, as often happens, the individual will suddenly imagine himself very wealthy, develop delusions of grandeur, changes in relations to friends and family. Gradually these symptoms become more and more aggravated. A sense of great hilarity will develop, perhaps he is suddenly possessed with ideas of great wealth, and, as is often the case, almost before his family and friends realize the danger the whole financial fabrication of his home and business is wrecked. Then here we have not only the economic loss in the earning capacity of the individual, but as is too often the case a small family of little ones cut off from the support of the father, left to fight life's battles without proper food, raiment, and the chances for an education.

Now this leads us to look at this thing a little while from a money standpoint. Let us look into the thing from the standpoint of a tax payer. We have touched on this before, but not as forcibly as I want to here.

We have said that 10 per cent. of our insane are in our hospitals because of syphilis. Three years previous to July 1st, 1918, we received down at the Central Oklahoma State Hospital at Norman, 1886 patients, and you have two other large hospitals for the insane of this State, besides the one at Norman. Now suppose all three of these institutions receive in the next three years four thousand, in addition to those already being cared for, and this is conservative, for we will receive more in the next three years than the estimate, but we will say that in Oklahoma there are today business and professional men and women, boys and girls of whom four thousand within the next three years will go to your State hospitals for the insane. Now 10 per cent. of these, or four hundred, will go because of syphilis, just as much a preventable disease as typhoid, and because of alcohol, another 10 per cent., making eight hundred who will go to your State hospitals from two preventable diseases.

Massachusetts in the last ten years received 26,000 new patients, costing the State over $35,000,000, 10 per cent. chargeable to syphilis and 10 per cent. to alcohol.   New York over 6000 new patients each year for past five, costing $37,000,000, 10 per cent. chargeable to syphilis, and 10 per cent. to alcohol. Ohio received 3000 new cases each year for past three, has expended $13,000,000, 10 per cent. of which were sent up from syphilis and 10 per cent. alcohol.

But all this talk about what syphilis is costing other States does not concern us, so much as what it is costing the people of Oklahoma. If my statement holds good as to the number of Oklahoma citizens who will be sent to our hospitals for the next three years, the cost to Oklahoma will run close to $1,000,000, 10 per cent. to syphilis, but this is three years in the future and that might be a little too far off to satisfy some of us, so we will pause long enough to tell you what our own State Legislature has appropriated for the care of the insane for the next biennium, which is $1,850,000, charge 10 per cent. to syphilis, don't forget that.

This sum is almost equal to the total appropriated for the entire State Educational system of the State, and in all this I have made no charges for the hundreds and hundreds of cases who have been sent to your School for the Feebleminded, your School for the Deaf, your School for the Blind, your Girls' Industrial School, your Training School for Boys, and your two big state prisons; if I should include all these I would not pretend to say where the figures would sum.

Time will not permit a discussion of the prophylaxis of this disease, but our people ought to be made to understand that insanity in this State is already costing us close to a million dollars per year, and fully one third of this cost can be charged to alcohol and syphilis, both preventable. Alcohol is gradually day by day sending fewer patients to us, and when people properly understand syphilis as they do smallpox and other contagious diseases and know it should be quarantined as smallpox and can be cured, the thing will be managed and not before.

SOME METHODS FOR THE TREATMENT OF SYPHILIS.

W. J. WALLACE, M. D.

PROFESSOR OF GENITO-URINARY DISEASES AND SYPHILOGRAPHY

UNIVERSITY OF OKLAHOMA

Mr. Chairman and Gentlemen of the Urological and Dermatological Section:

Our Chairman has assigned me the subject of the modern treatment of syphilis. That, in itself, would constitute a whole book, but I will try to make it very brief and yet give a clear and concise treatment according to my understanding of the pathology of this disease.

To make the treatment clear it should be divided into four stages. Each stage is permissible of variations according to the individual case, and it is important that each case be treated individually.

To treat these intelligently each case must be looked upon according to its own special pathology. Study carefully individual idiosyncracies and push the treatment according to the particular symptoms of each case.

In the first stage, the patient presents himself showing the chancre, and this, of course, will vary in degree as the symptoms in the other stages.

Briefly the pathology of the first stage is as follows:

A small cell infiltration and hyperplasia of the connective tissue, with an inflammation of the internal coat of the small arterioles and veins. This mass of cell infiltration is supported in a meshwork of thickened blood vessels. Some of the latter are obliterated by sclerosis. It is this condition which constitutes the typical induration, the amount of which will depend on the depth and circumference of the vessels which are affected.

This condition requires very intensive treatment, and three things are essential, namely, K.I., mercury and salvarsan. My treatment is as follows: A saturated solution of K.I., 15 drops in a glass of water, three-fourths of an hour before meals the first day; on the second day 16 drops the same way, and so on until we reach the point of iodidism. This symptom may occur at 25 to 50 drops and should it do so, do not make the mistake, as so many have, of discontinuing this very necessary medicine in the belief that the patient cannot tolerate same. All patients can take K.I. if the medicine is properly given. If at 35 drops this symptom manifests itself, I drop back to 25 drops. Begin in the same manner and gradually start up the scale again and usually the patient is able to take 50 drops before the symptom appears the second time. When it does, permit the patient to rest one day, then begin with 35 drops and start up the scale once more, and this time he will tolerate up to 75 drops without any untoward symptoms. Continue this until 100 drops are reached if possible, which will represent 300 grains a day.

We must give large doses, hoping by this means to liberate the spirocheta from its nest, and to absorb their protecting barrier, thus avoiding the old symptom chanco-reduc, or recurring chancre, which is caused by the spirocheta not being destroyed.

Beginning jointly with K.I., I have my patient use mercury by inunction. I prefer this method to any other form; but of course some patients cannot use it and some other form of administration must be used. To get best results, instruct the patient to steam himself with hot towels for 10 minutes to open the pores of the skin and then rapidly rub the mercury through the dermal structure until the entire contents have been absorbed. The first night he rubs the axillary region of the right side and the next night the other side in the same manner; the third night the entire inside of the right leg; fourth, the left leg; fifth, the back of the right leg, beginning in the popliteal space and rubbing the entire back of the leg; sixth, the left leg in the same manner. On the seventh night, I permit my patient to rest, and the eighth night he begins in the same way. Of course, other parts of the body can be used, but these are the ones I usually employ. I crowd this treatment, but it must not be used to the point of ptyalism.

The third essential is salvarsan or its equivalent, (one of the arsenical compounds which has been standardized) to begin at the same time.

For instance, the patient calls at my office for the first examination on Monday. He is first given the K.I. and mercury described above. Tuesday he is instructed to report prepared for the salvarsan treatment as follows: the patient has been thoroughly purged, no breakfast the morning of the treatment; as clean bowels and empty stomach are essential, urinary analysis and blood pressure are taken. If these are in good condition, he is given his first dose of the medicine, usually 4–10 gram intravenously. He is instructed to go home and remain in bed for six hours. At the end of that time he may have a soft diet and he should partake of light diet for the next 24 hours. One week from that day he must return for a similar treatment. This is repeated at weekly intervals until he has had at least seven doses of the salvarsan, being fortified all the time by the other medicine mentioned. At the end of the seven doses, the K.I. and salvarsan are discontinued, but mercury is given in the same manner for three months. At the end of that time I stop the mercury for thirty days. Then make another Wassermann and usually give one dose of salvarsan even in the case of a negative report. If the report should be positive, showing that all the germs have not been destroyed, I carry the patient through the same treatment as outlined in the beginning. This may seem rather intensive, but my experience shows that our patients must be very closely watched and the treatment must be crowded to the very utmost, and even then we may fail in a number of cases to entirely eradicate these germs. If at the end of this time the blood is negative, I instruct the patient to continue the mercury for a period of two years longer, rubbing three months, resting one month, and then report to me every three to six months for physical and serological examination.

The second stage of syphilis is one of generalization; with general and constitutional manifestations. The pathology in this is more profound and must be considered very carefully. Patients present themselves with various constitutional symptoms, such as respiratory, cutaneous, glandular and perhaps an invasion of the nervous system; hence very active treatment is necessary.

For this stage I adopt the treatment as outlined in the first stage with the exception of giving ten doses of salvarsan instead of seven. I do not mean to say that ten doses will cure, but the symptoms being slightly more profound, they require more intensive treatment and I take this for a standard and vary it according to the individual case. The tenth dose is given the patient in the hospital. Immediately following the administration of the salvarsan, a spinal puncture is made; for two reasons: first to test the serum collected, and second, to relieve the pressure on the cord, therefore, permitting an osmosis after the blood has been saturated with the salvarsan.

The next stage, commonly called tertiary, is localized in character.

Following the second stage the disease has been undergoing resolution and elimination in the greater part of the body, but certain localities have been attacked with the destructive process. The spirocheta seems to have a predilection or selective action for certain tracts which it affects to a greater or lesser degree. The treatment in this is somewhat different from the preceding stages, as it is no longer a generalized disease but is a localized, pocketed, thickening of the arteries, veins and gumma formations, hence more difficult to reach than the other stages.

It is best to begin with the K.I. and mercury as described above. Continue this for six to eight weeks until patient is taking 75 or 100 drops three times a day or until he is completely saturated with this diffusive iodine.

After this heavy dosage for the time mentioned I start the salvarsan treatment and usually give about ten doses ranging from 10 to 12 days apart, as in this the treatment does not have to be crowded quite as fast as in the preceding stages on account of the tracts involved, and too, I am trying to heal and reconstruct the damage done by these germs. So the doses are given at longer periods, the last one to be given in the hospital and a test made on the spinal fluid as described for the secondary stage. After the last dose has been given I discontinue both the K.I. and salvarsan but use the mercury for three months. Then rest a month. After thirty days another blood test is made and while the needle is still in the vein I give the patient one dose of salvarsan. If this test proves negative, all good and well; if positive, I continue the treatment as in the beginning until six doses of salvarsan have been given and then the same rest period as above mentioned. I alternate and continue the mercury for a period of three years, but have the patient return at each three to six months interval for tests and physical examination.

The next, which for the sake of classification of the treatment, might be called the fourth state, is the one with which there is marked central nervous system symptoms. Paraplegia, epilepsy, gumma of the brain, locomotor ataxia. In this class the K.I. and mercury are given as previously described. Lumbar puncture is made immediately, the spinal fluid, which is usually under great tension, is drawn off until the pressure is normal which is about 25 drops per minute, according to the size of needle used. While the needle is still in place, mercurialized serum containing one-twenty-fifth grain is injected into the dural cavity. In doing this, two things are accomplished. First, relief of a very great pressure in the spinal canal, and second, medication is instilled at the site most needed.

K.I. and mercury are continued. Every three weeks, mercurialized serum given in the spinal canal until four doses are given. By this time the patient is taking a large amount of K.I. At this stage a few doses of salvarsan will be of marked benefit, so I give a dose every ten days, alternating the treatment by injecting salvarsanized serum into the dural cavity. By this method the patient receives the benefit of both intravenous and intradural medication.

This is continued until about eight doses are given. The treatment is then discontinued for a period of four to six weeks, the patient observing the ordinary rules of hygiene, rest, diet, regular hours, etc.

Summary.

1. Each case must be treated individually, i. e., vary treatment according to the pathology.

2. Each stage must be treated separately and according to the amount of tissue involved.

3. Potassium Iodide is a most necessary adjunct.

4. Always test spinal fluid before releasing patient.

5. Give intradural treatment as soon as central nervous system is affected.

THE TREATMENT OF SYPHILIS.

J. W. ROGERS, M. D.
TULSA, OKLAHOMA

Before the advent of the Wassermann reaction in 1906, the demonstration of the spirocheta in 1905, and the introduction of arsphenamine in 1910, the treatment of syphilis had become fairly well standardized. The syphilographers of fifteen years ago were pretty well agreed that from three to five years of intermittent treatment with mercury and iodids would produce a cure in most cases. Since the discovery of the offending organism, the complement fixation test and arsphenamine, we have been experimenting with the expectation of getting a quick, sure cure and especially in preventing the morbid effects of syphilis on the nervous system. Necessarily, we are in the experimental stage at the present time, since it must take a generation or two in order to arrive at definite conclusions from the treatment of a disease that can lie dormant as long as syphilis does at times. On the other hand, we have seen re-infections which, in the light of our present knowledge, indicates that we have made progress and that syphilis can be cured. Since the introduction of the Wassermann reaction we have found that syphilis is much more·prevalent than was formerly supposed. Various authorities placing the syphilitic incidence in the United States at from 10 per cent. to 20 per cent. We have been elated and then disappointed in the effects of arsphenamine, we have abused the use of the Wassermann reaction and neglected the clinical aspects of syphilis, but on the whole, I feel that I am justified in saying that we have made progress in the treatment of syphilis. The conclusions that I have arrived at in the treatment of syphilis are based upon personal observations of a limited number of syphilitics, and a mass of literature which has appeared in the last five years. Apparent cures have been scarce in my practice, and an observation of only five years is rather too short to arrive at definite conclusions.

Primary Stage: Fournier, years ago, advocated the treatment of syphilis as soon as it was diagnosed; all modern syphilographers advise this, and yet we see men today who say "wait until he breaks out then he'll know he has something and will keep up his treatment." I can think of no more foolish thing than to wait. Syphilis should be treated as early as possible for if there is ever a time when we can give a favorable prognosis it is in the early stage. Personally, I find as many patients in the primary stage who will take their treatment and follow with the necessary tests as I do in the other stages of the disease, and much better than the latent and tertiary cases. A patient has more hope when it is gotten at early and he certainly doesn't have the depressing news of a positive blood test as often as does the man who doesn't begin treatment until the disease is well established.

It is in these early syphilitics where we can get the gratifying results. Where we can diagnose the disease during the first week, before the occurrence of adenitis, or a positive Wassermann, we can hope for a complete and speedy cure. In these cases, I give six injections of arsphenamine, and six injections of mercury—salicylate to the point of tolerance, wait a month, have another Wassermann, and if negative, as it usually is, I give a course of four weeks of arsphenamine and mercury, or occasionally, of mercury alone. In the few cases so treated, I think all are well. Sometimes a diagnosis during the first week is impossible. That is, the demonstration of the spirocheta in treated sores is often impossible, but if I am right in my belief that these early syphilitics can be cured in such a short time, one should at least tell the patient that the sore is suspicious and give him the privilege of taking the treatment or the responsibility of going until the Wassermann becomes positive.

The next class of patients are those who have the primary sore, adenitis, and a positive Wassermann. The results in this class have been encouraging to me. In these I give three courses of arsphenamine and mercury of six weeks each, giving the mercury, usually, after the arsphenamine, that is, the patient is under treatment twelve weeks at a time, with a months' rest between courses. I usually make blood tests before starting each course, but regardless of the fact that it is often negative after the first course, I insist that they take at least two more courses. I believe I have had one or two cures in this class with a year's treatment. If they should show up with a positive blood test the second year, I give courses of four weeks with a longer rest between courses. Sometimes I have to rely entirely upon mercury during the second year. Occasionally a patient won't take mercury, and I have seen at least one apparent cure from arsphenamine alone. By apparent cure, I mean one who has had repeated negative blood tests over a period of a year, and a negative spinal fluid, without any treatment during that time.

In these classes, a great many men advocate small doses of arsphenamine, given daily or every other day. I have never tried that method, but have been contented with the results of weekly injections of larger amounts. I believe the latter course is less dangerous and the results seem very good.

Secondary and Tertiary Syphilis: In this class, we can at the present time have no hope for a speedy recovery. I give in these cases, courses of arsphenamine and mercury of six weeks duration with a month's rest during the first year, the second year I give courses of four weeks' duration and six weeks' rest, sometimes with mercury alone. I usually have two or three blood tests made during the two years, but go on with the treatment regardless of the blood test. If, at the end of the second year, all laboratory findings are negative, I sometimes allow them to go without treatment, advising a blood test every three months, but many of these cases are not cured and have to take more treatment. In tertiary syphilis I usually give potassium iodid in moderately large doses, while giving the courses of mercury. I believe it helps to throw the spirochetes into the circulation, allowing the mercury and arsphenamine to destroy them. In tertiary syphilis, where the patient has had no previous treatment, I think four or five years of intermittent treatment should be given, of course this can be regulated somewhat by the laboratory findings and the clinical aspect of the patient.

Syphilis of the Nervous System: In this class of cases, except those early manifestations, we have a very difficult condition to cure, and in lots of these cases we can't even help relieve the symptoms. In syphilitic meningitis occurring during the secondary stage, and in a few cases of gumma of the brain, the symptoms rapidly disappear under the ordinary treatment, and if the treatment is carried out over a long enough period, no doubt permanent results can be obtained. In tabes and general paresis we have rather a discouraging field. In a few cases treated with intraspinal injections of salvarsanized serum or with the addition of mercury to the serum or neosalvarsan added to the serum apparent good has been done, but, I am still very pessimistic regarding the treatment of these conditions, and insist that early and efficient treatment should be given and prevent these later troubles.

Congenital Syphilis: In very young children I treat with courses of mercury, either by rubs or grey powder. In older children I treat the same as adults, but think the cure in later life requires a longer time than does even tertiary acquired syphilis, no doubt depending upon the number of years with the disease. The prevention of congenital syphilis seems very promising; when the mother is treated during the early months of pregnancy, she will usually give birth to an apparently healthy child.

In the treatment of syphilis, we all have patients whom we can't treat as we would like to treat. All can't report at your office at the times you wish, and in such cases one has to depend upon the administration of mercury by mouth or rubs. I believe the rubs are better, but many patients object to that, and insist on pills. In these I believe that five years should constitute the minimum time, though in the last two years very little need be taken. Finally, we come to the question of the patients whom we have hopes and reasons to believe are cured; in such cases I believe the advice Fournier gave years ago should be followed. He says, "To the question of 'Am I Cured?' 'Yes, I believe you are cured, as far as I have a right to believe so scientifically, but whatever may occur in the future, whatever disorder may effect your health, remember your former complaint, never neglect to inform your physician of your special antecedents. Tell him plainly, tell him ten times rather than once, that you have had syphilis. It is quite possible that this information may be of no value to him, but it is not impossible that the circumstances may occur in which this information may be of capital importance, both to him and to you, and on the confession of your antecedents may depend your chance of cure, or even your life'."

Conclusions: Syphilis treated early, before the advent of the positive Wassermann or secondaries, can be cured in a relatively short time, and all such should be given the benefit of the early or vigorous treatment, consisting of arsphenamine and mercury. Secondary, latent and tertiary syphilis is very refractory to treatment insofar as a cure is concerned, and requires at least two or three years of intermittent treatment of mercury and arsphenamine to produce a cure and should be watched carefully for at least ten years.

Tabes and general paresis may be helped by intraspinal medication, but when far advanced, seems to be hopeless.

THE CURABILITY OF SYPHILIS.

E. H. MARTIN, M. D., AND E. A. PURDUM, M. D.

HOT SPRINGS, ARKANSAS

Considering the curability of syphilis we take it as an accepted fact that we have in arsphenamine a real specific, one which will kill the mature treponema pallida whenever coming sufficiently into contact with it.

This is as much as can be said of any specific. For instance, you may find in certain drugs or combinations of drugs an efficient rat poison, one which will kill every rat which tastes it. That does not mean that rats are to be easily cleared out of the barn. In fact, circumstances requisite to the cure of syhpilis are very similar to those necessary when the tramp agreed to kill all the rats on a man's farm for a square meal. Having procured the square meal he secured a convenient killing instrument and posed with one foot on a log of the wood pile and said, "Now, Mister, bring on your rats."

And so when it comes to even a perfect specific eradicating a disease we must take into consideration the possibility of certain organisms having become inaccessible to the blood stream and of those organisms also having stages of development, like the spores of other germs, that are more highly resistent to the specific than are the mature organisms. Again, we wish to reiterate that we consider arsphenamine a perfect specific for the mature treponemata.

To consider the curability of syphilis intelligibly we must consider its curability in the different stages. Some years ago one of the writers defined the three stages of syphilis as follows: "The primary stage is the first colony. As inhabitants mature in this colony and begin to voyage through the lymph and blood streams of the unwilling host the secondary stage commences, and when other colonies are formed in the tissues of the body we have the tertiary stage. These three stages are based not so much on the lapse of time as on the activity of the treponemata. The tertiary colonies may be active, producing visible effects, or may settle down into latency to remain inactive for many years. These three stages of first colonization, voyaging and recolonization may be sufficient for clinical division, but under the head of treatment must be classed as fourthly, those tertiary colonies which have been formed in the inaccessible cerebro-spinal system."

To quote further from this article of Dr. Martin's: "The treatment of this disease in the first stage may be very disappointing to a patient who rushes to his physician and congratulates himself that he has come early and should, therefore, be most easily cured.   The organisms in a chancre are protected to a certain extent from the blood stream by the condition of induration in this new colony and there also may be present spirochetae in some stage of development when they are not killable by salvarsan.   In a few instances the induration of the chancre may disappear after one or two doses.   The healing is generally prompt, but in many cases the induration at the site of the chancre persists after healing.   The colony represented by this indurated spot continues to give off voyagers and the endotoxin reaction, while very slight, is positive.   Very few cases beginning treatment early during the initial stage lose the endotoxin reaction until after five or more full intravenous doses of salvarsan have been given.   By full doses I mean one decigram to each twenty pounds of the net weight of the patient.   By net weight I mean the ordinary weight of the patient less from seven to ten pounds allowed for clothing and less an estimated allowance for fat in the obese.   We are not intending to dose the patient, that is incidental, but we are drugging the disease-producing organisms.   Our object is to make a salvarsan solution in the blood of the patient strong enough to kill the spirochetae.   If one patient obviously contains twice as much blood as another, it will evidently take twice as much salvarsan to produce a 1-to-10,000 solution of salvarsan in his blood, and that is approximately what is necessary to obtain the best results.   So a full dose of salvarsan for a primary or secondary case in an adult may vary from 0.4 gm. to 1.0 gm., although usually the commercial dose of 0.6 gm. will be accurate enough for all patients weighing from 120 to 150 pounds in ordinary clothing.

"To return to our chancre case: the physician treating such a case and seeking to eradicate the disease has three courses to choose from.   He may excise the chancre and give salvarsan intravenously every week or ten days and then probably three or four doses will produce a cure.   He may leave the chancre to ordinary local treatment and give the five to seven doses of salvarsan.   Or he may give one or two doses to guard against the appearance of embarrassing secondaries and wait a month or two before resuming treatment, when usually the third or fourth dose of the next series will fail to produce even the slightest endotoxin reaction and the blood Wassermann will become negative.

"The question arises as to the doubtful cases.   Should a patient with apparently typical chancroids in which the spirochetae cannot be demonstrated be allowed to wait for secondaries or a positive Wassermann to prove the presence of a mixed infection before beginning the use of salvarsan?   This may be left to the physician's judgment.   The personality of the patient as well as his social condition would have great weight in making a decision.   As a rule one will be safe in considering all venereal sores as either chancres or mixed and in guarding against the possible appearance of secondaries by at least one dose of salvarsan.   If the Wassermann should be negative a month or two later, in such doubtful cases, no further treatment would be indicated.   If positive, the weekly dose of salvarsan should be given until not the slightest endotoxin reaction follows; until the blood has become negative and instructions have been given the patient how often and how long to remain under observation.

"The reason for giving salvarsan every five to ten days instead of at longer intervals is obvious when one considers that the shortest period of incubation in syphilis is about ten days.   While one dose of salvarsan may absolutely cure exceptionally favorable cases, it is not to be expected that all of the treponemata present are frequently in a killable stage of development at one time.   To get those escaping as soon as they are old enough to kill and before they are old enough to multiply, the five- to seven-day interval seems ideal.   Intervals of a month or six weeks might permit some cases to continue indefinitely.

"It is doubtful if the secondary stage of syphilis, during which all of the treponemata are in the circulating blood or lymph, ever exists alone for any great length of time. It begins before the primary lesion has healed and cannot last long before re-colonization takes place. So nearly all cases are either both primary and secondary or secondary and tertiary. We have seen the induration of the chancre still visible, a secondary eruption present and typical tertiary lesions beginning all at one time in the same patient. This is rare, but certainly the secondary stage cannot be measured in time.

"However, the early tertiary colonies, if forming in accessible tissues, are so active that they must be classed as secondaries for treatment.

"The absolute cure of a majority of, but not all, cases of secondary syphilis may be accomplished by weekly intravenous doses of salvarsan, continued until serologically negative regardless of the number of doses required. Do not give four or five doses and then lose what you have gained by discontinuing the salvarsan for several weeks and giving mercury. Maintain the early advantage you have procured and push it with all vigor until a successful conclusion has been reached which means, of course, a cure.

"The treatment of tertiary syphilis is the same as that of the secondary stage, except that here we have to repeat the doses until all of the colonies are broken up and killed. This usually requires from five to seven doses but no numerical limit should be fixed but doses should be repeated until the blood Wassermann becomes negative. If it is very difficult to render the blood negative, or to keep it so, examination of the spinal fluid should be made regardless of negative symptoms or signs referable to the cerebro-spinal system as frequently the blood is being re-infected from that source.

"Some cases of old tertiary ulceration of the skin are peculiarly intractable. One patient of this kind was given sixty-six (66) doses of salvarsan, and each dose was followed by an endotoxin reaction. These doses were not all given at weekly intervals, but at least half of them were given at intervals of ten days or less, once three weeks and twice four weeks elapsed between doses. The obstinacy of his case to treatment is due to the peculiar conditions present. He had many old tertiary ulcers on his arms and legs. The latter had made scar tissue, which had re-ulcerated repeatedly, of nearly all of the skin from his knees to his ankles. When first seen by us, both of his legs were masses of ulcerating tissue. This condition had for eight years resisted the most heroic treatment with mercury and the iodides that Hot Springs could offer. It would appear that so much normal tissue had been destroyed and so much scar tissue had taken its place that a cirrhosis of the skin existed. While always inflamed the scar-skin had really a very poor blood supply and colonies of treponemata remained more or less protected and it was difficult to kill all at the same time. While he became symptomatically well several times, it is probable that a cure in such a case as this would have been impossible, but our treatment was cut short by the patient's death from a gun shot wound.

"Such persistence in treatment is not often required in ordinary tertiary cases, but whenever the treatment of a case is begun it should be continued until the case is cured, or, if incurable, often enough to keep the patient free from symptoms.

"Inadequate courses of treatment with long intervals between will result in accidental cures occasionally, but the patient is apt to be in the same condition at the beginning of each course of doses if the interval is long."

The treatment of cerebro-spinal syphilis is really the great field for continued advancement and securing of good results at the present time. We do not usually experience any great difficulty in handling successfully and curing syphilis affecting other than the nervous system. Only during the past year have we personally begun to treat the various manifestations of nervous syphilis by any direct communication with the spinal canal, depending formerly upon repeated courses of intravenous injections over a long period of time to secure results equally as good as any appearing in the literature where a series of cases treated intraspinously was reported.

It has been evident since the beginning of intraspinal work that occasionally a brilliant result was obtained but by taking any series of cases for comparison, the results have often been no better and even worse than in properly repeated intensive intravenous treatment with arsphenamine alone. Our failure to adopt any form of intraspinal treatment earlier was prompted not only by the poor results often reported but by the frequent observation of patients coming under our care showing no better results following such treatment than might be secured as stated above and in addition, exhibiting lasting after effects or complaining of the severity of the reactions following each intraspinal injection.

Gradually during the past three years, articles have appeared showing that in many cases the serology of the spinal fluid is changed favorably by repeated courses of intravenous treatments and that this change is accelerated by the simple drainage or withdrawal of spinal fluid shortly after the intravenous injection, thus creating a rapid secretion of cerebrospinal fluid while the blood is highly impregnated with arsphenamine. And in those cases where the findings in the spinal fluid were not influenced by intravenous injections alone, the results following the combined treatment have been equally gratifying. One of the earliest reports which seemed to us to be a distinct advance was that by Corbus,[2] in 1917, and shortly after this we began withdrawing 25 c.c. of spinal fluid one hour after the intravenous injection. As it was often inconvenient to wait an hour, the time was gradually shortened and at present the fluid is drained immediately following the intravenous treatment. The change in the various tests is influenced just as rapidly when the spinal fluid is drawn immediately following the intravenous as when the interval is increased to one hour.

This observation has been confirmed by Williams,[3] of Toronto, and Koliski and Strauss,[4] of New York.

Where this work is done in the office it is quite a saving of time to get the patient back to his or her room shortly after treatment and it also avoids blocking the office with sometimes as many as three or four waiting to have the treatment completed. It is not necessary to go to the bedside to perform a spinal puncture for diagnosis or drainage unless the patient is quite weak or unable to walk without assistance. If they reside near the office, we allow them to walk home after treatment, but otherwise it is best to send them home in a car.

After giving several hundred treatments in this manner, we are thoroughly convinced that it is possible now to treat such cases as vigorously and as long as necessary to secure not only clinical improvement but negative serological findings. Of course, you have to do this by more than one series of doses and drainage if the patient cannot stand such strenuous treatment over a long period of time, but the point is that by keeping it up, either continually or in series, we have a method of producing results without endangering the life of the patient or without causing severe reactions.

At times the headache following spinal puncture is rather persistent, but if the patient is put to bed from 36 to 48 hours following, the percentage of headaches is small.

In all the reports we have read to date, there seems to be a lack of concentrated effort in the use of this method of treatment. By that, we mean the failure to use to full advantage spinal drainage after the intravenous injection of arsphenamine. If better results are obtained by doing so, why not proceed in this way after each injection instead of at the end of a series of intravenous injections or after several tests for arsenic in the spinal fluid show the necessity of doing so? Surely the after effects of the puncture are not sufficient to produce any contra-indication. If there is marked headache, you may do a spinal puncture after every other intravenous dose instead of each one. This has not been necessary over any great period of time in any of our cases so far. Once the need of intraspinal treatment is shown, the intravenous injection is given every seven days, followed each time by the withdrawal of 25 to 30 c.c. of spinal fluid so long as the patient stands it well. And it is remarkable how they do stand it now that we have perfected the technique by using a small spinal needle, sticking in the mid-line and getting the patient to bed shortly afterward.

It is also a remarkable fact that patients needing these punctures have less headache after a puncture than those whose spinal fluid proves serologically negative.

The results obtained by this method during the past year have been better than ever before and in two cases we have observed a negative spinal fluid in patients returning for observation three or four months following the time at which they were discharged with blood and spinal findings negative. We know that such results cannot be obtained probably for any length of time, and in some cases not at all, in paresis or pre-paresis, but apparently all of the other forms of cerebro-spinal lues can be handled successfully and if a diagnosis is made early enough, very likely the incipient pre-paresis cases can be influenced favorably or prevented from reaching the stage of incurability.

It is very fully established now that infection of the nervous system occurs during the secondary stage of syphilis and the colonization takes place then, only to become active months or years later. This more recent knowledge increases the responsibility of the physician many fold and he should not only persevere in the treatment of the early cases of syphilis until they are negative as to blood findings, but if there is the slightest suspicion of invasion of the cerebro-spinal system, an examination of the spinal fluid should be made before the patient is discharged as cured.

We believe that the time is not far distant when this will be done in every case and thus eliminate any doubt that might exist.

Why, then, should we not be optimistic regarding the curability of syphilis from now on? With full knowledge as to the proper cure of primary, secondary and tertiary cases not reaching the nervous system, and with the means at hand to either cure or prevent the progress of all but a small percentage of nervous system affections, it does appear that the results obtained in the future should be limited only by the lack of understanding on the part of the patient as to the necessity of following the plan of treatment and remaining under observation as directed.

Bibliography:

1. Martin, E. H., Treatment of Syphilis with Arsenical Preparations, Southern Medical Journal, 1917, Vol. X., p. 201.

2. Corbus, B. C., Jour. A. M. A., 1917, Vol. LXIX., p. 2087.

3. Williams, W. T., Amer. Jour. Syphilis, 1919: Vol. 3, No. 1, p. 139.

4. Koliski & Strauss, Am. Jour. Syphilis, 1918, Vol. 2, No. 4, p. 609.

CLINICAL REPORT OF MASTITIS.

Fred S. Clinton, M. D., F. A. C. S.

PRESIDENT AND CHIEF SURGEON OKLAHOMA HOSPITAL

TULSA, OKLAHOMA

A few months ago a prominent physician in a neighboring city called the writer in consultation with reference to the sudden serious sickness of his wife which developed about two weeks after her confinement.

Breast had been a little tender for a day or two but no record of pulse and temperature had been recorded at that time and little was known until patient had a very severe chill followed by temperature of 105 accompanied by delirium, frequent pulse, having all the general appearance of being profoundly ill.

Close examination revealed fissure in the nipple of affected side and considerable prominence of the breast with increased tenderness. Physician was advised that we were unable to tell the exact kind of mastitis, however, the most important thing was to have a definite, immediate, positive, active line of procedure in the management or treatment.

The writer employs a plan outlined by DeLee, which, when promptly and properly applied, is very satisfactory and is as follows:

(a) Remove the infant from the breast and from both breasts if the symptoms are not very mild; massage and pumping the breast are forbidden.

(b) Administer a brisk saline cathartic and repeat.

(c) Apply a tight breast binder.

(d) Put two or three ice bags on each breast.

There must be no hand contacting of nipple and it must be thoroughly cleansed at once and kept moist with saturated boric acid solution. The nipple is surrounded with a ring of cotton, a layer of same is laid between the two breasts; a rolled towel is placed to support the organ on the axillary side, and the breast lifted up or tightly bandaged. The ice packs must keep the breasts cool and nurse should be instructed to watch the skin for signs of freezing, which Dr. DeLee says he has never seen.

After temperature has been normal for twelve hours, bags are removed one by one and in twenty-four to thirty-six hours the child may be put back to the breast.

If the disease is recognized early and the above outlined treatment is promptly and energetically applied, the patient being kept in bed, will many times produce very gratifying results. This patient made a very satisfactory recovery. Improvement began within a few hours after treatment was instituted and forty-eight hours changed the whole scene. If an abscess forms it must be incised as soon as recognized; however, this is another story which will be covered by the report of a case at a later time.

August 12, 1919.

PROCEEDINGS OF ST. ANTHONY CLINICAL SOCIETY

DR. LeROY LONG, President   DR. LELIA ANDREWS, Secretary

DEATH REPORTS FOR APRIL, 1919.

Dr. Le Roy Long:—Carcinoma of the Cervix. Mrs. J., housewife, age 41. General examination almost negative. R. B. C. 4,750,000, W. B. C. 10,700, differential count normal. B. P. 136–80. Digital vaginal examination disclosed a mass attached to the cervix, diagnosed by one doctor as submucous fibroid.

Patient was taken to the operating room and given a general anesthetic. Examination with a speculum showed advanced carcinoma. I considered it an inoperable condition and put her back to bed. After much persuasion on the part of her relatives, I agreed to operate her the next day. At 2 p. m. she was given another anesthetic and I did a panhysterectomy. The cervix was the size of the fundus, the uterus was bound down with many adhesions and it was difficult to remove. Patient was not doing well. She was put in Trendelenburg position, warm saline was poured in the abdomen and she was given 15 min. of pituitrin. Patient improved and the operation was finished. She left the table with pulse 164, skin moist and warm.

The patient's collapse on the table might have been due to three things: (1) repeated anesthesia, (2) loss of blood, which was not great, (3) pulling on the uterus and surrounding structures.

At 9 p. m. the same evening her pulse had improved, her color was good and she was restless but not thirsty. A little later she had a stage of fright and a sense of impending death. She began choking and became unconscious. In seven or eight minutes she died.

Her death was from cardiac failure. The Trendelenburg position put more work on the heart and upset the balance between the arterial and venous system and might have indirectly been the cause of ther death.

Dr. S. R. Cunningham:—Osteomyelitis. H. B., laborer, age 19. Infected compound comminuted fracture of lower jaw. Pus discharging from sinus. Small fragments of necrosed bone palpable. History and physical examination negative except diseased jaw. Jaw was curretted and ends of bone wired, under general anesthetic. Patient left table in slight shock, pulse 150, but he soon recovered and improved rapidly.

Two weeks later patient was taken to operating room to do a bone graft from clavicle. On the evening before he had a chill and his jaw was tender. I decided to postpone the bone graft and do a bone curretment instead, although his heart and lungs were negative. He did not do well under the anesthetic and it was necessary to stop and perform artificial respiration even before he was relaxed. His color was not good and he did not relax but he had lost sensation to pain, so the ether machine was started and I made the first incision, liberating some pus. At this point he gave a spasm and his heart quit. He died a cardiac death in just fifteen minutes after he was put on the table.

Collapse occurs less often with ether than chloroform. If it does occur it is usually after prolonged anesthesia. Endocarditis and septic embolism are to be considered, but I think he died of cardiac and vascular dilitation.

Dr. J. W. Riley:—Endothelioma. Frank McG., age 37. Appendectomy and cholecystectomy, May, 1918. No other lesions discovered. Made good recovery. Three or four weeks after recovery he began to have cramping pains in abdomen not related to food. There were frequent stools and considerable gas formation.

On January 19, 1919, he came into the hospital with intestinal obstruction. There was a tumor twelve or fourteen inches from the ileocecal valve obstructing the ileum. An ileocolostomy was done in which the ileum was attached to the ascending colon. Exploration revealed no other evidence of tumor at that time.

April, 1919, he returned with pains in his back and a mass the size of two fists in the region of scar. He had intestinal obstruction and considerable fluid in the abdomen. W. B. C. 69,000, poly's. 5, lymph's. 95, resembling lymphatic leukemia. Exploratory incision showed large amount of serum in abdomen, large masses of glands at the root of the mesentery, and matting together of intestines in right abdomen involving abdominal wall. Abdomen was closed with drain. Patient left the table in some shock. Died that evening.

Autopsy showed all mesenteric glands enlarged and hard, causing contraction of the mesentery, large firm mass on inner side of ileum adherent to the ileum, and many adhesions in right side of abdomen.

Discussion.

Dr. L. A. Turley. This was a tumor from lymphatic tissue more often primarily in the mesentery but may arise from lymphatic tissue anywhere in the body. This endothelioma, once called large round celled sarcoma, springs from the endothelium of the lymph sinuses, has its own blood supply and is very malignant. It may metastasize anywhere in the body. It may be of two types:

I. Endothelioma.

II. Lymphoblastoma, which is a tumor of the blood stream either of the adult or embryonic type. The cells of the adult type resemble the adult lymphocyte while in the cells of the embryonic type the nucleus is not so dense and there is more cytoplasm.

When the first operation was done it was of the first type and the lymph nodes were not involved and there were no other tumor manifestations in the abdomen. At the time of the last operation it was of the embryonic cell type and the tumor cells had invaded the lymph nodes. Many of them were also in the blood stream, giving a blood picture which resembled lymphatic leukemia.

Dr. J. W. Riley:—Septic Pneumonia. Lymphatic Leukemia. Tom Mc., laborer, age 42. Entered the hospital April 10, 1919, muscle and mental condition weakened. Marked pallor, fever, cough and nausea. Rigidity of neck and spine, moderate distention of the abdomen. Patient was having chills and rigors followed by high temperature. Blood count: Hg. 38 (Sahli), R. B. C. 1,500,000, size, shape and color irregular. W. B. C. 180,000, poly's. 4, large mono's. 7, lymph's. 87.

Transfusion of 600 c. c. of citrated blood was done on April 11. On the following day 2 gm. salvarsan was given intravenously. No improvement. On the 12th, 800 c. c. of citrated blood. The Hg. was raised, and W. B. C. dropped to 56,000, but the patient was clinically no better. On April 22nd patient died.

Autopsy Report. Numerous petechial areas over body. Heart shows hemorrhagic areas along the blood vessels. Heart muscle pale. A few sclerotic areas in the aorta. Right lung solidified at lower border. Left lung contains dark yellow substance resembling pus. Numerous areas over the surface which resemble abscesses. Spleen twice the normal size. Lymph nodes not enlarged.

Cause of death septic pneumonia. Lymphatic leukemia.

CASE REPORT.

Dr. W..M. Taylor, Oklahoma City:—Hemorrhage in the Newborn. Baby H., female. Hosp. No. 21487. Born May 2, 1919, full term, weight 7 lbs., 12 oz. Fairly well nourished. Father in good health. Denies lues. Mother delicate and anémic. Baby made fair effort to nurse but nipples were inverted and it was unable to obtain any milk. On the third day it was given whole milk with 3 per cent. sugar. Its weight was 6 lbs., 7 oz. On the fourth day there was a large dark stool suspicious of blood. A few hours later there was bright red blood in the stool. The next day there were three hemorrhages from the bowel. Two intramuscular injections of whole blood, 15 c. c. each, were given with no results.

The baby was anemic, slightly jaundiced, and too exhausted to nurse. Milk containing 5 per cent. sugar and 1 per cent. fat was given by medicine dropper. May 6th four more hemorrhages. Two subcutaneous injections of whole blood and 10 c. c. of horse serum was given with no benefit. On the following day three more hemorrhages. Baby too weak to cry. Then 300 c. c. of citrated blood from the mother was injected into the superior saggital sinus. The lips changed from a pallor to pink while the child was on the table. The next stool was dark but contained no fresh blood. On the following day another similar injection was given. The baby took the bottle for the first time. May 10th, weight 6 lbs., 9 oz. Baby nursed the breast and cried. First gain noted. No more hemorrhages. The baby improved rapidly, the cry was more vigorous and there were two normal stools per day.

There has always been some controversy as to the etiology. We might have considered syphilis but there was no eruption, no snuffles and no enlarged spleen.

Hemophilia is more common in males and does not appear before the first year.

There must be some obscure infection that produces changes in the blood vessel walls which allows the escape of blood.

Discussion.

Dr. J. W. Riley. Hemorrhagic diseases of the newborn are interesting because they occur so early in life. The pathology is either in (1) the circulating blood, or (2) in the walls of the vessels.

Many things have been tried. Gelatin, adrenalin and coagulose have failed. The thing par excellence is blood. Typing is not necessary because the mother's blood is compatible. The citrate method is simple, harmless and easily controlled. In this case 3 c. c. of 2 per cent. sodium citrate solution in the syringe is sufficient to prevent clotting. The blood was taken from the mother to the operating room and injected into the superior saggital sinus of the baby. This has a great advantage over the saline injection because it raises the color index by supplying R. B. C., and it gives something for the heart to pump.

Dr. Fowler. In the New York Lying-in Hospital, Welch was able to save two-thirds of the cases by use of the serum. Two months ago I saw a case in which there was hemorrhage from the mouth, ears, nose, bladder and bowels. Parents showed negative Wassermann, but the father was almost a hemophiliac. Blood serum was given and the coagulation time was reduced from 21 minutes to 11 minutes, but the child died of general hemorrhage, because the coagulation time went back to 21 minutes. If they live through the first week they usually get well.

I think it is due to some obscure infection. It may be in the nursing or it may be from the placental site.

I consider the blood transfusion the most valuable treatment. If it is used at once the citrate may not be used.

Dr. Lelia A. Andrews. I have just read Pemberton's report of 1000 cases transfused in the Mayo clinic. In cases of hemophiliacs they are able to bring the coagulation time down from 21 minutes to 3 minutes, but it again goes up in a few days. They attribute their reactions to (1) foreign protein, (2) sodium citrate, (3) error in grouping. In the transfusion of the newborn the latter danger is eliminated because the mother's blood is compatible.

I wish to congratulate Dr. Taylor upon his success in handling the case.

Dr. De Roy Long. This condition must not be confused with hemophilia which comes on in the first or second year of life, most commonly in males. The citrated blood is very convenient. It can be transported from one place to another and it can be given after several hours.

Dr. Taylor (closing). In closing I wish to make two points:

I. This hemorrhagic condition is due to some obscure infection.

II. Blood transfusion is the standard treatment.

JOURNAL OF THE OKLAHOMA STATE MEDICAL ASSOCIATION

VOLUME XII   MUSKOGEE, OKLA., SEPTEMBER, 1919   NUMBER 9

PUBLISHED MONTHLY AT MUSKOGEE, OKLA., UNDER DIRECTION OF THE COUNCIL

DR. CLAUDE A. THOMPSON, Editor-in-Chief
308 SURETY BUILDING, MUSKOGEE

DR. CHAS. W. HEITZMAN, Assistant Editor
BARNES BUILDING, MUSKOGEE

ENTERED AT THE POST OFFICE AT MUSKOGEE, OKLAHOMA, AS SECOND CLASS MAIL MATTER, JULY 28, 1912

THIS IS THE OFFICIAL JOURNAL OF THE OKLAHOMA STATE MEDICAL ASSOCIATION. ALL COMMUNICATIONS SHOULD BE ADDRESSED TO THE JOURNAL OF THE OKLAHOMA STATE MEDICAL ASSSOCIATION, 308 SURETY BUILDING, MUSKOGEE, OKLAHOMA.

The editorial department is not responsible for the opinions expressed in the original articles of contributors.

Reprints of original articles will be supplied at actual cost, provided request for them is attached to manuscript or made in sufficient time before publication.

Articles sent this Journal for publication and all those read at the annual meetings of the State Association are the sole property of this Journal. The Journal relies on each individual contributor's strict adherence to this well-known rule of medical journalism. In the event an article sent this Journal for publication is published before appearance in the Journal, the manuscript will be returned to the writer.

Failure to receive the Journal should call for immediate notification of the editor, 307-8 Surety Building, Muskogee, Okla.

Local news of possible interest to the medical profession, notes on removals, changes in address, deaths and weddings will be gratefully received.

Advertising of articles, drugs or compounds unapproved by the Council on Pharmacy of the A. M. A. will not be accepted.

Advertising rates will be supplied on application. It is suggested that wherever possible members of the State Association should patronize our advertisers in preference to others as a matter of fair reciprocity.

EDITORIAL

A PERMANENT RECORD OF OUR MEMBERS.

If the Secretary-Treasurer-Editor of your Association meets with cooperation of the members in the undertaking, steps will soon be taken to secure an accurate record of the salient points and phases of the career of every member. The task is not light; the final results will show many meager histories, but the sum total will be of incalculable interest and after systematic rules for additions are in force the collection should become one of historical interest to all lovers of science and its progress with time.

The collection of data must come mostly from the physician himself, then his county secretary and other sources. The papers in the Association's office affecting the individual will be grouped, filed in permanent cases and thereafter everything arising will reach those concerned. In view of the important part taken by our profession in the War some means should be taken to permanently preserve the record and achievements of our men.

THE CHIROPRACTOR AT IT AGAIN.

Press dispatches from various centers of the State universally agree that there has been a systematic propaganda fathered by the ignorant aggregation styled "Chiros" against anti-typhoid vaccination timely suggested and inaugurated by State Health Commissioner, Dr. A. R. Lewis. Physicians do not need reminders of the efficiency of this preventative measure; they have only to recall the tragic days of 1898-1899 accompanying the Spanish War, its thousands of cases, its hundreds of fatalities mutely evidenced by draped coffins returned to the homes of American people who hoped for a happier termination of the service rendered by their sons—and then—contrast the record of today, and a war immeasurably greater in every respect.

Only an insane person can fail to appreciate the overwhelming lesson presented. Medical science, argument and fine fetched conclusions are swept aside, while common sense, weighing the two inevitably conclude that the results of prophylactic vaccination is hardly short of miraculous.

Scientists who have studied these matters are in a proper state of honest irritation at the foolish, ignorant onslaughts brought by these incomparable ignoramuses. There is a very general idea that possibly the layman should hereafter be presented with the record achieved and then allowed without hindrance to choose his course without further suggestion from those who know more about it than he does. Why not adopt the slogan, "Vaccinated Sanity vs. Unvaccinated Assinity"?

NEW RULINGS ON NARCOTIC LAW.

Attention of physicians should be directed to certain rulings by Federal Courts affecting the above law, which radically change some of the practices heretofore adopted as a rule. The important changes or court interpretations of the law are, in effect, as follows:

Practitioners dispensing or selling to any person from his stock are classed as retailers or wholesalers, as the case may be, and are subject to excess tax above that paid as a physician who only writes prescriptions or dispenses drugs in the course of his routine practice.

Office changes of physicians must be reported within 30 days.

Physicians may not prescribe narcotics to habitual users thereof merely for the purpose of satisfying their craving for such drugs, but the act must show good faith in every essential. Probably the only exception to this rule is that found in cases of sufferers from incurable or prolonged chronic diseases, in which the cases demand narcotics for relief. In such instances the prescription must, of course, indicate the reason for ordering what appears to be an unusual amount, and constant reordering for such patient. The explanation "Addict" would not be acceptable, and the prescriber lays himself liable to Federal indictment.

Prescribing of excessive amounts, with direction for gradual diminution of dosage, is indictable, unless the case can be shown to be under treatment in good faith; and the very plain rules of common sense will apply in the investigation of the cases. Mere technicalities and hair-splitting in efforts to explain the matter, are swept away by the various court rulings; the physician must show good faith and sincerity throughout.

SOME ASPECTS OF THE VENEREAL PROBLEM.

The subject of venereal infections is undoubtedly one of the most difficult of approach and efficient handling before the people today. Unfortunately these infections, biologically identical with all other infections produced by micro-organisms, have been considered by the public, scientists and physicians since its advent in Italy and France in the fifteenth century as different from other infections. Those suffering from them were subject to ridicule, ostracism and other atrocious injustices and ignorant misunderstandings. Instead of calling the diseases sicknesses or infections just as others were plainly labelled, the sufferer from long years of repeated reiteration of a system of mishandling, knowing the ignominy in store for him, often stoically suffered alone, untreated, until destruction was beyond repair. In this connection, it is a notable travesty on modern knowledge that we still have everywhere, loud mouthed reformers, "Social Uplifters," good intentioned, but sadly misinformed and ignorant publicists, who systematically spread the unsympathetic prejudices of a dark past.

It is regrettable that an unusually large number of the medical profession hold no, or chaotic views on the subject. A glance at the customary charges of physicians for treatment of the infections indicates that they consider the services unusual or difficult. It is common knowledge that these sufferers, more often than any other class, are the victims of outrageous charges from the dishonest physician, based on exaggerated representations of the dangers which are made to increase the mental suffering of the victim.

The clear duty of our profession, the only one having accurate knowledge of the matter, is to place the dangers, their avoidance and treatment sensibly before the people. Prudishness has no place in the problem. Such infections should be plainly and bluntly discussed and handled. The idea that acquiring easily preventable smallpox and typhoid infections is more a reflection on our boasted modern intelligence, should be constantly borne in mind by the physician. The duty of the State to disseminate knowledge to the students in our schools is clear and paramount to all false arguments of prudery and obsolete ignorance.

PERSONAL AND GENERAL NEWS

Dr. E. M. Poer, Mangum, has moved to Hobart.

Dr. H. E. Rappolee, Caddo, has moved to Madill.

Dr. E. J. Orvis, Blackwell, visited Montana in August.

Dr. H. H. Wilson, Shawnee, visited Colorado in August.

Dr. J. A. Jester, Elk City, motored to Colorado in August.

Dr. E. E. Darnell, Colony, is moving to Mt. Pleasant, Iowa.

Dr. J. M. Clifton, Norman, visited Colorado resorts in August.

Dr. D. Autry and family, Marietta, are motoring to California.

Dr. W. J. Melton, Shamrock, has moved to Desdemona, Texas.

Dr. J. H. Kay, Durant, has been appointed City Health Officer.

Dr. P. Rollins, Guthrie, has returned to his old location at Paden.

Dr. C. M. McCallum, Sapulpa, has returned from oversea service.

Dr. T. H. Flesher, Edmond, visited the Rochester Clinic in August.

Dr. J. F. Gorrell, Tulsa, visited Pittsburg and New York in August.

Dr. C. H. McBurney, Clinton, has been appointed mayor of that city.

Dr. W. E. Lamerton, Enid, has returned from Wyoming and Colorado points.

Dr. R. W. Holbrook, of Perkins, visited his old home in Kentucky in August.

Dr. W. R. Marks, Vinita, has returned from oversea service and is in his old location.

Dr. J. E. Walker, Earlboro, has been appointed County Officer of Health, Pottawatomie County.

Dr. A. P. Gearheart, Blackwell, has been discharged from army service overseas and returned to his home.

Dr. W. G. Ramsey, McAlester, has returned from oversea service and will take up work at his old location.

Dr. J. G. Janney, formerly of Lawton, has returned from oversea service and is located at Dodge City, Kansas.

Dr. C. E. Calhoun, Sand Springs, has returned from oversea service and will take up his work at the old location.

Dr. O. E. Templin, Alva, arrived in Philadelphia from oversea service early in August and will soon be discharged.

Dr. O. N. Windle, Sayre, is suffering from a broken arm. He undertook the role of cowboy and scored a failure.

Dr. R. R. Hume, Minco, Captain Medical Corps, U. S. A., has been discharged and returned from overseas service.

Dr. H. E. Huston, Cherokee, has been discharged from the Army and will take up eye, ear and nose work at his old location.

Dr. R. W. Williams, Anadarko, has been discharged from Army Service. He was assigned to points in the Orient and Siberia.

Dr. Hugh Scott, Holdenville, has re-entered the Military Service and has been ordered to Palo Alto, California, Naval Hospital.

Dr. C. L. Reeder, Tulsa, director of the Venereal Clinic, is securing pointers for his work by visiting similar clinics in the country.

DR. J. H. BARNES.

Dr. J. H. Barnes, Enid, died in Minneapolis, August 7th, after suffering for several weeks from endocarditis. He had been moved to Minnesota by his friends in hope that the cooler climate would benefit him. Br. Barnes was born near Beaver Dam, Ky., May 10, 1872, attended the common schools of Kentucky and afterward taught for several years, graduated from the Hospital College of Medicine, Louisville, in 1901. He afterward located in Chickasha, practised there and at Jet and Helena until 1904, when he took up eye, ear, nose and throat work in Chicago. The fifteen years he lived in Enid enjoying a large practice. He was a member of many special and technical societies and a persistent worker in the profession. His passing records a distinct loss to the medical profession of Oklahoma.

Dr. G. S. Baxter, Shawnee, had his vacation in Colorado marred by suffering from an infection of the jaw which necessitated operation.

Southwestern Hospital, Lawton, according to the press, has been purchased by Drs. E. B. Dunlap and G. S. Barber, Lawton, and others.

Dr. R. W. Higgins, Springer, narrowly escaped death when he ran his car off a bridge near Ardmore. He received painful but not serious injuries.

Dr. G. A. Waters, Pawnee, accompanied by his family spent some time in Colorado in August, incidentally taking in the Denver Clinic on the trip.

Dr. A. R. Lewis, State Commissioner of Health, is visiting New York and Washington to investigate the possibilities of securing prophylatic treatments for influenza.

The Oklahoma Tuberculosis Association will hold the Second Annual Oklahoma State Public Health Conference, September 23 and 24. At the time of going to press the programme was not available.

Dr. Guy McNaughton, Miami, has returned from oversea service. Dr. McNaughton was immediately re-appointed Health Officer on his return. Dr. J. A. De Tar who had acted in his stead, retired.

Dr. John W. Duke, Guthrie, has taken over the Municipal Baths of the city and will operate them in connection with his Sanitarium. He contemplates many improvements and announces that no pains will be spared to make the affair one of profit and benefit to the people requiring such hydrotherapeutic aids as may be indicated.

Mayes County Medical Society entertained the dentists, druggists, nurses and their families of the county at Locust Grove, August 14th. In addition to the dinner and refreshments served an elaborate program was presented. Many physicians from other localities were present. Dr. A. R. Lewis, Commissioner of Health, was on the program for an address.

Dr. P. P. Nesbitt, Muskogee, Major Medical Corps, U. S. A., has returned from France after more than two years in service. Dr. Nesbitt was examined for the service in May, 1917, ordered to Ft. Riley almost immediately and was one of eight men selected from forty volunteers for pioneer service with our developing army, going overseas in August. He was connected with the surgical service of the Base Hospital at St. Nazaire practically all the time after its establishment.

Dr. M. H. Foster was discharged from the U. S. Army August 1st at Ft. Sill, Okla., where he was serving as Chief of the Genito-Urinary Service. After spending the month of August in Washington University School of Medicine, St. Louis, he moved his location from Alderson (McAlester), Okla., to Alexandria, La., where opened an office in the Haas building, 4th and Johnson streets, September 1st. His practice will be limited to genito-urinary surgery, cystoscopy and dermatology.

MISCELLANEOUS

STATE HEALTH NOTES.

The typhoid inoculation campaign of the state health department under Commissioner Arthur R. Lewis, has been brought to a successful end. Commissioner Lewis estimates that through the free vaccine offered by the state in amount of 40,000 doses and through private vaccination, at least 120,000 persons have been immunized.

"The campaign brought many enemies of the serum idea and the medical profession generally to light," Dr. Lewis declared. "Chiropractors and members of a certain religious sect which professes to cure by faith alone, began hammering the minute the typhoid campaign was announced.

"In addition, a few members of the medical profession objected because they were asked to give a little time to administering this vaccine free to those who were too poor to pay for it. I met one of these objectors the other day and he told me that he had changed his views, that the advertising we had given the value of vaccine had sent three times as many pay patients to him for inoculation as he vaccinated free.

"The campaign was a big success, North Carolina being the only state in the union which has vaccinated more in one year than we have."

FRAUDULENT "CURES" FOR VENEREAL DISEASES SEIZED.

By order of the Federal Courts more than 450 seizures have been made recently in different parts of the United States of so-called cures for venereal diseases. They were made on information furnished by officials of the United States Department of Agriculture through its Bureau of Chemistry. A campaign to end the false labeling of such preparations is being conducted by the officials charged with enforcing the Federal Food and Drugs Act.

The goods seized include a great variety of compounds. Some of the labels bear the claim of the manufacturer that the contents are sure cures for venereal diseases. Some even contain statements that cures will be effected within definite periods, varying from three days to a few weeks. In others, indirect statements, suggestive names or deceptive devices are craftily used to make it appear that the use of the preparation will be followed by a cure of the disease.

In all the seizure actions the Government alleged the preparations to be falsely and fraudulently labeled, because the ingredients could not produce the results claimed on the labels.

The officials state that such preparations are sold largely because of plausible but false claims regarding their curative effect. Many sufferers with dangerous contagious venereal diseases are led to believe that cures will be effected by these preparations, and adequate treatment under competent medical supervision is neglected until permanent injury to health and even danger to life has resulted. Thus is created one of the greatest obstacles to the proper control and eradication by health officials of venereal diseases. In many instances had such sufferers secured competent advice, early and complete cures might have been effected.

Self-treatment with worthless concoctions causes not only continued suffering but sometimes permanent injury to the unfortunate victims and makes of them a menace to the public health because of the extreme danger of others contracting the disease from them.

Action under the Federal Food and Drugs Act in reference to venereal disease preparations coming under its jurisdiction and sold under proprietary names is limited by the terms of the act largely to the prevention of false or fraudulent labeling. The act does not prevent the sale of any mixture as medicine, however worthless it may be, if there is directly or indirectly no false or fraudulent labeling. The officials in charge of the enforcement of the act are of the opinion, however, that by causing the elimination of false labeling, upon which the sale of such preparations largely depends, the evils and dangers resulting from their indiscriminate use can be greatly checked, and substantial aid rendered to public health officials.

FOURTEENTH ANNUAL MEETING OF THE MEDICAL ASSOCIATION OF THE SOUTHWEST TO BE HELD AT OKLAHOMA CITY, OCT. 6, 7 AND 8.

The fourteenth annual meeting of the Medical Association of the Southwest, which is to be held at Oklahoma City, October 6, 7 and 8, is to be largely in the manner of a welcoming home to the very large number of its members who have been on active duty in the army.

Monday afternoon and evening the meeting will be given over to the Medical Officers who will have a reunion and in the evening a camp-fire smoker which will be a very enjoyable affair. Many will be there to tell their experiences and many will be there to tell their disappointments, but on the whole, every one will be there to renew acquaintances and have a good time.

Tuesday and Wednesday forenoons the profession of Oklahoma City will entertain the visitors with clinics; it is expected that every line of work will be well represented. A number of specialists who have large offices will plan to hold interesting clinics in their offices and of course all who do surgery will hold clinics in the hospitals.

A number of prominent physicians have been invited to be present to address the gathering and they will have something of interest to say.

The railroads will grant a fare of one and one-third fare for the round trip on the certificate plan so every one attending should purchase their tickets one way, paying full fare for the same and take a certificate from the ticket agent which will be countersigned at the meeting by the Secretary and will entitle the holder to a ticket to his home at one-third the regular fare.

The Lee Huckins Hotel will be headquarters and it will be advisable for all to make reservations as early as possible to be sure of accommodations.

It is hoped that this will be by far the largest and most enthusiastic meeting the association has ever held that it may properly celebrate the return of the Medical Officers who have done such valiant service to civil life.

There is still room for a few additional papers on the program and those desiring to present a paper should at once write the Secretary, Dr. Fred H. Clark, El Reno, Okla., and give him their name and the title of their paper.

VENEREAL DISEASE.

The work of the U. S. Public Health Service for the control of venereal disease in the military zone is described by C. C. Pierce, Washington, D. C. (*Journal A. M. A.*, Aug. 9, 1919). Special measures were necessary, based on the findings in other countries during the war. Epidemic disease is contracted, it had been shown, mainly in municipal areas with unsatisfactory sanitary regulations.

The inevitable relation between liquor and prostitution and venereal disease had been demonstrated and five-sixths of the infections found among troops were acquired in civil life before entering camp. Telegrams calling for a campaign of wisely conducted publicity, immediately followed by a letter containing a program of work, were sent to all state health officers.   The first step in the plan was the opening of clinics, and up to the time of writing fully 250 of these, where cases could be treated, have been established.   Legislation was also asked for, and the activity and cooperation achieved were greatly aided by the Chamberlain-Kahn Act of Congress, making appropriations for state boards of health and requiring the reporting of cases of syphilis and gonorrhea.   A further stimulus was given by the Presidential order of July 1, 1918, placing public health activities of civilian federal agencies under the Public Health Service.   The first year's work has emphasized the cooperation with state boards of health, and at the present time this cooperation is being carried out in forty-four states.   Investigations on the causes and prevalence of venereal diseases are being carried on along four lines, which may be generally described as, medical, educational, legislative and social.   Medical investigation is carried on largely in clinics and in hospitals.   Vocational work is also started in certain hospitals for venereal patients and carriers.   Thorough mental examination is included.   The follow-up work is also mentioned.   Public education on the subject is carried on frankly, without being necessarily frightful.   The consensus of opinion of teachers as regards sex hygiene is that the information should be given simply and unobtrusively in connection with courses on botany, biology, civics, history, etc.   The ignorant and wilful should be controlled by laws duly enforced.   The enforcement of sanitary measures should not raise an issue with educational and moral appeal.   The undertaking is a community undertaking— not merely a task for physicians.   In the beginning of the work a retail druggists' association, representing about one-sixth of the retail druggists in the U. S., offered its cooperation, and a card containing an appeal approved by these druggists, was sent to all the pharmacists in the country, asking their cooperation in the good work.   The response was most gratifying.   In closing, Pierce emphasizes the peculiar relation of the physician to this work.   It is he who must teach the people, and his duty often means the discovery of sources of infection, the tracing up of carriers, and the maintaining of high standards of the clinic in the hospitals.   He must be assured of the aid of an intelligent and appreciative public.   We face long established prejudice, which yields slowly, but the possibilities have been shown by what has already been done.

COUNCIL ON PHARMACY AND CHEMISTRY
AMERICAN MEDICAL ASSOCIATION

This report is limited according to the ideas and opinions as to its usefulness and practicability to Oklahoma physicians. A complete report is obtainable upon request from the Council, 535 North Dearborn St., Chicago.

NEW AND NONOFFICIAL REMEDIES.
(Abridged Report.)

Pituitary Solution-Abbott. Liquor Hypophysis U. S. P. A sterilized solution of the water soluble extract of the posterior portion of the pituitary glands of cattle. It is standardized by the method of Roth. (For a discussion of the actions and uses of pituitary preparations, see New and Nonofficial Remedies, 1919, p. 204.) The Abbott Laboratories, Chicago.

Ampules Pituitary Solution-Abbott, 0.5. Each ampule contains 0.5 c. pituitary solution-Abbott. The Abbott Laboratories, Chicago.

Ampules Pituitary Solution-Abbott, 1 c. Each ampule contains 1 c. pituitary solution-Abbott. The Abbott Laboratories, Chicago.

PROPAGANDA FOR REFORM.

Partola. A physician reports that a patient taking Partola as a blood purifier is now in a rundown condition with discoloration of the skin and a craving for the drug and that another patient took three tablets before going to bed, developed cramps and aborted the next day in her third month of pregnancy. Analysis indicated Partola to be tablets containing 2.64 grains phenolphthalein per tablet, sugar, starch and oil of peppermint (Jour. A. M. A., July 5, 1919. p. 55).

Commercial Therapeutics. The Merrell Proteogens present another attempt to foist on the medical profession a series of essentially secret preparations whose therapeutic value has not been scientifically demonstrated. It is the old story of exploiting physicians through commercial pseudoscience, of trading on the credulity of the profession to the detriment of the public. Sir William Osler says the remedy against the commercial domination of therapeutics is obvious: "Give ourst udents a first hand acquaintance with disease, and give them a thorough practical knowledge of the great drugs, and we will send out independent, clear-headed, cautious practitioners who will do their own thinking and be no longer at the mercy of the meretricious literature, which has sapped our independence.". Excellent! But must humanity wait a generation? Why not stop this evil at once? The American Medical Association has provided the means whereby this may be done, if physicians will only make use of it—The Council on Pharmacy and Chemistry (Jour. A. M. A., July 12, 1919, p. 109).

Tyree's Antiseptic Powder. An advertisemet appearing in the New York Medical Record, contains a bacteriologic report on Tyree's Antiseptic Powder by W. M. Gray, M. D., Microscopist,

Army Medical-Museum, and Pathologist to Providence Hospital. Every person who sees this advertisement and is not familiar with the facts will naturally suppose that this report, written on the stationery of the Surgeon-General's Office, War Department, is a recent report. As a matter of fact, the report was issued January 3, 1890, nearly thirty years ago. Furthermore, the product that Dr. Gray examined was a different substance from the present Tyree's Antiseptic Powder. All these facts were brought out in the Journal A. M. A., May 17, 1919, yet the Medical Record persists in publishing this inherently dishonest advertisement without explanations or apology (Jour. A. M. A., July 12, 1919. p. 129).

Protecting the Sick Soldiers. The Council on Pharmacy and Chemistry, aided by the A. M. A. Chemical Laboratory, did a great work in investigating and passing on the many medicinal products offered to the Surgeon-General for the treatment of the sick soldiers in the hospitals and in the field. Fakes of every description were offered the government and it is a well known fact that no matter how fraudulent, how fakish, or how ridiculous the wares might be, their promoters were able to get political influence, even certain congressmen and senators being secured to help them. Automatically all medicinal preparations offered to the Surgeon-General were referred to the Council and thus many worthless preparations were barred from use by the government. It has been well said that our soldiers were better protected than our civilians; for while the government does not take any chances on the acceptance of useless if not worthless medicinal preparations, yet there are any number of doctors who fail to profit by the findings of the Council on Pharmacy and Chemistry (Jour. Ind. State Med. Assn., July 15, 1919, p. 196).

Proteogens of the Wm. S. Merrell Co. The Council on Pharmacy and Chemistry report that Proteogen No. 1 (Plantex) for Cancer, Proteogen No. 2 for Rheumatism, Proteogen No. 3 for Tuberculosis, Proteogen No. 4 for Hay Fever, and Bronchial Asthma, Proteogen No. 5 for Dermatosis, Proteogen No. 6 for Chlorosis, Proteogen No.7 for Secondary Anemia, Proteogen No. 8 for Pernicious Anemia, Proteogen No. 9 for Goitre, Proteogen No. 10 f or Syphilis, Proteogen No. 11 for Gonorrhea, and Proteogen No. 12 for Influenza and Pneumonia inadmissible to New and Nonofficial Remedies because their composition is secret; because the therapeutic claims made for them are unwarranted; and because the secrecy and complexity of their composition makes the use of these preparations irrational. The Proteogens are said to be prepared "under the personal supervision of the originator, Dr. A. S. Horowitz," who also originated Autolysin (an alleged cancer remedy, exploited some years ago). At one time advertising for Proteogen No. 1 (Plantex) gave the impression that this was essentially the same as Autolysin. A study of the medical literature revealed no evidence establishing the value of the Proteogens; in fact, no evidence was found other than that appearing in the advertising matter of the manufacturer. The range of diseases in which Proteogens are recommended is so wide as to make obvious the lack of scientific judgment which characterizes their exploitation. Considering the grave nature of the diseases for which Proteogens are recommended, the want of a rational basis for the method of treatment and the general tenor of the advertising, it appears safe to conclude that these agents do not represent any definite advance in therapeutics (Jour. A. M. A., July 12, 1919, p. 128).

Dr. Miles' Heart Treatment. According to the Miles Medicine Company this is "a heart strengthening regulator and tonic for the weak heart." No information regarding the composition of Miles' Heart Treatment is vouchsafed by the manufacturer beyond the statement of the alcohol content (11 per cent.) as required by the law. However, quotations in the advertising suggest that the preparation contains digitalis and cactus. To determine the presence or absence of digitalis in Miles' Heart Treatment, physiologic tests were made. The question as to the presence of cactus was not considered of interest because cactus grandiflorus has been shown to have no physiologic action. The physiologic tests indicated that there were no digitalis bodies present in the preparation (in amounts that could have any therapeutic effects) in doses containing enough alcohol to induce narcosis. Examination in the A. M. A. Chemical Laboratory showed Miles' Heart Treatment to be a solution of a compound or compounds of iron representing about 0.12 gm. metallic iron in 100 c. c. A solution of iron glycerophosphate in 10 per cent. alcohol, with about 5 per cent. glycerin, and a little sugar or glucose had much the same chemical properties as Miles' Heart Treatment (Jour. A. M. A., July 26, 1919, p. 287).

"Accepted by the Council on Pharmacy and Chemistry." The Council on Pharmacy and Chemistry of the A. M. A. is the department of our national organization that has not received the plaudits and encomiums of a wildly joyous medical profession nor the grateful praises of the enthusiastic manufacturer of pharmaceutical articles. Perhaps the reason for this may be found in the character of its duties, for the Council must expose fraud, sometimes in high places, and protect the physician from being duped by avaricious persons and by persons who are themselves sometimes the victims of their own credulity. It thus happens that some proprietary article previously held in high esteem by the practitioner proves valueless, perhaps even fraudulent. The practitioner, however, may have credited much of his success in treating sick conditions to that preparation and the maker has had success in accumulating dollars from the sale, and both parties emit a loud and vicious roar against the Council because both lose money. Despite many obstacles the Council on Pharmacy and Chemistry has serenely pursued its allotted tasks and today stands as the only medium through which physicians may turn for information regarding proprietary articles. The words, "accepted by the Council on Pharmacy and Chemistry of the American Medical Association" should be printed on the label and on all advertising circulars of proprietary articles that have been admitted to New and Nonofficial Remedies. Then, when pamphlets and circulars are received by physicians, they will read the statements of manufacturers with sympathetic understanding and with full confidence of their verity of declarations (Jour. Mo. State Med. Assn., July, 1919. p. 223).

OFFICERS OF COUNTY SOCIETIES, 1919

County	President	Secretary
Adair	D. P. Chambers, Stilwell	J. A. Patton, Stilwell
Alfalfa	E. L. Frazier, Jet	J. M. Tucker, Carmen
Atoka-Coal	F. E. Sadler, Coalgate	W. T. Blount, Tupelo.
Beaver		
Beckham		J. E. Standifer, Elk City
Blaine	W F Griffin, Greenfield	J. A. Norris, Okeene
Bryan	H. B. Fuston, Bokchito	D. Armstrong, Durant
Caddo	P. H. Anderson, Anadarko	C. R. Hume, Anadarko
Canadian		W. J. Muzzy, El Reno
Carter	A G Cowles, Ardmore	Robert H Henry, Ardmore
Choctaw	C. H. Hale, Boswell	J. D. Moore, Hugo
Cleveland		D. W. Griffin, Norman.
Cherokee		
Comanche	A. H. Stewart, Lawton	E. B. Mitchell, Lawton
Coal-Atoka	F. E. Sadler, Coalgate	W. T. Blount, Tupelo
Cotton		
Craig	C. B. Bell, Welch	F. M. Adams, Vinita
Creek		H. S. Garland, Sapulpa.
Custer	K D Gossam, Custer	O H Parker, Custer
Dewey		
Ellis		
Garfield		L. W. Cotton, Enid.
Garvin		N. H. Lindsey, Pauls Valley
Grady	Martha Bledsoe, Chickasha	J. C. Ambrister, Chickasha.
Grant		
Greer	Ney Neel, Mangum	Fowler Border, Mangum
Harmon		
Haskell	T B Turner, Stigler	R. F. Terrell, Stigler.
Hughes		Hugh Scott, Holdenville
Jackson	J. S. Stults, Olustee	J. B. Hix, Altus
Jefferson	D B Collins, Sugden	W M Browning, Waurika
Johnston		H. B. Kniseley, Tishomingo
Kay	G. H. Nieman, Ponca City	D Walker, Blackwell
Kingfisher	Frank Scott, Kingfisher	C. W. Fisk, Kingfisher.
Kiowa		A. T. Dobson, Hobart.
Latimer	E. L. Evins, Wilburton	C. R. Morrison, Wilburton
Le Flore	C. H. Mahar, Spiro	Harrell Hardy, Poteau
Lincoln		C. M. Morgan, Chandler
Logan		O. E. Barker, Guthrie.
Love		
Mayes	J. L. Adams, Pryor	L. C. White, Adair.
Major		
Marshall	J E Reed, Madill	J L Holland, Madill
McClain	J. W. West, Purcell	O. O. Dawson, Wayne
McCurtain	A W Clarkson, Valliant	W B McCaskill, Idabel
McIntosh	S. W. Minor, Hitchita	W. A. Tolleson, Eufaula
Murray	A F Brown, Davis	W. H. Powell, Sulphur.
Muskogee	J. L. Blakemore, Muskogee	H C. Rogers, Muskogee
Noble		B. A. Owen, Perry.
Nowata	J. E. Brookshire, Nowata	J. R. Collins, Nowata
Okfuskee	C. C. Bombarger, Paden	H. A. May, Okemah.
Oklahoma	W. J. Wallace, Oklahoma City	J. N. Alford, Oklahoma City
Okmulgee	Harry Breese, Henryetta	W. B. Pigg, Okmulgee
Ottawa	A. M. Cooter, Miami	G. Pinnell, Miami
Osage	A. J. Smith, Pawhuska	Benj. Skinner, Pawhuska
Pawnee		E. T. Robinson, Cleveland
Payne		J. B. Murphy, Stillwater
Pittsburg	L. C. Kuyrkendall, McAlester	T. H. McCarley, McAlester.
Pottawatomie	E. F. Rice, Shawnee	G. S. Baxter, Shawnee.
Pontotoc	L. M. Overton, Fitzhugh	S. P. Ross, Ada
Pushmataha	H. C. Johnson, Antlers	Edw. Guinn, Antlers
Rogers	J H Haley, Chelsea.	F A Anderson, Claremore
Roger Mills		
Seminole	W. T. Huddleston, Konawa	W. L. Knight, Wewoka.
Sequoyah	V W Hudson, Salisaw	S A McKeel, Sallisaw
Stephens	J. W. Nieweg, Duncan	J. O. Wharton, Duncan.
Texas	W. H. Langston, Guymon	R. B. Hays, Guymon
Tulsa	G. A. Wall, Tulsa	A. W. Pigford, Tulsa
Tillman		J. E. Arrington, Frederick.
Wagoner	C E Haywood, Wagoner	C E Martin, Wagoner
Washita		A. S. Neal, Cordell.
Washington	O S Smerville, Bartlesville	J G Smith, Bartlesville
Woods		J. A. Bowling, Alva.
Woodward		

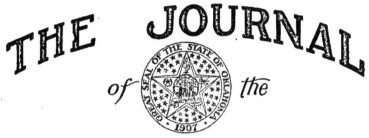

Oklahoma State Medical Association

| VOLUME XII | MUSKOGEE, OKLA, OCTOBER, 1919 | NUMBER 10 |

SYMPOSIUM ON SYPHILIS

(Continuation of papers read in Section on Genito-Urinary Diseases, Dermatology
and Radiology, Muskogee, May, 1919. See September issue
for papers previously published.)

LUES OF THE DIGESTIVE TRACT.

J. T. MARTIN, M. D.

OKLAHOMA CITY, OKLAHOMA

Constitutional syphilis involves practically all the various organs of the digestive
tract. Primary sores appear only on the exposed mucous surfaces, i. e., lips,
mouth, tongue, palate, anus, and rectum.

Chancres of the lip are relatively common. Nivet reports 260 cases out of
338 cases in his clinic during one year. The chancre of the lip oral cavity and
tongue result from direct contact or indirect contact by infected articles, e. g.,
spoons, plates, towels, etc.

Chancres are seen on the lips of a new born when the nurse's nipple is infected.
The chancre of the mouth is single and usually commences as a trivial lesion.
It is mistaken for a crack or scratch and most common at the commissures of the
lips. The movement of the mouth on the lips in partaking of food makes the
chancres bleed and often take on a form of indolent tumor. This form has usual
crust over it like chancre of the skin and shows a brownish top. The sore is
usually painless and when marginal accompanied by unilateral enlarged glands
and bilateral adenopathy with median chancre.

The secondary lesion of the lips appears as opal tinted erosion, and is very
contagious; it is most common in children. Tertiary lesion is rather rare on the
lips, more common on the upper lip than on the lower lip, and lesions are practically
without pain.

The primary sores occur frequently on the tongue and when found are usually
on the tip of the tongue and the glandular enlargement is the same as found in
chancres of the lip. These lesions are frequently found painful due to the irritation
by the movements of mastication and incessant contact with saliva, drink and food.

Mucous patch is a frequent tongue lesion of the secondaries. Mucous patches
may appear as ulcers, erosions, nipple-like projections, and smooth patches. Fissures, cracks, ulcers, especially on the back of the tongue, are common lesions.
Dieulafoy names the projecting form of syphilis on the back of the tongue "toad's

back." A common variety found is the smooth patch and known as varnished. These patches are fairly regular in contour and only found at the back of the tongue. These conditions are often called eczema of the tongue, lingual psoriasis, etc., and a careful examination is necessary to make a proper differential diagnosis.

The gumma of the tongue is divided into two classes, the superficial and the deep. The superficial involves chiefly the epithelial layers, and the deep are in the muscles and are nowhere as frequent as in the tongue. Gummata may cause the tongue to swell and extend from the mouth. A single gumma may so grow that the same phenomenon is exhibited. A frequent diagnosis of this condition is lingual cancer, sarcoma or tubercular ulcer.

Ulcerations may result from gumma here as elsewhere. Less frequently the ulcer appears without the gummatous swelling. The ulcer is deep, with clean cut edges and sloughing floor, grey to yellow green color and often covered with fungoid growth resembling cancer. These ulcers are neither bleeding like epitheliomata nor purulent like tuberculosis.

Syphilomata has a tendency to cicatrize and may cause permanent deformity of the tongue. Sclerotic glossitis or oral leukoplasia (Vidol) and other conditions about the mouth have syphilis as the common etiologic cause.

The common observation of all of us shows the frequency of palate infection in this disease. The patient with a hole in his mouth due to perforated palate ulcer is usually syphilitic. The ulcer is not oral, but more often nasal, in its origin. A syphilitic rhinitis most always precedes perforation of the palate.

Primary syphilis of the pharynx is rare, though cases of tonsillar chancre and even one of the preglottic has been reported. The pharynx is the favored spot for mucous patches and other manifestations of constitutional syphilis. They usually show symmetry in size and arrangement. A slight elevation of temperature usually occurs and the patient has a dry hacking cough. When these patches ulcerate, you have a well defined, highly elevated area with necrotic centers, discharging a foul greyish secretion. These patches are usually superficial, but frequently leave a fibrous scar.

The gumma is the characteristic tertiary lesion in this area and appears anywhere on the tissues of the pharynx. The gumma frequently breaks down, leaving a deep, gangrenous sloughing ulcer. The slough may contain necrotic bone and be accompanied by profuse discharge.

Syphilis is very rare in the oesophagus. In spite of its rarity, several cases of obstruction due to gumma of the oesophagus have been reported, according to Bower and Murphy.

The English medical literature record very few cases of syphilis of the stomach. The French report wide experience with this lesion. Dieulafoy classified these lesions anatomically as: erosions, ecchymoses, gumma infiltration, ulcerations, and cicatrices; clinically showing themselves by symptoms which resemble dyspepsia, gastralgia, ulcer, and cancer of stomach. Dieulafoy explains in detail many cases of clinical gastric ulceration that show syphilis as cause of the lesion. Murchison reports a post-mortem of syphilitic ulceration found by him in which the artery had been opened by ulcer.

The diagnoses of dyspepsia, gastralgia, and ulcers are so often only a subterfuge for an uncomplete examination of the case. Because the causative factor behind the conditions is not always plain, and syphilis can cause such conditions, it behooves us to exclude the spirocheta pallida from the etiology. This can readily be done by the Wassermann and the Hecht tests, and these tests should be routine in all gastric causes.

Cases simulating gastric ulcer by history, x-ray and by changed chemistry are frequently seen. As a type, I will cite one case diagnosed as ulcer shown by radiograph as clean cut rather than usual ragged ulcer and recurring semi-annually for five years. The man was found to be luetic and was properly treated. His ulcer has not returned for five years. These cases do not respond to the usual alkaline-milk treatment, as does simple ulcer, but do respond when anti-leutic treatment is added to ulcer management. Dieulafoy reports erroneous diagnosis of cancer of stomach in gumma, especially gumma about a pyloric cicatrix following ulcer or following gumma may by mechanical interference cause all the mechanical symptoms of obstruction and thus be diagnosed as cancer. Wassermann and Hecht observation of treatment will soon clear up diagnosis.

The small intestine is very rarely the site of known syphilitic lesions, although I see no reason why all the mucous membrane affections caused by this disease would not manifest themselves in the mucosa of the small bowel. It is true that diagnosis is very difficult without present means of study.

The duodenum is occasionally found involved with stomach and by the same type of lesions. The lower ileum is the more frequently involved portion, especially around the ileocecal valve. Chronic enteritis with enlarged lymph nodes and the deformities due to scars are the most common.

The colon is slightly more often involved than the small intestine and by the same type of lesions. Gumma also appears in walls of the colon.

Chancres of rectum are uncommon. Chancres of anal canal and anus are relatively common; women more often show this lesion than men, due to direct contamination from vulva; ulcers and strictures from the resulting scar are most common lesions. Hypertrophy of rectal walls, including mucosa and presence of ulcers without hard raised edges and feeling of a narrowing of cavity, are the usual findings. This, with positive Wassermann and positive history, will make your diagnosis clear. Only too frequently, on insufficient grounds, are rectal ulcers called syphilitic. This is a grievous error and comparable only to error in opposite direction, viz, overlooking the rational method is in all cases of doubtful etiology to work your case out completely. This applies most aptly to diseases of the gastrointestinal tract. No case of doubtful origin can be considered worked out without a Wassermann and history. Doing these two things routinely on vague gastrointestinal cases will give a beneficial light on an obscure subject.

URETER AND RENAL PELVIS.

W. F. Braasch, Rochester, Minn. (*Journal A. M. A.*, Sept. 6, 1919), devoted his chairman's address before the Section on Urology mainly to a discussion of the dilatation of the ureter and the renal pelvis. The mechanical obstructions were first noted, but greater space was given to the inflammatory dilatations. He finds that dilatation of the ureter and the renal pelvis may occur without mechanical causes, and the difference between the mechanical and the inflammatory dilatations, in their anatomy and pathology, and in the clinical signs, are quite definite. The clinical demonstration of such conditions may be of much diagnostic value. Cases have been described of what is called atonic dilatation, due to paralysis of the bladder from nervous disease; or occurring in some cases without known cause. Congenital constriction is so rare as to be almost negligible, and probably the cases described as such are often due to an acquired mechanical obstruction. The details of the condition are fully given, and the article is illustrated.

PROSTATIC AND VESICAL CANCER.

Frank Hinman, San Francisco, (*Journal A. M. A.*, June 21, 1919), describes and illustrates an instrument for the radium treatment of prostatic and vesical cancer, modified from the catheter method of Young, allowing the patient to move more freely than was the case with the unmodified method. The value of radium in these conditions has been confirmed, or at least reported on encouragingly, by eminent urologists, but most of the methods have their disadvantages. Hinman's description is too detailed to be given in an unillustrated abstract, but he reports its satisfactory use.

SYPHILIS OF THE EYE.

A. S. Piper, M. D.

ENID, OKLAHOMA

When I was invited by your chairman to read a paper on Syphilis of the Eye, I thought it futile to attempt a review of the various ocular manifestations, to which this infection may give rise.

In the first place, the changes induced by syphilis of the eye are so numerous and varied, that a dissertation dealing in full with the most important would consume much more time than you have been kind enough to place at my disposal.

The introduction of the Wassermann test and the treatment by salvarsan have, however, during the past few years added much to the certainty of our diagnosis of syphilis and our means of combating the disease, and while the value of both of these new diagnostic and theurapeutic methods have been largely recognized and appreciated, the almost constant appearance in the journals of new experiences with both, has caused me to attempt a review of some of the most notable of these publications, giving enough of the clinical pathology to crystalize our knowledge regarding these broad subjects of ocular syphilis.

In 1915, Finlay, reporting in the *Archives of Ophthalmology*, stated that in the literature at his disposal he was able to find about 100 cases of primary palpebral syphilis, and from different writers the total summing up of primary lesions of the eye seemed to be near 500.

It is therefore evident that most syphilitic eye involvements are either hereditary or acquired, secondary, or tertiary involvements, as is further shown by Spratt's investigation, and (Fournier cited by Spratt), *Journal A. M. A.*, 1913, that from six to ten per cent. of primary syphilitic lesions are extragenital, and that the eye ranks after the lip, finger, and breast in primary involvement.

We will now consider the part played by syphilis in the causation of diseases of the eye. Before the introduction of the Wassermann reaction and the existence of a sure method of diagnosis, figures estimating the frequency of syphilitic ocular affections were very variable. Since the introduction of this reliable test, a number of attempts have been made to arrive at some definite conclusions upon this point. Perhaps the most valuable of these is given in a paper by William C. Posey, of Philadelphia, *N. Y. State Medical Journal*, February, 1918, of a study by Mason, Mackie, and H. E. Smith, who made an examination of the blood of 250 patients, all of whom were suffering from diseases known to be sometimes caused by syphilis or else of uncertain etiology. With regard to some of the conditions, the numbers are too small to form a basis for any valid conclusions, but the following points may be noted.

In interstitial keratitis, the reaction was positive in 88.8 per cent. G. F. Harkness, Davenport, Ia., received 30 affirmative answers out of 92 replies from ophthalmologists, or approximately 33⅓ per cent., so it would seem that De Schweinitz's statement that 60 per cent. of the cases of parenchymatous keratitis as being due to syphilis is approximately correct.

Since a positive reaction is in itself conclusive evidence of the presence of syphilis (apart from a few diseases rarely found in this country), whereas a negative reaction is inconclusive evidence of its absence (the first named authors say that only 75 per cent. of cases in the tertiary stage yield a positive result), this percentage tends to prove that interstitial keratitis apart from syphilis must be very rare.

The majority of cases of interstitial keratitis are due to inherited syphilis, only about seven per cent. are due to acquired, according to Stephenson's investigation.

Keratitis cannot be considered an entity in itself but as part of a condition involving the uveal tract as well. The iris, ciliary body, and choroid, are always involved, and Marshall has demonstrated by microscopical studies that keratitis is really a manifestation of a uveitis.

The infiltrative stage is preceded by a punctate keratitis with subsequent vascularization and development of the salmon-patch as described by Hutchinson. It begins by watering of the eyes, followed in a few days by faint cloudiness, later by irritability, photophobia, and impaired vision, due to the opaque spots and vascularization. From three to twelve months are usually consumed in the development of the various stages of the disease, and it is most frequently observed between the ages of five and fifteen years.

The principal changes occur in the deeper layers of the substantia propria of the cornea, and consist essentially of dense infiltration of these areas. Ulceration rarely occurs, but nonetheless, ulcers of discoverable size are sometimes present. There is a difference of opinion as to whether the disease is primary or secondary to uveitis.

The local treatment with atropine to maintain mydriasis, prevent iritis, and allay inflammation, should be systematically employed, unless rise of tension appears. Dionin is of distinct service, as well as hot fomentations. The eyes should be protected by dark glasses.

In taking up the subject of iritis, it is interesting to note that the trend of opinion has, for a number of years, and particularly of late, been to reduce the percentage of such involvement as being due to syphilis.

First, De Schweinitz, quoting Alexander, states that from .42 to 5.37 per cent. of syphilitics suffer from iritis and that syphilis is regarded as the most common cause of iritis.

Jennings and Hill in 1909 reported 500 cases from Will's Eye Hospital, and gave 61.4 per cent. as due to lues.

In the 250 cases examined and reported upon by Mason, Mackie, and Smith, of the number having iritis, 54 per cent. were proved to be of syphilitic origin.

Out of 82 answers received by G. F. Harkness from members of the profession, the cases of iritis reported as being due to lues averaged 48.22 per cent. In a general way, those connected with the teaching centers gave a lower percentage.

Another contribution of great value in determining the frequency with which syphilis affects the eye, is a paper read before the American Ophthalmological Society in 1916, by Brown and Irons, of Chicago, giving the results of a careful analysis to determine the etiology of 100 patients suffering from iritis. Careful attention was given to the history, and a complete physical examination was made to detect the presence of syphilis, tuberculosis, gonococcal infection, and infections from teeth, tonsils, sinuses, prostate, pelvis, or other structures which might give rise to ocular lesion.

The laboratory examination included Wassermann tests which were conducted by two laboratories. From this comprehensive study, syphilis was found to be the cause of the iritis in 23 cases, and in eleven other instances it was associated with other coincident infections—a total of 34. In five other cases there was some reason to think syphilis should also be considered—a total of 39. In the remaining 61 cases, a searching examination failed to reveal any evidence of past or present syphilitic infection. In the words of the authors, "so far as one may draw conclusions from this number of cases, it would seem that the widely accepted statement that 50 per cent. or more of iritis is due to syphilis may have to be revised." Certainly in the absence of other evidence of active syphilis in a patient with iritis, the assumption that the iritis is syphilitic is more likely to be wrong than right.

William Lang, reporting in the *Lancet*, June 23, 1917, says that out of 200 cases of iritis in his private practice, that only six per cent. of the cases were caused by syphilis, but hospital figures would probably show an increase of this percentage. However, he believes the modern anti-syphilitic methods will cause it to become the rarest cause.

As a hereditary manifestation, luetic iritis rarely occurs, with the exception of the constant association of inflammation of the uveal tract with a parenchymatous keratitis. The involvement of the iris may at times become quite conspicuous, and to a lesser degree is always present.

Luetic iritis occurs as a secondary or tertiary manifestation, but the differentiation is not always easy. As Fuchs states, "Syphilitic iritis with the formation of nodules offers an easy diagnosis, but the syphilitic forms often resemble those due to other causes, and furthermore, it is difficult to differentiate the same microscopically."

When due to lues, both eyes are generally involved and the iris has more often a muddy appearance and the iritis assumes the plastic type.

Localized sphincter lesions always suggest the influence of syphilis, and with the development of papules a form of iritis appears which yields characteristic, if not pathognomonic, signs of its origin. These yellowish or reddish brown nodules, varying in size from a hemp seed to a small pea, are situated at the pupillary area or ciliary border, as Fuchs maintains they do not arise in the mid-breadth of the iris. Under treatment they are gradually absorbed without leaving very marked scars, although a certain amount of atrophy of the iris marks their former location.

Gumma of the iris occurs, according to Alexander, almost constantly at the ciliary border, the lesion is solitary, the size of a pea and grows toward the ciliary body. Such a manifestation, strictly localized in the iris, is extremely rare. It appears, if at all, in the so-called tertiary period of syphilis.

The most important local drug is atropine sulphate to obtain mydriasis which should be maintained until all ciliary irritation has subsided. Should atropine not be tolerated, scopolamine or hyoscyamine may be substituted.

Dionin is valuable on account of its lymphagogue and analgesic action, which is increased by the addition of a two per cent. holocaine solution. Hot moist compresses are also beneficial.

Almost all diseases of the choroid are symptomatic of general disease. It is to be doubted that lues affects the choroid, or the retina alone, but that at some stage the condition should more properly be termed a choriod-retinitis.

The ophthalmoscope is not to be relied upon for a positive luetic diagnosis, be the lesion localized or disseminated. Harkness, quoting Parsons, states that the changes due to lues are indistinguishable from those due to other causes.

Various classifications have been made according to the type of lesion present, such as diffuse, disseminated, or circumscribed. In Mason, Mackie, and Smith's report on 250 cases investigated, only five out of 26 cases of choroiditis and choroidal atrophy gave a positive Wassermann, although they state that the per cent. is decidedly less than might be expected. However, most writers class syphilis in the congenital or acquired forms, as being responsible in the majority of cases. Further investigation as regards focal infection will probably reduce the number of cases due to lues.

Both eyes are generally affected and particularly so in acquired syphilis, the lesions appearing from six months to many years after the initial lesion. Opacities in the vitreous is a common accompaniment, and some writers claim that fine dust-like deposits, with a cloudy retina and involvement of both eyes, is pathognomonic of syphilis.

Lubrick, Graefe, and others, claim to have established a genuine syphilitic retinitis, but as a primary condition it is extremely rare as compared to its involvement as a neuro-retinitis or secondary from the choroid.

There is a condition spoken of as retinitis-luetica in which the papilla is normal, but with a large exudate on one or more of the vessels, especially the veins, and a large scotoma passing across the field of vision; due to an occlusion of the cilioretinal artery.

Lues deserves first consideration in involvements of the optic nerve, be the condition a primary atrophy, an inflammation, or a secondary atrophy.

In Mason, Mackie, and Smith's investigation over half of the cases of optic atrophy studied proved to be syphilitic. In ten cases in which the atrophy was diagnosed as primary, all gave a positive reaction.

An optic neuritis due to hereditary lues is rare and usually associated with a meningitis. The syphilitic neuro-retinitis presents a large oedema often extending two papillary diameters.

It is important in primary atrophy to try to distinguish syphilis as a cause separate from tabes and paresis. Tabetic atrophy generally appears early and may for years be its only symptom.

Reflex immobility of the pupil with atrophy, indicates tabes, while absolute immobility with a dilated pupil, paresis or syphilis in some other form. Miosis only occurs in tabes.

Optic atrophy, the Argyle-Robertson pupil and absence of knee-jerk, establishes tabes.

The positive Wassermann test is absolute as regards the presence of syphilis, though it does not so establish this as a causative factor of the lesion present.

In muscular palsies, out of thirteen cases reported by Mason, Mackie, and Smith, seven gave positive Wassermann and six negative results. Of the positive cases, four were of the third nerve, one of the fourth, one of the sixth, and one of the sixth and third combined. The negative cases were all of the sixth nerve. This would tend to show that the external rectus, the eye muscle most subject to paralysis, is relatively immune to syphilitic disease.

The concensus of opinion of such men as Uhle, Mackinney, and Posey, of Philadelphia, Knapp, of New York, and others, is that early frequent small doses of salvarsan is very beneficial in combating the acute symptoms of most syphilitic eye involvements, but that most cases have to be followed up with some form of mercury. And Posey says that the combination of salvarsan with mercury and K.I. greatly augments the spirochaeticidal properties of each of these specifics, which has also been my own observation.

For a long time there was a general impression that salvarsan acted deleteriously upon the tissues of the optic nerve and especially in the presence of non-syphilitic diseases of the retina and optic nerve.

Gibbard, however, who investigated this phase of the subject, observed but two cases of cerebro-nerve disease out of 1200 cases in which salvarsan was used and an increase in dosage caused a disappearance of the trouble. Further search of the literature also indicates that there is no grounds for the belief that salvarsan has a poisonous effect on any of the ocular tissues.

That the administration of salvarsan does not prevent the appearance of new syphilitic symptoms during the period of administration is generally recognized, and is probably due, as Stephenson has pointed out, to the presence of nests of organisms which escaped the action of the initial dose.

Doctor Posey, of Philadelphia, says, that from his experience, it would appear that the toxic effects wrongly attributed to salvarsan may be avoided by trusting the administration of the drug to only those who are properly trained, a practice which I have followed for some time, being associated with Dr. Hays, the Chairman of this division, he devoting his time to genito-urinary and venereal diseases, and by his looking after the internal treatment and I the local treatment, we have never experienced any bad results from the use of salvarsan.

Fordyce insists that every case of secondary syphilis as a matter of routine should have an ophthalmoscopic examination from time to time. Marked evidence of pathologic changes may be present with slight subjective symptoms and impairment of vision and the condition may be completely overlooked unless one is on the alert.

Discussion.

Dr. Julius Frischer, Kansas City, Mo.: I have only a few words to say. We should commend the officers in this symposium for their most excellent work, and also to impress upon the general practitioner that group work is very necessary in this work on syphilis. Now, our laboratory diagnosis is very essential. We should go with our serological tests and pathologic laboratory for good work in syphilis. I have even seen the penis amputated for carcinoma and sent to the laboratory and found out to be specific. One certain point I wish to bring out concerning the period of incubation in syphilis. It is a mistaken idea that it takes six weeks before a person gets a chancre. I have seen the period of incubation vary from one week to six weeks. Now, the sore does not have to be typical. I believe ninety per cent. of the sores of the penis observed in a venereal way are syphilis, no question about that. The negative Wassermann does not necessarily mean that a patient does not have syphilis. I believe that a person who has a chancre will not have a negative Wassermann, will not have a positive Wassermann until one week or a few days before he has a secondary eruption. The very nature of the spirocheta varies as to the resistance of the individual, also as to the peculiar strain; by peculiar strain, I mean that the strain of spirocheta can cause a paresis and a certain strain of spirocheta that infects an individual will cause the paretic, will be more virulent than it will be in another individual, and the resistance of the individual will vary as to the infection.

Great stress has been placed on spinal puncture, which I think is very necessary, and it has to be eliminated from your cerebro-spinal system as well as from your blood stream and from your capillaries. Now, I wish to say that sodium cacodylate is absolutely no good in the treatment of syphilis. It has been proven Doctor Murphy made a great mistake when he advocated the sodium cacodylate and a great deal of time has been spent—lost—in taking care of syphilis. I mean a great deal more of valuable time can be saved by giving the everyday form of treatment, than when sodium cacodylate is used.

SYPHILIS.

J. F. Schamberg, Philadelphia (*Journal A. M. A.*, Sept. 13, 1919), says that there has risen in many minds the query of how we can be sure of the complete extinction of syphilis in a person. There is reason to believe that many persons treated intensively in the early stage are cured, as they remain free from symptoms and give negative Wassermann reactions, but these indications alone do not prove positive cure. Schamberg reports a case of a second attack, two years after the first. The man had had repeated negative Wassermann reactions during the interval after the treatment of the first chancre and before the contraction of the second. The case is more remarkable because the patient had evidence of early meningeal involvement; and there was no sign of immunity, as the second attack was severer than the first. The case has a bearing on the question of the curability of syphilis; the cure, in the first instance, is called indisputable by Schamberg. The criteria of cure are hard to establish, as negative Wassermann reactions are not conclusive. But the fact that the man could contract syphilis again, and again be cured, seems established in this case.

THE TREATMENT OF CHRONIC URETHRITIS.

T. B. COULTER, M. D.

TULSA, OKLAHOMA

As a result of the examination of several million of men in the past four years, the attention of the whole world, as well as the more careful attention of the medical profession, has been called to the prevalence of urethritis in all stages, and among all classes of people, and especially has our attention been called to the chronicity of Neisserian infection, and the many recurrences in apparently cured cases.

If the results of treatment of other diseases are compared with those obtained in the treatment of chronic urethritis, we are led to ask why is this essentially local condition so hard to treat successfully, and why do complications arise in spite of treatment.

Any condition causing inflammation of the urethra, whether it be trauma from the passage of a stone, or instrument, external violence, or bacterial infection, may lead to a chronic condition.

As bacterial infection is responsible for at least eighty per cent. of all chronic inflammations of the genito-urinary tract, it is with this type of chronic inflammatory trouble that we are chiefly interested.

There is probably no organism more difficult to eliminate from the tissues than the gonococcus,—an organism which shortly after implantation, buries itself in the urethral crypts and follicles, extending by continuity of tissue, or urged on by irrational treatment, resulting in only enough reaction to produce discharge, and local in character, an inflammation not extensive, or active enough to stimulate the formation of antibodies, so long as the condition is limited to the anterior urethra, as is shown by the fixation test on gonorrhoeal cases. We never get a positive finding early in a first infection, unless the posterior urethra has become involved, and even then nature's laboratory does not produce enough antibodies to produce even a temporary immunity.

This limitation of the local and systemic reaction I think explains to us one vital reason why gonorrheal infections are especially prone to become chronic in character, aside from the fact that a great many acute conditions only receive treatment until the discharge is checked,—the patient then, out of his great experience with such things, deciding that further treatment is not necessary, goes his care-free way until he is reminded by a fresh discharge that he still has, or again has, an infection.

Although time is an essential element in considering whether a given condition has become chronic or not, the state of inflammation is the deciding factor,—some infections being chronic in character from the start, while the most chronic infections, as to time and symptoms, may have acute exacerbations, each condition demanding appropriate treatment.

It is to be remembered that in chronic urethritis we are dealing with tissues that have already in a measure given up the fight to right themselves, or have been so changed that in themselves they predispose to further inflammatory changes; treatment, to be successful, must be carried out without further destroying this resistance, requiring gentleness, patience and time in its execution.

As with other chronic affections, so here we have a great diversity of symptoms, meaning much or little, as the case may be, but which have to be considered in treating the condition.

In order to arrive at a definite conclusion as to the character and location of the trouble with which we have to deal, it is well to ask ourselves a few questions:

1. What is the physical condition of the patient?
2. Is active infection still present?
3. What condition, natural or acquired, is responsible for persistence of symptoms?

4. Where is this condition located?

As no two conditions react the same to treatment, any more than two individuals are exactly alike, it is well not to limit the examination of our patients too closely to the history of the present condition, but to inquire carefully into his previous troubles, and especially his general habits; with this information at hand, we can safely progress to the more careful examination of the condition. I think it is well here, to adhere to a regular routine examination, so far as conditions permit.

1. Is there discharge present; if so, what is its character; does it contain gonococci?
2. Is the meatus normal in size; is the mucosa normal?
3. Are the external genitalia normal?
4. Is the urine normal?
5. Are the prostate and seminal vesicles normal?
6. Is there stricture present, or palpable folliculitis?
7. Is there any pain produced during the course of examination, similar to that complained of?

The presence or absence of gonococci is primarily of great importance in its bearing on treatment, as all treatment for underlying conditions should be held in abeyance until a thorough effort has been made to eliminate this infection, as very few chronic anterior infections are found, which are not dependent upon posterior infections for their persistence.

It is well to begin treatment by through and through irrigations, using solutions slightly stimulating in character, as 1–10,000 solution of Ag. No. 3, or 1–6000 potassium permanganate, supplemented by instillation of stronger medication, as 1–2 per cent. silver nitrate into the posterior urethra; these measures not only bring treatment to the true seats of urethral infection, but also cause a mild inflammatory congestion necessary to promote true healing.

Among the newer remedies for this type of condition, the mention of acriflavene should not be omitted, as in this preparation we have a very active germicidal agent, and one, while not entirely non-irritating, does produce a minimum of trauma.

Many cases are by these measures promptly and thoroughly cleared up, but a certain per cent. of cases are not so easily disposed of; these may be divided into two classes, according to the cause on which they depend.

One class is characterized by the fact that symptoms, whether they be discharge, morning drop, gluing of the meatus, or only filaments in the urine, remain little influenced by treatment; in the second class, symptoms are held in abeyance as long as treatment is continued, but return as soon as it is stopped, if inflammation has not been relieved.

The first are always due to infiltrative catarrh, causing a constant throwing off of pus cells from the wall of the urethra, while in the second, the glandular sexual organs, especially the prostate, are the seat of an inflammatory catarrhal process.

In about eighty-five per cent. of all cases of chronic urethritis, examination reveals some trouble in the prostate; this need not necessarily be of such a grade as to be discoverable on palpation, but may be only revealed by microscopic examination of prostatic secretion,—care being taken to have the urethra washed free of pus, either by urination, or by irrigation.

As it is very rare to find one single region responsible for the trouble, it is well while possibly paying the greatest attention to that region most at fault, not to neglect the minor sources of inflammation, so of necessity treatment has to be varied to meet all requirements.

The prostatic involvement should have systematic massage, ranging in frequency and severity, according to the results attained, some prostates responding wonderfully to the treatment, while others should be left alone, just as most urethral inflammations are benefited by treatment, while others do better without active treatment, requiring careful neglect, and rest, rather than treatment.

As a rule, massage should be given two or three times a week, usually including the vesicles in the first few massage strokes, then the prostate itself, massage being directed towards the urethral orifices of the ducts, pressure being directed to those areas surrounding the diseased areas, and avoiding too severe pressure, as I believe results of massage are not dependent on the amount of secretion obtained, but rather on the combination of *mild* stimulation, improvement in the circulation of the gland, and removal of abnormal secretion, massage to be followed by mild permanganate of potash, irrigation, and supplemented by occasional dilation with the Kollman dilator.

By these means, practically all inflammatory prostates can be brought to a condition where they cease to produce symptoms. If, however, the urethra has not been carefully treated at the same time, even with the prostate normal, discharge and symptoms of irritation may persist; to avoid this, it is well to make an endoscopic examination at as early a time in the treatment as it can be safely done, with the urethra anesthetized with four per cent. novocaine or alypin, very little pain is produced, and an accurate idea can be gained of the conditions present in the whole of the urethra, and especially the prostatic portion, and at the same time direct applications may be made to those areas requiring active treatment. It is especially in the posterior urethra that we may find marked signs of irritation, the whole posterior urethra may be oedematous, purplish in color; this will be wonderfully benefited sometimes, by a single light application of 10–20 per cent. silver nitrate; the veramontanum is of course included in this inflammation, and it is here that the trouble is liable to persist after the remainder of the posterior urethra has returned to normal,—inflammation in the utricle and ducts entering here, being slow to eradicate; here, if the inflammation is intense, I think the milder applications, as 10–20 per cent. silver nitrate, also give the best results, reserving the application of stick silver for those more chronic cicatricial conditions demanding great stimulation, or even partial destruction of tissue. At times the utricle alone may be the sole site of inflammation.

In these cases, the injection of one per cent. silver nitrate into the utricle by means of the utricle syringe is very helpful, care being taken to use very little pressure, otherwise an acute epididymitis may be added to your troubles.

Other conditions, such as infected follicles, may also be treated locally through the endoscope, treatment of these conditions resulting in a return to normal in the great majority of cases.

In those catarrhal infiltrative types, however, resulting in the laying down of scar tissue in varying amounts, we have changes more permanent in character to deal with, and demanding special consideration.

Varying from superficial scars, often producing no symptoms, to dense scar tissue, causing absolute retention, depending on the severity of the original infection, and its duration and location, forming slowly, and contracting so gradually that it may be months or years after the original infection before pronounced enough symptoms are produced to call the patient's attention to the condition.

All cases not actively infected, but showing signs of urethral irritation, either by morning drop, recurrent attacks of discharge, or pus or shreds in the urine, should be examined for stricture, the most satisfactory means of examination being the flexible bougie-a-boule, using the largest size that will pass the normal meatus, even the slightest thickening in the wall can be detected by using varying sizes, and the number, size and location of strictures may be ascertained.

No matter where the stricture may be, or its extent, the aim of the treatment is the same,—relief of constriction, and absorption of scar tissue, with the constriction alone removed, and the urine given free passage, catarrhal symptoms subside; this happy termination, however, is not easily attained, and the means to that end must vary with the condition encountered.

All inflammatory strictures located far back in the urethra should be dilated if possible; those anterior to the bulb should be dilated if possible,—otherwise cut.

Strictures that are very tight, filiform in calibre, usually yield to dilation with filiforms and followed up to 20–24 F., when it is as well to turn to ordinary sounds or the Kollman dilator, advancing not more than 2–3 numbers at a treatment, and repeating not oftener than every three or five days.

It is essential that all instruments be passed with a minimum of trauma, as injury only leads to further scar formation, absorption of old scar tissue being caused by slight pressure, and stretching. If the stricture is so dense, however, that dilation is hopeless, urethrotomy should be resorted to, the entire thickness of the constricting band being cut, if the ideal result is to be gained. After urethrotomy, sounds must be passed at intervals of a few days, to prevent the healing of the edges of the incision, and to promote further reabsorption of scar tissue, the passage of all instruments being preceded by irrigation with some mild antiseptic solution, leaving sufficient fluid in the bladder to slightly distend it, and serve as an irrigation after removal of the instrument.

One other condition coming as it sometimes does during the course of treatment, and causing considerable embarrassment to the physician, is epididymitis, although its occurrence usually has no relation to treatment, coming in almost all cases as the result of inflammatory extension from the posterior urethra. So long as inflammation persists here, it is a possibility to be reckoned with.

Premonitory symptoms, which may be heaviness in the perineum, a dull pain in the groin, if recognized, give a fair opportunity for abortive measures to be instituted; rest in bed, elevation of the scrotum, and laxatives, with stopping of all other treatment will in many cases stop further progress of the trouble.

If, however, the inflammation has already developed in the epididymis, with its attendant pain, swelling and constitutional symptoms, more active measures must be used.

While the older methods consisting of hot or cold applications, strapping and elimination still have a large field of usefulness, this leaves too much to the natural powers of repair, and is at best slow in relieving pain.

Much better results are obtained in my experience by incision and puncture of tunica vaginalis, or equally good and requiring less after care, puncturing the tunica vaginalis over the globus minor with a large sized hypodermic needle.

This, while it does not remove pus, does relieve the tension, allows the circulation to come back to near normal, and pain disappears almost at once; following this, strapping is still essential in aiding a return to normal; usually after ten days to two weeks, treatment of the original trouble may safely be continued.

Although we have many questions to decide during the course of treatment of chronic inflammation of the genito-urinary tract, there is none that places more responsibility upon us than that of deciding when it is safe for a patient to marry, and may only be decided in the affirmative if, after a reasonable length of time, and on repeated examinations, we have been unable to find any evidence of infection.

To sum up, the successful treatment of chronic urethritis is dependent upon accurate diagnosis, judicious selection of instruments and medication, used with great care, and thorough understanding of the results to be obtained.

Discussion.

Doctor J. H. Sanford, Muskogee: My experience in the army was that a great number of men entered the army with gonorrheal infection, and they proved to be upon examination, that about two-thirds of them had never been dilated, that had constricted areas in the posterior urethra, as well as in the anterior, and a great many of them had a small meatus that would not admit a No. 20 sound. Of course, in those conditions they have all had associated prostatic involvement as well as prostatic vesicles. Our routine treatment is becoming old; the standard of dilatation, irrigation of the size of the prostate with occasional endoscope in the posterior urethra, particularly at the villi, we find in a good many of those chronic persistent cases with recurrences we have had infections in the catarrhal difficulty and by local applications of the silver nitrate via the endoscope have cleared up very promptly; but the biggest impression that I got, with the treatment of gonorrhea with any number of people, was lack of dilation with the instrument, hard, indurated, and soft, and required continued dilations both with the Kollman dilator and with the sounds.   Of course we made prostatic examinations regularly and had the secretions microscopically studied, and as I say, I hardly saw any chronic gonorrhea where the old standardized treatment of massage, irrigation, and thorough dilation can be improved upon.

I think the doctor covered the subject in his paper very thoroughly.

Doctor W. J. Wallace, Oklahoma City: Mr. Chairman, there are just a few points I would like to mention.

Now, in the treatment of a chronic gonorrheal condition as the doctor has mentioned, meatotomy is necessary if you have a small meatus, then we have practically a routine treatment and it is almost a song that we sing, and that consists of practically three things.

It is a sound, absolutely, or a Kollman dilator (personally I prefer a sound), and beginning with the size that will be permitted without drawing blood and gradually increasing that sound, or we get a sound, then follow that by the massage. The sound opens up the ducts, the prostate and the meatus are involved; you have a little backing of the tissue so that opens the ducts first; then massage that out, both the vesicles and the prostatic trouble, and then follow that with a deep instillation.   I do not think an irrigation does one particle of good.

Permanganate of potash is absolutely worthless in a chronic condition of gonorrhea.   It is an astringent and you don't want an astringent, you want something that will penetrate the diseased ducts, and I prefer a deep instillation.   Now, if we have some complications of pus and blood that we want to wash out, then it is well enough to give a deep irrigation, or bladder irrigation, but for routine treatment it is worthless, in my opinion.

So it resolves itself, then, into, first: the sound; massage, and deep instillation. Now, in that case, we alternate, of course, according to the case, the patient and the condition.   Protargol is one of the favorites, once or twice a week, but the nitrate of silver, four and a half per cent. is my preference, and the argyrol varying in strength, depending entirely on the condition of the patient; but keep this up in a systematic way, with the general tonics and certain hygienic rules, why, in time, with the help of the good Lord, we will get our patient in condition.

Now, about the acute epididymitis of the chronic form, there is just a word I would like to say along that line.   Not that I do not believe in puncturing the epididymis, I think that produces a certain amount of adhesions, and we do irreparable harm, because the trouble will not be relieved, in my mind, in that way. So the rules we observe, and the rules that we have followed for several years in making an incision the size of the parietal area, never fail to relieve the fluid, because we will always find a little interstitial involving the parietal, always between the head of the globus major and the testicles; labor that thoroughly, you can do an inverse, or else you can cut a V-shaped piece of the tunica vaginalis. In that way, if there should be any more of the infiltration due to the epididymous condition, why, it will be observed in the smaller tissue and you relieve the contents without doing damage by going into the globus minor or into the globus proper.

Doctor Coulter (closing):   In regard to the sounds in preference to the Kollmans, or vice versa, personally I adhere to the Kollman, for, as a result of personal experience I believe that the Kollman stretching the mucosa in a longitudinal line rather than the way of the sound pressed apart in the transverse way, if we should get trauma you are less liable to have an excess of scar tissue formed, for the factors of the formation of the scar are less from a longitudinal stretching than from the transverse stretching of the urethra mucosa. I believe, in the epididymitis, that it is better to use the more radical measure. Many patients won't resort—won't subject themselves to a radical procedure; there, I believe that the puncture is permissible. I don't believe it is advisable, but I believe it is permissible, because it does give, in a great many cases, relief from the pain and lessens the time of the disability, but the more radical measure is undoubtedly the more to be preferred.

GONORRHEA IN FEMALE.

C. P. Linn, M. D.

TULSA, OKLAHOMA

When a man has gonorrhea he knows it. I do not deny the possibility of a symptomless or practically symptomless gonorrheal urethritis in the male, still such cases, if at all existent, must be extremely rare. This is not, however, the case with women. A woman may go through an acute gonorrhea from beginning to end without knowing it, may have a chronic gonorrhea for years without being aware of its existence, often sincerely believing that she is perfectly well. A man is not used to having pains or burning in his urethra, nor is he used to having any discharge from it. At the least pain or scalding, or the least appearance of discharge, he knows there is something wrong with him. The urethra when infected in women does not give as severe symptoms as inflammation of the urethra in men, and besides in many cases the female urethra escapes infection, the infection being limited to the cervix alone or to the cervix and Bartholin's glands.

A woman is used to pains, the premenstrual pains with which many of them suffer are severer than the pains caused by the gonorrheal infection; and they often have a leukorrheal discharge of greater or lesser degree. An increase in the amount of secretion or in its color and consistency does not attract their attention. It is for this reason that many women harbor the gonococcus for months before applying to a physician and some of them never apply at all. It is as a rule when the discharge is very profuse, offensive and irritating, when urination is painful and burning, or when there is a sharp salpingeal attack, that the doctor is consulted. I repeat that many women go through life with a chronic gonorrheal cervicitis, with a discharge containing gonococci, and use no treatment except an occasional douche because they are under the impression that they are suffering from lukorrhea or whites. I do not wish to be understood as claiming that gonorrhea in the female is always of a mild character, pursuing a subacute or symptomless course. I mean to say that such are the vast majority of cases which present themselves to the physician.

Because in them the infection, when it takes place, is usually the result of chronic gonorrhea in the husband; when the infecting man is suffering from a chronic gonorrhea, the infection in the woman usually pursues a subacute or chronic course. But when the man has an acute gonorrhea, then the infection in the woman may from the very beginning assume a superacute, even fulminant character. And the rapidity with which the infection may show itself is remarkable. While several days usually elapse between the infecting intercourse and the first symptoms, there are cases in which the latter show themselves in 24 hours. In short, the symptoms showed themselves in twelve hours after the infecting intercourse.

While it usually takes months for a salpingitis to develop as the result of gonorrheal infection, there are cases in which distinct symptoms of inflammation of the fallopian tubes may develop within a few days, or even within a few hours after an infecting intercourse. In such cases we are forced to believe in the suction action of the uterus. It is impossible to believe that the infection reached the fallopian tubes by continuous extension, within such a short period. It is more plausible to believe that the infection took place by the infecting gonococci—containing material being sucked up into the uterus and into the fallopian tubes. This appears to be more likely from the fact that a gonorrheal salpingitis may exist without an intervening endometritis or metritis.

The symptoms in an acute or superacute case of gonorrhea may be very severe. Within several days after an infecting intercourse, and sometimes within several hours, the latter particularly in young virgin brides and still more particularly if the act is performed stormily and repeatedly, the woman begins to complain— many of them do not complain until their condition becomes unbearable—of a burning and itching in the vulva and vagina, of frequent urination, accompanied by strangury, and a scalding sensation. A discharge soon makes its appearance, which, according to the severity of the case, may be creamy, cream-yellow or green- ish. It may possess little odor or be extremely offensive. It is often very irritating, eroding the skin with which it comes in contact and causing pruritis and intertrigo around the genitals, anus, thighs, etc. If proper cleanliness is not observed, the infecting discharge may invade the anus and gonorrheal proctitis be the result. There is usually an elevation of temperature, 100 to 102 degrees F., there may also be a chill, and the feeling of general malaise may be quite pronounced. If the in- fection involves also the fallopian tubes, then all the general symptoms may be greatly aggravated. The chill may be quite severe, the temperature may go up to 103 degrees or even 104 degrees F., the abdomen is tender, and the feeling of malaise may be so severe as to create apprehension of a general peritonitis.

The diagnosis of an acute or superacute case of gonorrhea in the female presents no difficulties. The history and the symptoms as related by the patient are alone sufficient. Inspection of the genitals, covered with pus, the introduction of a speculum, which shows us an inflamed eroded cervix, bleeding at the slightest touch, and bathed in pus which oozes from its external os, makes the diagnosis certain.

The great, the paramount point in treating gonorrhea in women is to prevent the disease from passing the internal os and spreading through the endometrium into the tubes, and from there into the ovaries and peritoneum. As long as we can keep the gonorrheal process limited to the cervix and the other external genitals, gonorrhea is not a terrible disease. We can handle it without great difficulty and cure it eventually, though the time required for a cure may in some cases be ex- asperatingly long. It is when the gonorrheal process is extended above the internal os, that we become helpless. For after the process has involved the endometrium and the fallopian tubes, there is no medical treatment; there is only expectant and surgical treatment, which is of course no treatment at all in the true sense of the word. Removing the tubes may be necessary to save the patient's life, but to cut out an organ is not to cure it. A large percentage of cases of endometritis and metritis, salpingitis, and peritonitis,—thousands of cases requiring surgical interfer- ence, are due directly to the physician's well-meant energetic treatment. The introduction of syringes and probes into the cervix, the scraping and cauterizing with strong caustic solutions, are in many instances directly responsible for the extension of the inflammation and for the aggravation of the patient's condition. Those who know anything about the treatment of gonorrhea in women know that we get the best results by the gentlest methods and mildest applications.

I consider these prefatory remarks of extreme importance, for until the phy- sician is imbued with the feeling, saturated with the conviction, that brutality is not a necessary element in the treatment of gonorrhea, that too energetic treatment is often injurious instead of beneficial, that the uterine cavity must at all hazards be protected from an extension of the inflammation, and that he at least must not be the causative factor of that extension, until he is convinced of all these things he is not a safe person to undertake the treatment of a case of gonorrhea in a woman.

The general treatment of acute gonorrhea in the female can be expressed in one word or phrase; rest, taking it easy—if we wish to avoid a salpingitis or ex- tension of the inflammation above the internal os. It is unfortunate that many women, and respectable married women at that, still must keep on doing their household work or other heavy work. Where it is unavoidable it is unavoidable, and that is all there is to it, but the proper thing would be to put the woman to bed, or at least keep her in her room for a couple of weeks and have her take things very easy.

Where there is a considerable rise of temperature or symptoms of salpingitis seem to be threatening, then putting the patient to bed is imperative and applying an ice bag to the abdomen is very useful.

Coitus must be absolutely forbidden. One can think of nothing more harmful, more dangerous, than coitus for a woman affected with gonorrhea. Intercourse is bad for a male with acute gonorrhea, but it is very much more dangerous for a female gonorrheic patient. It not only aggravates the existing condition, increasing the inflammation in the vulva, urethra and cervix, but it is about the surest way to cause a salpingitis. I have known cases which were progressing very nicely, which were on the point of recovery, but which became suddenly aggravated and in which symptoms of salpingitis became evident immediately after coitus. So this must be forbidden absolutely in all acute and subacute cases of gonorrhea. No exceptions can be permitted. Whether this extension of the inflammation is due simply to the engorgement of the uterus and other genital parts induced by the coitus or to a certain suction and peristaltic action of the uterus is immaterial. Both may be causative factors. The fact remains that coitus is a dangerous procedure which may lead to a fatal issue, for a woman suffering with acute or subacute gonorrhea. (A man who forces a woman in such condition to submit to intercourse is a criminal brute and the woman who submits to it is a pitiful slave. And still the woman is often forced to submit to it, the husband thinking that if he uses a condom, and is not too violent, he has done everything necessary to protect himself and her.)

As far as the diet is concerned, little or no change need be made in it if the urethra is not involved. Spices and alcohol, however, are best omitted, as they do perhaps cause congestion of the genitalia and thus aggravate the condition. But where there is a urethritis practically the same restrictions are indicated as in gonorrhea of the male.

As far as internal treatment is concerned, none is necessary unless the urethra is involved. When the urethra is involved and urination is painful, then we may give the same balsams, hyoscyamus and alkalies, as we do in urethritis of the male.

If the local treatment in male urethritis is important, it is much more so in gonorrhea of the female. In fact it is the only part of the treatment from which definite results can be obtained, the internal treatment being merely occasional and auxiliary. The treatment to be successful must be of two kinds; one administered by the physician, the other administered by the patient or to the patient in her home. The home treatment consists in the use of injections and suppositories. The medical treatment, that is the treatment on the part of the physician, consists in local applications, that is in swabbing and painting the parts, and occasionally in cauterizing. Both parts of the treatment are necessary, as they supplement each other.

As stated before, the home treatment consists in the use of vaginal douches and suppositories. The injections that I prefer to all others are iodine, lactic acid, and a combination of alum, zinc sulphate and copper sulphate. Where the discharge is very profuse, the injections should be given as often as four times a day. After the discharge becomes less profuse, twice a day and then once a day is sufficient. The iodine injections are made by adding one tablespoonful of tincture of iodine to two quarts of hot water. In some cases this is too irritating and we may commence with a teaspoonful to two quarts of water. The lactic acid is used in the strength of 1-500 to 1-1000. The alum, zinc, copper combination has the following formula:

Aluminis _ oz. iv
Zinci sulphatis _ iv
Cupri sulphatis, aa _ iv
Sig. Tablespoonful to 1 or 2 quarts of water.

The injections or douches should invariably be taken in the recumbent position, the patient lying flat on her back on a flat douche pan. It is better when the buttocks are raised, so that they are on a higher level than the rest of the body. The injection is given very slowly, the fountain syringe hanging, but high enough to permit the liquid to run out. After each injection the patient should remain for half an hour or at least fifteen minutes flat on her back. This permits some of the liquid that remains in the vagina to bathe the vaginal walls and the cervix. In the average case I order two vaginal douches a day; in the morning, either the iodine or the lactic acid solution, in the evening the astringent powder. Where three or four injections a day are ordered they are used in alternation. There is no doubt as to the good effect of these injections. Not only do they keep the parts clean and mechanically remove the discharge, which is such a good nutrient medium for the various saprophytic bacteria, but they also have a gonocidal effect, heal erosions and congestions and help materially the doctor's work.

In some severe cases I also order suppositories, one suppository to be introduced at night. The suppositories usually contain as their active constituent either protargol or the lactic acid bacillus.

The patient comes to the office always immediately after having taken a thorough douche. The only time the douche is left out is when the doctor wants to make a bacteriologic examination of the secretions. He wipes off the vulva, examines carefully for any inflamed points or erosions, and if there are any he touches them with silver nitrate 10 to 50 per cent., or even with the silver nitrate stick. The ducts of Bartholin's glands are examined carefully, an attempt is made to express any pus, and if found necessary they are cauterized with a thin probe, or a 10 per cent. silver nitrate solution is injected into them by means of a hypodermic syringe with a blunted needle. The urethra is next examined and if affected is swabbed with a 5 to 10 per cent. silver nitrate solution. As a rule the urethra responds to treatment very readily. I have no use for any urethral bougies or suppositories in women any more than I have for them in men. The vagina is next examined with a speculum and a good light, and erosions, if any, are touched with silver nitrate solution, 10 per cent., or tincture of iodine full strength. Lactic acid full strength is also a good application.

We then come to the cervix, which is the most important part of the treatment. We wipe it off as carefully as we can, introduce several cotton-wound probes and try to remove the cervical plug. The entire cervix is then painted with tincture of iodine, and a thin cotton swab dipped into tincture of iodine is gently introduced into the os. Care is taken not to pass the internal os, though if it should pass, the danger of extension of the infection would be nil or practically nil. Iodine is one of the best agents we have in treating gonorrhea of the female, and while I still use silver nitrate applications to the vagina, vulva and urethra, as far as the cervix is concerned I limit myself exclusively to iodine. My results have been much better since exchanging silver nitrate for iodine, because silver nitrate denudes the delicate surface of the cervix and may perhaps be influential in causing an extension of the inflammation. Instead of a probe, a thin long uterine syringe may be used and a few drops of tincture of iodine may be deposited in the cervix.

When the infection has spread into the endometrium and the tubes, then it really ceases to be a genito-urinary and becomes a gynecological case. But the gynecological surgeon can do medicinally no more than the ordinary physician, unless it is a case which demands operation. The proper treatment of endometritis and salpingitis is rest, hot or cold applications by means of compresses or poultices to the abdomen, and tampons of gauze saturated in glycerite of boro-glycerin or ichthyol-glycerin or thigenol-glycerin. That is all we can do and that is all we should do. Injecting or swabbing the uterus with caustic or strong antiseptic applications, scraping or curetting the uterus, all these are brutal and useless procedures; not only useless but injurious. They may do good in some cases, but the cases in which they do harm are so much in preponderance that no conscientious physician should employ them. We can never be sure of removing all the germs by these measures, while we are pretty sure to cause their further spread and development and to aggravate the inflammation. Curetting is not abused so much now as it was formerly, but it is still practiced ten times more often than it should be. Hot baths, particularly concentrated sea-salt baths, are useful in aiding the absorption of exudates. And I repeat that unless the case is a distinctly surgical case, demanding surgical intervention, this is all the gynecologist, genito-urinary surgeon or general practitioner can do.

Discussion.

Doctor W. B. Pigg, Okmulgee: Mr. Chairman, Gentlemen of the Society: In speaking to a paper that opposes my views I have much to say, or, if I am unable to say it by virtue of the fact that I cannot speak, I think a great deal, but in the paper presented to us today, I find it as Pilate did when Jesus was brought before him and he washed his hands, and he said, "I find no fault with this man." His ideas so accord with my own that, searching as I could for an avenue to enter a wedge of complaint, I have been unsuccessful. The paper is good and it is practical, it is an everyday paper, it is a paper that you doctors who have practiced in country districts can follow with success, and feel safe. As he says, they never apply until some pain announces itself, and there is really the only point I desire to emphasize. Right in your practice and in mine there are many women suffering from pelvic trouble brought about by an uncured gonorrhea of their consort that they never realized, nor do they believe that there is any infecting germ disturbing them. And in those cases, those unusual cases, you will find more often than not that the disturbing factor is the gonococci. Bear in mind the cases that come to your office with pelvic pain, and while they hurt as they go down the steps and the jolt will jar them on the left side, usually, sometimes on the right; you take a smear, it proves to you nothing; and yet those women have fistulas, those women have adhesions, and their husbands, if you know them—jitney drivers, barbers, carpenters, what not—will give a history of having had the gonorrhea a half a dozen times; but they are well now, the last they had was six months ago and they had a bottle of Big T or HGS or PGT, or whatever it is, and it cured them and they are not running, but though you can't find the germs by looking at their consorts, you can find a safe basis to predicate your opinion upon, that you have an infection caused by gonorrhea.

It is not the plain cases that the doctor has described that puzzle us; we all know those. He has told us the plain cases and I know them and you know them and the men on the street know them, everybody knows them, but it is those obscure cases, cases occurring in families in which you would not think, and yet at the basis there is a gonorrhea. Perhaps I am encroaching too much upon the section of gynecology, but even so, if I do, I am telling him the trees to look up for the squirrel.

Now, as the doctor has said, they never apply for the treatment until some acute pain drives them to the office, and when they do that, fellows, it is too late for you genito-urinary people to do any good. Just mark that down! Whenever a woman applies to you for the pain from which she has been suffering for a long time, and then she comes to you as a genito-urinary man, or as a man that knows how to fix the fixings of folks, it is too late for you to do any good. You are then on the border line of the gynecologist, and unless you want to go over the top and into the other domain, you had better call consultation then and there. That has been my experience, not only often, but painfully often and again.

He speaks of the suction of the uterus in drawing the inflammation up. I do not believe that, not a word of it. The suction of the uterus does not draw it up, there is no suction of the uterus except where there is a ———— on the part of the woman. If there is an inflammation by extinction it is either by continuity of service or by the lymphatics, so that the suction of the uterus is not there at all.

I have got some more notes, but I cannot read them, and as I have only got one minute more I will spend that by thanking you for your kind attention.

Doctor Linn (closing): In conclusion I will say that in regard to the suction action, that a great many authorities claim it is true, some claim it is not, but I think that there is considerable suction action of the uterus as a matter of course, and the female has an organ, it may happen in this case, in rupture, especially do you find it in virgins or in young brides more often than in any other class of people. You never find it in a woman that has been married any length of time, where you have this salpingitis so rapidly as last made mention of in this paper.

CLINICAL REPORT OF OPERATION ON PUERPERAL SUPPURATIVE MASTITIS.

Fred S. Clinton, M. D., F. A. C. S.

PRESIDENT AND CHIEF SURGEON OKLAHOMA HOSPITAL

TULSA, OKLAHOMA

Mrs. P. F., admitted to Oklahoma Hospital, February 21st, for confinement. On March 3, 1919, she developed rapid pulse, temperature of 104, with localized pain, heat, swelling and redness of right breast. These symptoms of mastitis responded promptly to usual attention. However, after returning home, and not being careful, about March 28th, she began to have chills, fever, rapid pulse, sweating, and pain, swelling, etc., in the right breast which was permitted to run along for two or three days and when admitted to the hospital for the second time on April 1st, a diagnosis was made of puerperal suppurative mastitis. Immediate operation was advised and assented to and thorough drainage was had through two incisions extending to the pus pockets and in a line radiating from the nipple, dressing being applied as hereafter described. Patient made an uneventful recovery.

The inflammatory process of the breast of a recently confined woman may be located as follows: In the: (a) Subcutaneous tissue of the areola, (b) Gland of parenchyma proper, (c) Retromammary space.

Early diagnosis is not always easy. In absence of local edema, fluctuation, etc., associated with history of recent confinement, appearance seven to twenty-one days thereafter of the following group of local symptoms subsequent to a fissure at or near nipple: (a) Pain, (b) Heat, (c) Swelling, and (d) Redness, and constitutional symptoms varying from slight malaise with increasing pulse and temperature to rapid pulse and high temperature with all appearance of profound sepsis.

Prompt attention should be directed to: (a) Emptying, (b) Cleansing, (c) Supporting the breast, and (d) Producing thorough saline catharsis.

If relief is not obtained in forty-eight hours, suppuration may be counted upon and found in one or more above locations.

The following technic was used:

As soon as diagnosis is made, after thorough aseptic preparation,

(a) An incision in a line radiating from the nipple must be so placed as to afford thorough drainage to each suppurating cavity in the breast.

(b) The drainage is facilitated by use of pure gum fenestrated rubber tubes, and dressing kept moist by saturated solution of boracic acid.

(c) Breast must be supported.

(d) Patient must be kept in bed until all acute symptoms have subsided.

(e) Nourishing food and usual attention to elimination.

(f) Avoid hand contacting while dressing.

(g) Get patient up and out soon as conditions warrant.

PROCEEDINGS OF THE ST. ANTHONY CLINICAL SOCIETY.

DR. LE ROY LONG, President.   DR. LELIA ANDREWS, Secretary.

DEATH REPORTS FOR MAY, 1919.

Dr. Lelia Andrews. I. *Broncho-Pneumonia, complicating Acute Intestinal Infection.*

Baby H., age 4. Acute infection followed eating a green banana. At the end of eight days pneumonia developed in the left lung. On the following day both lungs were involved. Patient was having thin watery stools streaked with bright blood. She was very weak and emaciated. The child died of exhaustion and toxemia.

II. *Cerebral Hemorrhage—Cardiorenal Vascular Disease.*

Mrs. H., age 72. Had been in good health up to a few weeks ago when she began to feel dizzy and have headache. The condition grew worse until she was brought into the hospital in semi-conscious condition. Blood pressure 256-98. Wassermann weakly positive.

Her condition gradually grew worse until her death. Just before death the temperature was 106 degrees.

Dr. S. R. Cunningham. I. *Meningeal Hemorrhage.*

Baby H. Mother had influenza a few weeks before the delivery. Slow labot but measurements were normal. No instruments used. The child did not breathe well, was pale and relaxed. Examination showed the occipital bone had been pushed under the parietal bones causing hemorrhage. The child died in 30 hours after delivery.

Dr. S. R. Cunningham. *Adenoma and Chronic Pyonephritis.*

Mrs. H., age 39. Complained of loss in weight, metorrhagia, pyuria and pains in the sides. Urine showed albumin four plus and many pus cells. Preoperative diagnosis: Chronic salpingitis, pelvic cellulitis, with involvement of the left ovary. Left salpingo-oophorectomy, Baldy-Webster, appendectomy and left nephrectomy were done by anterior incision. Rubber tube was inserted and stab was made posteriorly for drain. Two days later patient died.

Discussion.

Dr. L. A. Turley. Microscopic examination of the kidney showed a chronic pyonephrosis on a capsuloglomerular and intercapillary glomerular nephritis. The fibrosed glomerulae had undergone hyaline degeneration and the capsule was thickened. The proximal system was absent. In one end of the kidney was a yellow mass the size of an olive which proved to be adenoma. The distal tubules were firm and divided by septae except in places where there were degenerative masses.

Final diagnosis: Adenoma and chronic pyonephritis.

CASE REPORTS.

DR. W. A. FOWLER.

Case No. I. 21727. *Pregnancy Complicated by Eclampsia.* Mrs. D., age 39. Has had enlarged thyroid for five years which has made her nervous and often obstructing breathing. First three months of pregnancy accompanied by nausea and vomiting, the last period of gestation by thyroid enlargement.

June 2nd patient complained of headache which was followed by a convulsion. She was brought to the hospital in semi-conscious condition. B. P. 170-95. Eighteen-hour catheterized specimen showed 700 c. c. urine with ablumin acetone and diacetic, showing a condition of acidosis.

The treatment after a convulsion is always a question. The treatment in general was rest in bed, no food, free elimination and soda bicarbonate. I used morphine 1-8 p. r. n. for the nervousness, gastric lavage and soda bicarbonate solution for acidosis, 4 oz. castor oil, with one drop croton oil and 40 gr. of bromide were given through the tube followed by high enema. Then soda solution dram every two hours was given by mouth until the acidosis was clear. No food was given from the 2nd to the 7th, then milk and lime water, and finally malted milk was given. One June 4th, 650 c. c. of blood was withdrawn and the B. P. reduced to 160. Fetel heart tones were 168.

On June 8th, following the feeding, the B. P. was 200 due to auto-intoxication. The fetal heart tones were becoming irregular and less distinct. Her urine was free from albumin and diacetic and the quantity was normal. It was 2500 to 3000 c. c. when I first saw her on the day she came to the hospital. Her non-protein nitrogen was below normal, 17.5 mg. per 100 c. c. against 62.5 mg. when she came in. Since she was in good condition for labor, it was decided to terminate the labor the morning of the 9th, but nature anticipated our actions and pains began. She was given morphine 1-8 twice and scopolamine 1-300 once. Easy forceps delivery was accomplished under light anesthesia.

The child was stillbirth, small and undernourished.

Case No. II. *Pregnancy with Threatened Eclampsia.* Mrs. H., age 38. Enlarged thyroid with hyperthyroidism, considerable nausea and vomiting during the latter part of gestation. Morphine was given on several occasions to prevent miscarriage. Edema of hands and feet. Albumin and casts in the urine. The non-protein nitrogen was 85 mg. per 100 c. c. of blood. B. P. 175.

Under the treatment outlined in case 1, the patient improved considerably and is awaiting labor.

Discussion.

Dr. Lelia Andrews. Toxemia of pregnancy certainly is one condition in which we are rewarded by careful examination and supervision of obstetrical cases. The responsibility is grave but the condition may be controlled if we begin early. In New York Lying-In Hospital large doses of morphine are used. The soda is of great value in treating the acidosis. I agree with Dr. Fowler on his views about interrupting the pregnancy.

Dr. M. Smith. The cause of eclampsia is unknown. It is some toxemia due to faulty elimination. In toxemias we have been taught to remove the cause. Why not remove the cause in this condition? The next convulsion may end in death. The morphine quiets the nerves and gives the patient a chance to gain resistance for the labor. If pregnancy is the cause, terminate the pregnancy.

The thyroid undergoes some change during menstruation and is said to enlarge during pregnancy, but the hypersecretion in these cases made it more grave. The most essential thing to watch is the blood pressure. There may be severe cases with no albumin or there may be albumin with no convulsions, but the blood pressure is the guide.

Dr. J. S. Hartford. This is a case of a primipara 39 years old with a fetus apparently in good condition. Why not deliver? If delivery is attempted, use morphine to quiet the nerves. If you do not deliver, use no morphine because it ties up the secretions, 1-8 may cause anuria. By terminating the pregnancy the mortality is better for the mother and there is a possibility of saving the child. This late in life the child means a great deal to the mother.

Dr. J. F. Kuhn. In a case of this kind I think a hurried cesarean section does less harm than waiting. If there is some dilitation, use forceps and deliver the child.

Dr. Long. It is dangerous to base our opinions on all of our cases, but in any case of eclampsia I think it is best to empty the uterus. Give her a chance to get well if possible. I don't know of a single death to the mother with this procedure.

In case of a primipara with no dilitation, do a cesarean. The risk is no greater than any other surgical operation.

Dr. Fowler (closing). I wish to thank the gentlemen for their discussions. I deliberately brought them on because I wanted to hear the different views on the termination of pregnancy.

Why wait?

1. Because it gives a better mortality. Stroganov, from a large number of cases, reported 6.6 per cent. mortality by waiting, against 25 to 30 per cent. by the radical treatment.

Why wait?

2. Because it is more logical to wait. This condition is not due solely to pregnancy but to the altered metabolism and the absorption of toxins from the overworked alimentary system. The source of danger to our patients' lives in these cases is the pathological state, namely, degenerative processes in the vital organs, especially the liver and kidneys, acidosis and profound shock. It is true that immediate radical procedure will terminate the pregnancy but in so doing we may so increase this dangerous pathological state as to lose the lives of our patients.

Why wait?

3. Because the clinical course of these cases indicated an improvement in the pathological condition and it would seem wise to wait as long as the general condition was being improved. When I first saw case No. 1, she was passing 2500 to 3000 c. c. urine per day. At the time of delivery the quantity was normal, the albumin had disappeared, the acetone and diacetic was less, the non-protein nitrogen had dropped from 62.5 mg. per 100 c. c. of blood to 17.5 mg., and her general appearance was very much less toxic. According to every evidence the general condition was gradually improving.

As to the fetus—if there is a slight increase in the per cent. of babies born dead as a result of conservative treatment, let us remember that the babies in these cases of premature delivery are not physically 100 per cent., prematurity being one of the most frequent causes of death. While there may be a slightly larger number of babies born dead following conservative treatment, there will be as many live babies leaving the hospital as in the radical treatment. And if there is an increase, it is much less than the improvement in maternal mortality, and we should certainly say that the mother whose status in society is established, is entitled to at least as much consideration as the unborn baby.

In recent years there has been a great amount of discussion relative to the treatment of eclampsia. The opinion of authorities cannot yet be said to be agreed on any line of treatment. The tendency however, is very strong toward the conservative treatment. Edgar (*J. A. M. A.*, Apr. 27, 1918, page 1205) stands for conservative treatment. He believes that the cesarean section must be considered in primipara with long rigid cervix and in cases of disproportion between the size of the head and pelvis. McPherson, formerly one of the strongest advocates of the radical treatment, is now a strong supporter of the conservative treatment. He shows a marked improvement in the mortality at the New York Lying-In Hospital, (*J. A. M. A.*, Oct. 27, 1917, page 1467). Stroganov, in a series of 360 cases treated conservatively, reported a maternal mortality of 6.6 per cent., and a fetal mortality of 21 per cent. Tweedy, with a slightly less conservative treatment, reported a maternal mortality of 8.11 per cent. and a fetal mortality of 30 per cent. Davis (*J. A. M. A.*, Oct. 27, 1917, page 1466), reports 25 cases treated by cesarean section with a maternal mortality of 32 per cent., and a fetal mortality of 31 per cent. Austin Flint (*A. J. Obst.*, Nov., 1918, page 413) considers that a patient in eclampsia is in a condition of shock and that an attempt at operative delivery increases this shock. Tweedy and Wrench say the objections to accouchment force are that it leads to severe shock; if performed during the convulsive period, it increases the irritation of the poisoned nerve centers; sepsis is liable to arise after it; nor have any statistics covering long periods of time yet been published that show its superiority as a treatment over the treatment adopted at the Rotunda Hospital and elsewhere.

JOURNAL OF THE OKLAHOMA STATE MEDICAL ASSOCIATION

VOLUME XII   MUSKOGEE, OKLA., OCTOBER, 1919   NUMBER 10

PUBLISHED MONTHLY AT MUSKOGEE, OKLA., UNDER DIRECTION OF THE COUNCIL

DR. CLAUDE A. THOMPSON, EDITOR-IN-CHIEF
506-9 BARNES BUILDING, MUSKOGEE

DR. CHAS. W. HEITZMAN, ASSISTANT EDITOR
BARNES BUILDING, MUSKOGEE

ENTERED AT THE POST OFFICE AT MUSKOGEE, OKLAHOMA, AS SECOND CLASS MAIL MATTER, JULY 28, 1912

THIS IS THE OFFICIAL JOURNAL OF THE OKLAHOMA STATE MEDICAL ASSOCIATION. ALL COMMUNICATIONS SHOULD BE ADDRESSED TO THE JOURNAL OF THE OKLAHOMA STATE MEDICAL ASSSOCIATION, 308 SURETY BUILDING, MUSKOGEE, OKLAHOMA.

The editorial department is not responsible for the opinions expressed in the original articles of contributors.

Reprints of original articles will be supplied at actual cost, provided request for them is attached to manuscript or made in sufficient time before publication.

Articles sent this Journal for publication and all those read at the annual meetings of the State Association are the sole property of this Journal. The Journal relies on each individual contributor's strict adherence to this well-known rule of medical journalism. In the event an article sent this Journal fo publication is published before appearance in the Journal, the manuscript will be returned to the writer

Failure to receive the Journal should call for immediate notification of the editor, 307-8 Surety Building, Muskogee, Okla

Local news of possible interest to the medical profession, notes on removals, changes in address, deaths and weddings will be gratefully received.

Advertising of articles, drugs or compounds unapproved by the Council on Pharmacy of the A. M. A. will not be accepted.

Advertising rates will be supplied on application. It is suggested that wherever possible members of the State Associa tion should patronize our advertisers in preference to others as a matter of fair reciprocity.

EDITORIAL

OVERTRAINING THE NURSE.

More than fifty thousand deaths occurred during the influenza epidemic which might have been prevented had fairly efficient nursing been available, according to the estimate of a well known Chicago practitioner. Sharply criticising the short-sighted rules and regulations of law and health boards which require hospitals to admit only the super-trained nurse, the conclusion is reached that:

"The best class of nurses come from young women who have had good home training, grammar school education, and who are from bread-winning families." Another writer believes "Nurses are frequently retained in training schools who are incompetent and unsatisfactory, because they have had one year of high-school education in compliance with the requirements of the State Board of Nurse Examiners." Daughters of thousands of mechanics have been rejected from such schools because they have not been in position to obtain the one year preliminary, but are thoroughly qualified otherwise. It is pointed out that thousands of wounded soldiers obtained very efficient first aid, not from super-educated nurses, but from orderlies who had had very little except intensive training for a few weeks or months after they had been taken from the ranks.

We thoroughly agree that the trend of the times seems to point to a condition which will ultimately make candidates for the nursing profession fewer and fewer until the dearth of nurses will be felt throughout the country. There is no good reason why an intelligent woman should be required to give three years of her time in order to master the fundamentals necessary to carry out the orders of the attending physician. While thorough education of the nurse is to be encouraged and the completest information and instruction given her, it is not necessary to require a course of study substantially equivalent in time to that taken by the bulk of physicians under whom she must work. If the breaking-in process, drudgery, and similar time-wasting processes were eliminated from the three years course required, at least one year could be profitably saved to the nurse, which in turn could be given to the care of sick people who are suffering for the lack of care they should have. As the matter now stands, the creation of the nurse from raw material savors much of the apprentice system of unionism. Each one, regardless of mental and physical fitness, goes through the same, often silly, course of preliminary work, each demands the same remuneration before and after finishing, without reference to the amount of work performed or the superiority of the service rendered above that of her fellow worker.

The physician only requires his orders executed; to do this the nurse needs intelligence, energy and a sensible amount of training. That a course in anatomy and chemistry is necessary to this end is certainly debatable and much suffering could be obviated by instruction in the essentials, leaving the higher education of the nurse to postgraduate work as she develops taste and capability to receive it.

PERSONAL AND GENERAL NEWS

Dr. John W. Duke, Guthrie, was reported ill in September.

Dr. A. N. Lerscov, Claremore, was critically ill in September.

Dr. W. R. Leverton, Hobart, is doing post graduate work in St. Louis.

Dr. Fred Boso, Tulsa, is reported answering emergency calls by airplane.

Dr. W. P. Hailey, Haileyville, reported seriously ill in October, is improving.

Dr. J. P. Cowman, Comanche, returned from California points in September.

Dr. W. L. Knight, Wewoka, spent two weeks of October with the Mayo clinic.

Dr. D. E. Little, Eufaula, has been discharged from the army and returned to his home.

Dr. C. W. Tedrow, Woodward, has returned from the Philadelphia and New York clinics.

Dr. J. C. Breedlove, Sallisaw, suffered from a broken arm when he attempted to crank a car.

Dr. S. N. Chattergee, Norman, has located in Muskogee and opened offices in the Flynn-Ames Building.

Dr. L. M. Sackett, Oklahoma City, has returned from a Colorado vacation and trip to the clinics of New York.

Dr. J. C. Johnston, McAlester, has opened his new x-ray laboratory for the treatment of the diseases of the skin.

Dr. Walter Hardy, Ardmore, attended the meeting of the American Hospital Association held in Cincinnati, in September.

Dr. Frank P. Davis and Miss Athie Eliza Sale were married at Enid, September 25th. They will be at home after November 15th.

Dr. L. Haynes Buxton, Oklahoma City, delivered an address before the Colorado Congress, on Ophthalmology, which met in Denver in August.

Drs. Ben C. Harris and O. C. Coppedge, Bristow, have been appointed Superintendents of Health for the Eastern and Western Districts of the County.

Dr. J. Clay Williams, after trying to leave Oklahoma and reside in Mississippi, has seen the error of his ways and announces his return to Miami.

Dr. R. L. Westover, Okmulgee, has been discharged from the army after oversea service, and resumed eye, ear, nose and throat work at his old location.

Okmulgee County Medical Society met at Henryetta, October 13th, with the following program: Function of the Nose, Dr. Wm. Nagle, Muskogee; Influenza, Dr. E. C. Byram, Okmulgee; Sleeping Sickness, Dr. I. W. Bollinger, Henryetta; Literature and the Doctor, Dr. R. J. Crabill, Citra.

Iowa State Medical Society publishes the following condensed information relative to the operation of Medical Defense by the Society during the last ten years since its inception. Total amount of damages claimed in all cases, $1,669,398.00; judgments recovered against members, 4; aggregate amount of judgments, $5,275.00. This showing is an eloquent indictment of the class of litigants who bring such suits and their attorneys.

St. Louis Clinics. Some of the members of the Saint Louis Medical Society have organized a section of that body called the Clinical Section of the Saint Louis Medical Society, and have established a system of clinics to which members of our association are invited when they are in St. Louis. The advertisement appears in this issue under the heading Saint Louis Clinics. There is a large amount of clinical material in St. Louis which has never been organized, but now should afford splendid opportunities for physicians who desire to take advantage of the arrangement.

The Medical Association of the Southwest, meeting at Oklahoma City, held its election October 8th, with the following results: President, Dr. Ernest Day, of Arkansas City Kan.; Vice Presidents, Drs. Horace Reed, Oklahoma City; Wilse Robinson, Kansas City, Missouri; W. H. Deaderick, Hot Springs, Ark.; W. T. Wilson, Navosata, Texas; Secretary-Treasurer, F. H. Clark, El Reno. The principal feature of the meeting was the clinics held in various Oklahoma City hospitals.

Muskogee County Medical Society tendered returned army medical officers a banquet at the Severs Hotel, October 13th, Hon. N. A. Gibson acting as toastmaster on account of the linguistic modesty of the President, Dr. J. L. Blakemore. The eats were good, the preliminaries passably so, war time prohibitory measures considered. The speaking mostly confined to returned soldiers, varied from the most excellent to the usual level of scintillating after-dinner wit. The French offered up by the speakers was accepted at par and without question. The entire affair was voted a pronounced success by more than forty well entertained guests.

MISCELLANEOUS

THIRD SURVEY OF HOSPITALS.

The third survey of hospitals being made under the auspices of the American Medical Association is now well under way. Through an extensive correspondence and a third questionnaire, the association has collected a mass of information on the subject. Much of this material has been tabulated and forwarded to committees in each state representing the state medical associations. Most of the state committees have arranged definite lines of action and by inspection of the hospitals or by other methods are securing first-hand information by which the data collected by the Association is being carefully checked. The immediate end sought is to provide a reliable list of hospitals which are in position to furnish a satisfactory intern training. The investigation is not limited to intern hospitals, however, but will cover all institutions and the data obtained will be useful in any future action which may be taken in classifying hospitals. The work in Oklahoma is in charge of a committee of which Dr. Fred S. Clinton, President, Oklahoma Hospital, of Tulsa, is chairman and the other two members being Dr. M. Smith, Associate Professor of Clinical Surgery, University of Oklahoma School of Medicine, Oklahoma City, and Dr. C. A. Thompson, Secretary, Oklahoma State Medical Association, Muskogee. The closer relationship which the hospital now bears to the public in the community which it serves makes it all the more important that the service rendered by it shall be excellent in character.

INFLUENZA WARNING!

Even though the re-occurence of influenza this fall is still a matter of opinion, it behooves us all to be prepared in every way to crush the very first evidence of another epidemic. Thorough prophylactic measures should be put widely in force everywhere with the first case which appears. Only in this case can we prevent its rapid spread and consequent suffering.

Probably the greatest prophylactic measure developed during the last epidemic was Dakin's remarkable antiseptic, Dichloramine-T. Previous investigations by military medical men had demonstrated its power to prevent infectious diseases originating in the upper air passages, such as meningitis, diphtheria, etc., and had shown its ability to clean up diphtheria carriers.

Its use as a spray to the nose and throat to prevent influenza was therefore perfectly logical. Thousands of people, in some cases the entire working force of large industrial plants, received sprays twice daily to nose and throat of a 2 per cent. solution of Dichloramine-T in Chlorcosane. Also they were instructed to use as a gargle, Chlorazene, Abbott, 0.25 per cent solution every two hours and before entering street cars or other public places.

The results were gratifying. Wherever these measures were carried out the incidence of influenza was unusually small. Further information on the uses of Dichloramine-T and Chlorazene may be obtained upon request to The Abbott Laboratories, Chicago, Ill.

SOUTHERN MEDICAL ASSOCIATION, THIRTEENTH ANNUAL MEETING, ASHEVILLE, NORTH CAROLINA, "LAND OF THE SKY," NOVEMBER 10-13, 1919.

ANNOUNCEMENT.

Monday, November 10th: Section on Urology, Section on Pediatrics, National Malaria Committee (Conference on Malaria), Southern States Association of Railway Surgeons, Conference on Medical Education, Southern Gastro-Enterological Association, and at night a public meeting under the direction of the Section on Public Health.

Tuesday forenoon: The formal opening with the addresses of welcome, address of the President, Dr. Lewellys F. Barker, the Orations on Medicine, Surgery and Public Health, etc.

Tuesday afternoon, Wednesday and Thursday: Section on Medicine, Section on Public Health, Section on Surgery and Section on Eye, Ear, Nose and Throat. Also on these days the American

Child Hygiene Association (formerly the American Association for the Study and Prevention of Infant Mortality).

Tuesday night: A big general meeting early in the evening followed by a reception to the President at the famous Battery Park Hotel. Wednesday night: another general meeting.

A great program, delightful entertainment, beautiful scenery, balmy climate, fine hotels and plenty, reduced rates on all railroads—everything just ideal for this meeting.

SEALE HARRIS, M. D., Secretary,
Southern Medical Association.

INFLUENZA.

(Statement by Commissioner A. R. Lewis.)

To the Medical Profession of Oklahoma:

I am writing you in regard to the possibility of a recurrence of an epidemic of influenza this fall and winter, and also to give you the benefit of information accumulated while on a tour of inspection in the east.

According to statements made by officials of the U. S. Public Health Service, there will probably be a recurrence of this disease. Surgeon General Blue has issued a bulletin calling upon city officials, state and city boards of health to take steps to combat, and prevent as far as possible, such an epidemic, and states positively that influenza is spread by direct and indirect contact. The Surgeon-General, speaking of influenza, also says:

"It is not yet certain that the germ has been isolated or discovered, and, as a consequence, there is no positive preventive treatment except the enforcement of rigid rules of sanitation and the avoidance of personal contact. . . .

"Evidence collected during last winter's epidemic points strongly to infected eating and drinking utensils, especially in places where food and drinks are sold, as being one of the modes of transmission of this disease."

The medical profession is divided in opinion as to the use of vaccine. Dr. K. P. Pearson, of Atlanta, Ga., an influenza specialist, who has recently been in Washington conferring with health authorities, says:

"Despite the efforts of specialists and physicians the world over, there has not been found a cure for the disease. The germ has not been isolated, but authorities everywhere are working to that end. This is the time of year when most persons are susceptible to colds. If colds are neglected they may lead to serious consequences."

Dr. John F. Anderson, formerly connected with the Research Laboratories of the U. S. Government, and now at the head of E. R. Squibb & Sons' Laboratories, makes the following statement:

"It is the opinion of many men in public health work that the great mortality during the recent influenza epidemic was due, not to the influenza itself, but to pneumonia caused by pneumococci of either types one, two or three, or by the streptococcus. The statistics from some of the army camps, as well as from civil hospitals, show that the high mortality rate could be traced to the pneumococcus complication of the disease, and in many cases pneumonia could be prevented by the use of pneumococcus vaccine. There have been many men in public health work who have advocated the employment of a mixed or combined vaccine to be used as a preventive or prophylactic against influenza and its complications. Statements have been made by some such as Dr. E. C. Rosenow of the Mayo Foundation, that an administration of three doses of a mixed vaccine, seven days apart, greatly reduces the number of cases of influenza, and almost eliminates the pneumonias accompanying the disease. A very striking demonstration of the value of vaccine against pneumonia is that reported by Major Cecil and Captain Austin of the U. S. Army, in the *Journal of Experimental Medicine*, dated July, 1918. They reported that at Camp Upton, 12,519 men were vaccinated with pneumococcus vaccine. The number unvaccinated was 19,481. These men were under observation about ten weeks. Three or four doses of vaccine containing types one, two and three pneumococcus were given at intervals of five to seven days. During the ten weeks following no cases of pneumonia of the three types occurred among those who had two or more injections. During the same period there were 26 cases of types one, two and three pneumonia among the unvaccinated men. There were six cases of type four pneumonia and 106 cases of streptococcus pneumonia. In other words, there were seventeen cases of pneumonia from all causes among the vaccinated, and 173 cases during the same period among the unvaccinated. The death rate for the vaccinated troops was .83 per thousand, and for the unvaccinated, 12.8 per thousand. They conclude that prophylactic vaccination against pneumococcus of types one, two and three is practical, and apparently gives protection against pneumonia produced by those types.

"According to Surgeon General Gorgas, Major Lister vaccinated miners in South Africa in three different mines with pneumococcus vaccine types A, B and C. In one mine there were no cases of pneumonia of the types used, and in the other two mines the incidence and mortality rate from pneumonia showed a definite decrease. The miners were kept under observation from six to twelve months.

"I am firmly of the opinion that the greatest mortality in influenza is due to complications of the pneumonias, and that these pneumonias can be very much lessened and their occurrence very much decreased by the administration of a mixed or combined vaccine according to the formula originated by Dr. E. C. Rosenow, of the Mayo Foundation. This formula contains

Pneumococci	3000 million
Streptococci	1000 "
Influenza	500 "
Staphylo-Aureus	500 "

Dr. Eugene L. Fisk, Director of the Life Extension Institute of New York, of which Wm. H. Taft is Board Chairman, says:

"The fighting of the epidemic disease is not a matter of medical treatment, but prevention along definite lines which we cannot follow until we identify the enemy and know where his machine gun nests are located. Until the cause of influenza is located the disease is as dangerous an enemy as were the Germans."

In the *Denver Times* of September 26, 1919, Dr. Royal S. Copeland, Commissioner of Health of New York City, is quoted as saying:

"I have no doubt but that we will have another epidemic this year, though infinitely less violent than last year's, when practically every person was affected."

When asked what could be done to prevent influenza, Dr. Copeland prescribed soap and water and fresh air. He also said influenza was essentially a house disease, and apparently needed long contact to become infectious; that it was not like smallpox which you could get in a minute, but that you had to live with influenza to get it. Dr. Copeland further says:

"It naturally follows that out-of-door life, sleeping with windows open regardless of the weather, taking exercise and using common sense with regard to food, are the best preventives.

"Above all, avoid those who have influenza. In families, patients who have colds ought to be kept by themselves, they should not associate with others.

"Apparently the germs of influenza are conveyed by the hands more easily than other ways. Everyone should have clean hands. People should make it a rule to wash their hands and faces several times a day with soap and water.

"There is no cause for excitement since the Board of Health are watching symptoms of influenza the world over, and is co-operating with other Boards of Health throughout America.

"Masks are no good. This has been demonstrated to the satisfaction of scientists. We are old fashioned here and do not believe in closing schools and churches. We did everything unconventional here in 1918 and had the lowest death rate of all. Masks are filthy, preventing the patient from getting good air,and cause him to rebreathe bad air."

It is reported that in Australia at this time there is a wave of influenza of a particularly virulent type sweeping through New South Wales; that the fatalities are far higher in proportion than last year, and that in Sydney whole families in the congested areas are stricken down and many dying for the lack of nursing and medical attendance.

Because of the movement of troops from districts in Europe where influenza was generally prevalent and lingered long, there is considerable danger of its recrudescense in this country. It therefore behooves all health authorities, and especially those at ports of disembarkation, to be on the alert and to take ample preventive measures. If this plague again gets a foothold it will be next to impossible to bar its rapid progress. The health authorities of this country should therefore get together and suggest to the public at large such necessary precautions as in the premises seem advisable. Our people on the whole are well disciplined, and will follow when a lead is given them.

That influenza is coming back is also the opinion of scientists who have pledged support to Dr. O. P. Geir, of Cincinnati in his fight for a congressional appropriation of $5,000,000.00 for the study of the causes and means of preventive medicine section of the American Medical Association, the fight for it being led in Congress by Senator Harding and Representative Fess, both of Ohio.

Now, as you will see from above quotations from men of varied experience, and who were authorities on the treatment and handling of influenza in the last epidemic, that the profession is agreed upon no definite plan of preventive treatment, nor do we know very much about the disease. The only common points agreed upon seem to be sanitation and cleanliness, well ventilated sleeping quarters and the avoidance of crowded and congested places, and that we are almost certain to have a recurrence of this disease.

There, I earnestly ask the medical profession of Oklahoma to co-operate with me along these lines, giving me their hearty support, and to use their own judgment in regard to the use of vaccine.

I also desire that all physicians in the state keep me posted as to any outbreak of influenza in their communities. This is necessary not only from a statistical standpoint, but that I may be in a position to render aid or relief where necessary and desired.

I am in receipt of the following letter from Surgeon General Blue:

"Dr. A. R. Lewis, Commissioner,
  Department of Public Health,
    Oklahoma City, Okla.
"Dear Doctor:

"In order to be prepared for the possible recurrence of influenza in epidemic form, the Bureau desires to have lists of physicians available for emergency epidemic duty in each state.

"May I ask you to secure and forward to this Bureau a list of 100 physicians in your state who would be willing to serve under your direction in such an emergency.

"The salary will be $200 per month, a per diem of $4.00 for subsistence, together with railroad fare. The Bureau will utilize these men in their own state, and in so far as possible, in their own communities.

"An early reply will be appreciated.
                                        Yours very respectfully,
                                            (Signed) RUPERT BLUE,
                                                Surgeon General."

Trusting that I may have the hearty support of the entire profession in this state; that fully 100 doctors will write me at an early date signifying their willingness to serve in the event of an epidemic, and that all county health officers will start a clean-up campaign and instruct the people along that line, I beg to be,

                                        Yours fraternally,
                                            A. R. LEWIS,
                                                State Commissioner of Health.

COUNCIL ON PHARMACY AND CHEMISTRY
AMERICAN MEDICAL ASSOCIATION

This report is limited according to the ideas and opinions as to its usefulness and practicability to Oklahoma physicians. A complete report is obtainable upon request from the Council, 535 North Dearborn St., Chicago.

PROPAGANDA FOR REFORM.

Arsenoven S. S. and Solution of Arsenic and Mercury not Accepted. The Council on Pharmacy and Chemistry reports that Arsenoven S. S., sold by the S. S. Products Co., Philadelphia, and Solution of Arsenic and Mercury (formerly called Arseno-Meth-Hyd) of the New York Intravenous Laboratory, New York, are inadmissible to New and Nonofficial Remedies because unwarranted therapeutic claims are made for them and because the names are not descriptive of the composition of these preparations. Arsenoven S. S. is claimed to contain dimethylarsenin 15.4 grains, mercury biniodid 1-10 grain, sodium iodid 1-2 grain. Dimethylarsenin is asserted to be similar to sodium cacodylate, but with a more pronounced therapeutic action. Solution of Arsenic and Mercury comes in three dosages, 2 gm., 1.5 gm., and 0.7 gm., respectively. The 2 gm. form is claimed to contain 2 gm. (31 grains) of sodium dimethylarsenate (cacodylate), U. S. P., and mercury iodid 5 mg. (1-12 grain) in 5 c.c. of solution. Both preparations are advised for the treatment of syphilis, intravenously. The report of the Council reminds physicians that cacodylates have been found inefficient as spirocheticides and warns against the abuses—often dangerous—to which patients are frequently subjected when "intravenous therapy" is employed (Jour A. M. A., Aug. 2, 1919, p. 353).

Hormotone and Hormotone without Post-Pituitary. The Council on Pharmacy and Chemistry reports that Hormotone of the G. W. Carnrick Company is advertised as "A pluriglandular tonic for asthenic conditions." The same firm also advertises Hormotone Without Post-Pituitary for use "in neurasthenic conditions associated with high blood pressure." These preparations are sold in the form of tablets for oral administration. Each tablet of Hormotone is said to contain 1-10 grain desiccated thyroid and 1-20 grain of entire pituitary together with the hormones of the ovary and testes—the amounts and the form in which the latter are supposed to be present are not given. From this it is seen that the only definite information given the medical profession regarding the composition of Hormotone is that it is a weak thyroid and a still weaker pituitary preparation. Hormotone without Post-Pituitary is said to contain in each tablet 1-10 grain desiccated thyroid, and to "prevent" "hormone bearing extracts of thyroid, anterior pituitary, ovary and testes." The Council declared these preparations inadmissible to New and Nonofficial Remedies, because: (1) Their composition is semisecret, (2) The therapeutic claims are unwarranted, (3) They are sold under names not descriptive of their composition, but suggestive of their indiscriminate use as "tonics" (4) In the light of our present knowledge, the routine administration of pluriglandular mixtures is irrational (Jour. A. M. A., Aug. 16, 1919, p. 549).

Bromide and Acetanilid Compound. The period of acceptance having expired for Granular Effervescent Bromide and Acetanilid Compound-Mulford, the Council of Pharmacy and Chemistry directed its omission from New and Nonofficial Remedies because an examination of the available evidence demonstrated that mixtures of this kind are inimical to rational medicine and the public. The use of mixtures of bromide and acetanilid in fixed proportions is irrational and prone to induce their indiscriminate use by the public—and this despite the perfectly frank declaration of the composition of this mixture by the manufacturer (Rep. Coun. Pharm. Chem. 1918, p. 58).

Pollen Antigen. Pollen antigen-Lederle is a pollen extract which represents the pollen of plants blooming in spring and in fall. The Council on Pharmacy and Chemistry declared these preparations inadmissible to New and Nonofficial Remedies because there appeared no warrant for complex pollen preparations representing both spring and fall pollens. In consideration of the essentially experimental status of the use of pollen preparations for the prevention and treatment of "hay-fever," such products should be as simple as possible. Hence pollen protein preparations prepared from the pollen of two or more species of plants are accepted for New and Nonofficial Remedies only if there is evidence that the given combination is rational (Rep. Coun. Pharm. Chem.. 1918, p. 65).

Restoria. "Restoria for Bad Blood" is sold by the Restoria Chemical Company of Kansas City, Mo. It is sold as a sure cure for syphilis, but is also recommended for rheumatism, kidney trouble, lumbago, eczema and catarrh. The A. M. A. Chemical Laboratory reports that Restoria contains no mercury or arsenic but does contain iodid, probably as potassium iodid, equivalent to 1.693 gm. per hundred cc. It also was found to contain much vegetable extractive, some alkaloidal drug and a bitter oil or oleoresin (Jour. A. M. A., Aug. 9, 1919, p. 438).

Cinchophen: formerly Atophan. The Chemical Foundation, Inc., which has purchased some 4,500 German-owned patents, many of them for synthetic drugs, proposes to continue the wise policy of the Federal Trade Commission by requiring that those who receive licenses for the use of patents for synthetic drugs must use a common designation for each drug selected by the foundation. Cinchophen has been selected as the designation for the substance introduced as atophan (also described in the U. S. Pharmacopoeia under "phenylcinchoninic acid"). In consideration of this action on the part of the Chemical Foundation and also because physicians found it difficult to use the pharmacopoeial name, phenylcinchoninic acid, the Council on Pharmacy and Chemistry has recognized the contracted term cinchophen as the name for the drug introduced as atophan (Jour. A. M. A., Aug. 9, 1919, p. 427).

The Council on Pharmacy and Chemistry. The profession should recognize that the most important factor in the clearing up of the advertising pages of medical journals has been the Council on Pharmacy and Chemistry of the American Medical Association. The Council has been criticized both by the manufacturer and the profession, but it has gone on doing the work for which it was created. Sometimes the practitioner feels that his clinical experience justifies the use of a preparation which the Council has not found reason to accept. While apparent clinical results may be misinterpreted, the carefully conducted examinations of the Council are likely to be definite and dependable. We are becoming more and more convinced of the unreliability of reports of clinical use by physicians. Practitioners should avail themselves of the Council's investigations by frequent reference to the reports of the Council. If they would keep on hand a copy of New and Nonofficial Remedies for ready reference and prescribe only of the new preparations those that have been accepted by the Council, they would aid materially in the establishment of a scientific and reliable therapeusis (Jour. Kansas Med. Soc., Aug. 1919, p. 193).

S. S. S. The state of Louisiana has a law prohibiting the sale of venereal disease remedies, except on the written prescription of a licensed physician. In May of this year, the Bureau of Venereal Diseases of the Louisiana State Board of Health notified the druggists of Louisiana that the sale of "S. S. S." ("Swift's Syphilitic Specific" or "Swift's Sure Specific") would meet with the same law enforcement measures as were being waged against any venereal disease nostrum. The result of this notice was a letter sent to various drug stores of Louisiana by the sales manager of the Swift Specific Company declaring that "S. S. S." is not recommended or advertised as a venereal medicine. A few years ago, "S. S. S." was boldly heralded in newspaper advertisements as a "cure" for syphilis. (Jour A. M. A., Aug. 30, 1919, p. 707).

NEW BOOKS

Under this heading books received by the Journal will be acknowledged. Publishers are advised that this shall constitute return for such publications as they may submit. Obviously all publications sent us cannot be given space for review, but from time to time books received, of possible interest to Oklahoma physicians, will be reviewed.

THE SURGICAL CLINICS OF CHICAGO.

The Surgical Clinics of Chicago. Volume III, Number 4 (August, 1919). Octavo of 287 pages, 116 illustrations. Philadelphia and London; W. B. Saunders Company, 1919. Published Bi-Monthly. Price, per year: Paper $10.00; Cloth $14.00.

This issue contains many articles dealing with the problems of war. Peripheral nerve surgery, bone injuries, bone transplant, ununited fractures, old dislocations, nerve injuries, and similar results of the traumas of war are given a leading position. "Methods of Examination in the Diagnosis of Abdominal Tumors," by Dr. Daniel Eisendrath, Chicago, is a profusely illustrated article based on his clinics at Cook County and Michael Reese Hospitals. "Technic of Abdominal Section," is presented by Dr. Edward H. Ochsner, Augustana Hospital; the subject, certainly an old one, is still fraught with faults and imperfections when executed in the many hands of operators. This proposes to further systematize and simplify the steps.

THE VENEREAL DISEASES.

An Outline of Their Management, Prepared Under the Direction of the Surgeon General of the Army for the Use of Medical Officers.

Revised for Use of Civilian Physicians, Third Edition, Printed for the United States Public Health Service, Rupert Blue, Surgeon General. Cloth, 159 pages, Price 25 cents. Chicago: American Medical Association, 535 North Dearborn Street.

Distributed by the State Board of Health of Oklahoma, Oklahoma City, and without question contains the last word on the treatment of venereal diseases, bearing in mind practically the unanimous opinion of authorities, able clinicians and research workers.

The book is most fitting at this time for it is generally agreed that the conception of the problem and treatment of these diseases by the general practitioner is woefully short of accepted standards. It is admitted without question that diagnostic abilities and effort for their control have improved little or none, despite the constant reiteration of lessons and well established principles appreciated by the average practitioner. It is the desire of the Public Health Service that this work be widely distributed. Oklahoma physicians are requested to communicate with Dr. J. C. Mahr, U.S.P.H.S., Oklahoma City, if they wish copies of this work.

"WHAT WE KNOW ABOUT CANCER."

A Hand-book for the Medical Profession. Prepared by a Committee of the American Society for the Control of Cancer, American Medical Associated Press, Chicago, 1918.

The American Society for the Control of Cancer has been in existence and working effectively for a number of years. The sole object of the society, at present at least, is the "dissemination of facts in regard to cancer to the end that its mortality may be reduced by a wider knowledge of the disease."

The effort represented by the present pamphlet has perhaps the most far reaching possibilities for good of any single attempt to lessen cancer mortality undertaken in this country.

It is no longer necessary to argue the point that delay is the one great factor in cancer mortality. At least four-fifths of cancer deaths could be prevented by early recognition. The conditions necessary for recognition of cancer in ample time for cure are not ideal but distinctly practicable. Public education is one important pathway of improvement, but education of the medical profession itself is of equal if not greater importance. Statistical studies have shown that in the majority of cases the doctor has had the cancer patient "under observation" over a year before efficient curative treatment is instituted. It is needless to state that during this year the majority of cases have changed from curable to incurable. As the pamphlet itself somewhat mildly puts it, "The conditions call for a far keener appreciation of responsibility for the mortality from cancer than now generally exists in the medical profession."

It is not possible here to abstract this pamphlet which is already so condensed. The general facts concerning cancer are outlined and then each important type and site of cancer is taken up in detail and the forms, symptoms, standard treatment, and results to be expected for each type.

The chief point we would make here is that if every medical man would study and seriously apply the teaching in this pamphlet, which he can read in an hour, the question of delay in cancer would be solved in so far as it is referable to the medical profession. The ultimate possible good obtainable from the wide spread dissemination of this pamphlet is so great that we would urge every possible means to get it into the hands of as many medical men of all classes as possible. It can be had from the American Medical Association, 535 N. Dearborn St., Chicago, for 10 cents. If you are a trained surgeon, get it. It will interest you. If you are further afield, get it and study and apply it. If you feel misgivings that some of your cases in the past might have been saved had you been more sure and acted more promptly (and who of us does not have such misgivings), get it. It will help you in future cases.

We would especially beg the assistance of Boards of Health, both state and municipal, and of medical societies in distributing the pamphlets. It can be bought cheaper in quantities and sent out with your other mail matter with almost no extra cost or trouble. When such a simple means for such far reaching good is in our hands it is a pity to let it lie neglected.

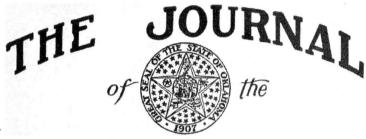

Oklahoma State Medical Association

VOLUME XII   MUSKOGEE, OKLA., NOVEMBER, 1919   NUMBER 11

SYMPOSIUM ON PNEUMONIA*

PNEUMONIA.

W. W. RUCKS, M. D.

INTERNIST, WESLEY HOSPITAL, OKLAHOMA CITY

FORMERLY INTERNIST OKLAHOMA METHODIST HOSPITAL, GUTHRIE, OKLA.

LATE MAJOR MEDICAL CORPS, U. S. ARMY, AND CHIEF OF MEDICAL SERVICE, U. S. ARMY,

BASE HOSPITAL, FORT SAM HOUSTON, TEXAS

The past two winters have been so fraught with tragedy that when one stops to review his activities he is surprised at the magnitude of it, and is at a loss to know how to correlate his labors into a comprehensive story.

The country has been afflicted by a series of epidemics of respiratory infections, concerning which much has been written and published in most all medical periodicals. And, too, there is not a physician practicing medicine in any nook or corner of this country, nor on this globe, who has not had practical experience. Each and every one has formed some original idea and has put into practice some original thoughts. The sum total of which will be the step forward in the management and treatment and prevention of respiratory diseases. It would be out of place at present to endeavor to review the thought so far recorded by the profession, but I will briefly call your attention to the various forms of pneumonia resulting from these various air passage infections.

The first epidemic or wave of infection came in September, 1917. I was then at U. S. Army Base Hospital at Fort Sam Houston, Texas, where I had been assigned to the Medical Service in July. I was put in charge of the first pneumonia ward. All pneumonias admitted and all occurring in the hospital were transferred to my ward. The result was that I was soon in charge of several full wards of pneumonia. These were truly pneumococcic pneumonias, running true to type, beginning with a chill, high temperature, rapid breathing and rapid consolidation of one or more lobes. They were studied from every angle. A routine of culture of sputum and blood, and examination of stools for parasites, blood count and pneumococcic type determination was carried out. So truly typical of lobar pneumonia was this first epidemic that a department order was issued that a diagnosis of pneumonia must not be made unless the soldier had a temperature of at least 102, a respiration of 30, and white blood count of 18,000, and it was usually possible to have all three requirements, the white count often going much higher, unlike the last epidemic, when a pronounced leukopenia prevailed. These patients recovered by crisis with the few exceptions of those slowly resolving conditions and those

*Read in Section on Surgery and Gynecology, State Medical Association, Muskogee, May 21, 1919.

in whom fluid developed. The incidence of empyema in the first epidemic was small, not larger than would be found in the same number of cases in private practice. Endeavor was made to determine the type in each case. Type one and type four predominated. Type two was not uncommon, and type three occasionally occurred. Type one anti-pneumococci serum was used in all type one cases, and there is no doubt that the mortality in patients suffering from that type was much reduced. From the early use of serum, and large doses, the best results are obtained. After desensitizing the patient, 100 c.c. of serum with 100 c.c. of normal salt solution are given in the vein, slowly by gravity, and repeated in six, eight, or twelve hours. The results at times are extremely gratifying. The mortality in this epidemic was about 12 per cent. By clinical observation, laboratory reports, and post mortem findings, these cases were truly pneumococcic lobar pneumonia. Also the small per cent. developing fluid showed a pneumococcic infection, and I think Major Blesh will bear me out in stating that these first cases respond nicely after operation, and the mortality was small.

The second lap of this 1917-18 infection gives us two distinct classes of pneumonia. One is the lobar, which we have just discussed, reinfected with the streptococcus hemolyticus, and the other is the broncho-pneumonia in which the streptococcus hemolyticus was so common that it seems to have been the causative factor. The streptococcus hemolyticus apparently made its advent with the appearance of measles. And there got to be many carriers, healthy and otherwise of that organism, and in that way, and also from cross infection in the ward, we have the second variety of pneumonias in my list, i. e., lobar re-infected with streptococcus hemolyticus. From December 1, 1917, to March 1, 1918, there were admitted 319 cases of primary lobar pneumonia, 44 or about 14 per cent. of these became re-infected with streptococcus hemolyticus. This does not include a certain small group of primary streptococcic infections affecting the chest. These 319 cases of pneumonia were all originally pneumococcic infections proven either by sputum culture, blood culture, lung puncture, or tissue culture at autopsy. Clinically, they looked and acted like lobar pneumonia up to a certain point in the progress of the disease. The streptococcus was grafted upon a lobar pneumonia. It made itself evident in a very short time. Often a pleural exudate, containing streptococcus, occurred in 24 or 48 hours after admission to the hospital. The exudate was a peculiar dirty brownish fluid containing streptococcus. Of the total number of lobar pneumonias occurring between these dates, 97 developed fluid; 22 of these were pneumococcic empyemas, of which 5 died; 33 streptococcic, of which 17 died. One showed both pneumococcic and streptococcic infection and was a fatal case. In 41 cases the fluid was sterile or undetermined, of which number, 9 died; no doubt some of these were streptococcic infections. The high incidence and high mortality of streptococcic infection is at once apparent; the mortality in these re-infected cases was over 60 per cent.

The third group of pneumonias I wish to mention is broncho-pneumonia, following measles. During the winter of 1917-18 we had 618 cases of measles, with 89 pneumonias and a mortality of 47 per cent.; 80 per cent. developing fluid in the chest.

The symptoms usually began within a few days after the onset of measles, or a few days after convalescence from that disease, with a pain in the chest, sore throat, cough, chill, fever, and general malaise. The physical signs are indefinite, but there is usually some vague dulness over the chest and rales are heard scattered widely throughout both lungs, especially at the bases posteriorly. After a few days, dulness is pronounced and usually the exploratory needle reveals the presence of a turbid fluid in the pleural cavity. This accumulates rapidly and re-accumulates with extreme rapidity when removed. This fluid invariably shows the presence of the streptococcus hemolyticus. Other complications than empyema were not uncommon, otitis media, mastoiditis, sinusitis, and generalized infection resulting in furunculosis, arthritis, and meningitis occurred.

The fourth variety of pneumonia is that which has differed from any pneumonia with which this generation of doctors has had to deal. I refer to the pandemic of pneumonitis which has invaded the entire world and has been designated Spanish influenza. I cannot give the exact number of cases treated at Base Hospital, Fort Sam Houston, but this I know, that in the latter part of September, 1918, it came like an avalanche filling the entire hospital, and every other available space. Every precaution was taken to prevent cross infection, beds were spaced ten feet apart and separated by sheets; head to foot sleeping was ordered; doctors, nurses, and corps men were gowned and masked and all sanitary precautions taken. Nevertheless, about one in six developed demonstrable physical signs of pneumonia, and it ran so true to type that it led me to believe that a potential pneumonia existed in all cases and that we might not be far wrong when we refer to the epidemic as one of pneumonitis, and that a special cause existed—bacteriological study of nose and throat swabs and culture from the sputum in the recent cases did not reveal the influenza bacillus. Neither was it found in the study of the cases that had fully developed pneumonia. In a very complete record of the bacteriology of one hundred cases of fully developed pneumonia treated in one ward by Capt. Henry J. John, the bacillus of influenza was found in three instances, in culture of sputum once, and in culture of swab from throat, twice.

Bacteriological Data on First 100 Cases Admitted.

	Sputum	%	Throat	%	
Streptococcus Hemolyticus	16	16	15	15	
Micrococcus Catarrhalis	11	11	11	11	
Bacillus Influenza	1	1	1	1	
Pneumococcus:					
Type I	1	1			
Type II	1	1			
Type IIa	5	5			
Type III	2	2			
Type IV	16	16			

	Positive	%	Negative	%	
Blood Cultures	7	7	95		

	Sterile	%	Organism	%	Type
Fluid in Chest (Total No. tapped, 24)	6	25	18	75	Streptococcus hemolyticus 13. 1 Streptococcus viridans. 3—IV —Pneumo- 1—III —coccus.

	Sterile	%	Organism	%	Type
Lung Punctures:					
Antemortem	7	50	7	50	Streptococcus
Postmortem	2	100			hemolyticus.

	Sterile	%	Organism	%	Type
Heart Punctures: (Postmortem)	2	50	2	50	Streptococcus hemolyticus. IV. Pneumococcus

As per the above chart it would seem that the old organisms with which we had been dealing were the causative organisms, but the clinical manifestation did not bear this out, and it seems that they are implanted upon the field prepared by the specific infection. Whether or not this specific infecting agent is the old influenza bacillus, many investigators are in doubt. Interesting investigations on animals have been carried out by Dr. A. J. Heinkleman, in Wesley Laboratory, Oklahoma City, and reported in the *New York Medical Journal*, April 26, in which he states that he has found a motile bacillus which he believes is a higher organism than the old influenza bacillus, but of the same family, but has changed its morphology by evolution, just as the typhoid bacillus may have evoluted from the colon bacillus. Be this as it may, we are dealing with a specific infection causing a peculiar pneumonia. I agree with Riesmon when he states that to him it appeared that pneumonia was not an accidental complication, but an integral part of the epidemic.

The symptoms of the onset of influenza are too familiar to everyone to need any reference here. The insidiousness of the beginning pneumonia is significant. Any influenza running a temperature unduly long usually does so because of involvement in the lung, and you only have to search to find it, usually in the base of one of the lungs posteriorly and is heard as a fine shower of rales at the end of a deep inspiration. This may last for a few days and the pneumonic spot clear up. And again it may rapidly spread until a great wide area of lung is consolidated, spreading to the other lung, and frequently bubbling rales appearing throughout the whole lung, announcing the fatal pulmonary edema.

The accumulation of fluid in these cases was comparatively small, but the number of slowly resolving pneumonias was comparatively large, and aspiration of these consolidated areas frequently resulted in a dry tap. These were essentially broncho-pneumonias resembling lobar, in that they became massive in their consolidations, and this term describes them best, massive bronchos.

As to treatment, that is a matter of personal preference with one or two exceptions. In the first class mentioned, pneumococcic pneumonias, in type one infection, type one anti-pneumococcic serum properly given is specific. In the measles pneumonia, treatment was very unsatisfactory and was symptomatic. We digitalized our patients, fed them and stimulated them and quieted them with sedatives. In the influenza type our only change from the general accepted ideas was in the use of glucose. We gave 250 c.c. of a 10 per cent. solution intravenously and I am satisfied with good results. The acidosis suggested its use and the results were that, after its administration, several hours of quiet rest ensued, the cyanosis was diminished, the evidence of edema lessened, the heart strengthened and elimination increased. To avoid the chill that sometimes followed, we almost habitually added 1-8 grain morphin to the solution, also if digitalis was indicated we added that; in my opinion this is our one big advance in the treatment of pneumonia. As to empyema there is a selective time to operate. We tried early operation, delayed operation, aspiration, and let-alone policy, with no material difference in results, except that those operated very early died from immediate toxemia and shock. It came to be my personal belief that three of four days' delay gave time for the patient to react and develop some degree of resistance. I am satisfied that I am correct in this.

SURGICAL COMPLICATIONS OF PNEUMONIA WITH SPECIAL REFERENCE TO EMPYEMA.

A. L. BLESH, M. D.

CHIEF OF STAFF AND SURGEON TO WESLEY HOSPITAL,
OKLAHOMA CITY.

FORMERLY MAJOR AND CHIEF OF SERVICE, U. S. ARMY, BASE HOSPITAL,
FORT SAM HOUSTON, TEXAS, AND BASE HOSPITAL,
CAMP SHERIDAN, ALABAMA.

GENERAL CONSIDERATIONS:

It has been familiar knowledge for many years that the pneumococcus will give rise to surgical infections of many kinds, in different locations, that no tissue can be said to be exempt from its invasion. What can be said of the pneumococcus with which we are all familiar, may be said with greater force of the streptococcus hemolyticus. These various surgical complications may have to do with any part of the body. Metastatic abscesses have been found in joints, in the abdomen, in the mastoid cells, etc. In this paper we shall deal alone with that complication known as empyema and incidentally with lung abscess.

Of especial interest to us at the present time because of the recent epidemic which had its origin in the base hospitals, and because it is new to us, is the streptococcus hemolyticus. This germ runs true to the streptococcus type, in the character of the pathologic changes to which it gives rise. In its clinical course it is rather sub-acute than acute. Very rarely indeed is it acute. Almost as rarely is it chronic.

The chronic clinical symptoms which have been observed in streptococcus hemolyticus infections are those of empyema, and are due to badly drained abscesses. It is prone, like its cousins, to form matastases. Multiple abscesses are common. When the pleural cavity is infected it more often gives rise to localized abscesses than does the pneumococcic. It is rare to find the pleural cavity one large suppurating cavity, as is so often the case in pneumococcus infection. On account of the tendency to multiple abscess formation the surgery of it is less satisfactory, and presents a higher mortality than does the surgery of pneumococcus empyema. In the beginning of the streptococcus hemolyticus epidemic in the U. S. Army Base Hospital, at Fort Sam Houston, Texas, it was the custom to post-mortem every fatal case. This taught us that the cause of death was the inadequacy of the surgery, that is, there were foci consisting in abscesses about the crux of the diaphragm and other surgically inaccessable localities which had not been tapped. The thoroughness of the post-mortems done at this time at this hospital can be attested because they were done by a detachment from the Rockefeller Institute. One of the characteristic actions of this germ is its hemolytic action upon the red blood cells. It is this hemolysis that causes the profound illness of these patients. This is so striking that it was not a difficult matter in merely walking through the wards to be able to point out those suffering from this infection.

For the reason that Dr. Rucks has gathered and accurately presented the statistics as to mortality in the paper which he has just read, we shall not enter into this aspect of the subject very deeply.

DIAGNOSIS.

Around the question of the elective time for operation has waged a considerable controversy. For that reason, if for no other, the early diagnosis of pleural empyema, whatever its source, becomes very important. In the base hospitals, as in private practice, this was in the beginning often made late, consequently these early cases were submitted late, to surgery. In these the course was not unlike that familiar to us in civil life. The lung was collapsed, and bound down by dense adhesions to the root of its tree. The ribs raftered over an enormous cavity. The lung could not come out to the chest wall, consequently the surgical indication was to cave the chest wall into the lung. No matter where the simple drainage was placed the cavity would remain and drainage keep up indefinitely. For reasons later to be mentioned in this paper, early diagnosis in this type of infection has a special significance.

In addition to the ordinary diagnostic methods, such as percussion, auscultation, and the exploratory needle, the x-ray not only proved to be an extremely valuable means of early diagnosis, but pointed out the site for drainage as well.

OPERATIVE INDICATIONS.

Aside from a few anatomical conditions the old rule of the early evacuation of pus holds true in suppuration of the pleural cavity, whether as a whole, or in circumscribed abscesses, here as elsewhere.

The fact that the floor of the abscess is yielding and collapsible, and the roof fixed, must be borne in mind in admitting atmospheric pressure in making a drainage opening. An abscess, the walls of which cannot collapse, will not get well. Also if in making an opening to such a cavity, the bottom falls out, i. e., the lung collapses, a new danger, that of spreading the infection over wide uncontaminated areas, must be borne in mind. Also the danger of adhesions fixing the lung in this collapsed position must not be forgotten. The fact that hemolytic infections are sub-acute in their course, and that the abscesses are inclined to be localized, gives us the cue as to the elective time to drain them. That time should be when the visceral pleura has been anchored by the inflammatory process to the parietal so that the lung will not collapse under the forty pounds atmospheric pressure admitted when an opening is made.

All streptococcic adhesions are firm and hard, and leave no line of demarcation, but amount to what is practically a fusion of the tissues involved. In this respect the hemolytic acts as does its cousins. If an abscess is opened before these adhesions are firm enough to resist the atmospheric pressure, and the lung collapses in response thereto, adhesions will immediately begin forming about it which will forever hold it in its collapsed state. For the formation of these protective adhesions to the chest wall we found that from four or five days to a week or ten days was required. This then constituted the time of election for operating the hemolytic cases. The neglect of this point, or rather the failure to comprehend it, gave us both a much higher mortality and morbidity in the early cases than we had in the later.

Just exactly the opposite was found to be true in the pneumococcus infections, that is, the earlier the operation, after pus was detected, the better the result. The reason for this was that though the lung collapsed immediately upon the admission of air to the pleural cavity, it invariably expanded again. Often this could be seen to occur while the patient was on the operating table. If not then, it could be demonstrated that it had occurred within a few days of the operation. Adhesions in this type of inflammation are not so firm, nor extensive nor so early formed, as in the hemolytic type.

I disagree with Dr. Rucks as to the cause of primary mortality, which he attributes to the shock of operation. The operation per se under a local anesthetic was absolutely shockless. Lung collapse, however, could, and probably did, contribute to the mortality in the early cases. In the streptococcus cases where death did not immediately follow lung collapse, morbidity was greatly increased, as well as subsequent mortality from prolonged suppuration. As to the time of operation I am in agreement with the writer of the previous paper. This selective time, and the reasons for it I have pointed out above. It is based upon our experience in approximately four hundred cases, operated upon by either Captain Stout, or myself. These cases were placed under the ward care of physicians selected by the Chief of Service, and the opportunities for observation could not be excelled.

To meet this collapse of the lung, due to atmospheric pressure, several types of operation and several instruments have been devised. This fact remains, however, that the mortality under all has been about the same. There is a difference, however, in the morbidity. The mortality ranged between twenty-five and thirty per cent. As pointed out by Dr. Rucks, the early epidemic which was due to a pneumococcic infection furnished a much lighter mortality. Our surprise came at the high mortality of the second epidemic. This set us studying the causes, and we found it due to a new type of infection—the streptococcus hemolyticus, the clinical course of which we had yet to learn. We soon found that early operation, that is, operation as soon as the fluid showed germs, or pus, would not do in this type as in the former. The proper thing to do in these cases, as indicated above, is to wait a sufficient time for the abscess to localize, and for adhesions to form, but not sufficiently long to encourage metastases. What is true of the hemolytic infections is also true of those following measles.

As to the time of operation, the main fact to remember, in our experience is, that in the pneumococcus type of infection very early operation is indicated. In the hemolytic type it is best to wait till firm adhesions have anchored the visceral to the perietal pleura. In the determination of this time the x-ray picture is invaluable. It is important also to remember that in the hemolytic variety of infection a collapsed lung never again expands. I say, never again, because I never saw one do so. The selective time to operate in the hemolytic type, therefore, is not so much a matter of days, not so much a matter of shock, but is a matter of the time when we know the lung is fixed. In the hemolytic type the infection more often runs to circumscribed abscess formation, in the pneumococcus, more often to true empyema.

THE RELATION OF LUNG ABSCESS TO EMPYEMA AND VICE VERSA.

Is empyema or abscess of the pleura primary, or is it secondary to a primary lung abscess caused by the pneumonic process perforating into the pleura, or involving it by extension? The post-mortems done at the Base Hospital at Fort Sam Houston, throw no especial light upon this question. They demonstrated that pulmonary abscess and pleural abscess, or empyema quite often co-existed. There are those who believe that an interlobular pneumonic abscess is the commonest source of pleural abscess and empyema. We know that empyema and pleural abscess may exist without a demonstrable abscess of the lung, and indeed without the previous existence of a pneumonia. It is rational to believe that either may cause the other, or that either may exist alone. This view coincides exactly with the facts as demonstrated by post-mortems. A lung abscess, small, sub-pleural, may easily extend itself or perforate into the pleural cavity, and thus be the beginning of the pleural process. This is probably more often true than the converse. An abscess of the lung may, or may not, be an extremely serious complication. If it is deeply situated and on this account does not fix the visceral pleura to the perietal it is surgically a grave problem. This is said even in view of the fact that so great an authority as Moynihan considers the lung as surgically accessible as the abdominal viscera. To suddenly deprive the patient of one half of his breathing capacity cannot be considered as without its danger. There can be no question in the writer's mind that it is to the patient's interest at times to take this risk, but it should not be debonairly done. It is true that lung abscesses frequently spontaneously recover by rupture into, and emptying through, a bronchus. No doubt many small abscesses complicating pneumonia are sequestrated, sterilized and absorbed by natural processes. Lung abscesses are rarer without a complicating empyema than the converse. In this statement I have the support of the Chief of the Medical Service as well.

TYPE OF OPERATION.

Based on the work at some of the base hospitals, the closed method of operating has become quite popular of late. The sole reason being to avoid collapse of the lung with its sequellae. This is a desirable thing, provided, in securing it, first surgical principles are not violated. In any of the methods so far devised it cannot be said that this is true. Drainage is inadequate and not continuous. Practically we find that the mortality in the series of cases reported is not lowered perceptibly. As to morbidity, crippled lung function, I do not believe the last word has yet been said for this method. My reason for this statement is this; if the pleural cavity is not continuously drained there will be times when the positive pressure of the filling abscess will compress the lung. The question of returning lung expansion will then depend altogether upon whether the lung is fixed by adhesions in its compressed position. If a better functional result is not obtained, and the mortality is as high, the open operation, involving rib resection, has such distinct advantages that it should be the operation of choice. In my work, when following the indications for operations outlined above, I am quite sure that the open operation, with incision, and rib resection placed at the bottom of the abscess, giving as it does the best drainage, has proven to be the most satisfactory. In these very ill patients, a general anesthetic of any kind will contribute to the mortality. Ether the most, gas the least, but each will have a distinct mortality of its own. The incision and resection of the rib can be made absolutely without pain under local anesthesia, the patient being prepared, and soothed by a preliminary hypodermic of morphine. I have done the operation without the patient knowing that I was operating at all, the manipulations necessary to the operation being explained under one or another pretext. Psychic shock is an element which must be taken into account.

THE CARREL-DAKIN SOLUTION.

My experience with this has not convinced me that it has contributed materially to the recovery of my patient. In the cases in which drainage was not properly placed it was of value in taking the place to a degree of a proper surgical operation. When the surgery was adequate it did not hasten convalescence. I had as good results from normal salt solution. Upon the whole, my army experience has not made me more a friend of the Carrel-Dakin solution, in surgery. Since this portion of this paper will be attacked, I will reserve further remarks for the closing discussion. Suffice it to say, that when anything goes wrong with the complicated machinery necessary in its use, everything goes to pot immediately, and often disastrously. There is nothing surer than that the Carrel-Dakin solution will never be a substitute for correct surgery, nor an excuse for slovenly surgery.

THE SIMULATED SURGICAL ABDOMEN OF PNEUMONIA.

By the surgical abdomen we mean the typical syndrome associated with inflammation of the peritoneal cavity. This is of more frequent occurrence than we formerly believed. The immense number of cases of pneumonia, with pleural complications gathered together at one time, and in one service, demonstrated this fact. In one thousand cases it approximated five per cent. In several cases the abdomen was so characteristic, and the lung findings so negative, that an immediate operation was performed for ruptured appendix, only to find the appendix normal and a condition of intestinal paresis. The clinical picture of these cases was typical, in that the temperature would range from 103 to 105, there would be pulse acceleration, and of course, leukocytosis. The abdomen would be excessively hard, and very painful to pressure. The pain was so great that one quarter of a grain of morphine would have no effect upon it. In many of the cases the lung findings would be absolutely negative in the beginning. The urgency of the abdominal symptoms made immediate operation seem imperative. Mistakes were made, of course. Experience made us later very cautious.

In analyzing the symptoms, after having had the experience, it seems relatively easy to make the differentiation. It can usually be done on the following facts: 1. Excessive elevation of the temperature; 103 to 105 is not an abdominal temperature but is typically a lung temperature. Experienced surgeons know that a temperature of 103 and over is rarely found in abdominal surgical conditions.

2. The leukocyte count. This is always too high for a beginning inflammatory condition in the abdomen. To have a leukocyte count running from fifteen to thirty thousand would designate suppuration, if it had to do with the abdomen. Just as is the case with the temperature, this is also typical of pneumonia. 3. Pain. This is out of all proportion. Pain having its origin in a peritoneal inflammatory lesion is usually relieved with one-quarter grain of morphine. I have never seen this pain, when due to pneumonia, relieved by this dose.

By carefully considering the above three points we finally became able clinically to eliminate most of these cases of simulated peritonitis. Within twenty-four hours as a rule, the pneumonia would become frank. Probably what happened here was a central diaphragmatic pneumonia, the inflammation touching the peritoneum of the attic of the belly, and thus setting adrift the whole peritoneal syndrome, because wherever an inflammatory process touches the perietal peritoneum the muscular reflex is immediately excited. Even with the experience we have had, none of us are as yet sure that we are able always to differentiate sufficiently to postpone operation in what seems to be a terrific abdominal catastrophe. I would yet say when in doubt, open the abdomen, for I know of no case in which this was done, under mistaken diagnosis where life was lost because of the operation.

THE ETIOLOGY AND PATHOLOGY OF THE SPANISH INFLUENZA.

Louis A. Turley, M. D.

NORMAN, OKLAHOMA

PROFESSOR, PATHOLOGY AND HISTOLOGY, ASSISTANT DEAN,
UNIVERSITY SCHOOL OF MEDICINE

When we approach the subject of the etiology and pathology of the "Spanish influenza," commonly known as the "Flu," we are met with a voluminous literature by a multitude of authors, for there has never been a disease that has been attacked by such a large number of trained men armed with such complete facilities for the study of a condition in all of its phases as has been the case with the pandemic that spread over the world in 1917-19. And yet one cannot pursue his studies far by the conflicting, not to say opposing, conclusions of the many, many workers who have attacked this problem. In fact, scarcely any two of them agree in general, let alone in particular, either as to the etiology or the pathology. Part of this disagreement is due to the fact that many men rushed into print early when they had either not made sufficient observations, or were inexperienced in such matters so that there was soon a considerable literature on the subject, and later investigators, many of them, spent their time in either proving or disproving the contentions of these early observers.

Another fact that appears to me to have added to the confusion, is the fact that, as is always the case, when an epidemic is raging there are many similar conditions that are called the same thing. Or in other words, there were many cases of disease that were called "Flu," because of the similarity of some of the symptoms, that were really not the entity that gave the name to the epidemic.

The consideration of all of the cases as "Flu" has necessarily given a complexity to the reports. One man reports that the characteristic pathological finding was emphysema, another says, "in 50 autopsies I saw no emphysema." Some men say that the pathology was an extensive bronchopneumonia, while other studies show that the bronchi are open and that what might be called areas of exudation are in reality infarcts. So we are forced to the conclusion that either the "Flu" is met with in many forms, or that in reality, instead of having a pandemic of a single disease entity, there were many epidemics of respiratory tract involvement that occurred at the same time. So that it is very possible that in one section of the country there was an epidemic of bronchopneumonia with a few cases of "Flu"; in another section there was an epidemic of "Flu" with a good sprinkling of bronchopneumonia; and in another there was an epidemic of pernicious bronchitis with a few cases of "Flu" and bronchopneumonia. If this is true, and it is not only possible but highly probable, it is easy to see why careful observers and students would disagree in their findings and yet all be equally right, except in calling the cases "Flu." From my own studies, I am convinced that the general run of cases that were met during the pandemic, were in few cases what could be called uncomplicated "Flu." And in looking over the report of at least one observer it would seem that there were about ten cases out of a series of over fifty that could be so considered. They were often a true pneumonia superimposed on a "Flu," or "Flu" on pneumonia, or on bronchitis. But it also seems to me that the characteristic "Flu" pathology is distinctive enough that it can be detected even in these complicated cases.

Keeping these facts in mind, non-"Flu" cases called "Flu," complicated "Flu" and pneumonia, or bronchitis and "Flu" bronchitis alone all called "Flu," we can review the reports of the various observers with more confidence and sympathy. But at the same time, if one wishes to discuss intelligently the etiology and pathology of the "Flu," he must have a series of autopsies in which the pathology corresponds, and the bacteriological studies also agree. Then if he can take these bacteria or organisms and produce the same pathology as occurred in the original case, he will be in a position to speak with authority on the etiology and pathology of the disease. But where one has a series of cases in which the bacteriological studies gives "n" per cent. of one bacillus and "m" per cent. of another bacillus and "x" per cent. of still a third, if he cannot divide the autopsy findings so as to say, so and so are the findings when "n" bacillus is in pure or almost pure culture, and such and such are the findings when "m" bacillus are in the ascendancy, he is in a poor position to speak with much exactness. And this latter is the case with two exceptions with the present reports. They all report a variety of bacteria in each case and a variety of autopsy findings without correlating the two studies and without satisfying the biological postulates. Unfortunately for the purposes of this discussion so far as I am concerned I have not had the time nor opportunity to make bacteriological studies from "Flu" cases so that what I say in that regard will be my conclusions from the reports of competent observers in other parts of the country. And I will say that we are now in a position to really begin a study of the etiology rather than to close the discussion.

It may be asked, why should we have such a variety of epidemics involving the respiratory tract at the same time, if it is true that so many of the cases called "Flu" were either not "Flu" or were complicated "Flu"? The answer to this question gives one of the etiological factors of the pandemic if not of the "Flu" itself, for it must be remembered that the infecting agent is only one of the etiological factors in any infectious disease.

Therefore, we must consider the general conditions that prevailed throughout the world at the time the epidemic started and raged. It will be remembered that a large part of the population were living under suddenly altered conditions of life, in camps, training schools, or districts, or in some form of service, or for other reason in an unusual geographical location. And it was among such camps or groups that the disease first made its appearance in any community where there was such a camp. It will also be remembered that the whole population were living on an altered diet, in many cases and in many ways an insufficient diet. These conditions always predispose to infection. It will also be remembered that during the period from 1917 to 1919 the meteorological conditions were unusual, that throughout almost the entire world there was an unusual amount of moisture in the air and an unusually low temperature prevailing, so there were an unusual number of summer colds even before the "Flu" began. These meteorological conditions are themselves predisposing or favorable to respiratory tract infections. Thus we have a population predisposed to infection and an environmental condition favorable to respiratory tract affliction so there was a fertile field and a determining factor as to what the crop would be.

If we turn from the subjects of infection to the infecting agent, our answer is not so plain. That the "Flu" is an infectious disease no one will question. But as to the nature of the infection we have many answers, more or less conflicting, and all more or less unsatisfactory.

Japanese observers made extensive bacteriological studies in the Kitasato Institute, from "Flu" cases and they reach the conclusion that the "Flu" is caused by the bacillus influenza, although they admit that in almost all cases there were also found pneumococci and streptococci. Haasteen at the Ulleval Hospital, Christiana, Norway, reports that in the cases studied by him, bacillus influenza was rarely found but streptococci were very common. Munro, in England, examined 150 "Flu" sputums by smear and culture and in about half of them he found a short gram-negative bacillus: but he adds, "there was never wanting plenty of gram-positive diplococci and streptococci, and micrococcus catarrhalis." His conclusions are that the "Flu" is started by bacillus influenza and that pneumococci and streptococci are responsible for the pulmonary conditions. A summary of the bacteriological studies made in this country would agree with this decision with possibly one exception. Wolbach, of Boston, and Goodpasture, of Charleston, conclude that bacillus influenza is responsible for the uncomplicated "Flu," admitting that the picture is almost always confused by the invasion of pneumococci and streptococci. The Italian observers succeeded in isolating a very small streptococcus, called by them, "streptococcus pandemicus." They were able to produce "Flu" symptoms in guinea pigs inoculated on the nasal musosa, with these organisms. They also found that animals died when inoculated with cultures passed through a Chamberland filter, also with cultures that had been heated for an hour to 55 degrees centigrade. This would kill the vegetative forms but would not kill the toxin. These experiments would tend to prove what the symptoms indicate, that part of pathological effects or conditions of the disease is produced by toxins.

Early in the discussion of the etiology of the "Flu" it was suggested by many that the real etiological factor or rather the infective factor was a virus, meaning one of the ultramicroscopic organisms, and would class it with the cause of measles, typhus fever and other diseases for which the exact etiological organism has not been found. The experiments of the Italian investigators above referred to would seem to answer this question, at least that the organism was a very minute one and might easily be overlooked by any observer. Right along this same line, Gibson, Bowman, and Conner in England grew a minute filterable micrococcus from filtered sputum and lung tissue of "Flu" cases and also from the kidneys of infected animals. They also produced typical "Flu" lesions in animals inoculated with these organisms and recovered the organisms from the animals. This organism is probably the same as the streptococcus pandemicus of the Italian observers and is an organism that might easily have been included in the cultures of other workers and be responsible for the results they obtained. And while these results require further study and confirmation, they come nearest to answering the question as to the infecting agent of the "Flu" for the reason that in the reports of all of the other observers there is such a catalogue of bacteria listed that we must come to the conclusion that either the specific organism has not yet been found, or that there is no one disease that can be called the "Flu," but rather that the condition that has been called by that name is in reality a mixture of conditions, caused by a variety of organisms acting at the same time.

If we turn from the etiology to the pathology of the "Flu," we find not much more agreement among the pathologists as to the changes that take place than we find among the bacteriologists as to the organisms causing the changes. As was said before, this is, to my mind, because there have been a great many pneumonias and bronchitises that have been called "Flu." And it is impossible to separate the "Flu" from the non-"Flu" cases until we have established the fact that there is a true "Flu" and just what is its pathology.

Personally, I believe that we are justified in saying that there is a condition that is so unlike the pneumonias and bronchitises or mixtures of these as we ordinarily meet them, that we must consider it a different disease entity even if it proves to be caused by the same organisms. I base this belief on the autopsies that I have studied during the past year. And I shall limit my discussion to the characteristic changes on which I base this belief for the time will not permit me to go far into detail with all of the changes found. I shall further consider the subject of the pathology of the "Flu" under two heads: first, the pathology of the fatal cases, and second, the pathology of the cases that recover. And I will take them up in the order named.

In the first place, the "Flu" cadaver is markedly cyanosed, especially about the head and neck. This is so marked and to a degree that frequently it cannot be obscured by the colored injections of the undertaker. This condition is noticeable in the living and clinicians have remarked that it will not yield to any means now known for relieving this condition, even the administration of oxygen. Why this condition should occur will be brought out later.

When the thorax is opened there is usually found more or less fluid in the cavity. Sometimes this is scant and sometimes it is enough to cause atelectasis of the unconsolidated portions of the lung. There is extensive lung involvement. This may be confined to one side or involve both lungs, and is usually more pronounced in parts of the lobes, and but rarely involves all of the lobes. Even in the most involved lobes there are usually air containing areas, especially along the anterior margin, rarely scattered about as would be the case of confluent bronchopneumonia. The involved areas are markedly congested, dark reddish in color, and usually there are areas of smaller or larger size outlined by grayish lines. Some of these are almost microscopic in size while others are several centimeters in diameter. There are numerous ecchymoses in the visceral pleura, even on the air containing regions. When cut, fluid runs out of the interior of the lung. This is sometimes blood stained and sometimes almost clear. The bronchi contain more or less frothy material, rarely pustulous liquid. The roentgenologist at St. Anthony's Hospital injected several "Flu" lungs through the bronchi and took roentgenographs of them, and anyone would be astonished to see how free the bronchi were. Even the smallest twigs are plainly visible, showing that they were open at the time of death.

The pathological changes in the other organs of the body were similar to the changes met with in death from other infectious fevers. That is, there was nothing unusual that distinguishes the "Flu" kidney or the "Flu" liver from those organs in other diseases of similar nature. The lymph nodes were swollen as was the spleen. The kidneys showed acute tubular nephritis, and there was little change in the heart. So that the lesions that are typical of the "Flu" are largely confined to the lungs. That is, so far as the gross findings are concerned.

A microscopical study of the involved areas of the lung showed a double picture. In general the alveoli were filled with a hemorrhagic or a sero-hemorrhagic exudate instead of the white cell exudate of pneumonias. The bronchi were for the most part open or contained a small amount of cellular exudate, the epithelium being little if any changed, except in certain localities there was a more or less dense cellular infiltration of the bronchi and a cellular exudate in the lumen. In the areas above referred to as outlined by grayish lines, there was a dense infiltration of endothelial cells and polymorphonuclear leukocytes. These areas did not correspond always to lobules of the lung, or to areas supplied by a single bronchus, and the condition of the bronchi in these fields seemed to be secondary to the alveolar condition. Another thing that was common and striking was the condition of the smaller blood vessels. They were filled with thrombi. So that it would appear that the denser areas of cellular infiltraiton were infarcts rather than lobules consolidated by exudate as is the case in bronchopneumonia, and explains the gray outlines of these areas seen in the gross.

I want to emphasize the blood vessel conditions of the lungs, for right here is seems to me is the characteristic pathological change in true "Flu." The characteristic exudate of the "Flu" is hemorrhagic. There are numerous ecchymoses of the pleura. There are frequent thrombi in the smaller blood vessels. A hemorrhagic exudate means an increased permeability of the vessel walls, also this is one of the causes of excessive edema. Thrombosis indicates injury to the intima of the vessel walls. And the consequent interference to the circulation due to the thrombosis would account for the unyielding cyanosis that is characteristic of the "Flu." Also the infarction of the lungs would account for the frequency of lung abscesses and empyema in those cases that survive the first acute stages of the disease. So that it appears to me that it is the vascular system, not the parenchyma of the lungs, in which the typical lesions of the "Flu" occur and that instead of dealing essentially with a pneumonia as we ordinarily speak of it, we are dealing with a pulmonary phlebitis. Dr. W. W. Lyon, of Washington, is the only other observer whose report I have seen who emphasizes the blood vessel condition and he suggests the name Hemorrhagic Pulmonitis instead of influenza as more descriptive of the conditions found.

To summarize, the true "Flu" differs from lobar pneumonia in that it is rare to find a whole lobe involved, in the numerous ecchymoses, in the character of the exudate, and in the extensive thrombosis. It differs from bronchopneumonia, even of the confluent type, in the extent of the area involved, in the nature and location of the air filled areas, in the character of the exudate, and in the thrombosis and infarcation. It differs from extensive pernicious bronchitis in the freedom of the bronchi, in the lack of extensive bronchiectasis and emphysema and in the points above named for the other ordinary lung involvements. Personally, I did not find a single bronchiectasis as spoken of by some others as being so common, nor did the x-ray studies above mentioned reveal any. And I agree with Lyon in that I did not find emphysema, either interstitial or parenchymatous, except in the air filled areas. This condition is emphasized by some as one of the characteristic lesions.

As to the pathology of those who survive and apparently recover from the "Flu," there are several conditions that are met with. It frequently happens that patients are left with heart trouble of the nature of asthenia, which indicates that there are changes such as cloudy swelling of the heart, although I did not find this condition in the hearts of the patients who died in the acute stages of the disease. Another set of pathological conditions are in the nervous system. These vary all the way from impaired memory and mental acuity to various forms of insanity. But the exact nature of the changes back of these symptoms can only be determined from autopsies a few years hence in known cases of "Flu." As a boy during the epidemic of 1889-90, I was struck by the various cases of spastic paralysis of parts of the body, and by reported softening of the brain in my neighbors, following an attack of the then called Russian influenza.

CONCLUSIONS:

1. There is a separate disease entity commonly called the Spanish influenza, but is more properly a hemorrhagic pulmonitis or a pulmonary phlebitis.

2. The infective etiological factor is most probably a very minute or ultra-microscopic organism, possibly streptococcus pandemicus or the filterable micrococcus of the English investigators.

3. The characteristic lesions are in the vascular system of the lungs rather than in the parenchyma of those organs and the picture seen at autopsy can best be explained on this basis.

Discussion.

Dr. F. M. Sanger, Oklahoma City: As has already been said, the past winter and past fall at times it looked as if fully one-third of the people with whom we had to deal were affected more or less with this influenza, or as I sometimes think, the grippe. I know where I was one-third, thirty-five per cent. of the cases—thirty-five per cent. of the nurses were brought down with it and about thirty-eight per cent. of the corpsmen, not to say anything of the others that were brought into the hospital. Doctor Blesh spoke of this as being a pneumonic infection and of the different kinds of infection we have in the pneumococcus and streptococcus.

I wish to speak particularly on one or two points he spoke of there as to the operative condition, and at first as to the time to operate.

We know some of the text-books have told us before, and even those that were written during this war, that the sooner we operate for empyema with all cases, the better it is.

As has been brought out in the remarks and addresses, in the pneumonic type if you will operate early it is the better. We found out that we didn't always get these cases as early from the medical ward as we wanted to. They were diagnosed and we advocated the early operation of these cases, but sometimes the chief of the medical service wanted to delay for two, three, four and five days—even until the patients, one or two, at least, became so moribund that it seemed an operation was beyond any benefit to them. I wish to say this: That all of the cases we had, something near ninety-nine of those empyema cases, I believe every one of them would have died if they had not been operated on. That is my conviction, and we had them when they seemed so far gone, or rather were so weak, that they would not be able to undergo any shock or any pain or any effects of an operation at all, and, as Doctor Blesh said, in so many of these cases when the lung was collapsed after operation it would expand again. I have seen that lung before I got through with the operation, begin to expand, before I would get the patient off of the table he would say that he felt better, and nearly always could breathe better and often within an hour would be able to smile at you. Now, gentlemen, when we see these conditions, when we see how, after repeated aspirations, the patient will not improve, we must confess that the open operation is a remedy for this condition. I know that at one time I got from my commanding officer, Major Chidester, who was Chief Surgeon at the Letterman General Hospital in San Francisco, instructions to use the aspiration instead of the open operation, but when he saw the result of this open operation he was convinced that in favor of the open operation.

Now, Doctor Blesh spoke of the multiple infections of the streptococcus hemolyticus. I believe in the army—in fact, I know—we had a better and clearer chance of observing these cases from the inception to the very end than we had anywhere else, unless it is in big ward hospitals or municipal hospitals; and even there we do not get them as much as we do in the army, because in the army when a man becomes ill we tell him what he must do and he does it. He stays there until we get ready to dismiss him, makes no difference whether he is an officer or a private.

Now, in many of these cases we noticed the abscess in the lung; that is, in the streptococcus hemolyticus. Many of them we had to open up. I remember one case in particular, a young man who was gassed in France. He was in the hospital several weeks in Paris and, it seems, he did not improve. He was sent over to the United States and kept in one of the hospitals in the east for about three weeks and was finally sent to the hospital where we were. He was able to be up and since his sister was living in San Francisco he was sent to us. X-ray showed abscess in lung. We operated him, and he made an uneventful recovery. This is only one of many that I might cite.

Doctor Blesh said that in these serious cases in going through a ward you could tell those who are going to get well. Gentlemen, those of you who have been through these wards—the pneumonia and influenza wards—especially when you have been O. D., if you didn't get down with the grippe or something else, you had a pretty strong heart. As the doctor said, you could pick them out. I believe we can prognosticate those who are going to get well and those who are going to die. I remember in more than one instance in the influenza wards that I told the surgeon in charge or the chief of the service, "That man will not get well." I hated to say it; but it looked like those of us who went through those conditions could look at the patients and say whether they would get well or no. I remember very particularly one man that later developed empyema and we operated on him and he lingered for two weeks and then died, and I told the ward surgeon when I first saw him that it was a fatal case. He was one of four. We operated on him and he was one of those who did not get well.

The Symposium on Pneumonia was also briefly discussed by Dr. R. I. Allen, Nowata; Dr. Livermore, Chickasha; Dr. Goodman, Kansas City; Dr. Ross Grosshart, Tulsa.

Dr. W. W. Rucks, closing: I have been very much interested in the discussion of these papers. There are one or two things to which I wish to refer in closing. One is the quinine treatment. I know it was used quite extensively in Camp Travis, and has many strong adherents. At Fort Sam Houston our results with it were not so good and we discontinued its use. We also used the convalesence serum. We used the serum of recovered patients, taking the blood as soon after recovery as we thought it was safe to do. A Wassermann was made of each donor, and then the serum pooled and the Wassermann re-action of the pooled serum taken. This we used quite freely, with apparently good results. The objection to it is that the blood of the donor and the recipient were not typed, and therefore there was danger of hemolysing the blood of the recipient.

Dr. White referred to the fact that you should not use glucose in less than five per cent. solution. That is quite true. Less than five per cent. produced hemolysis. It is safe to use a twenty-five per cent. solution. Our habit was to use a ten per cent. solution, given in doses of 250 c.c.

Dr. Turley's paper quite coincides with the pathological findings of Fort Sam Houston, and I think also with the clinical manifestations.

In the last epidemic, when you consider the great number of people who suffered from it, the percentage of mortality was not so great. The mortality in bronchial pneumonia, following measles, was much larger.

Dr. A. L. Blesh, closing: There are only two or three points in the discussion of this paper that I wish to dwell upon for a few moments. One speaker called attention to the fact that I could have gone farther in my remarks upon the abdominal types of pneumonia and with this I agree. The point that I wish to bring out is this; that in my opinion wherever we find the abdominal inflammatory syndrome there is inflammatory contact with the parietal peritoneum; that it is a reflex due to a local diaphragmatic peritonitis which in no manner differs from the syndrome of any peritonitis, except in the degree of its intensity. The upper abdominal zone seems to be far more sensitive to irritation than is the lower, and it therefore responds by a more intense muscle reflex. In a few instances supradiaphragmatic abscesses followed in these cases still further supporting the view mentioned above.

Another fact to which Dr. White called attention still further confuses the diagnosis in this class of cases; that is the presence of a co-existing appendicitis. Such cases do exist and when they do the diagnosis is indeed very confusing. The only safe course is, when in doubt open the abdomen. In looking over the past I have some vain regrets where I did not do this because some of those patients are dead. None are dead where I did it.

Relative to the streptococcus hemolyticus, I mentioned in my paper that these patients are very sick from the beginning. This is due to the tendency to early acidosis which is always present. This germ is very appropriately named hemolyticus.

The glucose treatment, as pointed out by Dr. Rucks, is extremely valuable in combating this tendency. It is the hemolytic action of this germ upon the blood that leads to this pronounced and early acidosis. This acidosis is the cause of early death in practically all of these cases. Acidosis can only be truly antidoted by rest-producing sleep. These patients have a tendency to sleeplessness from the start. Unfortunately we have no drug that will produce this acidosis-preventing sleep. Morphine is the nearest approach to it but even it, to a degree, increases this tendency. The glucose mixture used intravenously is a geat help and therein exists its value.

Dr. Turley, closing: The remarks of Doctor Goodman illustrates what seems to me to have clouded the whole subject of the etiology of the "Flu." He says that at the hospital in which he was serving they made cultures from the naso-pharynx of every case of "Flu." To my mind, the study of the bacteriology of the naso-pharynx in a case of lung involvement is about as valuable as the study of the bacteriology of the back of the mouth to determine the specific bacillus causing a case of appendicitis. It is necessary to study the bacteriology of the lesions themselves.

SOME OF THE SEQUELAE OF EPIDEMIC INFLUENZA.*

A. B. Leeds, A. B., M. D.
CHICKASHA, OKLAHOMA

The suggestions submitted, today, are based on a series of 1037 cases, of the "flu," treated and seen during the present epidemic, and 274 cases seen lately, in which sequelae have developed following an attack of the "flu."

Full laboratory data, careful and painstaking examination and the results obtained, in the treatment of these cases by the form of sero-therapy used, have convinced the author that we have had a mixed infection epidemic.

With but two cases of the "flu" developing after 1182 prophylactic doses (of the mixed infection phylacogen combined with the pneumonia phylacogen or the influenza serobacterin combined with the pneumonia serobacterin) had been given and these two cases, of a very mild nature and without complications, makes the author feel that his mixed infection epidemic was of a very definite nature.

The "flu" bacillus, pneumococcus, staphylococcus, streptococcus hemolyticus and viridans, as well as other micro-organisms, were found more or less constantly.

We found that the streptococcus was the predominant micro-organism, particularly in all cases of a serious nature, or those cases having serious complications.

The treatment of this number of cases of the "flu," and those cases developing sequelae following an attack of the "flu," convinces me that all persons contracting the "flu" had a lowered resistance, from some cause, even if they were in apparently good health.

Where there had not been loss of sleep, chilling, exhaustion, insufficient or irrational feeding, etc., *there was a definite history of a chronic focal infection, as a predisposing cause, in all cases.*

There was not one serious case of the "flu," or a case with serious complications, which came under the author's observation but what had a definite history of a chronic focal infection.

An attack of the "flu" being superimposed upon a serious chronic focal infection frequently, if not always, was responsible for the serious complications as well as the fatal terminations.

Diseased tonsils, teeth, sinuses, antrums, and prostates were the principal chronic focal infections observed in this series of cases.

In the series of 274 cases, seen lately, in which sequelae have developed fol-

*Read in Section on General Medicine, Annual State Meeting, Muskogee, May, 1919.

lowing an attack of the "flu," we have been able in each case to demonstrate a definite foci of infection.

In our series of 274 cases of sequelae, we have found that the ages most affected were between 20 and 45 years, though we had one case nine years and one 68 years old.

While men were more often affected than women, yet we found that nearly all the cases of involvement of the nervous system were in women.

We had 74 cases involvement of the heart; 22 cases involvement of respiratory tract; 2 cases involvement of brain; 28 cases involvement of frontal sinus; 2 cases involvement of ethmoidal sinus; 12 cases involvement of antrum; 87 cases involvement of nervous system; 21 cases involvement of kidneys; 4 cases involvement of long bones; 8 cases involvement of bladder; 9 cases involvement of prostate; 5 cases of exacerbation of chronic discharging ears.

We found in the 74 cases of heart involvement, that we had four varieties. Either a toxic weakening of the heart muscle; an involvement of the valves; a cardio-nephritic involvement, with a high per cent. of albumin and definite edema, or a vasomotor depression.

Palpitation, shortness of breath, easily tiring after ordinary exertion and asthmatic breathing, accompanied by annoying cough, with or without expectoration, usually brought this class of patients to the doctor for relief.

The removal of the chronic foci of infection cleared up all the heart cases, except one in which there was permanently damaged tissues. In this case, there was an improvement but not entire relief.

In the 22 cases of respiratory tract involvement, we found either pulmonary congestion (due to cardio-vascular or vasomotor paralysis, partial if not total), delayed resolution, empyema (with or without bronchial connection), some pus pockets not in contact with the chest wall, apparent flaring up of symptoms of clinical tuberculosis and annoying irritation of the bronchi.

In all of these respiratory tract cases, the x-ray findings were indefinite and in only one case, of those simulating a tubercular infection, were we able to demonstrate t.b., but, in all these cases, we did find the streptococcus and the staphylococcus.

The removal of the chronic foci of infection, in these respiratory tract cases, gave relief from all the symptoms.

In the two cases of brain involvement, one was apparently the so-called epidemic lethargica encephalitis while the other was a meningeal type (associated with clinical pyelitis).

In the 28 cases of frontal sinus involvement, we had a persistent, obstinate and annoying train of symptoms but in only two cases did we have any difficulty in relieving the condition, after the chronic foci of infection had been removed.

In the two cases of ethmoidal sinus involvement, we were very fortunate in finding the chronic foci of infection, and the removal of these foci gave relief.

In the 87 cases of nervous system involvement, we had a regular three-ring circus type of symptoms and conditions.

From congested fundus oculi, vertigo, lack of co-ordination, mild type of paralysis of one side, arm and leg to the so-called neurasthenia train of symptoms, confusional psychoses and acute mania of the depressional form.

It was certainly very gratifying to see the improvement that followed the removal of the chronic foci of infection, in this class of cases.

We were very much impressed with the severe constitutional symptoms which accompanied the twelve cases of antrum involvement, as they were unusually severe for antrum infections.

Besides removing the chronic foci of infection, in some of these antrum cases, it was necessary to institute thorough drainage before much relief was obtained.

Clearing up the five cases of exacerbation of chronic discharging ears was accomplished by the removal of the chronic foci of infection.

In the 21 cases of kidney involvement, we had a condition of general congestion as well as streptococcus infections, of all types. One very interesting case, in this series, had both a streptococcus and staphylococcus infection.

The improvement, after the removal of chronic foci of infection, in this class of cases, was more tardy in appearing than in the other types of cases seen.

The four cases of long bone involvement were severe, aggravated, and all had a grave systemic disturbance. In one case, the entire shaft of the bone was involved and an amputation was necessary.

Drainage, in two cases, in addition to the removal of the chronic foci, was necessary for clearing up the condition.

In the eight cases of bladder involvement, we had acute cystitis, involvement of the cut-off muscle or retention of the urine as the reasons for this class of patients coming to the doctor.

Irrigation, in addition to the removal of the chronic foci, in some of these cases, cleared up the condition.

The nine cases of prostate involvement usually complained about a sudden onset, congestion, pain in the back, a feeling of fullness in the thighs which radiated down the limbs.

Staphylococcus aureus, as well as streptococcus, infection was found predominating in this class of cases.

Removal of the chronic foci, followed by massage after the acute stage had subsided, and the use of the sero-bacterins cleared up these cases.

The investigation and the results obtained, in this series of cases of sequelae of epidemic influenza, has certainly been gratifying and interesting to the author and we feel that finding and removing the chronic foci of infection is the paramount consideration in the treatment of these cases.

INFLUENZA AND PREGNANCY.

Fernando Calderon, Manila, P. I. (*Journal A. M. A.*, Sept. 27, 1919), describes the effects of influenzal epidemics on pregnancy. In two cases, quinin was considered also a cause, together with the influenza, for the interruption of pregnancy. In twenty-seven other cases, however, in which influenza was considered a complication, quinin was not given and so could not be considered responsible. Abortions occurred in seven cases in which the influenza was complicated by bronchial or lobar pneumonia. He asks, as a question of scientific interest, "Is pregnancy interrupted by the cough and asphyxia that are usually associated with the disease, or does the toxin of the Pfieffer bacillus act as an ecbolic? The fact that coughing and asphyxia were not prominent symptoms in some of the cases tempts me strongly to believe that the toxin acts directly on the uterus. Its selective action on this organ is further supported by the early appearance of menstruation when the women contracted the disease." Calderon summarizes his observations as follows: "1. Influenza exerted a pernicious influence on pregnancy. This pernicious influence was direct and independent of the broncho-pneumonia and lobar pneumonia complicating the disease. 2. Influenza caused untimely appearance of menstruation. 3. Lobar pneumonia complicating influenza was responsible for the high mortality of this ordinarily benign disease in pregnancy. 4. Broncho-pneumonia produced by influenza caused 100 per cent. mortality when it occurred in the course of the puerperium. 5. Influenza caused a deleterious effect on the product of conception."

PREVENTION OF INFLUENZA AND ALLIED DISEASES.*

WALTON FOREST DUTTON, M. D.

TULSA, OKLAHOMA

Influenza is a communicable disease of serious import and of more serious sequence. It has been epidemic and pandemic at periods down through the centuries. At each outbreak the toll in deaths has been large. It is classed among the most dangerous of communicable diseases.

The pandemic of influenza during the year 1918 cost the world approximately two million lives. The sequelae of influenza will, conservatively speaking, involve five million more.

A disease which causes such direful results certainly demands the earnest attention of both the medical profession and the laity. It shall be my endeavor in this paper to set forth the salient principles governing the prevention of influenza and allied diseases.

Diseases of the respiratory system are common the world over, where crowded conditions prevail or unsanitary conditions exist. In South Africa, diseases of the respiratory tract are common. On the Rand, prevalence of these infections is aggravated by the dry, dusty climate and rapid changes of temperature. In the tenements of cities, crowded conditions, poor food, low resistance of individuals tend to cause rapid spread of communicable diseases. The crowded conditions in military camps together with the many carriers furnish potent sources for the spread of infections of the respiratory tract.

As Chief Surgeon for a number of large industrial concerns in Western Pennsylvania for ten years, my various duties brought me in contact with the serious problems of communicable diseases of the respiratory tract. In addition, my researches into bacteriological and pathological conditions of typhoid, pneumonia, and tuberculosis have proven invaluable. My work in diagnosis and internal medicine of recent years has enabled me to attack the problem of prevention of respiratory disease with a certain degree of accuracy.

During the epidemic of influenza, in 1918, I had the unusual opportunity of observing preventive measures used in municipalities and in army camps. The far more important and far reaching work has been that of pursuing my own methods in private practice. From the beginning to the end of the epidemic vaccines were used. At first, only the smaller dosage was used, as follows:

Four Syringes	A	B	D	C	
Bacillus Influenza	12.5	25	50	100	million per mil.
Staphylococcus aureus	50	100	200	400	million per mil.
Staphylococcus albus	50	100	200	400	million per mil.
Streptococcus	12.5	25	50	100	million per mil.
Pneumococcus	12.5	25	50	100	million per mil.
B. Friedlander	12.5	25	50	100	million per mil.
M. Catarrhalis (group)	12.5	25	50	100	million per mil.

Later the larger dosage, as suggested by Hitchens, was used as follows:

	A	B	C	D	
B. influenza	125	250	500	1000	million
Staphylococcus aureus	125	250	500	1000	million
Staphylococcus albus	125	250	500	1000	million
Streptococcus	125	250	500	1000	million
Pneumococcus	125	250	500	1000	million
B. Friedlander	125	250	500	1000	million
M. catarrhalis (group)	125	250	500	1000	million

When a bacteria appeared to be predominating or to have hemolytic character-

---

*Read in Section on General Medicine, Annual State Meeting, Muskogee, May, 1919.

istics, a therapeutic dose sufficient to overcome that advantage was used. Compound vaccines were used as preventive and curative measures with most excellent results. The results were so entirely satisfactory that my confreres adopted these measures and have reported results that give conclusive evidence of the effectiveness of properly selected and prepared vaccines.

I shall digress further in the field of therapeutics in answer to the advocate of autogenous vaccines to say that often before the vaccine can be prepared the patient is dead. Therefore, the *standardized stock vaccine, in acute infections of the respiratory tract, will be the potent therapeutic measure of the future.*

My work in typhoid, pneumonia, and tuberculosis has taught me not to minimize the importance of anaphylaxis. This factor applied in the employment of vaccines and sera for the prevention and treatment of infective diseases serves as a governor or guide. *Anaphylaxis is in reality not due to idiosyncrasy. It is the measure of the therapeutic effect of a vaccine or sera. Anaphylactic shock can be prevented by the administration of small doses of the indicated serum. This preparation of the patient is as necessary as the preparation for a major surgical operation. It is the common sense application of physiological and therapeutic principles.*

The anaphylactic phenomena in respiratory diseases is more evident and important than in any other group of diseases. In an individual with acute respiratory catarrh a moderate dose of mixed vaccine will cause a marked local and general reaction. The individual free from such infection shows little if any reaction after the administration of a moderate dose. The activities of the causative infection develop an anaphylaxis. This phenomena is almost always present and diagnosis can be made without any clinical evidence by noting the results of the inoculation of an applicable dose of mixed vaccine made from cultures found in respiratory infections.

The local and general symptoms found following the administration of mixed vaccine in an individual suffering from a respiratory catarrh are similar to those in pulmonary tuberculosis following a dose of tuberculin. This anaphylactic phenomena serves as a valuable guide as to dosage and interval in vaccine theraphy.

Symbiotic activities of micro-organisms is much more appreciated now than formerly. The preparation of an autogenous vaccine for respiratory infections from the sputum should incorporate all micro-organisms commonly found. By this method all pathologic organisms developing on human blood agar should be given proper consideration. All cultures and subcultures should be kept under observation for five or six days in order to provide for the organisms of slow growth. A mixed vaccine prepared after this manner gives more satisfactory clinical results.

The individualistic factor should always be under observation. Some persons go through life entirely free of respiratory infections while others are affected from time to time with some one of the diseases until they become chronic. Acute exacerbations may occur and the spread of infection by means of droplets sprayed into the air in sneezing, coughing, and other expulsive actions is not uncommon. It is from these carriers that, in many instances, epidemic and even pandemic respiratory diseases have a beginning. This is best illustrated by the recent pandemic.

It is undoubtedly true that the initial infection in this pandemic was B. influenza, but other organisms as streptococcus, M. catarrhalis, streptococcus mucosis capsulatus, streptococcus hemolysins, and pneumococcus rapidly became of considerable etiological importance. The majority of cases diagnosed as influenza were not true influenza, but due to mixed infection. A most interesting point in the influenza epidemic in the United States was the fact that the most serious cases did not occur in the young, old, and feeble, but in the robust adults in their prime. As evidenced in our army camps, physical fitness did not insure against attack from respiratory infections. The use of prophylactic vaccines against infective respiratory diseases has proven that specific immunization can be established successfully.

Whenever and wherever individuals are closely associated and mingle in social and commercial intercourse, virulent organisms, in the air from coughing, sneezing, expectorating, etc., are always present. They gain ready access to the respiratory tract through inspiratory currents of air, and to vulnerable points. The lung tissues richly supplied with blood are readily attacked because of their delicate structure. Irritant and noxious vapors, bacterial toxins, or foreign bodies constantly attacking these tissues predispose to respiratory diseases and incidently to constitutional weakness. This weakness or acquired susceptibility can be successfully overcome by specific immunization against air breathed pathogenic bacteria.

Influenza is probably due to an organism which was described by Pfeiffer and others in 1892. It is present in lachrymal, nasal, and bronchial secretions, and is also found in the lung when pneumonia complicates the disease. It is one of the smallest bacilli known. This organism is always associated with other infections as, the M. catarrhalis, pneumococcus, etc. Influenza is endemic in Northern Central Asia, and at intervals travels westward from this region by the principal trade routes. It spreads at a rate corresponding to the most rapid means of transportation. It is a communicable disease which attacks a large proportion of the population within a short time.

Epidemics of influenza have occurred at various times in North America since 1627. The pandemic of 1889-90 was of unusual virulence. The pandemic of 1918-19 surpassed that of 1889-90 in virulence and varied complications. The peculiarities of this disease during the last pandemic were such as to place the etiology in the uncertain class.

Bacteriological findings have not proven whether the disease is due to a filterable virus or to ordinary bacteria.

I shall call attention again to the individual factor in this disease. Some authorities have found the influenza bacilli predominating, others the streptococcus viridans, streptococcus hemolyticus, M. catarrhalis, diplococcus mucosis, and often pneumococcus. Some individuals have a natural or acquired immunity to these bacteria, others a low resistance. The inoculated individual recovers, if attacked at all. The non-inoculated individual of low resistance when attacked succumbs or slowly recovers, and here lies the secret of high or low mortality.

Most all authorities disagree concerning the number of the various bacteria isolated, but agree on the fact that in practically all severe cases of influenza, pneumococcus, streptococcus, staphylococcus, M. catarrhalis, bacillus mucosus capsulatis, and streptococcus viridans are found.

The prophylactic measure may be summarized as follows:

1. Keep the system in good condition.
2. Avoid needless crowding.
3. Walk instead of riding in street cars, when possible.
4. Retire early, rise early.
5. Remain in open air and sunshine as long as possible.
6. Avoid poorly ventilated places.
7. Breathe through the nose, and do not allow the mouth to be a gateway for infection.
8. Clothing should be loose, warm, and the feet kept warm and dry.
9. Avoid talking, sneezing, coughing, spitting, and snuffling persons.
10. Avoid cooking and eating utensils, etc., used by others, unless properly sterilized.
11. Avoid houses and districts where there is influenza.
12. Wear face masks to protect nose and mouth, and goggles to protect the eyes in hospitals, sick room, or other places where liable to infection.
13. Isolation and treatment of carriers.

14. Destruction or isolation of animal carriers.

15. Proper sanitary measures in the care of those ill with influenza in order that the infection will not be spread.

16. Keep secretions of the body neutral or alkaline by the use of sodium bicarbonate, or other suitable alkali.

In 1880, Pasteur and Sternberg described a coccus found in human sputum which was called coccus of sputum septicemia. Fraenkel, in 1884, published an accurate and detailed description of the characters of the pneumococcus. Since that time the pneumococcus has been recognized as the chief factor in the etiology of acute pneumonia. The knowledge of today, however, from a bacteriological and clinical standpoint, considers various factors as the cause of pneumonia. It is my purpose to show that our present viewpoint is the most logical.

A series of cases of acute lobar pneumonia selected as typical cases were investigated. The sputum was carefully collected and within two hours inoculated into white rats. In each case, cultures were made upon human blood. Cultures from the heart blood of rats that died, were made on human blood agar. Cultural examination revealed pneumococci, staphylococci, streptococci, M. catarrhalis, streptococcus mucosis capsulatus, B. influenza. In 47 per cent. of the cases, the pneumococci were a negligible quantity.

In pneumococcal infections, there is no constant lesion in the lung. The pathological lesions vary from lobar, or broncho-pneumonia to indefinite distribution of pathologic processes. Bacteriological examination does not corroborate the evidence that the pneumococcus is the sole etiological factor.

The majority of pneumonias diagnosed as typical are as a matter of fact atypical. The stereotyped diagnosis of a catarrhal pneumonia, or a broncho-pneumonia is as false as it is obsolete. The fact also remains that the diagnostician is not, as a rule, the clinician.

Many years of experience has taught me that all infections are more or less mixed infections. I refer here again to my observations in such infections as typhoid, tuberculosis, and colonic infections. Our so-called pneumonias may exist, with or without pneumococci. The organisms commonly found in atypical pneumonias are, staphylococcus, M. catarrhalis, streptococcus, streptococcus hemolysins, B. Friedlander, B. influenza, pneumococcus.

The prima-facia evidence as to the etiological factors of pneumonia gives therapeutic value to mixed vaccines prepared from numerous strains of prevailing organisms. Prophylactic inoculation has reduced the mortality. The mortality has been enormously reduced by therapeutic inoculation.

The prevalence of pneumonia in our army camps, in 1918, and in cities in the United States in which influenza raged for months, was much more marked than in previous epidemics. The appalling mortality was almost entirely due to the so-called pneumococcic infections. The "follow-up" examinations of sputum and lungs demonstrated that the conditions were due to mixed infections. This infection in the greater number of cases increased in virulence until a septicemic type developed.

As soon as the epidemic started requests from all points of the compass came to the profession for a vaccine to prevent and combat this disease. These requests were met with numerous vaccines of questionable value. Some had stable potency while others had no preventive or therapeutic worth. In November, 1918, several biological laboratories produced vaccines of value. The employment of these compound vaccines produced highly satisfactory results. The use of a compound or mixed vaccine for the treatment of pneumonia and other respiratory infections is of material aid to the physician who does not have the aid of an experienced bacteriologist. Further, regardless of the respiratory disease, the keen and observing clinician can apply a vaccine prepared along the above lines. The simplicity of therapeutic application of mixed vaccines commends them to the physician.

The valuable experimental work carried out in this country by Cole, Rosenow, and others; the work in South Africa by F. G. Lister, J. P. Johnson, and others, has proven to be the foundation of preventive and curative measures in pneumonia and other respiratory diseases.

I shall not discuss the laboratory problems of prevention carried out by the many investigators, but refer briefly to the strains of pneumococcus. Recent advances in bacteriology have, in a measure, made the subject more complete and difficult. During the years 1904-8, in my work on "Insect Carriers of Typhoid," I isolated 24 strains of bacilli between the typhoid and the colon, thus establishing a connecting link. This connection was disputed at the time. Since then we have been forced to accept typhoid A, B, etc., and various strains causing dysentery, pneumonia, etc. I have always believed in the phenoma of "mutation." My observations in noting the changes of the specific characteristics of the typhoid micro-organisms have been confirmed. I also have every reason to believe that the phenomena of mutation holds in most, if not all, micro-organisms. Bacteriologists may not, at this time, be able to classify all the changes, but in due time will be able to do so. It is not for the clinician to wait until this is accomplished, but to devise a means for the prevention of such infections. The recognition of the different strains has been of much practical value in enabling the preparation of vaccine from individual and mixed virulent strains.

It has been the tendency, in recent years, when success has not been achieved by a vaccine theraphy or prophylaxis to attribute, this lack of success to an unidentified strain of micro-organism. This was noted in the experiments carried out on the Rand in South Africa and more recently in our army camps. It has been proven beyond a reasonable doubt, that therapeutic and prophylactic vaccines cannot be prepared from one individual micro-organism as a basis.

My experience has taught me that in the preparation of various vaccines the problem of variation in bacteria is practically solved by the preparation of vaccines and sera from a large number of unidentified strains. The number of strains employed does not affect the potency of the vaccine provided each strain is a virulent organism exhibiting the chief characteristics of the particular organism and is recently isolated from a definite pathological condition.

The preparation and dosage of a particular vaccine should be limited to that vaccine and not applied to other vaccines.

Dr. G. D. Maynard, Johannesburg, reports the investigation of experimental inoculation carried out by the Rand mines with Lister's vaccine, in which 55,900 natives were employed, with the following conclusions:

1. That the attack rate from pneumonia is apparently lessened by inoculation, a small positive correlation being obtained.

2. That there is little or no evidence that the case mortality is favorably affected by inoculation.

His report is at variance with that of Wright and Johnson. Major Johnson, in discussing this report, says, "he is unable to give any satisfactory reply as to whether the vaccine prepared by Lister from identified strains offers any advantage over the vaccine previously prepared by Wright from non-identified strains. On the face of it these conclusions are paradoxical. To claim protection against a particular disease, at the same time to admit that the mortality among the inoculated is not favorably affected, is entirely at variance with the experience gained of preventive inoculation in other diseases. It has been the universal experience that among the individuals previously inoculated against typhoid and paratyphoid fevers, who in spite of inoculation developed the disease, *the mortality is considerably reduced*, the disease tending to be mild and free from complications."

Johnson discusses at length the results obtained at Kimberley and on the Rand by Lister. He states that "these results are in accordance with bacteriological findings as pneumococcus alone has been a comparatively unimportant factor in the heavy mortality during the prevailing epidemic." "In conclusion," he says, "it is necessary to state that the failure in the present method of prophylactic inoculation against pneumonia is due not to the presence of an unidentified strain or strains of pneumococcus, but to the fact that the etiological importance of other organisms, especially M. catarrhalis, streptococcus, streptococcus mucosus capsulatus, B. influenza, B. Friedlander, B. septicus, and staphylococcus has not been appreciated. The employment of a highly multivalent vaccine prepared from numerous recently isolated virulent strains of the above organisms enormously reduces the incidence of pneumonia and other respiratory diseases (excluding tuberculosis) and markedly reduces the mortality of these diseases. It is also significant that the individuals inoculated prophylactically with the mixed vaccine shortly before the prevailing influenza epidemic appeared in South Africa have escaped infection or only suffered from mild attacks free of complications."

During the epidemic in Tulsa and environs, I gave 685 prophylactic inoculations of influenza vaccine. Five of those who had been inoculated were attackd with influenza but the disease was mild and free from complications. Eighty per cent. of those inoculated had severe reactions following each injection, fifteen per cent. mild, and five per cent. had no reaction.

In conclusion, I should like to place on record my appreciation of the valued assistance and loyal support of the members of the medical profession in Tulsa, C. H. Hubbard, Mayor of Tulsa; the Tulsa Health Department, Dr. C. L. Reeder, County Health Officer, Dr. John W. Duke, former State Commissioner of Health, in their noble efforts, in the prevention of influenza and allied diseases during the epidemic of 1918-19, that gave Tulsa the lowest mortality rate of any city in the southwest.

Suggestions relative to prophylactic measures as a means for the control of influenza:

1. Knowledge should be disseminated, at appropriate periods, to the laity by means of school texts, and other literature, laying particular stress upon the gravity of communicable respiratory diseases.

2. Laws providing for the control of influenza and other infectious diseases which often become epidemic and pandemic.

3. Incorporate in our medical texts facts in regard to influenza based upon clinical evidence, and not clinical evidence based upon obsolete texts.

4. Statistics on various forms of prophylaxis in influenza and allied conditions available for physicians.

Summary.

1. Anaphylactic and anti-anaphylactic phenomena are valuable guides in vaccine theraphy of influenza and allied diseases.

2. Symbiosis is an important factor in bacterial infections of the respiratory tract.

3. In a diathesis brought about by constitutional weakness, specific immunization with a highly multivalent mixed vaccine prepared from numerous recently isolated virulent strains of pathologic bacteria commonly found in the respiratory organs will reverse the resistance.

4. Approximately 47 per cent. of cases diagnosed as pneumonia in practice are traceable, primarily, to infection with pneumococcus. The percentage is often found much less in many series of cases.

5. In all cases of pneumonia mixed infection with M. catarrhalis, streptococcus, B. Friedlander, streptococcus mucosus capsulatus, staphylococcus, B. septicus, are found as important factors.

6. Clinical results in practice from prophylactic and therapeutic inoculation for influenza and pneumonia with a mixed vaccine give prima-facie evidence of undoubted value.

7. A mixed vaccine prepared from recently isolated strains of virulent

bacteria of the respiratory tract, in curative therapeutic, or prophylactic dosage, the actual dose should be a little less than that of a particular organism used separately.

8. These views were confirmed during the last epidemic of influenza, 1918-19. The heavy mortality was due to pneumonia. The mortality from pneumonia has been greatly reduced by the use of mixed vaccines. Prophylactic inoculation with larger doses of mixed vaccine has reduced the incidence of influenza and prevented pneumonia.

9. The failure of preventive vaccination against pneumonia with various pneumococcus vaccines is due to inadequate knowledge of the etiology of the disease so often diagnosed as pneumonia. A purely pneumococcic vaccine is of no value unless the pneumococci predominate. Then it should only be used in connection with the mixed vaccines.

10. The failure of various vaccines during the last epidemic was due to inaccurate and incomplete knowledge of the etiology of pneumonia. The hard-shelled clinicians whose ego has cost the lives of thousands and tens of thousands will have to leave their darkened cells and get out in the sunlight and fresh air with the pathologist, bacteriologist, and sanitarian, in an endeavor to work together for the benefit of progressie medicine and mankind.

11. Prophylactic inoculation with mixed vaccines prepared from pneumococcus, M. catarrhalis, streptococcus, streptococcus mucosus capsulatus, B. Friedlander, staphlococcus, B. influenza, B. septus, with such other strains as deemed necessary, will enormously reduce the incidence of influenza, pneumonia, and other respiratory diseases (excluding tuberculosis), and largely reduce the mortality from these diseases.

12. The actual composition, proportion, and dosage must be governed by a close and comprehensive study of the micro-organisms found in the respiratory tract.

Discussion.

Dr. H. T. Price, Tulsa: It seems to me, that we have first of all to combat the decided opinions of the people. We have to educate them that the health authorities must do with them as they see fit, and along that line we would have to do again approximately what we did during the last epidemic. We would not have to have our people close the picture shows, churches, etc. We would have them educated to keep away from each other when epidemics get into our midst. When this influenza epidemic was among us, our people were not aroused as they were later, and it was very hard to keep a case of influenza isolated. I recall one case that was very severe. One day when I called on him he was very ill, the next day he was in the barber shop being shaved with the same razor used on others. Now our cities have not the money to do all they could. They should have a full time health officer. That would be a tremendous help to us. The wearing of gauze masks is very good and is sometimes successful, but it must be done properly. When you say to an entire city, "You must wear a mask on the street," that does not count much because they may wear it wrong, and that is no prevention. Now, the fact can be accounted for that the youth of the country was stricken for the reason that they got out more. So far as the bacterial prevention is concerned we do not know yet what the cause of influenza is. We positively do not know. The use of vaccine in some cases has proven of worth, and in others no use at all. With any stock vaccine we will probably not have any success. It must be a specific vaccine because in controlling an epidemic in certain cities of certain states it would seem that first of all we must have knowledge of the bacteria prevailing in that vicinity. There is a difference in different localities. The question of vaccine immunity has not yet been solved so far as I can see.

Dr. Lea Riley, Oklahoma City: This has been a very absorbing subject for the last nine months and there are lots of things we have done and thought they were absolutely right that did not do the work. It seems that an epidemic of poliomyelitis preceded this in other countries. We have never effectively found the bacteria for poliomyelitis. The same way with this. I personally think there must be a germ. There are things we do not understand about this epidemic. For instance the city of San Francisco closed all their public gatherings early; everyone had to use a mask, and San Francisco was hit as hard as any other city. On the other hand, New York, one of the most thickly populated cities of the world, was less hard hit and they did not hardly use masks. There are lots of things about this I do not know.

Dr. W. R. Leverton, Hobart: I enjoyed the doctor's paper very much. I think when we study the condition more a great deal of good will be brought out. I want to agree with Dr. Price on the use of vaccine. I was located where we had 250 influenza patients. We did not use any vaccine, only the ordinary measures, plenty of fresh air and the enforcement of a mask. Our percentage of infection was probably a great deal lower than in some localities. We cannot say that the use of vaccine is going to absolutely prevent or even relieve, because we did not use these things. I think our rate was 35 per cent. of what it was in the rural districts.

Dr. A. B. Leeds, Chickasha: I had quite a little experience with the influenza, having had a "Flu" jaunt over the state in the U. S. Public Health work, and fortunately for me my last location happened to be among the full blood Indians. You perhaps all realize the tendency of Indians to succumb to repiratory disease and lack of sanitation. The two cases I saw happened to be a case of influenza pneumonia. I gave this Apache woman the serotherapy. I went back to see her the next day. She was lying on the floor as they all do when they are sick unless they think they are going to die. We had 360 cases of "Flu," 64 cases pneumonia, with four deaths, among those Indians. Previously they had been dying at the rate of six or eight a day at that agency. My other experience with the serotherapy convinced me there was more in that than in any form of treatment. Within six days the epidemic among these Indians was entirely stopped.

Dr. J. W. Duke, Guthrie: I think perhaps there has been enough said upon this subject, but I am constrained to say just one word to you gentlemen on the public health matter. Your best interest in these matters is to co-operate with the Board of Health. I had quite a number of experiences as former commissioner. We decided to put on a state-wide quarantine. The co-operation came from quarters least expected. I know you all agree that ignorance is the worst enemy we have to overcome, but the rank and file co-operated more fully with the State Board of Health in maintaining quarantine than the high-brows. The greatest trouble we had in maintaining quarantine came from the institutions. The other came from the churches. They insisted on maintaining services. I cannot think of a picture show that did not co-operate with the State Board of Health in closing their doors. Those people need education. The city of Tulsa gave the State Board of Health absolutely no trouble at all. On the other hand everyone there from the mayor, health officer, city police and everybody did everything they could to carry out the instructions of the State Board of Health. Do you know how many died in Oklahoma during this epidemic? Something more than 4000 people died in Oklahoma in 90 days. More than 400,000 died in the U. S. from this disease. So in the prevention of influenza the best means at our hands today is to combat that disease by isolation, scattering the crowds, eating wholesome food and walking to and from home instead of using public conveyances, until some bacteriologist makes a vaccine that is a specific for these cases. I wrote the Government for a good supply of vaccine and I distributed it as intelligently as I could where I thought it would do the most good, and the reports received from those using this serum were all encouraging. My personal experience is about 25 persons. Eight of those persons contracted influenza, but none had pneumonia. None of them died and I am inclined to believe that some vaccine or serum will be evolved soon that will be all right. There must be more scientific work done than has been done. My personal experience with those who had pneumonia was they all died. They died all over Oklahoma. Our physicians did as well as they did elsewhere. The quarantine carried out by the State Board of Health did not do much good.

Dr. L. J. Moorman, Oklahoma City: I was very much interested in Dr. Dutton's paper and I think he deserves credit for the energetic part he took in regard to the treatment of this disease in the city of Tulsa. From all the stress which has been brought about by this influenza, it seems to me that only one therapeutic measure stands out as unquestionable in its value. After all the experimentation and study of this disease there is no uniformity of opinion in regard to the treatment except as I stated awhile ago, not one thing, and I believe every doctor in this room will agree to that one thing, and that is rest. I am sure everyone who has had anything to do with the disease has seen the result of rest. I want to refer to the point Dr. Duke made awhile ago, I think we might say this, that many of these cases of influenza had pneumonia. It is not always easy to discover it. Many cases of pneumonia in epidemics recover.

Dr. Dutton, closing: I desire to thank those who have discussed this paper so freely and fully. I have been using the vaccines for a number of years. I believe my first experience was in the year 1910, which was advocated by most authorities, to use the pneumococcus alternately with streptococcus. The experience I had was not very satisfactory and I have been treating my cases as many do, in the best way as symptoms developed. I believe it was at the meeting we had at Medicine Park that I got into an argument with Dr. Leeds in regard to mixed vaccines, and since that time I have had considerable experience.

MENINGITIS AND INFLUENZA.

F. H. Stangl, Chicago (*Journal A. M. A.*, Oct. 4, 1919), notices in the reports of the pandemic of influenza references made to toxemia and to the symptoms of shock and meningitis, and quotes a number of authorities who have specially mentioned such conditions. He has, therefore, reviewed again the records utilized by Keeton and Cushman, with the addition of those which have accumulated since their report, a total of 3,400 cases, and finds that nearly 1 per cent. of the total showed symptoms suggesting meningitis or cerebral involvement, ranging from slight neck rigidity and bilateral or lateral Kernig reactions to deep delirium and marked stiffness of neck, and in one case to opisthotonus. Eight fatal cases, variously diagnosed as epidemic meningitis, uremia, tuberculous meningitis, apoplexy and polyarthritis, proved, on necropsy, to be influenza with marked lung involvement. The polyarthritis case is reported, the meningeal symptoms being most prominent. Another group of cases diagnosed as influenza-pneumonia or meningism, comprising twenty-one cases, including seven deaths, is tabulated. In all, rigidity of the neck was noted, the Kernig sign was positive in thirteen, and in six the Brudzinski sign was positive, and opisthotonos was present in one. The necropsy findings showed the usual influenzal lesions. The brain and its membranes presented only congestion and edema. The author summarizes as follows: "A severe toxemia and active delirium with definite meningeal manifestations such as is encountered in systemic infection and the acute exanthems occur in some patients suffering from influenza and influenzal pneumonia. The clinical picture in some instances closely simulates that of an actual meningitis or other intracranial causes of delirium and unconsciousness, and postmortem examination fails to reveal any inflammation of the brain or its membranes."

CLINICAL REPORT OF TWO CASES OF TRAUMATIC ASPHYXIA.

FRED S. CLINTON, M. D., F. A. C· S.

PRESIDENT AND CHIEF SURGEON OKLAHOMA HOSPITAL

TULSA, OKLAHOMA

In October, 1918, Mr. and Mrs. S., about 35 and 30 years of age respectively, while riding in a Ford touring car collided with an automobile resulting in their car being overturned, pinioning both of them underneath it. Their bodies remained between the car and the pavement for some time until the car was lifted from them and they were removed to the Oklahoma Hospital.

The most interesting feature connected with the recognition of the group of symptoms, which has been designated as that of *traumatic asphyxia*, is the comparative rarity of the disease.

The marked cyanotic discoloration of the skin of the head, face and neck terminating abruptly about an inch internal to the edge of the trapezius muscle, following the squeezing or severe injury of the chest and abdomen, has been graphically depicted in Plate 8, Page 908, Vol. I, Keen's Surgery.

The cyanotic color of the man was typical but the discoloration was not so marked in his wife. The thoracic compression resulted in fracture of ribs, a lung penetration and consequent emphysema in both cases. The sub-conjunctival hemorrhage was more marked in the man.

Treatment: The patients were given the customary emergency attention on arrival at the hospital, made comfortable, fractured ribs immobilized, morphine given to control pain, plenty of air and supported in an upright position in bed as this seemed more satisfactory than any other. In fact, the patients insisted upon the sitting or half reclining posture during their entire convalescence, which lasted some three weeks. Both patients recovered.

This report is presented because of the comparative rarity of the condition and the very striking appearance of one who has sustained such an injury.

FOREIGN PROTEIN IN PNEUMONIA.

C. W. Wells, Camp Travis, Texas (*Journal A. M. A.*, June 21, 1919), reports the results from the intravenous injection of a foreign protein in eleven cases of influenzal pneumonia. Nine of the patients were critically ill, and the prognosis, grave. "The protein used consisted of typhoid bacilli, macerated and exposed to the soluble action of alcohol for 12 hours, washed free of alcohol and suspended in physiologic sodium chlorid solution, the concentration being the equivalent of approximately three million bacilli per cubic centimeter. The dose employed was sufficient to produce a definite so-called protein reaction, as a rule 1 c.c. Leukocyte counts were made previous to the injections, and from four to twelve hours following the reaction. In several cases blood chemistry determinations were made before and after the injections." Thirty to forty-five minutes after the injections a typical protein reaction occurred, with severe chill and moderate cyanosis, followed by profuse sweating and a marked elevation of temperature. Shortly after this the patient felt decidedly better and seemed improved. In several cases there was a rapid crisis after the fever with no subsequent rise of temperature. Several cases are reported and a table of blood examinations given. Wells also reviews the literature of similar treatment by others. So far as can be determined, the intravenous injections of typhoid protein had no deleterious effect as regards increased retention of the products of catabolism. It is his opinion that the method is efficacious in selected cases, but should not be used as a routine by the general practitioner.

PROCEEDINGS OF THE ST. ANTHONY CLINICAL SOCIETY.

DR. LE ROY LONG, President.   DR. LELIA ANDREWS, Secretary.

DEATH REPORTS.

Dr. LeRoy Long. *Atropic Cirrhosis.*

Mrs. P., housewife, age 50. Influenza in December, 1918. Patient came to the hospital with edema of extremities and fluid in the abdomen. 5,000 c.c. of straw-colored fluid of sp. gr. 1.006 was removed, but it reaccumulated rapidly.

Six days later, Talma's operation was done in order to establish compensatory circulation by the formation of new blood vessels in adhesions between the omentum and the abdominal wall.

In making the incision to the right of the median line, an abnormally large vein the size of a little finger was injured. The liver was retracted and contracted much above the rib margin. It was about one-fifth the normal size and "hob-nail" in character. The fluid was removed from the abdomen and the peritoneum rubbed with gauze and the omentum sutured to it.

The patient left the table in good condition but sixty hours later she developed Cheyne-Stokes' respiration and seventy-two hours later she was unconscious. At the end of eighty-two hours she died in a convulsion.

In this case, in my judgment, death was due to several factors:

1. The liver, on account of disease, was not able to perform its function. Urea and other waste material was stored up in the blood.

2. The portal circulation was greatly embarrassed on account of the damage done to the already existing compensatory circulation.

3. There was poor kidney function—as shown by the very scant urinary output.

4. There was undoubtedly edema of the brain as manifested by Cheyne-Stokes' respiration. This may have developed in connection with the decreased kidney function.

Dr. J. F. Kuhn. *Strangulated Inguinal Hernia. Post-operative Pneumonia.*

Mr. M., age 60. Very large and obese. Patient came to the hospital with intestinal obstruction, severe abdominal pain and temperature 102.4 degrees. His heart and lungs were negative. There was a left inguinal hernia which had become strangulated. On incision, the bowel was found to be very dark, but when the hernia was reduced, it regained its color and the patient left the table in good condition.

Two days later he developed a condition resembling influenza pneumonia with gradually deepening cyanosis and rales which began as crepitant clicks and extended from base to apex. He died as a result of the extensive involvement of the lung.

Autopsy showed the right lung adhered to the diaphram. It was all dark red and infiltrated except at the apex. The bronchi were filled with a thick white viscid material.

CASE REPORTS.

Dr. Horace Reed. *Gastric Carcinoma causing pyloric obstruction.*

Mr. John F., age 66. The patient, a very emaciated old man, came into the hospital complaining of: (1) Intestinal obstruction, (2) marked loss in weight.

The obstruction came on about three weeks ago and was located at the pylorus. He would vomit within two hours after eating. The vomitus is sour and lately has become "coffee grounds" in appearance. He has not been able to retain any food for three weeks, during which time he has not had a bowel action. He had taken laxatives but they were vomited. He has lost fifty pounds in weight in the past two months, and is very weak and emaciated. Fluoroscopic examination showed an empty duodenal cap, very inactive peristalsis, and retained food and gas. X-ray with barium showed filling defect in duodenal cap and retention.

This was a case in which there was not time to work out thoroughly the details of the case. The history and physical examination point to malignancy, but it was evident that something had to be done immediately or he would die of starvation. There was clearly a pyloric obstruction which was due, we thought, to a malignancy.

In a man of his age with marked arteriosclerosis and a mitral systolic murmur, we thought it best to use local anesthetic. Local infiltration with one-half per cent novocain solution made a satisfactory anesthetic.

Posterior gastrojejunostomy was done and the abdomen closed without drain. There was such extensive growth of the malignant mass that its removal was impossible.

The patient improved nicely and you see him here tonight, three weeks after the operation, with a healed abdominal incision. Recent x-ray plates show that food is passing through the new opening.

We could not even hope for a cure in this case. The operation only gave him a little more time in which to arrange his affairs to meet the fatal issue which surely cannot be very far away.

Dr. Lea A. Riley. *Gastric Carcinoma.*

Mr. H., age 64, Austrian, occupation, farmer. Patient came into the hospital complaining of jaundice, general weakness and marked loss in weight. He has lost fifty pounds in weight in the past six months and has gradually become very jaundiced, but his exhaustion has come on in the last four weeks. Since that time he has had considerable nausea and vomiting.

He is very emaciated and his skin is of a lemon yellow, the pigment being evenly distributed over his body. Liver palpable 3 c.m. below costal margin. Veins of abdominal wall distended but no "caput medusa." R. B. C. 3,200,000. W. B. C. 7,400. Poly's 72. Lymphs 28. Pancreatic efficiency tests showed 20 units in the urine and almost 0 units in the feces, indicating some obstruction to the outflow of pancreatic enzymes.

X-ray shows a prepyloric indentation, a distorted caput and retention at the end of forty-eight hours.

This is a case which conforms nicely to Courvoisier's law. That is; a painless persistent jaundice with a distended gall bladder points to obstruction probably due to malignancy.

By keeping him in bed and giving him good diet, his condition was slightly improved and he was transferred to surgery with a diagnosis of gastric carcinoma involving the pancreas with possible metastasis in the liver.

Incision showed a mass on the posterior wall of the lesser curvature of the stomach, a hard friable pancreas surrounded by a mass of enlarged lymph glands, and enlargement of lymph glands along both borders of stomach extending to the cardiac region. Gall bladder greatly distended with nodules at the juncture of the cystic and common duct.

The involvement was so extensive, the operation was impossible and he was closed without drain.

The mass near the pylorus which was also shown by the x-ray accounts for the persistent vomiting. The enlarged pancreas shut off the duct as was indicated by the pancreatic efficiency tests. No doubt, this with the nodules about the liver caused the obstructive jaundice.

Very little can be done for this case and the final result will be death from exhaustion and toxemia.

JOURNAL OF THE OKLAHOMA STATE MEDICAL ASSOCIATION

VOLUME XII   MUSKOGEE, OKLA., NOVEMBER, 1919   NUMBER 11

PUBLISHED MONTHLY AT MUSKOGEE. OKLA., UNDER DIRECTION OF THE COUNCIL

DR. CLAUDE A. THOMPSON, EDITOR-IN-CHIEF
508-9 BARNES BUILDING, MUSKOGEE

DR. CHAS. W. HEITZMAN, ASSISTANT EDITOR
BARNES BUILDING, MUSKOGEE

ENTERED AT THE POST OFFICE AT MUSKOGEE. OKLAHOMA, AS SECOND CLASS MAIL MATTER, JULY 28, 1912

THIS IS THE OFFICIAL JOURNAL OF THE OKLAHOMA STATE MEDICAL ASSOCIATION. ALL COMMUNICATIONS SHOULD BE ADDRESSED TO THE JOURNAL OF THE OKLAHOMA STATE MEDICAL ASSSOCIATION, 308 SURETY BUILDING, MUSKOGEE, OKLAHOMA.

The editorial department is not responsible for the opinions expressed in the original articles of contributors.

Reprints of original articles will be supplied at actual cost, provided request for them is attached to manuscript or made in sufficient time before publication.

Articles sent this Journal for publication and all those read at the annual meetings of the State Association are the sole property of this Journal. The Journal relies on each individual contributor's strict adherence to this well-known rule of medical journalism. In the event an article sent this Journal for publication is published before appearance in the Journal, the manuscript will be returned to the writer.

Failure to receive the Journal should call for immediate notification of the editor, 307-8 Surety Building, Muskogee, Okla

Local news of possible interest to the medical profession, notes on removals, changes in address, deaths and weddings will be gratefully received.

Advertising of articles, drugs or compounds unapproved by the Council on Pharmacy of the A. M. A. will not be accepted.

Advertising rates will be supplied on application. It is suggested that wherever possible members of the State Association should patronize our advertisers in preference to others as a matter of fair reciprocity.

EDITORIAL

THE "NEW" REMEDIES FOR MALARIAL CONTROL AND TREATMENT.

Offering nothing new, but strikingly reiterating that which almost every physician thought he knew and understood, is the issuance by the International Health Board to its medical officers a statement or concensus of opinion as to the above matter. The work of Dr. C. C. Bass (see page 168, Journal Oklahoma State Medical Association, June, 1919), is noted and summarized as follows: The study was for control by sterilization of patients and carriers and concludes that quinine sulphate is the best form for routine use, oral is preferred to intravenous or intramuscular application, daily doses over long periods disinfects more cases than when the treatment is broken into a few days of the week. Ninety per cent. of all can be disinfected by oral administration of 30 grains daily, divided into three doses in the acute stage, to be followed by ten grains daily at bedtime for eight weeks. Children under fifteen are given the same drug, but in doses of one-half grain for the infant under one year, 1 grain for one year old, 2 for two years old, 3 for three to four years old, on to eight grains for children up to eleven to fourteen years of age.

The studies of Lieutenant Colonel J. W. Stephens of the Liverpool School of Tropical Medicine and his associates made in Asiatic countries and at Salonika note "useless drugs" which neither controlled temperature paroxysms nor destroyed parasites, as: Tartar Emetic, administered intravenously; Amylopsin and Trypsin, intramuscularly; Quinotoxin by the mouth; Colossol manganese and Liquor arsenicalis.

"Palliative drugs," which partly controlled but allowed relapse were: Novarsemobilin, Disodoluargol intravenously, and Quinine sulphate (3) grains daily or under, administered either intravenously, intramuscularly or orally.

"Curative drugs," which controlled the acute attacks and prevented relapse; 1st, Quinine sulphate orally, 90 grains daily for two days, 60 per cent. cures; 45 grains daily for three to eight weeks, 64 per cent. cures; 45 grains Satuday and Sunday for eight weeks, 72 per cent. cures.

Quinine hydrochloride, 15 grains intramuscularly for two days followed by liquor arsenicalis B. P. by mouth for eight weeks, omitting treatment for entire third and sixth weeks. Combined quinine-arsenic treatment yielded 87.8 per cent. cures.

These conclusions seem to be worthy of more than perfunctory trial. They are based on unusual observation in many thousands of cases by experienced observers who took nothing for granted. Their promise held out to the physician is that exact and painstaking administration will cure most cases. We know fro m experience that half-hearted methods result only in half hearted cures, so it behooves those having this very crippling infection to deal with to insist on thorough and painstaking administration of the only drug yet known to be effective—quinine— and in proper form to effect a permanent cure.

PERSONAL AND GENERAL NEWS

Dr. W. O. Thompson, Kusa, is moving to Hanna.

Dr. W. A. Aitkin, Enid, has returned from overseas service.

Dr. C. L. Hill, Haskell, is arranging to open a hospital in that city.

Dr. S. A. Welch, Dacoma, attended the New York Clinics in October.

Dr. W. E. Rammell, Bartlesville, is recovering after an operation for gall stones.

Dr. S. P. Strother, Holdenville, announces that he will move to Oklahoma City.

Dr. W. G. Omer, Thomas. is taking steps to have the Thomas Hospital enlarged.

Dr. Julian Field, Enid, has been doing special work at Harvard for some time past.

Dr. A. G. Cowles, Ardmore, is visiting clinics in Cleveland, New Orleans and Chicago.

Drs. Wallace and Boiend, Oklahoma City, announce the dissolution of their partnership.

Dr. C. E. Calhoun, Sand Springs, has returned from army service overseas and is at his old location.

Dr. J. G. Edwards, Henryetta, is moving to Okmulgee and will form a partnership with Dr. W. M. Cott.

Dr. A. L. Stocks, Muskogee, attended the meeting of the Southern Medical Association in Asheville in November.

Dr. R. O. Early, Ardmore, announces that he will open a clinic for the treatment of eye conditions in Ardmore children.

Dr. Thos. H. Flesher, Edmond, and Miss Margaret Elizabeth Cherry, Ardmore, were married in the latter city, October 18.

Drs. H. C. Weber and A. North, Bartlesville, representing Washington County Medical Society, will formulate plans for the establishment of a laboratory.

Dr. and Mrs. L. T. Strother, Nowata, celebrated the anniversary of their golden wedding October 21st. Dr. Strother was formerly one of the Councilors for the State Medical Association.

Drs. J. H. Scott and **W. M. Gallaher,** Shawnee, and **C. S. Pettey** and **E. O. Barker,** Guthrie, attended the meeting of the American Railway Surgeons Association in Chicago in October.

Tulsa County Medical Society, on motion offered by Dr. Fred S. Clinton, offers a reward of $500.00 for the arrest and conviction of any Tulsa County physician found guilty of performing criminal operations.

Armour and Company has taken precautions among plant employes against a return of the "flu" epidemic in Chicago and other cities where the Armour plants are located. All employes have been notified that without charge they may have the influenza vaccine administered according to the formula of Dr. E. C. Rosenow. In addition to offering this vaccine free to employes, a general educational campaign along health lines and particularly with reference to the "flu" is being carried on among the workers in the plant. Dr. Volney S. Cheney, medical director of Armour and Company, reports that the employes are taking an interest in the campaign and that as a result no serious recurrence of influenza is looked for among Armour workers.

DOCTOR C. D. ARNOLD.

Dr. C. D. Arnold, El Reno, died in that city October 27th after a short illness.   Dr. Arnold had not been in good health for many years, but continued his work until a short time ago.

He was born in Hardin County, Kentucky, in 1845, and after common school and college courses, graduated from the Medical Department of the University of Louisville in 1876.   Dr. Arnold came to Oklahoma, locating at Kingfisher, April 22, 1889, on the date of the opening to settlement of Oklahoma Territory, soon after that he moved to El Reno which had been his home since that time.   In 1894 he was appointed Superintendent of Public Health for Oklahoma Territory, which position he held for two terms.   He is survived by his wife and one married daughter.   Interment was had in the El Reno cemetery.

The United States Railroad Administration announces that local surgeons hereafter will be supplied transportation on foreign lines to attend medical meetings when application for transportation is made showing the meeting or clinic they expect to attend.   The transportation so issued will not be available to families of local surgeons.

University Hospital, Oklahoma City, was formally dedicated Thursday, November 13; the exercises taking place in the House of Representatives Chamber, State Capitol, 2:00 P. M.   On the program Honorables J. W. Kaysor, State Board of Affairs; Samuel W. Hayes of the University Regents; Dr. Stratton D. Brooks, President of the University; Dr. Le Roy Long, Dean of the Medical Faculty; J. B. A. Robertson, Governor; Dr. A. R. Lewis, State Commissioner of Health; Dr. L. J. Moorman, President of the State Medical Association, and Jabez N. Jackson of Kansas City, who delivered the Dedicatory address.   The invitation to the exercises recites the purpose of the institution as follows:

The State University Hospital is established primarily to serve those citizens of Oklahoma who would otherwise be unable to secure satisfactory hospital service.   On order of the County Commissioners, such patients are received at a nominal cost to the county.   Owing to the connection of the hospital with the State University School of Medicine, excellent medical and surgical service is available free of cost.

Persons of limited means will be admitted on certificate from their physician or from the county health officer on payment of cost of hospital service.   Such patients receive medical and surgical service free of charge.

A limited number of rooms are available for pay patients at standard rates.

and contains the following information as to capacity, etc:

The State University Hospital contains 175 beds, of which 25 are in private rooms. There are five large sun porches which can be used for additional cases in emergencies. The eight wards include separate wards for men and for women, and for white people and for negroes.   The five operating rooms include one for emergency use, one for eye, ear, nose and throat, and three for general surgery.   There are ample laboratories for diagnostic purposes.   In addition to the main kitchen there is a diet kitchen with a dietitian in charge on each floor.   The x-ray room and equipment includes the latest improvements.   The entire equipment of the hospital is absolutely the best and most modern that can be obtained.   Every convenience for the treatment of special cases is available.   The spacious roof garden will be serviceable in the treatment of certain types of cases.   A wing of one of the floors has been set aside for teaching and for research laboratories.

A banquet for physicians and their guests was tendered at the Lee-Huckins Hotel at 7:00 p. m.

CORRESPONDENCE

Oklahoma City, Okla., Nov. 12, 1919.

Dr. Claude A. Thompson, Editor in Chief,
Journal of the Oklahoma State Medical Association,
Muskogee, Okla.

Dear Doctor:

I have read the editorial, "Overtraining the Nurse," Journal of the Oklahoma State Medical Association, Vol. XII, No. 10, pp. 295-6, October, 1919.

That editorial and any other article inviting remedial measures for the rapidly declining number of available nurses is most timely.   I believe this is one of the most important problems confronting the Medical Profession today and, like yourself and other doctors, am anxious to learn the cause of this dearth of nurses and learn what means may remedy it.

The matter is of sufficient gravity to be thoroughly investigated by an organization with adequate scope and means to perform such a task—the United States Public Health Service, the Rockefeller Foundation for Medical Research, or some similar body.

It is likely such an investigation would disclose many factors responsible for the shortage, and the cause and remedial measures necessary in one locality different from those in another.

Further than drawing attention and thought to the matter we will not get, by theorizing; especially when misleading and partial truths form the basis of our logic.

If it is true (which I much doubt) that "More than fifty thousand deaths occurred during the influenza epidemic which might have been prevented had fairly efficient nursing been available," the "well known Chicago practitioner" should present facts and figures substantiating his statement.

The second paragraph of your editorial suggests the necessity of careful collection of information to determine essential qualifications of the candidates in training and possibly a necessity for revision of entrance requirements, retention requirements, and requirements for graduation and practice, but such sweeping assertions as the following, without presentation of facts on which based, will not achieve the desired end: "Daughters of thousands of mechanics have been rejected from such schools because they have not been in position to obtain the one year preliminary but are otherwise qualified." I know that statement does not apply to the country in general. If such a condition exists locally it surely should be corrected and the correction would seem to be needed elsewhere than in the training schools.

No one has a greater affection for, or appreciation of, services rendered by the medical corps men of the U. S. A., than the writer; my opportunity of comparing their work with that of trained nurses has been as complete as most doctors and I cannot refrain from remarking, in the interest of medicine and on behalf of the wronged, that the insinuation in the last sentence of paragraph two of your editorial, that medical corps men rendered nursing service equal to that rendered by trained nurses in the recent war, is not in conformity with the facts.

With an institutional experience second to no man's in Oklahoma and experience equal to the large majority in work in patients' residences, I have observed the work under both conditions, of nurses real and alleged; those learned through experience only, those "graduated" after a six weeks training in a correspondence school, those graduated after six months intensive training in a hospital conducted by mediocre doctors, those who quit training after one or two years in a first-class school, and real graduate nurses.

Occasionally one finds an excellent nurse who had little or no scholastic training and I recollect two such who were illiterate, but those are rare exceptions.

As a group, the graduates of schools with a three year course of training; schools where training is actually given, are far superior to their less fortunate sisters and the patients who fall to their care fare best.

Speaking of what a physician requires of a nurse, a physician who "only requires his orders executed" is incompetent to practice medicine. He lacks a proper conception of his duty to his patient; he does not know the value of remedial measures such as dexterous handling of patient, bed and bed-clothing and the many trivial activities of a nurse that are conducive to recovery, or the reverse, that go on continuously during the absence of a physician; he does not realize the necessity of a guard for his patient who is competent to quickly recognize critical changes and meet emergencies during his absence.

As a matter of fact, few physicians know how to make a bed and fewer know how to prepare articles of diet or give a bath, much less instruct a nurse how to do so, and it is therefore quite as essential to have thoroughly trained nurses as thoroughly trained chemists.

Let us refrain from correcting a deplorable condition by creating a worse.

Fraternally yours,

John A. Roddy,
612 American National Bank Bldg.

MISCELLANEOUS

ADROITNESS IS CORRECT.

Gentlemen who are engaged in the chiropractic trade—we use the word "trade" advisedly—are furnished Helpful Hints for Ambitious Advertisers by an Indianapolis concern that makes a specialty of this line. In one of the numerous leaflets sent out from this source to "Chiropractors" they are urged to "employ an advertising man," and not attempt to write their own copy. It is pointed out that there are in many states laws prohibiting fraudulent advertising, and "today the liar in print is soon run to earth." While we are unable, regretfully, to agree with the last statement, the conclusions drawn from this premise are more easily accepted:

". . . to advertise inside the chiropractic, medical and truth laws, requires some adroitness, some ingenuity of expression, some more than common ability as a wordsmith."

We'll say it does!—*Jour. A. M. A.*, Aug. 23, 1919.

INFLUENZA AFTER-EFFECTS.

F. C. Gram, Buffalo (*Journal A. M. A.*, Sept. 20, 1919), gives an account of the influenza epidemic of 1918 which struck Buffalo with the suddenness of a cyclone. The disease appeared October 1, with twenty-one reported cases. By October 14, they had the highest number reported in one day, namely, 1,886 cases with forty-eight deaths from influenza, seven from pneumonia and seven from broncho-pneumonia. From that date on there was a gradual decline. It was a physical impossibility for physicians to see most of the patients more than once, hence many cases of pneumonia were reported only as influenza. It was only after the crest of the epidemic wave had passed that anything like accuracy in morbidity statics was possible. Gram gives an account of the measures taken by the health authorities; the prohibition of assemblages, etc., and the temporary increase of hospital facilities. "Our influenza was like a prairie fire—short and drastic. Every influenza patient was either convalescent or dead within five days from the onset of the attack." Exact knowledge is wanting as regards the sequels of the epidemic, and an after survey was undertaken, follow-up cards being distributed to every influenza victim under an appropriation by the city authorities. The field work occupied about two months, and the results are shown in tabulated form. On the first examination, 748 cases were found reporting after-effects—501 have since recovered, and 216 are reported as recovering. Four deaths have occurred, but whether they were due to the after-effects or not is hard to say. Only one death out of the four was caused by tuberculosis. There were 220 cases of respiratory disorders, and twenty-seven of these at least were tuberculosis. Out of the twenty-seven, eleven were already on their records as reported cases of tuberculosis before the influenza epidemic, and could not be charged to it. Only eight cases could be positively diagnosed. Several were in families with tuberculous records. The first important observatoin is the small number of sequelae as compared with the total number of influenza cases, and the high percentage of recovery. It seems definitely established that there is nothing to be feared as regards tuberculosis as a sequel. The results also show the value of the early and vigorous measures employed for prevention.

SPORTING NOTE.

"Nuxated Iron put added power behind my punch and helped to accomplish what I did at Toledo."—Jack Dempsey.

Thus the new world's champion, in large advertisements appearing in last Sunday's papers—at least in such papers as need the money from such sources. The secret is out. We feel that an apology is due to those of our readers who rely on this department for their knowledge of sporting events. We admit to a lack of enterprise in not discovering earlier what was going on behind the scenes in Mr. Dempsey's training camp. But three short years ago, Mr. Willard was telling the public—at the expense of the manufacturers of Nuxated Iron—that that marvelous "patent medicine" was the secret of his easy victories over Jack Johnson and Frank Moran. Now the Honorable William Harrison ("Jack") Dempsey—also at Nuxated Iron expense—"tells the secret" of his training and explains how "Nuxated Iron" helped him to whip Jess Willard! Ain't science wonderful!—*Jour. A. M. A.*, July 19, 1919.

RECURRENT EMPYEMA.

F. A. Stevens (Boston), Takoma Park, D. C. (*Journal A. M. A.*, Sept. 13, 1919), says that final results of operations for empyema can be ascertained only after a considerable period, varying in length according to the infection, the size and the shape of the cavity, and the treatment followed. The minimum of recurrences occurs when the sinus has been completely obliterated after treatment, and they are more frequent when a cavity containing air is left. If the Carrel-Dakin treatment is used to sterilize the cavity, the chances against recurrence are better. Two other possible causes of recurrence are mentioned, namely, isolated and undiscovered pus collections or sequestration of a part of the original cavity by contraction of its walls. Stevens has had the opportunity to complete the records of 123 cases, first observed at Camp Lee, Va., and later at General Hospital No. 12, at Biltmore, N. C. These fall into two groups, one of 100 treated by simple drainage, and the other twenty-three treated by preliminary aspiration until the first infection had subsided, and later by thoracotomy and use of a surgical solution of chlorinated soda. Forty-four of the first group were persistently and obstinately chronic until the Carrel-Dakin method was used. In only ten of these was the thoracoplasty of moderate extent finally indicated. Among the cases healed under simple drainage, there were recurrences within eight months in fourteen. Ten of them were due to the hemolytic streptococcus, the original infection. Among the cases healed under the Carrel-Dakin treatment there were eight recurrences. The efficacy of this treatment was shown by the higher percentage of the good results, and the group treated by this method showed that the pus pockets discovered were usually at some distance from the original focus. In these secondary foci there were two symptoms of value: (1) the failure to regain the normal weight or even the loss of weight, in spite of treatment, and (2) hte rapid pulse rate and the moderate fever that accompanied all cases of recurrence with pus secretion. These points are illustrated by two case reports. The details of the findings in these cases are given. Stereoscopic plates were usually necessary in diagnosing the condition. The treatment depended on the character of the fluid. When it was clear and sterile, aspiration was all that was needed. In all the cases of recurrence, with the exception of one, in which the cavity was completely evacuated at the first aspiration, all the purulent fluids were drained by thoracotomy. In many instances in which there were repeated recurrences at the original site, necrotic bone fragments were found, and there was required the greatest care, and the cooperation of surgeon, internist and roentgenologist.

GROWING OLD.

A little less anxious to have our way;
A little more tired at close of day;
A little less ready to scold and blame,
A little more care for a brother's name;
And so we are nearing the journey's end
Where time and eternity meet and blend.

A little less care for bonds and gold,
A little more zest in the days of old;
A broader view and a saner mind
And a little more love for all mankind;
And so we are faring a-down the way.

A little more love for the friends of youth,
A little less zeal for established truth;
A little more charity in our views,
A little less thirst for the daily news;
And so we are folding our tents away
And passing in silence at close of day.

A little more leisure to sit and dream,
A little more real the things unseen;
A little nearer to those ahead,
With visions of those long-loved and dead;
And so we are going to where all must go,
To the place the living may never know.

A little more laughter, a little more tears,
And we shall have told our increasing years;
The book is closed, and the prayers are said,
And we are a part of the countless dead.
Thrice happy, then, if some soul can say:
"I live because he has passed my way."

                                    —*New York Times.*

COUNCIL ON PHARMACY AND CHEMISTRY
AMERICAN MEDICAL ASSOCIATION

(The following articles produced by advertisers in this Journal have been accepted for inclusion with New and Non-Official Remedies by the Council on Pharmacy and Chemistry.)

Abbott Laboratories: Tablets Cinchophen-Abbott, 7½ grains.

Hynson, Westcott & Dunning: Acriflavine (Boots) Proflavine (Boots).

PROPAGANDA FOR REFORM.

Formaldehyde Tablets. During the recent influenza epidemic a variety of tablets or lozenges were advertised which were claimed to owe their asserted value to the fact that they contained formaldehyde and liberated it on contact with the saliva. Tablets containing hexamethylenamine or other formaldehyde compounds can neither cure respiratory infection, nor even confer a protection against such infection. To be effective, formaldehyde would need to be supplied to the entire respiratory tract continuously for some time, or else in concentrations that would be distinctly irritant and damaging to the tissues. Some years ago, the Council reported on the inefficiency of Formamint, which was said to be an efficient germicide by virtue of the liberation of formaldehyde on contact with the saliva. To call attention to the inefficiency of this form of medication, the Council on Pharmacy and Chemistry now reports that the following were found inadmissible to New and Nonofficial Remedies: Hex-Iodin (Daggett and Miller Company, Inc.), Formotol Tablets (E. L. Patch Company) and Cin-U-Form Lozenges (McKesson and Robbins), (Jour. A. M. A., Oct. 4, 1919, p. 1077).

Solubility of Intestinal Ipecac Preparations. T. Sollman reports that in the administration of ipecac preparations against intestinal amebas, salol coated pills are not always satisfactory, although with due care, it appears quite feasible. He reports that emetin bismuth iodid, which is described in New and Nonofficial Remedies, is only slightly soluble in water and dilute acid, but dissolves quite freely in one per cent. sodium bicarbonate solution. It is somewhat soluble in the stomach and produces some digestive disturbances. Alcresta ipecac, an absorption of ipecac and fuller's earth, though sold with the claim that the alkaloids are "physiologically inert as long as they remain within the stomach, and are rendered active when set free in the alkaline media of the intestine," was found by Sollmann not to be decomposed with liberation of alkaloid by solutions having the alkalinity of the intestinal fluid. Ordinarily, it would not be expected that a substance which is quite insoluble in the intestines should still be effective on amebas. The findings of Sollmann demand a careful examination of the clinical evidence on which the use of alcresta ipecac is based (Jour. A. M. A., Oct. 11, 1919, p. 1125).

The William A. Webster Company and the Direct Pharmaceutical Company. The Direct Pharmaceutical Company of St. Louis is apparently merely a sales agency for the William A. Webster Company, of Memphis, Tenn. In government bulletins issued in October, 1913, there were reported some cases of adulteration and misbranding on the part of the William A. Webster Company. In a similar bulletin issued in August, 1914, there were reported several more cases of adulteration and misbranding charged against the William A. Webster Company. In a government bulletin issued in June, 1917, the same company was charged with adulterating and misbranding Aspirin tablets (Jour. A. M. A., Oct. 18, 1919, p. 1231).

An Uncritical English Endorsement of Collosols. Under the auspices of the English Association for the Advancement of Science, there has appeared a report on the present status of colloidal chemistry. A chapter on the "Administration of Colloids in Disease" is devoted largely to the "Collosols" proprietary preparations made by the Crookes Laboratory. In it, the advertising "literature" of the Crookes concern appears to have been considered ample source of information. In the United States the medical profession has been informed by the Council on Pharmacy and Chemistry that a number of the "Collosol" preparations were not colloids at all and "if . . . injected intravenously as directed, death might result, making the physician morally if not legally liable." The Council also reported that in cases in which the therapeutic claims were examined, the claims were improbable or exaggerated and that "Collosol Cocaine" did not contain the claimed amount of cocaine (Jour. A. M. A., Oct. 18, 1919, p. 1218).

The Patenting of New Therapeutic Agents. Enterprising pharmaceutical manufacturers have usually been ready to appropriate the results of scientific research by investigators or therapeutic measures suggested by practicing physicians. Not infrequently, in such cases, the desire for financial gain has caused the marketing of such products with extravagant, if not false, claims as to their value. Therefore, though it is unethical for physicians to receive remuneration from patents on medicines or instruments, it is important that new therapeutic agents discovered in our research institutions be protected by patenting them and thus to so control them that they may be available without subordination to commercial interests. In 1914, the House of Delegates of the American Medical Association passed a resultion to the effect that the board of trustees of the Association should accept at its discretion a patent on a medicine or surgical instrument, as trustee, for the benefit of the profession and the public, provided that neither the Association nor the patentee should receive remuneration for this patent. The Rockefeller Institute for Medical Research has solved the problem in a similar manner. Certain products discovered there have been patented. It is proposed to permit the manufacture of such discoveries under license by suitable chemical firms and under conditions which will insure the quality of the drugs and their marketing at reasonable prices. It is further announced that the Institute will not receive any royalties or pecuniary benefits from the licenses it issues (Jour. A. M. A., Oct. 18, 1919, p. 1219).

Anasarcin Advertising. Dr. Louis Heitzman reports that charts and part of the text of a book by him is being used as advertising by the Anasarcin Company, and that his publishers think that, in spite of the violation of copyright, nothing can be done. Knowing the standards of ethics the Anasarcin Company adopts in the exploitation of its ridiculous squill mixture "Anasarcin," the appropriation of copyrighted material is not surprising. However, something can be done by those who hold the copyright (Jour. A. M. A., Oct. 18, 1919, p. 1232).

An Insidious Influence. A knock at the door. A gentleman with a grip full of samples and literature is ushered in. After a pleasant chat in which you are "informed" about the action of the particular remedies in which he is interested, he leaves you samples and departs. You turn to New and Nonofficial Remedies and find no mention of his remedy. Why? Because the Council on Pharmacy and Chemistry of our national organization has investigated the article and found sound reason why it should not be used by the profession, or else, the manufacturer did not deem it advisable even to submit the article (Minnesota Medicine, Sept. 1919, p. 355).

A Pharmaceutical Clearing House. The Council on Pharmacy and Chemistry of the American Medical Association is carrying on a work of great usefulness to doctor and layman. Actuated by no selfish interests, condemned by designing sharks who wish to exploit their frauds, and ridiculed by the jealous manufacturers of pharmaceuticals, the Council pursues the even tenor of its labors, playing no favorites, exposing frauds wherever found, and awaiting not the stamp of approval, of praise, or of gratitude from anyone. This "clearing house" is the medium through which physicians may learn the unvarnished, straightforward truths about proprietary products. A plea of ignorance of proprietary articles used does not excuse the physician, since it is his duty to follow the course of instruction offered by the Council and to appeal to this clearing house for information (Southern Medical Journal, Sept., 1919, p. 581).

OFFICERS OF OKLAHOMA STATE MEDICAL ASSOCIATION.

President—Dr. L. J. Moorman, Oklahoma City.
President-elect—Dr. John W. Duke, Guthrie.
1st Vice-President—Dr. Jackson Broshears, Lawton.
2nd Vice-President—Dr. G. Pinnell, Miami.
3rd Vice-President—Dr. J. A. Hatchett, El Reno.
Secretary-Treasurer-Editor—Dr. Claude Thompson, Muskogee.
Assistant Editor and Councilor Representative—Dr. C. W. Heitzman, Muskogee.
Delegates to A. M. A.—1919-1920, Dr. LeRoy Long, Oklahoma City. 1920-1921, Dr. L. S. Willour, McAlester.
Meeting place, Oklahoma City, May, 1920.

COUNCILOR DISTRICTS.

District No. 1. Texas, Beaver, Cimarron, Harper, Ellis, Woods, Woodward, Alfalfa, Major, Grant, Garfield, Noble and Kay. G. A. Boyle, Enid.

District No. 2. Dewey, Roger Mills, Custer, Beckham, Washita, Greer, Kiowa, Harmon, Jackson and Tillman. Ellis Lamb, Clinton.

District No. 3. Blaine, Kingfisher, Canadian, Logan, Payne, Lincoln, Oklahoma, Cleveland, Pottawatomie, Seminole and McClain. M. E. Stout, Oklahoma City.

District No. 4. Caddo, Grady, Comanche, Cotton, Stephens, Jefferson, Garvin, Murray, Carter, and Love. J. T. Slover, Sulphur.

District No. 5. Pontotoc, Coal, Johnston, Atoka, Marshall, Bryan, Choctaw, Pushmataha and McCurtain. J. L. Austin, Durant.

District No. 6. Okfuskee, Hughes, Pittsburg, Latimer, LeFlore, Haskell and Sequoyah. Vacant.

District No. 7. Pawnee, Osage, Washington, Tulsa, Creek, Nowata and Rogers. N. W. Mayginnis, Tulsa.

District No. 8. Craig, Ottawa, Delaware, Mayes, Wagoner, Cherokee, Adair, Okmulgee, Muskogee and McIntosh. J. H. White, Muskogee.

CHAIRMEN OF SCIENTIFIC SECTIONS.

Surgery and Gynecology—Chairman, Dr. Ralph V. Smith, Tulsa; Secretary-Vice Chairman, Dr. Ross Grosshart, Wright Building, Tulsa.

Pediatrics and Obstetrics—Chairman, Dr. C. V. Rice, Barnes Building, Muskogee; Secretary-Vice Chairman, Dr. J. Raymond Burdick, Ketchum Hotel, Tulsa.

Eye, Ear, Nose and Throat—Dr. L. C. Kuyrkendall, McAlester.

General Medicine, Nervous and Mental Diseases—Dr. Jas. T. Riley, El Reno.

Genitourinary, Skin and Radiology—Dr. J. Hoy Sanford, Muskogee.

Necrology Committee—Drs. C. W. Heitzman, Muskogee; John W. Duke, Guthrie; L. C. Kurykendall, McAlester.

Legislative Committee—Dr. Millington Smith, Oklahoma City; Dr. J. M. Byrum, Shawnee; Dr. J. C. Mahr, Oklahoma City.

For the Study and Control of Cancer—Drs. LeRoy Long, Oklahoma City; Gayfree Ellison, Norman; D. A. Myers, Lawton.

For the Study and Control of Pellagra—Drs. A. A. Thurlow, Norman; L. A. Mitchell, Frederick; J. C. Watkins, Checotah.

For the Study of Venereal Diseases—Drs. Wm. J. Wallace, Oklahoma City; Ross Grosshart, Tulsa; J. E. Bercaw, Okmulgee.

Tuberculosis—Drs. H. T. Price, Tulsa; C. W. Heitzman, Muskogee; Leila E Andrews, Oklahoma City.

Conservation of Vision—Drs. L. A. Newton, Oklahoma City; L. Haynes Buxton, Oklahoma City; G. E. Hartshorne, Shawnee.

Hospital Committee—F. S. Clinton, Tulsa; M. Smith, Oklahoma. City; C. A. Thompson, Muskogee.

Committee on Medical Education—Drs. A. L. Blesh; A. K. West; A. W. White, Oklahoma City

State Commissioner of Health—Dr. A. R. Lewis, Oklahoma City..

STATE BOARD OF MEDICAL EXAMINERS.

W. E. Sanderson, Altus; W. T. Ray, Gould; O. N. Windle, Sayre; J. E. Farber, Cordell; D. W. Miller, Blackwell; J. M. Byrum, Shawnee, Secretary; J. E. Emanuel, Chickasha; H. C. Montague, Muskogee.

Oklahoma reciprocates with Georgia, Kentucky, Mississippi, Nevada, North Carolina, Wisconsin, Kansas, Arkansas, Virginia, West Virginia, Nebraska, New Mexico, Tennessee, Iowa, Ohio, California, Colorado, Indiana, Missouri, New Jersey, Vermont, Texas, Michigan.

Meetings held on first Tuesday of January, April, July and October, Oklahoma City. Address all communications to the Secretary, Dr. J. M. Byrum, Shawnee.

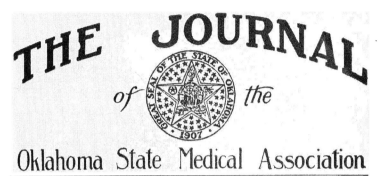

THE JOURNAL of the
Oklahoma State Medical Association

VOLUME XII   MUSKOGEE, OKLA., DECEMBER, 1919   NUMBER 12

THE TUBERCULOSIS DISPENSARY.*

HORACE T. PRICE, M. D.

TULSA, OKLAHOMA

Following so closely the conclusion of the War and of the influenza epidemic, it is but natural that our thoughts, medical, should be directed toward the prevention of disease, and so we find a number of the papers presented at this meeting to be along that line. This one follows the same course and is presented in this Section of General Medicine rather than in the Tuberculosis Section, because they who are especially interested are awake to the necessities of prevention along that line, while those in General Medicine may not be giving the desired attention to the subject, and it is hoped that by this discussion, you will all give greater thought to the end of preventing tuberculosis and diseases leading thereto.

The subject of dispensaries is peculiarly apropo just now, inasmuch as the state legislative bodies have so recently provided for the establishment of tuberculosis dispensaries in various parts of the state, to be chosen later, as well as three sanatoria, all of which will be of extreme value as tending toward the reduction of the incidence of this disease.

The State Tuberculosis Association has done most effective work toward bringing this about and has also directed the opening of eight dispensaries, all of which are thriving, so far as patients are concerned, and these special dispensaries will no doubt in time lead to the opening of general dispensaries, which are much needed and would do great good.

Historically, according to Davis and Warner,[1] the first recorded dispensary was opened in London in 1687. In the United States, in Philadelphia in 1786, the same building still being in use for that purpose. In 1827 the dispensary was first used to teach students. At the present time some four million persons in the United States, or one in twenty-five of the population, go to the general and special dispensaries.

There are various types of dispensaries—general, covering all diseased conditions, and special, limited to certain branches as, tuberculosis, children, eye, ear, nose and throat, venereal, etc.

The motive for establishing dispensaries is of interest, such as the teaching motive, where the dispensary is a part of a school and used to instruct the students, the medical experience motive, as the examination of large numbers of those afflicted with a certain ailment is of immense value to the medical man handling

*Read in Section on General Medicine, Annual Meeting, Muskogee, May, 1919.

1. Davis and Warner, Dispensaries 1918.

them; the public health motive, i.e., the education of the public, directly, at the dispensary and through distribution of advertising leaflets, Red Cross seal sales, lectures, and moving picture films and through the visiting nurse, all through the agency of the dispensary. Another motive is for the increase of facilities for the diagnosis and treatment of diseases. The two latter motives are more in connection with tuberculosis dispensaries, though they may be used in venereal as well.

It is the demand of the National Tuberculosis Association that dispensaries be opened in every city and county, so that any one who suspects he has tuberculosis may be examined and treated. This Association was organized in 1905 for the purpose of the study and prevention of tuberculosis and has organized since then fifty state-wide associations with over 1400 local organizations.

It is probable, and to be desired, that these locals will combine with like activities, forming a United Health Center, under a directing head, so avoiding duplication of effort.

The tuberculosis dispensary is quite a different proposition than the general or other special dispensaries. It is first of all, free of charge for most of its service, but because of the great desire to prevent incipient disease becoming more advanced, to prevent contact of the diseased with the healthy, to teach prevention of spread by care in coughing, and of sputum, by general cleanliness of person and home, it seems necessary to not entirely exclude those who can afford to pay, at least for the initial examination, especially so since the diagnosis here is of more importance in the majority of cases than the after medical treatment, a fact which does not obtain in other dispensaries where the drug or surgical treatment is of equal importance. And since it is well established that an early diagnosis of tuberculosis is often most difficult, to say the least, it follows that in many communities there is no physician paying special attention to this condition and people go to the dispensary as the only available place and the physician in charge can hardly decline to examine them, except at his own office, in other words, cannot refer cases to himself.

Other dispensaries, however, can very fairly refuse treatment at once, except only emergency, to those able to pay, as all the physicians are handling the type of work, and the educational and preventive endeavors are lacking.

It is, even so, essential that advantage be not taken of this privilege to too great an extent and the visiting nurse may be instructed to judge of financial capacity when making her calls at the home, which should be done in every case, and if it is found that one can afford to consult a physician for further advice or treatment, they should be advised to do so. City ordinances should also make it a misdemeanor to take such advantage.

It is also true that there are many families with its wage earner working steadily, earning enough for ordinary use and usual doctor's bills, who absolutely could not pay for a long course of treatment or some special, high priced treatment, or for competent consultants, such as x-ray, various laboratory work, special surgical and genito-urinary examinations. To those it seems necessary to extend the privilege of the dispensary, where all these may be secured at the expense of the dispensary or at greatly reduced rates by the dispensary consulting staff—all in the great effort to lessen the tremendous incidence of tuberculosis. But in spite of this, the dispensary should be conducted as nearly as possible as an institution for the care of the indigent, as it is essential that the incomes of physicians, often meager enough, should not be further depleted by his losing patients to the dispensary. On the other hand, he should be encouraged to send his poor tuberculosis cases there, or at least allow the visiting nurse to call on them at their homes and help to see that they are living correctly, in which work she will be found of great value, going into the details of housing, sleeping, fresh air, food, cleanliness, etc., right on the ground, with improvement suggestions which the busy physician might overlook or not have time to go into. The dispensary to be of full value must have every physician as its friend and co-worker and must be so conducted that no jealousy or other ill feeling may arise toward the staff.

This staff should consist of one or more examiners giving such time at such intervals as may be required to the general physical examination, paying special attention to the lungs, attempting to establish a diagnosis and having the privilege of referring cases to other members for special examination or treatment. There should be a genito-urinary man to look after the kidneys, bladder and pelvis, a surgeon for the diagnosis of joint troubles and treatment of spinal tuberculosis, an aurist and oculist to take care of the tuberculous condition in his field, and of great value should be a pediatrist to assume the care of children, of whom very many should be found in the ranks of those visiting a tuberculosis dispensary. An x-ray picture should be taken of every case and comparison made with the results of physical examination, much of value thereby accruing to both patient and examiner, so that a roentgenologist sould be a member of the staff. It is of course necessary to be in close touch with other laboratories so that examinations may be made of sputum, urine and blood in order to, if possible, exclude other than tuberculous conditions. In order to reduce the expense either to clinics or patients for these various and necessary laboratory aids, it seems that the dispensary should be closely affiliated with or a part of a hospital having such facilities, or be operated by the state, county or city with its own laboratories, otherwise the expense of needed routine laboratory work will be too great, and consequently only occasionally used and much valuable information not obtained, owing to a lack of a complete examination.

The tuberculosis dispensary is peculiarly a public health institution, being educational in character to a very great degree, advertising its service as other dispensaries do not, distributing literature, putting up posters, holding lectures and exhibits at public places, such as county fairs, etc., carrying on health, clean up, anti-spit and like campaigns, aiding other organizations in pure water and pure milk efforts, encouraging and aiding in the establishment of open air schools for children who are below par, not necessarily tuberculous but might be very soon without such assistance, encouraging general inspection of school children and all such efforts related to the prevention of tuberculosis or diseases leading thereto.

While the examining physician is an important "adjunct" to this dispensary, yet it must be positively stated that the visiting nurse is the one who is doing the real good work. She takes the histories, prepares the applicants for examination, aids during the examination, visits the home at frequent intervals, giving the necessary instructions, there on the ground, at subsequent visits determining if those instructions were followed in detail, judging the amount of material relief needed in each case, studying the social position of families, acting as agent between the sick and hospitals, sanatoria or other relief agencies, and sometimes even bringing patients to the dispensary building. So it behooves the dispensary management to look well into the qualifications of this specially trained public health nurse before employing her.

Many of the cases come to the dispensary through the agency of the printed matter, newspaper articles and other advertising features, others are referred by patients already attending, others through like organizations, while many may be secured through the industrial first aid stations, now to be found in many large business establishments, while school inspection will furnish many more.

The tuberculosis dispensary will not reach that point where it is doing even nearly all that may be desired until public and private sanatoria are available for all classes of cases. At the present time there are not a sufficient number of private pay sanatoria in each section of the country to afford admittance to all those applying who may be classed as curable cases, and no provision for those hopeless advanced cases which are so dangerous in the spread of the disease.

Public sanatoria, state or county, are wofully lacking, and cannot begin to admit all who should have institutional treatment, either in the endeavor to cure or to protect other members of the community. There should at once be established in each county in each state a sanatorium, so arranged as to be able to care for both pay and indigent, early and advanced, white and colored cases of tuberculosis, using the dispensaries as feeders for these institutions and to follow up the cases as they are discharged.

One more manner in which the dispensary may be useful to the public and to the medical profession, is to make of it a tuberculosis center, to which anyone may go with certainty, to consult the literature on the subject, which should be found there covering the various aspects of tuberculosis, its history, cause, prevention, treatment, location of dispensaries, pay and free sanatoria, with estimates of cost, possibility of immediate admission, and other information along public health lines which might be sought and be of great value.

In these and many other ways the tuberculosis dispensary may be an aid in advancing the health of its community, lowering general mortality rates and reducing the terrific loss incident to tuberculosis.

A REVIEW OF TUBERCULOSIS.*

J. W. NIEWEG, M. D.
DUNCAN, OKLAHOMA

Tuberculosis may be diagnosed with reasonable surety at a very early stage of its incipiency: though incipient tuberculosis of the hilus may be very difficult to diagnose. There are signs often found in examining a perfectly healthy lung that very closely simulate those found in both active and non-active tuberculosis.

Before attempting to describe some of the signs of tuberculosis, I will mention, rather vaguely, some signs that might easily lead a casual examiner to erroneously diagnose as tuberculosis what is a healthy condition.

Slightly harsh breath sounds and slightly prolonged expiration, at the apex, above the clavicle anterior and down to the third dorsal vertebra posterior, on the right side and the extreme apex on the left side, must not be considered diagnsotic unless other signs are present. Also the right second interspace near the sternum, due to the close proximity of the main bronchus. Immediately below the center of the left clavicle we get slightly harsh breath sounds with increased vocal resonance in the normal lung. There may be a slightly prolonged expiration at the left base posteriorly and harshness of respiratory sounds with prolonged expiration in the lower paravertebral regions of both lungs, most marked at the angle of the scapula, may be more marked on one side than the other, usually the left. The foregoing are the most common causes for an erroneous diagnosis of inactive tuberculosis.

In civil practice we are not much concerned about healed lesions. The thing that concerns us most is active lesions. The signs that may easily mislead us and cause us to make an erroneous diagnosis of active tuberculosis may be set forth as follows: When the stethoscope touches the edge of the sternum, fine crepitations may be heard, closely simulating crepitant rales. Clicks at the costosternal articulation are often heard that are transmitted for a short distance along the rib. Atelectatic rales heard at the apices may be mistaken for crepitant rales. They are not constant but disappear upon taking a deep breath. Marginal sounds, heard on inspiration, most marked in the right axilla, and the lingual sounds, heard at the apex of the heart, closely resemble crepitant rales. A crackling sound heard in the apical region, usually, especially in muscular subjects, so closely resembles crepitant rales that, if due caution is not used, the diagnostician will be led to make a diagnosis of tuberculosis. So far as I have been able to ascertain, this crackling sound is not mentioned in the text books, though my survey has

*Read before Stephens County Medical Society, June 25, 1919.

been very limited.   Lieut. King, of the Tuberculosis Board at Chickamauga Park, reports this crackling present in upwards of two per cent. in cases tabulated at that station.   At Camp Sherman we made no tabulation of adventitious sounds, but I am confident had tabulations been made, they would have run fully as high, especially among the recruits.   It appeared to be more common in recruits than in troops examined at the Remedial Hospital for classification and for over-seas. The calisthenics that are intended to exercise every muscle in the body probably overcame the condition that is responsible for the crackling.   It is more common in cold than warm weather.   If the patient be directed to hold his breath and exercise the muscle over which the examiner is auscultating and the crackling sound is still heard, it is a crackling of the muscles and not crepitant rales in the air cells.

Formerly it was thought tuberculosis always began as an apical tuberculosis. If the examiner had thoroughly examined the apices and found them intact he could assure his patient that he was free from tuberculosis without further examination.   Now we know that apical tuberculosis is rarely ever primary but most always secondary.   Incipient tuberculosis is generally first manifested in the bronchial glands at the hilus, as a tubercular lymphangitis, especially in children under two years of age, then invade a series of the peribronchial parenchyma, converting a tuberculous lymphangitis into a peribronchial tuberculosis.   If the process does not become arrested by immunity, or as Wright would call it, a high opsonic index, it may boil over, so to speak, and be conveyed to some other part of the lungs by the lymph channels—usually to the apices, or may instead, produce superficial lesions at the summit of the lower lobe; or to the opposite side, being either a peribronchial or superficial lesion.   Rarely, there is an extension to the lower .lobe resulting in extensively disseminated deep foci.

Owing to the obscurity of the physical signs, in minute deep lesions, peribronchial tuberculosis is very difficult to diagnose.   If crepitant rales (a sound like that produced by rubbing a lock of hair near the ear) are detected, if they are in showers, during inspiration only, all of the same size and constantly present, a diagnosis of active tuberculosis can be made without any other physical signs. In tubercular lymphangitis, the common mode of onset in children and the very incipiency of peribronchial tuberculosis, crepitant rales are not yet present.   Most of the diagnosticians doubt very much if a diagnosis can be made before the advent of the characteristic crepitant rales.   The feeble breath sounds may be caused by other conditions, so are not trustworthy.   The high pitched, short duration, slight tympanitic percussion note is of very little value only, to the expert with a trained ear.   There are so many things that will cause a variation in the sounds, such as not using the same force in the strokes, not percussing at the same stage of respiration, percussing over bone part of the time and over soft parts part of the time and many other causes.   Do not understand me to mean that this sign is of no significance.   What I wish to convey is, that it is difficult to detect by other than those who are thoroughly familiar with percussion and have an opportunity for extensive daily observation.

So far, the radiologist has not been able to assist us very materially in arriving at a diagnosis of incipient tuberculosis of the hilus.   It is true, that radiographs showing shadows with marked outlines aid very materially in establishing the diagnosis of fibrosis and calcification in old lesions and the fuzzy outline of active inflammation or an excess of blood in the part, but in the very incipiency there may not be sufficient.inflammation or congestion to interfere with the penetration of the x-ray.   If there is feeble respiration, high pitched, short duration, slightly tympanitic percussion note, and a slight shadow on the radiograph, incipient tuberculosis may be suspected.

A chronic non-advancing tuberculosis is readily recognized.   An accurate line may be drawn around the area of dullness.   Rales can be heard anywhere within the line, but never beyond it.   The moist rales are coarser than the crepitant rales heard in incipient active tuberculosis, and of the indeterminate variety. There is a broncho-vesicular breathing, prolonged expiration, transmission of the voice, due to fibrosis, as fibrous tissue is a better conductor of sound than air. As a rule, the greater the chronicity the more abundant the fibrous tissue and the more distinctly is the voice transmitted. If the lesion is extensive, there will be diminished expansion, or may be retarded expansion, or lagging on inspiration. Another sign rarely mentioned in text books and hitherto observed by very few tuberculosis men, is the subclavian murmur. This murmur is caused by the tortuosity of the subclavian artery due to either a fibrosis or an adhered. pleura. Narrowing of Kronig's isthmus is significant.

If the patient possesses a sufficiently high immunity to overcome the ravages of the bacilli, an incipient active lesion instead of becoming a chronic lesion will become an inactive dry-healed lesion. The signs are the same as in chronic active lesions, minus the rales. There are no rales in dry healed lesions. I wish to emphasize this, for sometimes we hear writers speak of dry rales. Sometimes moist rales may be heard in non-active healed lesions not due to the lesion itself, but due to external causes that stimulate an effusion of moisture into the air passages. Certain drugs are capable of increasing the osmosis of fluid into the air passages; women, during the menstrual flow, may have a slight effusion of moisture into the air passages. At Ft. Riley we found troops having lesions with moist rales during reaction from typhoid prophylaxis that proved to be dry healed lesions after the reaction ceased. If there is any reason to suspect the rales are due to other causes than tubercular activity, it is best to defer a diagnosis until after such causes can be eliminated. We may have recrudescence in which there is a healed lesion, beyond this a chronic active lesion, then an acute active lesion, each with its pathognomonic physical signs.

At the Base Hospital at Camp McClellan, all cases convalescent from measles were examined for tuberculosis by a special tuberculosis examiner before they were sent back to duty; then again one month afterwards. I think this would be a good procedure to follow in civil practice. We might add also whooping cough, influenza, and pneumonia, where the convalescence is long drawn out.

So far, no specific has been found for the cure of tuberculosis. Drugs must be limited to the combating of certain symptoms that may arise. Rest, fresh air and feeding is the tripod upon which we must build our patients. Even this often falls hopelessly short of our expectation. By rest we do not mean merely refraining from labor or active exercise, but mean that the patient must lie in bed perfectly relaxed—no rolling about or sitting up in bed and reading. Deep breathing must be prohibited; also exercising the upper limbs. Any kind of exercise of the lungs will cause an increased lymph flow in the lymph channels that are adjacent to the diseased portion of the lung. The diseased portion having lost its elasticity and the elasticity of the adjacent healthy portion being increased will excrete an excess of lymph presumably, pregnated with tubercular bacilli, is carried through the lymph channels to the healthy lungs. The two essentials to arrest an active lesion, are; the creation of sufficient antibodies to combat the tubercular bacilli, and the promotion of cicatrization and encapsulation. Both are enhanced by rest.

Fresh air, the second leg of the tripod, is perhaps as essential as rest. The blood must be thoroughly oxygenated to enable it to properly perform its function. It is not necessary to sleep out of doors, but may be permissable for the strong. The weaker should sleep in a well ventilated room and avoid the exposure to the vicissitudes of the weather. The windows should be so arranged as to admit of the free passage of air, sufficiently high to prevent exposing the patient to a draft. Cover rather light, as too much cover will invite an undesirable perspiration.

The third leg of the tripod, feeding, requires greater judgment than either of the two preceding. Sufficient food must be allowed to make up the deficit in nutrition. Hyperalimentation is highly undesirable and must be avoided. A perfect nutrition is desirable for the success of the difficult problem of furnishing sufficient antibodies to overcome the tubercular bacilli. Foods possessing the highest caloric value are desirable, as the nerve energy is usually below par in these cases.

A routine food can not be used successfully if we expect to get the best results. Different articles may be required to meet the constitutional peculiarities of different patients.

Tuberculin is dangerous in acute active lesions. May be beneficial in nonactive lesions. An accurate diagnosis is indispensible, or great harm may be done with this agent.

ACUTE MILIARY TUBERCULOSIS FOLLOWING PUERPERAL INFECTION.*

M. H. NEWMAN, B. Sc., M. D.

OKLAHOMA CITY, OKLA.

The subject of acute miliary tuberculosis following puerperal infection, which I choose for discussion, is to show that ofttimes a doctor is carried away in treating one disease, and fails to recognize the complications which arise that are of more importance than the original disease. I shall not attempt to discuss the subject of tuberculosis, but just to emphasize the importance of recognizing that disease in treating puerperal fever.

Acute miliary tuberculosis is an acute infectious disease due to the rapid eruption in various parts of the body of miliary tubercles; and is characterized by high fever, fast pulse, hurried respiration, pains in some parts of the body, particularly the chest, cough, and rapid prostration. The causes leading to that disease are various. In the majority of cases it is the result of an autoinfection, arising from either an active or latent tuberculous focus. Cases develop in which no apparent cause can be assigned. It often follows the fevers of childhood, as measles, whooping cough, variola, and influenza, or any other run down condition. It is well known how tuberculosis progresses much more rapidly after child bearing, due undoubtedly to the overwork of the various organs. Now, in case of puerperal fever, in which the system is saturated with toxemia, if the woman is susceptible to tuberculosis, it would only be natural to expect her to contract that disease. It is therefore necessary, in every case of fever after childbirth, to make an accurate and complete physical examination, utilizing all the aids which the recent advances in microscopy and bacteriology have placed at our command.

The first case of an acute miliary tuberculosis, following puerperal infection, which came under my observation, was in Omaha, while being in the hospital. An Indian woman from the reservation was sent to the hospital with the following history: She gave birth to a child two weeks prior to her coming to Omaha, which died on the third day. The mother attended the funeral on a cold and rainy day. When she got back home she had a chill, vomited, and had high fever. The doctor there treated her for puerperal fever for over a week, without results, and finally decided to send her to Omaha, probably for an operation. The surgeon at the hospital gave the case over to the medical man for further study. The case was then referred to me to make a report.

The history of the case as as follows: She was an Indian woman thirty-six years old, a mother of three children, well built, weighing about 180 pounds. She knew nothing of her family. On physical examination I found the heart normal, left lung normal, but in the right one, the percussion note lacked resonance in one place about the center. The breathing in that locality was tubual. There was also some subcrepitant rales over the same area. She coughed some at night, but she did not expectorate much. Her stomach and bowels were normal but tender. Her kidneys were normal. She passed twenty-four ounces of urine on the day of examination. The urinalysis was as follows: Color, brownish-red; sp. gr., 1028; reaction, acid; no albumen and no sugar. The microscopic examination was

*Read in Section on Pediatrics and Obstetrics. Annual Meeting, Muskogee, May, 1919.

also negative. The blood examination revealed only a high leucocytosis of 15,000. Her uterus was enlarged and tender on pressure, and the right ovary was also tender. The right leg was swollen and tender. The vaginal discharge was scant and had some odor. The microscopic findings of the discharge were only a few pus cells, but no T. B. Her tongue was coated and dry in the center and red at the edges. The temperature chart showed that her fever varied from $99\frac{1}{2}$ to 104, pulse from 100 to 140, and respiration from 36 to 50. She complained of headache, some pain in her chest and abdomen and right leg. She coughed quite a bit during the examination, probably due to disturbing her. I made a number of smears from her sputum for microscopic examination, but could not find any T. B., only a few pus cells, the same found from the vaginal discharge, were present. Though I recognized the lung involvement, but the history of the case, the negative microscopic findings, as well as the symptoms of puerperal toxemia, were so clear that I failed to give the proper importance to the pulmonary condition, and diagnosed just puerperal fever. It was clear that the infection had extended to her right leg, producing phlegmasia alba dolens, and it had affected even her lung on the same side. But I attributed the entire infection to the puerperal fever, to the absorption and circulation of pathogenic bacteria. However, that woman suffered from acute miliary tuberculosis, as the diagnosis was verified two weeks later at the post-mortem table. She undoubtedly had had puerperal fever to start with, but since then a more serious trouble had developed—acute miliary tuberculosis.

Several other cases have come under my observation since, almost similar in character, and if not for the first case in mind I would have probably made the same mistake again. I shall briefly report two more cases.

Mrs. H., thirty-seven years old, a mother of five children; father and mother living and well; having five brothers and five sisters living and in good health and one brother dead of tuberculosis; went to a doctor to produce an abortion, came back the following night and went out to her ranch several miles in the country. When she came home she had a chill, fever came up, perspiration was profuse, and she complained of pain all over. Her husband told me that she aborted, what seemed from his description, about a three month fetus, the following day. But she kept on having fever and pain all over. I was called out to see her about a week from her initial chill. I did not get much satisfaction as to the abortion, but she did admit that she had had a miscarraige several days ago, and that she had contracted a cold. On physical examination I found her heart normal, her left lung normal, but some dulness over the right lung, with bronchial breathing over the same side, also some rales. The pulmonary involvement, however, was less striking here than in the first case. Her abdomen was enlarged and tympanitic; her uterus enlarged and tender; both ovaries were also enlarged and tender. Her flow was rather profuse, but no odor. There was an area, the size of a silver dollar, about the middle of the calf of the right leg, which was very tender and painful, although there was nothing to see. Her kidneys were normal. The urinalysis showed nothing of importance. She looked very emaciated, although she had not been sick very long. Her tongue was coated like in typhoid. Her temperature was 104, pulse 130, and respiration 36. I told her husband that she was in a very serious condition; that she may have started with puerperal fever, brought on, undoubtedly, by the abortion and the exposure, but now there was a more serious condition—her lung condition, which looked like acute miliary tuberculosis. I made a number of smears from her sputum and also from her vaginal discharge, and finally obtained tubercle bacilli in the former, and only some streptococci in the latter. She gradually kept on getting worse, though she had had a number of other doctors, who did not agree with my diagnosis, and she finally died.

Mrs. N., the third case, twenty-four years old, had one child two years old; gave birth to another without event. She got up on the sixth day to help her mother with the work. On the eighth day she had a chill, fever camp up, and had pain all over. Her flow also increased considerably. I was told that she passed a blood clot the day she got up and her mother examined her vaginally to ascertain if there were not more clots. She kept on getting worse and I was called to see her. I found her with a terrific headache, pain in her abdomen, and her right leg tender. Her discharge was profuse, and had some odor. On physical examination I found the abdomen hard and tender, the uterus enlarged and so were the ovaries and the inguinal glands, and her right leg very tender. Her heart and left lung were normal, but the apex of her right lung was dull on percussion. There was tubal breathing over the right side, and also some rales. Her temperature was 103, pulse 115, and respiration 30. Her tongue was coated and her breath was foul. She looked very emaciated and was listless. She coughed some at night and in the morning, and the sputum was tenacious and had a bad smell. I examined her sputum a number of times before I found only a few T. B. She passed eighteen ounces of urine the day of examination. The urinalysis only showed a trace of albumen, otherwise normal. The vaginal discharge was also examined and only a few pus cells were found. She perspired some at night.

The seriousness of this case was apparent to everyone who saw her. Moreover, the surroundings were so bad that I had to make three to four calls a day and work with some old woman who helped to take care of her. The puerperal fever symptoms, however, gradually subsided, after two weeks of treatment, but the lung involvement kept up for several months. She was under my care for about a year, and even when discharged she still showed signs of tuberculosis.

The three cases reported are enough, I believe, to emphasize the importance of having acute miliary tuberculosis in mind in treating puerperal infection. Whether it is just a coincidence that the two diseases exist at the same time. or there is something in puerperal fever which starts up a miliary tubercle, has not definitely been settled. I am of the opinion, however, that a woman in puerperal infection, while the system is full of poison and the bodily resistance is the lowest, could easily be overtaken with another infection. An old or latent tubercle could start up to life again and disseminate through the whole system. Even if the symptoms of puerperal fever subside and the patient is gradually improving, we should still have in mind the gravity of the complication, if it exists, and institute the proper treatment, if it is not too late.

I am presenting this paper to bring before your attention the importance of having that disease in mind in taking care of puerperal infection, as it will save many a doctor the embarrassment in making a wrong diagnosis and a prognosis.

HEAT AND TUBERCULOSIS.

Harry Gauss, Chicago (*Journal A. M. A.*, Oct. 11, 1919), has studied the effects of high temperature during the hot spell of July, 1916, on the patients in Cook County Hospital, with special reference to the effect in tuberculous cases. The normal man is supposed to stand the excessive heat strain. For heat stroke it is not unlikely that heat, pure and simple, is the chief factor. During July, 1916, there were admitted to Cook County Hospital 158 patients suffering from heat stroke and exhaustion. But independent of those admitted as frank heat cases, rises of temperature were observed in other patients, greater than might have been expected in the ordinary course of their diseases. In the tuberculosis ward seven patients had temperatures 2 to 3 F. above that due to the usual course of the disease which corresponded in time with the principal heat wave. Similar observations were made in other diseases, but the tuberculous were taken for special study. Most of them had chronic advanced tuberculosis, and their fever tended to run an even protracted course without marked irregularities. The history of every case in this ward was examined and their temperature records were noted for the hottest five days, and the five days preceding and following. Fifty-six cases were thus observed, and their morning and afternoon temperatures for each day were averaged and plotted. "It is thus seen that in the five days preceding the heat wave, July 20 to 25, the average afternoon temperature varied between 99.5 to 100 F., in the five days of the heat wave, July 26 to 30, the afternoon temperatures varied from 100.5 to 100.8 F., and in the five days after the heat wave the afternoon temperatures varied between 99.7 and 100 F. The striking factor is that during the heat wave the average afternoon temperature was 100.62 F., as compared to 98.8 and 99.86 F. for similar periods preceding and following it." Gauss concludes that the increased temperature during the foregoing period was probably caused by the high air temperatures and unfavorable air conditions.

NEWER METHODS OF DIFFERENTIATING EFFORT SYNDROME, TUBERCULOSIS, AND HYPERTHYROIDISM.

RAY M. BALYEAT, M. D.

OKLAHOMA CITY, OKLA.

I wish to recite briefly the history of three cases, and discuss the recent methods of differentiating between the Effort Syndrome, Tuberculosis, and Hyperthyroidism:

CASE NO. 1: Miss A., age 25, nurse by occupation. The patient first entered St. Anthony's Hospital Feb. 15, 1918, complaining of fever. F. H. was negative, except that one brother has tuberculosis at the present time, and one brother died several years ago of tuberculosis. She was associated with the brother. P. H. was essentially negative. Except for an eruption on the body the physical examination was negative. Blood pressure was not recorded. Urine examination was negative. A diagnosis of measles was made. From this time until June, 1918, the patient was apparently in fair health. June, 1918, she was admitted to the hospital complaining of nervousness, fatigue, irritability, insomnia, and a slight loss of weight. Physical examination: Blood pressure, systolic 144, diastolic 95, eyes were normal. The chest examination revealed slight impairment of resonance at the right apex, but no moisture could be detected. There was a fine tremor of the fingers. She showed evidence of being very nervous. There was a trace of albumen and sugar in the urine. Her temperature varied from 98.6 to 100 and the pulse rate from 72 to 120. With rest in bed for a few weeks her sypmtoms had subsided to some extent. She then spent four months in Chicago in training, during which time she was rather nervous and at times ran a temperature above normal. Her third admission to the hospital was October 11, 1919, with symptoms similar to the ones she complained of on her previous admission. At this time she had no fever. Pulse rate varied from 72 to 120. The blood pressure was 115 systolic, 70 diastolic. The chest signs were not changed. The urine examination was entirely negative. The x-ray plate of her chest showed some decrease in radiance at the right apex, marked peribronchial thickening and rather heavy hilus shadows. The patient left the hospital before an adrenalin test was made. A diagnosis of pulmonary tuberculosis with a question of hyperthyroidism was made.

CASE NO. 2: Mrs. B., 25 years old, housewife. The patient entered the Peter Bent Brigham Hospital, of Boston, Mass., while I was a house officer in that institution, complaining of heart trouble, shortness of breath, weakness, dizziness, precordial pain and palpitation of the heart. F. H. was essentially negative. P. H. was negative. The patient was a healthy woman until two years previous to her entrance to the hospital at which time her symptoms began and have persisted. About thirteen months out of the last two years she spent in bed but without improvement. Her physical examination showed a nervous woman with a slight tremor of the fingers, a palpable assymmetrical thyroid gland. No eye signs were present. The lungs were clear. The heart beats were strong, regular and of a good quality. The pulse rate varied from 76 to 120. Laboratory findings, x-ray of heart and lungs, and electro-cardiogram of the heart were all negative. Basal metabolism was +4. She showed a typical positive adrenalin test.

A diagnosis of Effort Syndrome was made by the house staff of that institution and confirmed by Dr. Francis Peabody. Dr. Goetsch of Johns Hopkins Hospital saw the case and considered her a typical case of hyperthyroidism of atypical symptoms due to the adenoma of the thyroid gland, and advised operative search for the adenoma and if found, its removal.

CASE NO. 3: Mrs. N. F. B., age 38. Came to our office complaining of cough, loss of strength, choking attacks, and palpitation of the heart. F. H. and

P. H. were essentially negative, except that for the last twenty years she has had an enlarged thyroid gland. Her present trouble dated back three months, at which time she had what she calls an attack of bronchitis, associated with a sensation of choking. She has lost a slight amount of weight, has gradually lost strength and is very nervous. Physical examination reveals a normal temperature, a tachycardia and a blood pressure of 130 systolic, 80 diastolic. There was no exophthalmus, no tremor, but evidence of vaso-motor instability. She appeared very nervous and frequently coughed. There was a large symmetrical thyroid gland, which according to chest findings seemed to be partly intrathoracic. There was a slight impairment of resonance at the right apex with a few moist rales—a few moist rales could be heard over the right lower back—otherwise physical examination was practically negative. Clinical pathology showed nothing remarkable. The x-ray plate of her chest showed a partial intrathoracic thyroid. There was slight decrease in the radiance of the right apex. Moderate peribronchial thickening and very heavy trunk shadows. On account of her marked asthenia and rapid pulse an adrenalin test was done to find out if there was any over activity of the thyroid gland. She showed no hypersensitiveness to adrenalin. A diagnosis of questionable pulmonary tuberculosis with pressure from the enlarged thyroid gland, causing a chronic bronchitis was made.

These three cases represent conditions that the general practitioner comes in contact with frequently and the diagnosis many times is very difficult to make, but with the aid of the adrenalin test a great deal of our difficulty has been overcome.

The symptom complex known as neurocirculatory asthenia, irritable heart and effort syndrome was first observed by Da Costa during the Civil War. At that time no attempt was made to determine its etiology. During the recent war a very large number of such cases were observed both in American and English armies. Hyperthyroidism has been held by many to be the cause of the symptom complex. Many of these cases resemble very closely a condition known as the "forme frusti" type of Graves' disease. At the General Hospital No. 9, at Lakewood, N. J., the cause of the symptom complex was investigated by Major Francis Peabody,[1] and his co-workers. Many patients were sent into the hospital complaining of nervousness, fatigue, slight loss of weight, dizziness, precordial pain and palpitation of the heart. With the assumption that hyperthyroidism should cause abnormal increase in basal metabolism, these cases were studied.

On a large number of cases sent to the hospital with symptoms as mentioned, and with a positive adrenalin test, the basal metabolism was within normal limits. Few cases with but few signs of the hyperthyroid state were definitely positive to adrenalin. Means, of the M. G. H., of Boston, Mass., Du Bois, of Cornell University Medical School, and Peabody, of the P. B. B. H., of Boston, Mass., who have studied the basal metabolism on a large series of Graves' disease, have observed that the severity of the symptoms run parallel with the increase in basal matabolism. Peabody concludes that since the nervousness and tremor in the effort syndrome cases are so marked compared with definite cases of Graves' disease, that one would almost be certain that the basal metabolism would be increased and that if cases of mild hyperthyroidism were so common it would be almost inconceivable that frank cases would remain comparatively rare, and he points out that the whole picture is clinically different from that of Graves' disease.

Many of his cases gave a history of life-long nervousness associated with weakness and lack of energy. Many of them did not give a history of an acute attack of nervousness with loss of weight. The nervous activity with push, the restlessness, the physical and mental energy, as seen in Graves' disease, is often replaced by physical, sometimes mental inertia and a desire to evade the strain of life. He believes that the thyroid gland does not play a significant role in the symptom complex known as the "Effort Syndrome."

Major Harlow Brooks,[3] at Camp Upton, N. Y., makes the following statement:

"In regard to the etiology of the effort syndrome, I do not believe that any one can study these cases, at least those which have fallen into my service, without being at first strongly of the opinion that the condition is one of hyperthyroidism. There is no symptom in the N. C. A. which may not be caused by hyperthyroidism, nor which is not observed at least in analogy in young women afflicted with Graves' disease. On the other hand, a more careful study has shown me that this assumption is not satisfactory." So far as reported neither adrenalin nor metabolic studies were done in that camp.

Major Goodman,[4] a member of the Cardio-vascular Board at Camp Jackson, S. C., reports that out of 656 heart cases referred to them, they considered 48 cases to be suffering from hyperthyroidism.

During the last three years Emil Goetsch,[2] formerly associate surgeon at Johns Hopkins Hospital, and recently elected Professor of Surgery at Long Island College Hospital at Brooklyn, N. Y., has made an extensive study of the functional activity of thyroid adenomata, as indicated by the cellular content of the mitochondria and the adrenalin hypersensitiveness in clinical states of hyperthyroidism. He has found from a study of a large series of frank cases of hyperthyroidism that they all give a definitite hypersensitive reaction to adrenalin. He also found that many cases giving the same symptoms as seen in the Effort Syndrome gave a definite positive adrenalin reaction.

The adrenalin test is based on experimental evidence that thyroid secretion sensitizes the sympathetic nerve endings to the action of adrenalin. The technic of the adrenalin test is in brief as follows: The patient remains in bed several hours previous to the test and is assured that the procedure is in no way to be painful or dangerous. This is very important as fear might increase the nervousness which would interfere with the correct interpretation of the test. Readings are taken at five minute intervals of the blood pressure, systolic and diastolic, pulse rate and respiration until they are practically constant.

A note is made of the subjective and objective condition of the patient. This includes the state of subjective nervousness, manifested by throbbing, heat and cold sensations, asthenia, and the objective signs, such as pallor or flushing of the hands or face, size of the pupils, throbbing of the neck vessels or precordium, tremor, temperature of the hands and feet, perspiration, and any other sign or symptom noticed. Five-tenths of a cubic centimeter of one to one thousand solution of adrenalin chloride (Parke-Davis & Co.) is given in the deltoid region subcutaneously. Readings are then made every two and one-half minutes for fifteen minutes, then every five minutes up to one hour, and then every ten minutes for thirty minutes. At the end of this time the reaction has usually completely passed off.

In positive cases the blood pressure will rise, within the first fifteen minutes after the adrenalin is given, at least ten points and simultaneously there is an increase in pulse rate of at least ten. In course of thirty minutes there is a moderate fall with a second slight rise and a second fall to about normal within one and one-half hours. The following symptoms and signs, either all or in part, may be noticed: Increased tremor, apprehension, throbbing, vaso-motor changes, such as early pallor of the face, lips and hands, followed by flushing and sweating in fifteen to thirty minutes. In some of the positive cases the changes in blood pressure and pulse rate may be the most prominent feature, but there must also be present some accentuation of a majority of the signs and symptoms mentioned.

Goetsch has concluded from his investigation that no normal individual, or none of the conditions similar to hyperthyroidism, such as psychasthenia, hysteria, neurasthenia, or tabagism, will give positive reaction. He believes that all cases with a definite positive adrenalin reaction are cases suffering from hyperthyroidism. He divides goitre cases into three classes: (1) single colloid goitre; (2) adenomata; (3) exophthalmic goitre. He finds in the simple colloid goitre, where there are no symptoms the adrenalin test is negative. The plasma of the cells of such a gland show no increase in the mitochondria. In the cases of adenoma of the thyroid gland there is no increase in the mitochondria of the cells of the parenchyma of the gland itself, but markedly increased in the cells of the adenoma. There is always a marked increase in mitochondria of the plasma of the cells of the thyroid gland in cases of exophthalmic goitre. He has operated a very large series of cases which do not show the classical signs and symptoms seen in Graves' disease, but who show definite hypersensitiveness to adrenalin. In most of these cases adenomata were found and removed.

The symptoms in most of the cases promptly cleared up. In some cases adenomata were not found and the symptoms did not subside. On a second search when the adenoma would be found and removed the symptoms would promptly disappear. It is most interesting to note that cases suffering from an adenoma of the thyroid gland who show a definite adrenalin reaction will have a very weakly positive one or a negative one when the adenoma is removed. Also after lobectomy in exophthalmic cases the adrenalin reaction which has previously been strongly positive will become either weakly positive or negative.

In the past there has been a great deal of difficulty in differentiating early tuberculosis and the mild forms of hyperthyroidism. There is a large group of patients who complain of asthenia, fatigue, loss of strength and weight, nervousness, tachycardia, vaso-motor instability, and a slight elevation of temperature. On hearing such a story one immediately thinks of tuberculosis but in many cases the physical signs, laboratory and x-ray findings will not justify a positive diagnosis of tuberculosis. In many cases anti-tuberculosis therapy has been thoroughly tried without improvement of the symptoms. Other cases have been seen with similar symptoms and with physical signs and x-ray findings that would justify the diagnosis of early tuberculosis. Long continued anti-tuberculosis measures will largely clear up the signs of the chest but the symptoms, such as tachycardia, fatigue, and possibly a slight rise in temperature, will remain very little changed.

Only a few months ago Goetsch[5] studied a series of 40 cases at the Trudeau Sanatorium. The adrenalin test was done on these cases, by which means he divided them into three groups: In the first group there were 18 cases in which clinical tuberculosis was questionable. Ten of these cases gave definite positive adrenalin tests. In the second group of 16 cases a diagnosis of inactive tuberculosis was made, nine of this group showed a positive adrenalin test. In group three a diagnosis of moderately advanced tuberculosis was made and in all of these the adrenalin reaction was negative.

SUMMARY

One can at once see the importance of differentiating between hyperthyroidism and tuberculosis. In the uncomplicated cases of active adenoma of the thyroid gland the treatment is surgical while it is strictly medical in tuberculosis.

In many of the cases of active adenoma complicating inactive tuberculosis surgical procedure would be justified.

The complication of hyperthyroidism with tuberculosis will explain why the symptoms in many cases of tuberculosis do not clear up after persistent anti-tuberculosis treatment.

Considering the extensive work that Goetsch has done and being familiar with the work that Peabody has done along with my personal observation of adrenalin and metabolism studies on series of both the frank and atypical hyperthyroids, and the cases diagnosed as Effort Syndrome, I am made to believe that a majority of cases diagnosed as Effort Syndrome are cases of active adenomata of the thyroid gland, which do not raise the basal metabolism above the normal limits.

Knowing the attitude that the Staff of the Trudeau Sanatorium have taken towards the value of the adrenalin reaction in determining whether a patient is suffering from tuberculosis, tuberculosis complicated with hyperthyroidism or hyperthyroidism alone, has made me believe that the test will be of great diagnostic aid.

We are using the adrenalin test in differentiating between early tuberculosis and hyperthyroidism but have not yet made a sufficient number of tests to justify any conclusions.

BIBLIOGRAPHY.

1. Peabody, Francis W.: "The Basal Metabolism in Cases of the Irritable Heart of Soldiers." *The Medical Clinics of North America.* Sept., 1918, p. 507.

2. Goetsch, Emil: "Newer Methods in the Diagnosis of Thyroid Disorders." *N. Y. Medical Journal.* Vol. XVIII, No. 7.

"Functional Significance of Mitochondria in Toxic Thyroid Adenomata." *Johns Hopkins Bulletin,* Vol. XXVII, p. 129.

3. Brooks, Harlow: "Neuro-circulatory Asthenia." *The Medical Clinics of North America,* Sept., 1918, p. 477.

4. Goodman, Edward H.: "Results of the Examination of 23,943 Drafted Men by the Cardiovascular Board at Camp Jackson, Columbia, S. C." · *The Medical Clinics of North America,* Sept., 1918, p. 399.

5. Goetsch, Emil, and Nicholson, Norman C.: "The Differentiation of Early Tuberculosis and Hyperthyroidism by Means of the Adrenalin Test." *The American Review of Tuberculosis,* Vol. III, No. 2, April, 1919.

MERCUROCHROME-220

Impressed with the probable value of using dyes as a basis for the development of therapeutic compounds, H. H. Young, E. C. White and E. O. Swartz, Baltimore (*Journal A. M. A.,* Nov. 15, 1919), have devoted some of their researches in the James Buchanan Brady Urologic Institute to the production of an efficient urinary antiseptic, and have investigated a large number of compounds. The possibilities of one of these as such are described. It was sought to combine the following properties: "(1) ready penetration of the tissues in which the infection exists; (2) lack of irritation of the drug to tissues; (3) high germicidal activity; (4) ready solubility in water and stability of the solution; (5) freedom from precipitation in urine, and (6) sufficiently low toxicity to avoid systemic effects from the small amount of the drug that may be absorbed." The result was a preparation to which they give the name "mercurochrome-220"—a substance obtained by substituting one atom of mercury in a molecule of dibromfluorescein. "Chemically it is dibrom-oxymercury fluorescein, or its sodium salt. The latter contains about 26 per cent. of mercury . . . The free acid is a red powder insoluble in water, but readily soluble in sodium hydroxid solution, with the formation of a deep cherry red color, showing fluorescence on dilution. The dry salt forms iridescent green scales, slightly hydroscopic and readily soluble in water. The solution is stable and is not affected by moderate heat or exposure to the air. Strongly acid urine (ph equals 5.0) gives a slight precipitate *of the free dye*; but if the acidity is *p*h equals 6.4 or less, no precipitation occurs. There is entire freedom from precipitation when a one per cent. solution of the drug is mixed with an equal volume of medium rich in protein, such as hydrocele fluid." The tests as to penetration, irritating effects and bactericidal action are given, together with the methods used in the administration of mercurochrome-220. Its effects are illustrated by reports of cases. The authors summarize the results of their research in the following: "1. Mercurochrome-220 is experimentally a drug of great germicidal value, a solution of about 1:1,000 killing *B. coli* and *Staphylococcus aureus* in urine in one minute. It has practically fifty times the germicidal strength of acriflavine in urine medium for exposure of one hour. 2. In a strength of one per cent., the new drug is tolerated by the human bladder for from one to three hours without irritation. Injections of one per cent. solution of the drug into the renal pelvis are likewise free from pain, even when held in situ by plugging the catheter. 3. That mercurochrome-220 has a remarkable germicidal value is shown by the rapid sterilization accomplished in a series of cases of cystitis and pyelitis of long standing and refractory to other treatments. Now for the first time we feel that we have a method fo quickly curing certain chronic infections of the bladder. The rapidity with which a few cases of old purulent cystitis disappeared was surprising, becoming free of pus and bacteria in a few days. 4. Studies of the comparative value of acriflavine and mercurochrome-220 in gonorrhea are not yet complete, but it has been demonstrated that with both drugs, methods of great value in the treatment of the disease have been produced. Mercurochrome-220 has proved to be eminently satisfactory in the treatment of chancroids and as a dressing for buboes after incision. Other drugs developed along the same lines have been produced and are being experimented with by us."

PROCEEDINGS OF THE ST. ANTHONY CLINICAL SOCIETY.

Dr. Le Roy Long, President.   Dr. Lelia Andrews, Secretary.

DEATH REPORTS.

Dr. Geo. LaMott. *Pernicious Anemia. Otitis Media.*

Mr. E., age 67. This man came into the hospital complaining of weakness, shortness of breath, loss of appetite, and a discharging ear. His skin was a pale, lemon yellow, but he was apparently well nourished. His R. B. C. was 1,400,000. Hemoglobin index +1, many microcytes, and poikilocytes. W. B. C. 7,500, Poly's 70, L. 30.

A diagnosis of pernicious anemia had been made several months previous and he was sent to the hospital at this time with the intention of doing a transfusion. We were unable to do this, however, because of the acute otitis media. His temperature reached 105 degrees and he lapsed into a state of semi-consciousness.

On the third day of his illness there were intervals of twitching on the right side of his face. Pulsation on the right side of his neck was more marked than on the left. On the following day he began to develop a hypostatic pneumonia. The next day there was no venous pulsation on the left side, which I think, was due to venous thrombosis. Following this he lapsed into a state of coma and died.

This death should have been reported by the surgeon and not by the medical department because he died as a result of the middle ear infection. No doubt the pernicious anemia lay down the gap for infection, but it was not the immediate cause of his death.

I am very much in favor of transfusion in these cases when there are no complications and where other measures have failed. Yet arsenic in the form of Fowler's solution seems to prevent hemolysis of the R. B. cells which is brought about by the anti-bodies produced in the individual.

Bloomfield, from the Medical Clinic of The Johns Hopkins Hospital, reports a number of cases treated by transfusions and a number treated by the arsenic preparations, and the patients treated by the latter method seem to outlive those treated by transfusions.

Dr. Antonio D. Young. *Gastric Carcinoma.*

Mr. John F., age 66. This case was reported by Dr. Reed at the last meeting. The patient came to the hospital with an acute pyloric obstruction and very marked loss in weight. X-ray showed a filling defect and retention at the end of 48 hours.

His abdomen was opened under half per cent. novocain anesthesia and a posterior gastrojejunostomy was done. There was a large mass obstructing the pylorus and it had so involved the surrounding structures that it was not removed.

The incision was closed without drain and the patient was up in three weeks. He went home and stayed just 31 days. His appetite improved a little and he was able to walk around but there was no gain in weight.

He came back to the hospital under the medical service complaining of edema of the feet and eye-lids, nausea and vomiting and extreme weakness. Two days later he died of exhaustion and toxemia.

Autopsy Report. Incision showed almost absence of subcutaneous fat, the muscles were very pale and the omentum, which was adhered to the parietal peritoneum, was almost devoid of fat.

The opening made by the surgeon in the posterior gastrojejunostomy would admit two fingers and the pylorus was completely closed by a large white irregular mass occupying the pancreas, duodenum, tranverse mesentery and under surface of the liver, adherent to the liver and hepatic flexure of the colon. The pancreas was hard and friable and enlarged.

The pathological report of the tumor will be ready at the next time.

ABSTRACT

OF

AN INVESTIGATION INTO THE EFFECTS OF WAR NEPHRITIS ON KIDNEY FUNCTION
WITH OBSERVATIONS ON METHODS FOR ESTIMATING THE
EFFICIENCY OF THE KIDNEYS

By

H. McLEAN AND O. L. V. WESSELOW
CHEMICAL PATHOLOGICAL DEPT., ST. THOMAS HOSPITAL, LONDON

Read by MARIE BUMP

The article is a report of correlated chemical and clinical studies of a large number of cases of nephritis, from the onset of the acute stage until the termination.

Five types of cases are included: 1. Primary acute nephritis; 2. Acute nephritis occurring in kidneys, previously affected with chronic nephritis; 3. Acute nephritis terminating in recovery with regeneration; 4. Acute nephritis terminating in subacute; 5. Acute terminating in chronic.

The chemical tests that were found most valuable were blood and urine urea, urine diastase and urine chlorides.

Urea in a normal individual ranges from 20 to 40 mg. per 100 c.c. of blood. When renal function begins to fail, the kidney deals with urea and other nitrogenous waste with some difficulty and as a consequence is retained by the blood. The blood urea is, therefore, a good indication as to the efficiency of the kidney. Urea values that are within normal limits are noted in a type of chronic cases. When high values, in acute cases, tend to increase, the prognosis is unfavorable as are values above 300 mg. per 100 c.c. Mild cases show a decrease in amounts of urea.

Diastase or amylase in urine is determined in the same way that we do in our pancreatic efficiency tests. It was found that normal urine contains from 6.6 to 30 units per c.c. The lower the amylase content the more serious is considered the condition of the kidney. This value, of course, must never be taken alone.

Since urine urea determinations are valueless unless the blood urea, non-protein nitrogen, urine nitrogen and nitrogen intake are known, doses of urea amounting to 15 to 20 gms. of urea were given in a little water by mouth and the percentage of urea in the urine passed some time afterward was estimated. Results showed that the percentage decreased with increased retention.

Urine chlorides were found very low in cases showing high retention.

"During the early stages of an acute attack of nephritis there appears to be more or less interference with the renal activity in general. Thus, in a severe case there may be marked retention of nitrogenous products in the body with the usual abnormal ingredients in the urine; edema may be more or less distinct and the chloride content may be very much diminished. Sometimes the diastatic value is very low, while in other cases it may be normal. After the first few days the condition is often succeeded by a copious diuresis by which the retained products are eliminated. In favorable cases this phenomenon is associated with a marked reduction or disappearance of edema and gradually the patient becomes convalescent; in course of time, varying from a few weeks to a month or two, the protein disappears from the urine and the renal function seems to be completely restored.

"In other cases, however, there may be some early diuresis but the patient does not progress very rapidly and feels unwell; on examination it is found that the blood still contains excess of urea, a condition which may persist for several months after the onset of the trouble. Such patients are often quite free from edema and may pass only a comparatively small amount of protein in the urine, but the high blood urea figure persists, sometimes slowly decreasing and in other instances actually increasing. In such cases we have found that the diastatic reaction is of low value and remains low for a considerable time after the blood urea has returned to normal. In some patients, on the other hand, there is no increase whatever in blood urea, and the diastatic reaction is found to be high, but the case is characterized by a persistent edema and perhaps ascites."

Cases passing from acute to subacute and chronic show two distinct types of nephritis. There are cases with some of the characteristics of both types, but the majority clearly belong to one or the other of two types, referred to as azotaemic and hydraemic forms, the chief distinguishing features of which are shown on the chart.

IN THE URINE

Azotaemic Form
(azo and nitrogen radicals in the blood)
1. Oedema absent.
2. Hematuria frequent.
3. Epithelial and granular casts.
4. Urea concentration decreased.

Hydraemic Form
(water in the blood)
1. Oedema present.
2. Hematuria absent.
3. Small hyaline casts.
4. Urea normal.

IN THE BLOOD

5. Increased urea and nitrogenous products.
6. Heart enlarged and tendency to arteriosclerosis.

5. No nitrogen retention.

6. Heart not enlarged.

"The most obvious clinical difference between the two types is the edema and marked albuminuria in the hydraemic type, while the azotaemic type shows no edema but is often associated with cardiovascular changes."

—*The Quarterly Journal of Medicine*, Vol. II., No. 48, July, 1919, pp. 347-371.

TUBERCULOSIS

G. T. Palmer, Springfield, Ill., (*Journal A. M. A.*, Sept. 27, 1919), notes the progress that has been made in combating tuberculosis. Experience has taught that it cannot be measured by the standards of other contagious or infectious diseases. Failure has resulted in a seach for curative or preventive vaccines, and we must conclude that active tuberculous disease is not the result of a simple infection. Anti-spitting measures have not given results that inspire confidence. The relations between infection and disease have been shown to be very remote, dormant infection is so general that perhaps 80 per cent. of adults may be classified as tuberculosis carriers. The development of the disease is dependent on some factor or factors that reduce individual resistance, and such exist everywhere in any community. Palmer does not mean to say that we should abandon the methods now employed to restrict the disease. Open cases should be isolated. Coughing and spitting should be restricted, and care be taken to keep children from contact. Success in the past has been promising. During the twenty years following the first volunteer tuberculosis association tuberculosis mortality has decreased 30.25 per cent., while a comparison of five-year periods during the past fifteen, shows a tuberculosis decrease of 22.2 per cent. —a more gratifying showing than that of any other communicable disease for which science has not provided a specific remedy, with the single exception of scarlet fever. "But, a further observation of statistics causes us to become somewhat skeptical. During the twenty years from 1872 to 1891, the twenty years preceding the nation wide educational movement and including ten years preceding the discovery of the tubercle bacillus, the mortality from tuberculosis decreased from 339 per hundred thousand of population to 245 per hundred thousand, or a decrease of about 27.5 per cent. In fact, Hoffman has pointed out, from such statistics as were available, that tuberculosis mortalities have steadily decreased for a period of over a hundred years, from 1812, when the rate in New York, Boston and Philadelphia was close to 450 per hundred thousand. This steady increase in mortality, which had assumed interesting proportions years before the discovery of the bacillus, obviously cannot be attributed to battle against the germ, and yet it seems readily explainable and in perfect harmony with our present conception of the tuberculosis problem." It is generally agreed now that the disease in the adult is usually due to childhood infection plus some other factor of lowered vitality, thus the causes of tuberculosis become indefinitely multiplied and every sanitary factor has its part in prevention. For hundreds of years living conditions have steadily improved, cleanly habits have increased, fear of fresh air and other superstitions have been largely abandoned. Sewage disposal, water supply, safe milk and food supplies, ventilation, etc., have all come into more general use. In fact, Palmer is ready to believe that the improvement of general health through better milk supplies has done as much as anything else to stay the ravages. The general improvement in housing has been more far-reaching than supervision of infected premises. Antituberculosis associations have done good, and if their policy was narrow it was no narrower than that of others in a day of bacteriologic enthusiasm, and their practical performances have been broad and helpful. The author does not question the value of special antituberculosis activities or the good they have done.

JOURNAL OF THE OKLAHOMA STATE MEDICAL ASSOCIATION

VOLUME XII   MUSKOGEE, OKLA., DECEMBER, 1919   NUMBER 12

PUBLISHED MONTHLY AT MUSKOGEE, OKLA., UNDER DIRECTION OF THE COUNCIL

DR. CLAUDE A. THOMPSON, EDITOR-IN-CHIEF
508-9 BARNES BUILDING, MUSKOGEE

DR. CHAS. W. HEITZMAN, ASSISTANT EDITOR
507-8 BARNES BUILDING, MUSKOGEE

ENTERED AT THE POST OFFICE AT MUSKOGEE, OKLAHOMA, AS SECOND CLASS MAIL MATTER, JULY 26, 1912

THIS IS THE OFFICIAL JOURNAL OF THE OKLAHOMA STATE MEDICAL ASSOCIATION. ALL COMMUNICATIONS SHOULD BE ADDRESSED TO THE JOURNAL OF THE OKLAHOMA STATE MEDICAL ASSSOCIATION, 308 SURETY BUILDING, MUSKOGEE, OKLAHOMA.

The editorial department is not responsible for the opinions expressed in the original articles of contributors.

Reprints of original articles will be supplied at actual cost, provided request for them is attached to manuscript or made in sufficient time before publication.

Articles sent this Journal for publication and all those read at the annual meetings of the State Association are the sole property of this Journal. The Journal relies on each individual contributor's strict adherence to this well-known rule of medical journalism. In the event an article sent this Journal for publication is published before appearance in the Journal, the manuscript will be returned to the writer.

Failure to receive the Journal should call for immediate notification of the editor, 307-8 Surety Building, Muskogee, Okla.

Local news of possible interest to the medical profession, notes on removals, changes in address, deaths and weddings will be gratefully received.

Advertising of articles, drugs or compounds unapproved by the Council on Pharmacy of the A. M. A. will not be accepted.

Advertising rates will be supplied on application. It is suggested that wherever possible members of the State Association should patronize our advertisers in preference to others as a matter of fair reciprocity.

EDITORIAL

OUR OWN BUSINESS.

Should Organized Medicine Assume the Function of Prosecutor of Infractions of Public Health and Medical Laws?

Are we to interpret the generally accepted principle that man is his brother's keeper, to the extent that we personally make it our business to prosecute or insist on prosecution of flagrant violations of laws bearing on matters of disease, simply because our technical study of such matters puts us in position to see the fallacy and danger of uncurbed interference on sick persons by people so wholly unprepared by lack of education and experience that often their pretended efforts amount to murder by omission; in every case they are potentially dangerous as possible murderers of the ignorant sick, who are helplessly in their hands.

These thoughts are stimulated by a letter from a County Secretary, stating they were interested in the prosecution of a Chiropractor for treating until death, from diphtheria, a child; what would the Medical Association do to aid in the matter, etc.? The letter produced a variety of speculations on different phases. We answered the letter immediately, suggesting only a part of opinion aroused by the question, the features of which were, after pointing out that we did not mean to appear uninterested or callous on the matter:

> The State Society has never entered into prosecution of such cases; no policy has ever been adopted, but the general idea seemed to be that such offenses were as much violations of law as any other statutory matter, should be handled by county attorneys charged by law to handle them, just as he handles any other infraction; that he should advise complainants as to the course, if any, to follow, the evidence necessary and admissible and such other examination incident to the preliminaries.

We wonder why we should concern ourselves about this murder—that is all it amounts to—more than any other murder committed on some innocent and helpless citizen of ——— county? True, this was a little infant, more helpless than most people, but, we had to suggest why was it necessary to have to stimulate to activity a county attorney under solemn oath to handle such matters, any more than in any other case. Was it necessary for physicians to hold mass meetings, point out the infraction, produce evidence and give more time than any other good citizen of ——— gave? We assumed, as laymen, not as lawyers, that if this murder was a violation of the law, it was clearly and specifically provided for in the law books; if it was not provided for, even though it was in fact and essence murder, there was no use to concern ourselves about it.

Another feature not mentioned, but clearly recalled by all physicians who have concerned themselves in that past with such matters, with matters of improved public health legislation, quarantine, prevention of disease, etc., is this:

The physicians of ——— county, when found prosecuting this case, will promptly be charged with ulterior motives, with jealousy of the accused, with being a "Trust" perpetuating their own interests, wanting all others out of the way. People interested in other murders as witnesses, good citizens, etc., are not so charged by the public; why are we?

Many thinkers of our profession are becoming unanimous in opinion that we might do more good by attending strictly to our own business; they say that when we, in the best of faith, with intent to do no one harm, attempt to prevent dangerous disease by any manner or plan, our efforts are questioned as if we only acted with a dark motive in view. One of the largest daily papers in the important city of Tulsa opposed school inspection because it was proposed by physicians; the editorial suggested salaries for inspecting physicians was the end in view. A few months later one of the costliest herds of Holstein cattle in the State a few miles from Tulsa was *destroyed* because of the outbreak of disease among them; *inspection* might have prevented that costly destruction. A legislative Ass from Muskogee County opposed school inspection urging that it would frighten the children; he proved to be a Christian Scientist with a *motive* of his own.

The whole thing produces such a variety of irritating thoughts that one may be justified possibly in throwing up his hands and allowing ignorance to follow its course until the destructive result is so obvious to all that the victims themselves will demand repression of the destructive agent just as they repress other forms of destruction.

THE NORTHEAST MEDICAL SOCIETY.

When the war broke out this society was one of the best societies in the state, and since our return to peace it has been in a state of innocuous desuetude. Latterly it has been suggested that steps be again taken to resurrect it but no one seems to have given it any thought. The writer feels that some of the most valuable meetings he has ever attended were held by this society, and the goodfellowship which prevailed was well worth the time spent in attending them. We can only hope for results by cooperation, and cooperation can only be gotten by meeting each other and getting acquainted. By close association with one another we see our faults and those of the rest of us, and we finally come to the conclusion that we are no better than our colleague, and many times we are not nearly so good. Close acquaintance makes close friends, and friends are far more ready to overlook our failings than are our enemies, or those who do not know us at all.

Let's find a way to reorganize this society, and once more enjoy its valuable meetings. I am sure we can find a way if we only try. LET'S GO.

G. A. Wall, Tulsa.

MEMBERS PLEASE REMEMBER.

Our membership is earnestly requested to co-operate on the usual December or early January reorganization of their county medical society. Aside from the routine necessity for prompt reorganization, the placing of every member in good standing for 1920 during the month of January; the coming year is likely to hold more of import to our profession than any heretofore of our history.

Attendance at the annual meeting of the county society and consideration of the matters to be presented by your county secretary is of extreme importance at this time. Intelligent co-operation of our membership over the State will produce gratifying results. Neglect of detail and delay will bring discredit on the society most surely.

It is most important that officers, especially county secretaries, should be carefully selected with a view to their fitness and executive ability. Selection of any except those who are systematic and efficient will mean that that particular section of our membership will lag behind in the coming year at a time when every one is needed to do his bit.

PLEASE REMEMBER to attend your annual meeting. If your society is disorganized, do not allow it to remain so. Make it your personal affair to reorganize it. Any five members may call for a meeting in the absence of officers, or failure of them to call a meeting. This procedure should be taken if necessary.

PERSONAL AND GENERAL NEWS

Dr. E. B. Walker, Belzoni, has moved to Ida.

Dr. P. E. Wright, Antlers, has moved to Sasakwa.

Dr. T. W. Brewer, Miami, has moved to Okmulgee.

Dr. J. C. Dunn, Bartlesville, visited New York in November.

Tulsa Baptists are laying plans to erect a hundred thousand dollar hospital in 1920.

Dr. D. R. Aves has been discharged from the army and has located at Hearne, Texas.

Dr. G. W. Goss, Pawhuska, has been appointed superintendent of health for Osage County.

Dr. Levi Murray, Depew, has moved to Wellston and is associated with Dr. H. M. Williams.

Dr. F. B. Fite, Muskogee, is being urged to run for Mayor. Dr. Fite was formerly Mayor of Muskogee.

Dr. J. T. Martin, city physician of Oklahoma City, attended the New Orleans Public Health Conference.

Dr. H. H. Cloudman, Oklahoma City, attended the public health conference in New Orleans in November.

Dr. J. A. Deen, Ada, health officer of Pontotoc county, is engaged in a "Clean-up Campaign" of his jurisdiction.

Dr. R. A. Workman, Woodward, who underwent a serious surgical operation in Wichita recently, is reported as recovered.

Drs. M. K. Thompson, H. T. Ballantine and Sessler Hoss, Muskogee, attended the Asheville meeting of the Southern Medical Association.

Dr. L. E. Emanuel, Chickasha, visited the Rochester Clinics in November, incidentally attending the American Legion meeting at Minneapolis.

Dr. S. J. Bradfield, Bartlesville, has been placed in charge of the Venereal Clinic at that point. Dr. Bradfield recently was discharged from the army.

Dr. H. C. Antle, Chickasha, has returned from oversea army service. He has been doing special work in northern clinics for two months since discharge.

Dr. John Fewkes, Alva, has moved to Hot Springs, Ark., and is located in that city. He formerly resided there for several years before locating in Oklahoma.

All Saints' Hospital, McAlester, has received $23,000.00 for improvements, available January first. A further sum of $52,000.00 will be available within three years.

St. Anthony Hospital Staff, Oklahoma City, held memorial services October 9th for Drs. Robert L. Hull, Frank B. Sorgatz and Nurse Miss Caroline Walsh, who died while in army service. Addresses were made by Drs. Robert M. Howard, A. B. Chase, John Riley, George LaMotte, and Miss Lina Davis, Superintendent.

DOCTOR ANDREW LERSKOV.

Dr. Andrew Lerskov, Claremore, died in Kansas City, Mo., in November after several months illness from tuberculous peritonitis. His remains were interred at Claremore under auspices of the Masonic lodge.

Dr. Lerskov was a citizen of the Cherokee Nation, a relative of the prominent families of that country. He was born December 29, 1883, at Red Fork, Indian Territory, receiving his medical degree from Vanderbilt University in 1907. He is survived by a wife and one child.

Muskogee County Medical Society elected the following officers for 1920: President, Dr. P. P. Nesbitt; Vice-President, J. Hoy Sanford; Secretary, J. G. Noble; Censors, C. V. Rice and H. L. Scott, Muskogee.

The State Hospital at Norman is being enlarged by legislative appropriation. Approximately $300,000.00 is being expended in new buildings, which consist of receiving wards, laundry, ice and refrigeration plants.

Dr. G. A. Wall, Tulsa, who has placed Tulsa County Medical Society decidedly on the map by his activities, communicates to the Journal an editorial in this issue on the reorganization of the Northeast District Medical Society.

Dr. and Mrs. A. H. Stewart, Lawton, entertained the meeting of the Comanche County Medical Society, October 28th. After the scientific program, Mrs. Stewart served a dinner for the members present. It is planned to have several such meetings during the winter.

Muskogee business men will be asked to contribute a fund necessary to establish a hospital for additional accomodation of the sick at the School for the Blind until the legislature may appropriate money for the purpose. The Rotary Club will take charge of the raising of the fund.

Abbograms is the designation of a recently established organ of The Abbott Laboratories, Dept. 44, Chicago, Ill. It contains not one line of advertising, but is filled with clean, wholesome humor with not enough of "Shop" to tire the reader. It will be sent to anyone interested on request.

Indian School Property between Shawnee and Tecumseh has been offered to the State, according to press dispatches, by Commissioner of Indian Affairs, Cato Sells, for the purpose of a tuberculosis sanitarium. The property comprises ten buildings and eighty acres of land. The buildings will be converted at once. It is estimated that from one hundred to three hundred patients may be accommodated.

Jane A. Delano Post of Graduate Nurses, Muskogee, by resolution condemned the recent action of the Registered Nurses Association of Muskogee in raising rates for nursing service. "Profiteering" is the way the action was denominated by Miss Helen E. Barclay, P. and S. Hospital, who declared that many people had difficulty enough to pay the old rates, that needy people would suffer by reason of the raise.

Shawnee physicians have organized a clinic which is in full operation at this time. Office space sufficient for all purposes including private rooms, waiting rooms, laboratory, etc., has been secured in one building. The personnel is composed of Drs. G. H. Applewhite, G. S. Baxter, W. C. Bradford, M. A. Baker, J. M. Byrum, E. E. Goodrich, H. M. Reeder, E. E. Rice, T. D. Rowland, T. C. Sanders, J. H. Scott, H. A. Wagner and J. A. Walker.

Dr. C. W. Tedrowe, Woodward, holds the palm as the Early Bird among county society secretaries. He reports complete organization of his society with the following officers for 1920: President, Dr. R. A. Workman, Woodward; Vice-President, P. G. Eiler, Quinlan; Secretary, C. W. Tedrowe, Woodward; Censors, Drs. J. L. Patterson, C. J. Forney, Woodward, and E. Danse, Fargo; Delegates, Drs. J. M. Workman, J. L. Patterson, Woodward, and T. B. Triplett, Moreland. Thirty members are already accounted for as in good standing for 1920.

CORRESPONDENCE

December 4, 1919.

Dr. John A. Roddy,
612 American National Bank Building,
Oklahoma City.

Dear Doctor: I should have acknowledged receipt of your letter of November 12 earlier, but as it contained much of interest to the profession I took the liberty to publish it, reserving reply until my work allowed more time.

The quotations cited in the October Editorial were taken from a communication by Dr. H. J. Haiselden, Chicago, Chief Surgeon to the German-American Hospital, etc. I think it should be understood at the outset that they were probably estimates based on his personal observation and experience during the epidemic.   I take it there would be no practical way to gather accurate statistics on deaths possibly due to neglect, lack of nursing, no nursing or improper nursing incident to that epidemic, but every physician having to do with civil practice, I think will recall, not only as to the epidemic, but long before the war, that there was a serious shortage of nurses in Oklahoma.   They were commonly unobtainable in the larger centers and unknown in most of the smaller places.   This situation now exists.

We are agreed that a highly educated nurse is a better nurse than one with less education and training.   I refer in this to the two classes, there are exceptions on both sides of the question, just as we sometimes see a brilliant doctor with horse sense outclass the highly or over-educated doctor, who had not the capacity to appreciate the practical application of his study to the given case.

The hurriedly prepared "doughboy" nurses alluded to certainly did very well.   No one expected them to act with the precision and goodness of a highly specialized nurse, no one questions the service each rendered in their sphere.

I do not think that my communication can be interpreted to read that I favor giving the nurse anything but all the training she has the capacity and time to receive.   That is suggested in the last clause providing for postgraduate work.

As to what a physician requires of the nurse, "His orders executed"; I believe that is a matter of judgment.   Personally, and I believe for many physicians, general execution of orders is what they want, what they give them for, and what the family employs the nurse to do.   There is no greater danger or pest than the nurse who "practises" medicine on the patient in the physician's absence.   On peril of being classed as "incompetent to practice" I shall retain that opinion.   It is implied, of course that the nurse be well grounded in the basic fundamentals, that she be taught how to appreciate the danger signals, etc., but I recall with pleasure the most thoroughly made bed of my memory was the creation of an undergraduate nurse at Michael Reese, while my most painful memory is that of fourteen years before when a *graduate* incompetent misfit bumped the four corners of my bed every time she attempted to walk around and then with pleasure again I note the skill and deftness of her *undergraduate* successor who replaced her.   The graduate was a misfit, never to be efficient and skilfull, the last a jewel, held back by a "course" laid out to fit the dullest and most inept.   This experience could be multiplied many times, but it gets us no nearer the solution.   We will have no improvement until the system is changed in some respects.   As there is no use in useless railing without at least attempting amelioration, I should say that hospitals might try accepting the young women who are:

Healthy, vouched as being energetic, intelligent to the point of receiving training, and who would likely (probably) finish the course.

That as much of the drudgery as possible be eliminated.   This phase is not appreciated likely by those who have had to do only with the larger institutions.

That a degree or diploma be issued after a minimum time, on evidencing certain knowledge of the course, from both the theoretical and practical standpoint.   This would place a premium, and properly, on energy, intelligence, aptitude and work.

There is no reason on earth why, now that we have graduated our young woman that she should not be useful to the people in almost *all* practical demands made.   There is no reason why she may not continue the study in all its higher intricacies, if she has taste and capacity for it, either in some special school of instruction for her or as is done at present in postgraduate work.

As the matter now stands they are much in the same sorry plight as the Osteopath.   Under incessant stimulus he takes up a three-year "course" only to sadly realize in the end that he has a useless smattering of medicine which he is prohibited from using, and possibly a lot of "Osteopathy" which he knows is inapplicable.   As reform is my slogan, I have already taken the liberty to suggest to these gentlemen that they study medicine four years, become doctors, then take a postgraduate course in their refined manipulative science.   They nearly never do that.

Assuring you of my personal appreciation of your letter, which I know was dictated in a constructive sense, permit me to invite you to write again as often as you like.   Constructive letters from our members not only aid the Journal but are of interest and worth to our members.

Sincerely,

C. A. THOMPSON, Editor.

MISCELLANEOUS

THE IMPORTANCE OF THE RURAL HOSPITAL.

The importance of the rural hospital to the rural community—and not only to the rural community, but to the urban as well, for the health of the farmer is necessary for the feeding of the nation —is set forth in a study of conditions in rural hospitals, appearing in *The Modern Hospital*, Chicago.

The first thing to ask of any hospital is not whether it conforms to this or that specific requirement, but whether, in view of the sum of its services to the community, it deserves to exist.   Would the community be better off with or without it?

Many à rural hospital which would make a very poor comparison with the average city hospital is yet indispensable to the well-being of its community. Such hospitals need not to be suppressed but to be helped.

A general study of several communities has brought out the fact that the health and hospital problem of a small community is often rendered exceedingly complex in proportion to population by the multiplication of small hospitals. Often certain classes of cases are not adequately provided for. In many places the community has not learned to rely on the hospital as much as it should. The rural hospital really has a field of its own and a function distinct in many ways from that of the urban hospital.

ADVENTURE NUMBER TWO—DOCTOR YOUNG DOCTOR.

A short time after arriving, Young Doctor was called in to see a case which presented the features that we are accustomed to associate with appendicitis. There were pain, first general and later localized to the right groin, nausea and vomiting, fever and the white count showed about 10,000 leucocytes. It looked like a clear case to Young Doctor but he was unwilling to assume responsibility. He called in Friend Consultant. Consultant could not come at the moment but would be free in about an hour. That suited Young Doctor very well for he had a call down the valley to attend to. He told Consultant then to come along when he could and that though he was sure of the diagnosis and thought that he ought to remove the appendix at once, he saw no harm in waiting an hour or so. Young Doctor made his call and on returning he went to the house of his patient. There he was told that the girl had been taken to the hospital. He thought that he was really being treated better than he deserved. Here was an older man taking as much interest in his case as he took himself. It was mighty nice of Consultant, thought Young Doctor, to go to all that trouble just to help him out. He arrived at the hospital and bustled in, enjoying in anticipation his first appendectomy for a fee, he asked for his patient and was told that she was doing nicely, thank you. Yes, Consultant had made the most of his opportunity and patient was now coming out from under the anesthetic.—*Southwestern Medicine*.

DIAGNOSIS OF TUBERCULOSIS.

Thomas McCrae and E. H. Funk, Philadelphia (*Journal A. M. A.*, July 19, 1919), say that, while the recognition of chronic pulmonary tuberculosis is usually regarded as a simple matter, with small chance for error, this is not always the case, as can be readily seen by men with large experience. The authors report the results of a study of the 1,200 consecutive admissions to the Jefferson Hospital, Philadelphia, with the diagnosis of advanced pulmonary tuberculosis. In this series, seventy-two, or six per cent., were found to be nontuberculous, and out of 134 necropsies in this series, no tuberculosis was found in seven, which is fairly close to the percentage given above. In five of these cases there had been a correct diagnosis made before death. They refer to the work of Ash (*The Journal*, Jan. 2, 1915, p. 11), who found in 198 necropsy cases, twenty-three nontuberculous, only seven of which had been correctly diagnosed before death. In the authors' own series, "the various conditions which were wrongly diagnosed as advanced pulmonary tuberculosis are: cardiorenal, 19; pneumonic sequelae, 9; bronchiectasis 8; abscess of lung, 8; chronic bronchitis, 6; neoplasm, 5; syphilis, 4; aneurysm, 2; anthracosis, 2; bronchial asthma, 2; empyema, 2; diabetes mellitus, 1; cancer of rectum, 1; foreign body, 1; malingering, 1." The various disorders mistaken for tuberculosis are described in brief detail. The cardiac cases seem to be wrongly interpreted, partly through carelessness. The chronic inflammatory conditions of the lungs are generally more difficult problems. Six of the nine were atypical cases of bronchopneumonia; three were unresolved lobar pneumonia. The influenza epidemic had undoubtedly something to do with the origin of these cases, and most of them came in last winter. Bronchiectasis is easily mistaken for tuberculosis if the sputum is not examined. Sputum examination was evidently neglected in the eight cases of pulmonary abscess. Sputum, persistently purulent without tubercle bacilli, is strong evidence against tuberculosis. Emphysema and chronic bronchitis were mistaken for it by reading symptoms and signs alone, and the same remarks apply to cases of new growths in the lungs. Syphilis was conservatively diagnosed in the four cases, but seemed thoroughly proved. Aneurysm, bronchial asthma, and empyema may need the roentgen ray to confirm a nontuberculous diagnosis. Anthracosis is more frequently the cause of mistake than the figures indicate, and many such cases are early recognized in the dispensary and sent to the general wards. Lack of thorough examinations with hasty conclusions, and neglect of sputum examinations are probably the main causes of mistakes. The authors consider that the ordinary six negative sputum examinations in early cases are not enough to exclude tuberculosis. In the apparently advanced cases of tuberculosis, a diagnosis without positive sputum examinations should never be made, and physicians in tuberculosis hospitals should give particular attention to this point.

COUNCIL ON PHARMACY AND CHEMISTRY
AMERICAN MEDICAL ASSOCIATION

(The following articles produced by advertisers in this Journal have been accepted for inclusion with New and Non-Official Remedies by the Council on Pharmacy and Chemistry.)

During September the following articles have been accepted from our advertisers for inclusion in New and Non-Official Remedies:

Cinchophen-Abbott. The Abbott Laboratories have adopted the name cinchophen for the product accepted for New and Non-Official Remedies as phenylcinchoninic acid-Abbott (see New and Non-Official Remedies, 1919, p. 227).

Chlorazene Surgical Gauze. Gauze impregnated with, and containing approximately five per cent. of chlorazene. For a description of chlorazene, see New and Non-Official Remedies, 1919, p. 137. The Abbott Laboratories, Chicago.

NEW AND NONOFFICIAL REMEDIES.

Albutannin.—Tannin Albuminate Exsiccated. A compound of tannin and albumin, thoroughly exsiccated and containing about 50 per cent. of tannic acid in combination. It was first introduced as tannalbin. The use of albutannin is based on the assumption that the tannin compound passes the stomach largely unchanged and thus the astringent action will be exercised in the intestine where the compound will be decomposed by the intestinal fluid, slowly liberating the tannic acid. Albutannin is used in diarrhea, particularly in that of children, and in phthisis.

Albutannin-Calco. A nonproprietary brand complying with the standards for albutannin. The Calco Chemical Co., New York.

Albutannin-Merck. Merck and Co. have adopted the name albutannin for the product accepted as tannin albuminate exsiccated-Merck (see Supplement to New and Nonofficial Remedies, 1919, p. 12) (Jour. A. M. A., Nov. 1, 1919, p. 1363).

Acetannin.—Tannyl Acetate. The acetic acid ester of tannin.—Acetannin was first introduced as tannigen. Acetannin is claimed to be practically non-irritant to the stomach and to pass unchanged into the intestine, there to become effective as an astringent. It is used in diarrheal affections.

Acetannin-Calco. A brand of acetannin complying with the standards of New and Nonofficial Remedies. The Calco Chemical Co., New York.

Antipneumococcic Serum, Combined Types I, II and III—Gilliland. Prepared by immunizing horses with dead and living pneumococci of the three fixed types and standardized against Type I culture. Marketed in 50 Cc. gravity injecting packages and also in 50 Cc. and 100 Cc. vial packages. The Gilliland Laboratories, Ambler, Pa. (Jour. A. M. A., Nov. 8, 1919, p. 1442).

Tablets Cinchophen-Abbott, 7½ grains. Each tablet contains 7½ grains of cinchophen-Abbott. Cinchophen was first introduced as atophen and is in the U. S. Pharmacopeia as *Acidum phenylcinchoninicum.* The Abbott Laboratories, Chicago.

Acriflavine and Proflavine. These are dyes derived from acridine, a base found in coal tar. Their use in medicine is proposed on the claim that they have high antiseptic power, together with comparative freedom from toxic or irritant action and without inhibiting effect on the phagocytic action of leukocytes or on the healing process. They have been used as wound antiseptics, and acriflavine has also been proposed for the treatment of gonorrhea. The reports on the value of the two preparations are contradictory and conflicting. In the treatment of wounds, solutions of 1:1,000 in physiologic sodium chloride solution are commonly recommended. In gonorrhea, a strength of 1:1,000 in physiologic sodium chloride solution is used for an injection into the urethra, and weaker solutions have been used for lavation.

Acriflavine. This is 3:6 diamino acridine sulphate. For a discussion of the actions, uses and dosage, see above. Acriflavine is a brownish-red, odorless, crystalline powder, soluble in less than two parts of water and in alcohol, forming dark red solutions which fluoresce on dilution. It is nearly insoluble in ether, chloroform, liquid petrolatum, fixed oils and volatile oils.

Proflavine. This is 3:6 diamino acridine sulphate. For a discussion of the actions, uses and dosages, see the preceding article, Acriflavine and Proflavine. Proflavine is a reddish-brown, crystalline powder. It is soluble in water and alcohol, forming brownish solutions which fluoresce on dilution. It is nearly soluble in ether, chloroform, liquid petrolatum, fixed oils and volatile oils (Jour. A. M. A., Nov. 8, 1919, p. 1443).

Pituitary Solution-Hollister-Wilson,—Liquor Hypophysis. A sterilized solution of the water soluble extract of the posterior portion of pituitary glands of cattle, preserved by the addition of chlorbutanol. It is standardized according to the method of Roth and complies with the U. S. P. standard. The Hollister-Wilson Laboratories, Chicago.

Ampoules Pituitary Solution-Hollister-Wilson 1 c.c. Each ampoule contains pituitary solution-Hollister-Wilson 1 c.c. (Jour. A. M. A., Nov. 29, 1919, p. 1699).

PROPAGANDA FOR REFORM

American Made Synthetic Drugs. P. N. Leech, W. Rabak and A. H. Clark report on the work which was done in the A. M. A. Chemical Laboratory in the efforts to overcome the shortage of synthetic drugs during the recent war. In particular they report on the examination of and the establishment of standards for procaine (novocaine), barbital (veronal), phenetidyl-acetphenetidian (holocaine), and cinchophen, or phenylcinchoninic acid (atophan), manufactured under Federal Trade Commission licenses. They report that the shortage of German synthetics was not felt seriously in most cases because the demand for them had been artificially created, and that the few which were in great need are being rapidly replaced by American made drugs. The report explains how the Federal Trade Commission granted licenses to American firms for the manufacture of German synthetics which were protected by U. S. patents, and how these licenses were issued only after an examination of the firm's product in the Association's Chemical Laboratory had demonstrated that its quality was satisfactory and equal to that of the drug formerly imported from Germany. It is interesting to observe, the report declares, that of all the synthetic drugs imported into this country from Germany and on which American patents had been issued, the demand was sufficient only to make it commercially profitable to manufacture four of them on a commercial scale, namely, arsphenamine (and neoarsphenamine), barbital (and barbital sodium), cinchophen and procaine. The chemists caution that, in view of the agitation to found an institute for co-operative research as an aid to the American drug industry, it will be well for the American medical profession to be on its guard against new and enthusiastic propaganda on the part of those engaged in the laudable enterprise of promoting American Chemical industry (Jour. A. M. A., Sept. 6, 1919, p. 754).

Benzyl Benzoate. Although the benzyl esters have been known only a short time in medicine, the possibilities of their usefulness in certain fields of practice is becoming apparent. Benzyl benzoate has already been accepted for New and Nonofficial Remedies. The therapeutic applicability of benzyl esters arose from the investigation of opium alkaloids by D. I. Macht. The study demonstrated that opium alkaloids may be divided into two classes: the pyridin-phenanthrene group, of which morphin is the type, and the benzyl-isoquinolin group, to which papaverin belongs. The former was found to stimulate contractions of unstriped muscle, whereas the papaverin-like alkaloids inhibit the contractions and lower the muscle tone. A search for simpler, non-narcotic compounds of the latter which might still act in inhibitory manner on smooth mulculature led to the use of benzyl acetate and benzyl benzoate. Ureteral colic and excessive intestinal parietalsis have been found to yield to the tonus lowering action of these two drugs. Apparently satisfactory results from the use of benzyl benzoate in aysmenorrhea have recently been reported (Jour. A. M. A., Sept. 6, 1919, p. 770).

Iodin Tinctures, Water Soluble. T. Sollmann has investigated the claim that certain proprietary iodin preparations are superior to the official tincture of iodin and to compound solution of iodin (Lugol's solution). The claim of superiority is based on the allegation that the potassium iodid in the official preparations causes local irritant action. Since the proprietary preparations have been shown to contain free hydrogen iodid, this claim seemed improbable to Sollmann, and he surmised that apparent decrease in irritant effects was due to a lower iodin content of the proprietaries, such as Burnham's Soluble Iodin and Sharp and Dohme's Surgodine. From experiments which he conducted with the various iodin preparations, all diluted to the same iodin strength, Sollmann concludes: The presence of potassium iodid in the official tincture of iodin does not seem to render this preparation more irritant. On the contrary, it is somewhat less irritant to the skin and much less precipitant to protein than the simple alcoholic tincture or the secret and nonsecret "miscible tinctures." The more even spreading and the more rapid coagulation of proteins render the simple alcoholic solution of iodin probably the best for the "disinfection" of the skin, while the delayed protein precipitation of the U. S. P. tincture would probably render this somewhat superior for the disinfection of open wounds (Jour. A. M. A., Sept. 20, 1919. p. 899).

Case's Rheumatic Specific. More than five years ago, *The Journal A. M. A.* exposed Case's Rheumatic Specific, the A. M. A. Chemical Laboratory showing that its essential drug was sodium salicylate. Now comes the United States Post Office and interferes with Mr. Case's presumably lucrative quackery by denying him the use of the mails. In recommending the issuance of a fraud order, the solicitor of the post office department declared: "Mr. Case, the respondent herein, is not a physician and has had little opportunity for study along medical lines. . . . He knows nothing of the effect of drugs and he is incompetent to prescribe their use. When he sells one form of treatment for all forms of rheumatism, irrespective of the superintending cause or causes of the trouble, he well knows that it is mere guesswork on his part—a hit or miss chance of recovery, and when he calls such a treatment a 'Specific for Rheumatism,' and solemnly urges its use as a cure for practically all forms of rheumatism, he knows that he is not acting in good faith, and his scheme for obtaining money through the mails by such means should be suppressed." (Jour. A. M. A. Sept 13, 1919, p. 852).

The Lucas Laboratory Products. The products put out by the Lucas Laboratories, New York City, are for intravenous use, and the method of exploitation indicates that the concern is less interested in the science of therapeutics than in taking commercial advantage of the present fad for intravenous medication. The composition of the products is essentially a secret, which in itself should be sufficient to deter physicians from using them. Even the hieroglyphics that used to be palmed off on the medical profession by nostrum exploiter under the guise of "graphic formulas" are outdone by the "formalus" of the Lucas Laboratories: " 'Luvein' Arsans (Plain)" is said to be, "Di hypo sodio calcio phosphin hydroxy arseno mercuric iodide." The first part of this "formula" might stand for sodium and calcium hypophosphite. The remainder is meaningless except that it suggests (but does not insure) the presence of arsenic and mercury iodide. " 'Luvein' Arsans, Nos. 1, 2 and 3,"—"Meta hydroxy iodide sodio arsano mercurio dimethyl benzo dosio arsenate, ai oxy sodio tartaria sulpho disheuyl hydrazin." Who can venture even a conjecture as to the possible significance of this? The proposition offered to physicians by the Lucas Laboratories, Inc., is an insult to the intelligence of the medical profession. Physicians should heed the warning of the Council on Pharmacy and Chemistry that intravenous therapy should be employed only when most positively indicated. Further, because of the inherent danger of intravenous medications, physicians should use the products of firms of unquestionable public standing only (Jour. A. M. A., Sept. 20, 1919, p. 927).

Case's Rheumatic Specific. The post office authorities announce that the fraud order against Jesse A. Case has been revoked because Case has agreed to discontinue the sale of his Rheumatic Specific (Jour. A. M. A., Sept. 20, 1919, p. 928).

Secret Remedies and the Principles of Ethics. There are on the market today and used by members of the American Association, dozens, yes scores, of widely advertised proprietaries that are, to all intents and purposes, secret. The physicians who prescribe them do not know and cannot know what they are giving their patients. On this point Section 6, Chapter II., of the Principles of Medical Ethics of the American Medical Association says: ". . . unethical to prescribe or dispense secret medicines or other secret remedial agents, or to manufacture or promote their use in any way." The inherent and basic reasonableness of the various requirements of the Principles of Medical Ethics needs no exposition or defense (Jour. A. M. A., Sept. 27, 1919, p. 902).

The Direct Sales Co. The Direct Sales Co., Inc., Buffalo, sells its drugs to physicians by mail, and features a "profit sharing rebate." The concern has guaranteed its products to be in accordance with the Food and Drugs Act and to be equal, if not superior, to any on the market. One of the Quarterly Bulletins of the State Board of Health of New Hampshire, issued last year, announces that the following preparations of the Direct Sales Company were found substandard: "Tablets salicylic acid, 5 grains (1.72 grains found); Tablets acetylsalicylic acid, 5 grains (2.31 grains found); Tablets acetanilid, 3 grains (1.88 grains found); Tablets codein sulphate, 1-6 grain (1-15 grain found); Tablets nux and pepsin No. 2, claiming pepsin 1 grain, extract nux vomica 1-10 grain (found to have a gross average weight per tablet of only 1.17 grains, 0.54 grain of which was represented by sugar and other medicinally inert material; Tablets Infant's Anodyne (Waugh) showed serious discrepancy from formula." Subsequently the federal authorities examined the products of the Direct Sales Company, and Notice of Judgment No. 6193 describes cases of adulteration and misbranding of some of the drugs put out by the Direct Sales Company (Jour. A. M. A., Sept. 27, 1919, p. 1001).

Pinoleum. A postcard advertising Pinoleum implies that Alexander Lambert, President of the American Medical Association endorses this nostrum. Dr. Lambert has never used the Pinoleum products, and protests against the dishonest method of advertising them. Pinoleum has long been advertised to the public via the medical profession. Its life history is that of the typical nostrum. Epidemics are utilized as opportunities for pushing the product. As the Pinoleum Company now misuses the name of Dr. Lambert, so it made the false use of the name of Dr. George W. McCoy, of the U. S. Public Health Service (Jour. A. M. A., Nov. 1, 1919, p. 1380).

Lavoris. In recent years, Lavoris has been widely advertised as "*The Ideal Oral Antiseptic*," particularly to the dental profession. In 1913, a card was sent out according to which each pint of Lavoris contained zinc 'chloride, 1.040; resorcin, 0.520; menthol, 0.400; saccharin, 0.195; formalin, 0.195; cl. cassia zeyl., 0.780; cl. caryophyl., 0.195. Advertisements now appearing repeat the "formula," except that resorcin is omitted. The formula is indefinite and misleading in that no denomination of weight is given for the various constituents. Analysis in the A. M. A. Chemical Laboratory demonstrated that the Lavoris now sold contains no resorcin and that the zinc content is equivalent to 0.1 gm. per 100 c.c. (about one-half grain to the ounce). As the analysis shows that the "formula" is not only meaningless because no denomination of weight is given, but that the zinc content is inaccurate for any denomination which might be assumed, the Council on Pharmacy and Chemistry declares the composition of Lavoris essentially secret. The Council also reports that Lavoris is advertised to the public indirectly with claims that are unwarranted and objectionable from the standpoint of public safety. Further, the Council reports that the name is objectionable in that it does not indicate the composition or potent ingredients of the mixture and that the composition is irrational in that the user is likely to ascribe a false and exaggerated value to it. (Jour. A. M. A., Nov. 1, 1919, p. 1380.)

Olive Oil as a Laxative. In order that digestible oils may act as laxatives, it is necessary to give more than can be digested and absorbed. In the case of an infant, this may be one or more teaspoonfuls daily, beginning with small dosages and increasing them until the desired effect is obtained. For adults, one or two tablespoonfuls may have to be given three times daily, either an hour before meals or two hours after meals. Olive oil may be taken mixed with hot milk or floating in fruit juice. Olive oil might be particularly serviceable in spastic constipation in an emaciated individual. The use of olive oil as a laxative would be contraindicated in obesity, diabetes, gastric atony and in hypochlorhydria, as well as in those inclined to biliousness (Jour. A. M. A., Nov. 8, 1919, p. 1441).

Some More Misbranded Nostrums. The following preparations have been found to be misbranded under the federal Food and Drugs Act: Fruitatives, sold under the false claims that the laxative properties were due to the fruit extract; Tubbs' Bilious Man's Friend, a water-alcohol solution of sugar and plant extractives (rhubarb) with a very small amount of aromatics; Deerfield Water, consisting in part of a filthy, decomposed and putrid animal and vegetable substance; Mederine, a water-alcohol solution of sugar, potassium iodide, methyl salicylate, salicylic acid, glycerin and laxative plant extractives, and Robinson Spring Water, falsely claimed to be effective in Bright's disease, diabetes, gout, rheumatism, indigestion, etc. (Jour. A. M. A., Nov. 8, 1919, p. 1458).

Acriflavine and Proflavine. Tentative descriptions and standards for acriflavine and proflavine are published in New and Nonofficial Remedies for the information of manufacturers, pharmacists and physicians. In view of numerous inquiries regarding the therapeutic properties of these dyes which have been received by the Council on Pharmacy and Chemistry, the Council has prepared an abstract of the available literature on the subject. From this review, it is evident that the use of the dyes is in the experimental stage and that their value cannot be definitely judged. Of the thirty-four reports which are abstracted, twenty-five may be considered as favorable; seven are distinctly unfavorable and two are in the doubtful class (Jour. A. M. A., Nov. 15, 1919, p. 1542).

Medinal. Medinal is a proprietary name applied to barbital sodium (sodium diethylbarbiturate), the sodium salt of barbital (diethylbarbituric acid, first introduced as veronal). The Council on Pharmacy and Chemistry reports that Medinal was omitted from New and Nonofficial Remedies in 1916 because the advertising issued by Schering and Glatz (who then acted as agents for the German manufacturer) contained misleading and unwarranted therapeutic claims. The Council further reports that Medinal, said to be manufactured in the United States, is now marketed by Schering and Glatz, Inc., but that the claims which are made for it are still unwarranted and prevent the acceptance of it for New and Nonofficial Remedies (Jour. A. M. A., Nov. 15, 1919, p. 1542).

Phylacogens. A circular letter devoted to singing the praises of "Pneumonia Phylacogen," contains this: "Pneumonia Phylacogen has been found to be a dependable means of preventing and treating pneumonic complications of influenza. In one large city it became a routine measure to give all persons affected with influenza an injection of Pneumonia Phylacogen as a prophylactic of pneumonia. The results were remarkable. Not only did the cases improve rapidly but in a majority of them the pneumonia did not occur." The injection of Phylacogens is simply the administration of a mixture of the filtered products of several bacterial species. The results that follow represent the reaction of the bacterial proteins—a reaction for good or evil. There is no scientific evidence to show that they possess any specific prophylactic virtue. To recommend their use in patients with influenza, as a prophylactic against pneumonia, is unwarranted; and the physician who acts on the advice of the manufacturer must assume the responsibility of the results. In case of mishap, he cannot fall back on the manufacturer. He will find no scientific evidence to support him (Jour. A. M. A., Nov. 15, 1919, p. 1442).

Vaccines in Influenza. The efficacy of vaccines in preventing influenza or of preventing or decreasing the severity of secondary infections is unproved. In view of the varying preponderance of the different organisms isolated from influenza cases, it is evident that even if a certain mixture is found efficacious in one locality, it may not be effective in another. Thus far, hope and imagination have exceeded scientifically controlled facts. Many vaccines come highly recommended by their manufacturers; but very little dependable evidence is submitted to show how much, if at all, the patient will profit therefrom (Jour. A. M. A., Nov. 15, 1919, p. 1544).

The Eli Products of Eli H. Dunn. Physicians are receiving advertising matter from a concern that seems to operate under various names, such as "E. H. Dunn & Co.," "Eli H. Dunn," "Eli Laboratory," etc. The concern is located in Kansas City, Mo. It advertises "Eli 606 Capsules," "Eli Vaginal Capsules," "Eli 'Vim' Restorative," and an intravenous nostrum, "Ampoules Eli Venhydrarsen." "Dunn's Intravenous and Restorative Treatment" is advised for the treatment of hysteria, and a price to the patient of three hundred dollars is suggested. The gross commercialism that permeates the advertising again illustrates the fact that the fad for intravenous medication offers an attractive field for those who would exploit our profession (Jour. A. M. A., Nov. 22, 1919, p. 1628).

Cotarnin Salts (Stypticin and Styptol). The Council on Pharmacy and Chemistry announces the omission of cotarnin salts (Stypticin and Styptol) from New and Nonofficial Remedies. Salts of the base cotarnin have been used as local and systemic hemostatics. The hydrochloride was first introduced as "Stypticin" and is now in the pharmacopoeia as cotarnin hydrochloride. The phthallic acid salt of cotarnin—cotarnin phthallate—was introduced as "Styptol." In 1918, Stypticin was omitted from New and Nonofficial Remedies because the former American agents were no longer offering it for sale. Styptol was retained and is described in N. N. R., 1919. As was pointed out in the description (N. N. R., 1919), the evidence for the usefulness of the cotarnin salts has been contradictory and unsatisfactory. Now P. J. Hanzlik has made a thorough investigation of the efficiency of hemostatics and has shown the inefficiency of cotarnin salts. The evidence was so definite that the Council has directed the omission of the general article on cotarnin salts and the description of Styptol from New and Non-official Remedies (Jour. A. M. A., Nov. 22, 1919, p. 1628).

Uri-Na Test. The Uri-Na Test, sold by the Standard Appliance Co., Philadelphia, bears a strong family resemblance to Capell's Uroluetic Test. Both are said to permit the detection of syphilis by an examination of urine. There is no method known at the present time by which the absence or presence of syphilis can be determined by a simple color test of the urine (Jour. A. M. A., Nov. 22, 1919, p. 1630).

Micajah's Wafers and Micajah's Suppositories. The Council on Pharmacy and Chemistry reports that "Micajah's Medicated Wafers" (formerly called "Micajah's Medicated Uterine Wafers"), and "Micajah's Suppositories," sold by Micajah and Co., Warren, Pa., are inadmissible to New and Nonofficial Remedies because: (1) their composition is essentially secret; (2) the name of neither of these mixtures is indicative of its composition; (3) of unwarranted and exaggerated therapeutic claims, and (4) the therapeutic advice which accompanies the trade packages constitutes an indirect advertisement to the public. The "wafers" were analyzed in the A. M. A. Chemical Laboratory in 1910 and found to consist essentially of dried ("burnt") alum, boric acid and borax. The suppositories were recently examined in the A. M. A. Chemical Laboratory and, like the "wafers," were found to contain alum, boric acid and borax—and these substances practically alone—incorporated in cocoa butter. The company claims that "to these have been added Ammonii Ichthyosulphonate, Balsam of Peru, Ext. Belladonnae." The A. M. A. chemists report, however, that if extract of belladonna is present at all, it is in amounts too small to be detected by the methods commonly employed in the chemical examination of alkaloidal drugs.

The chemists report further that while ammonium ichthyosulphonate and balsam of Peru both have a decided odor and a dark color, the suppositories have but little color, and the odor of cocoa butter which forms their base is not covered by these drugs. Obviously, therefore, if ammonium ichthyosulphonate and balsam of Peru are present at all, the amounts are utterly insufficient to exert any therapeutic effect (Jour. A. M. A., Nov. 29, 1919, p. 1715).

NEW BOOKS

Under this heading books received by the Journal will be acknowledged. Publishers are advised that this shall constitute return for such publications as they may submit. Obviously all publications sent us cannot be given space for review, but from time to time books received, of possible interest to Oklahoma physicians, will be reviewed.

MISCELLANEOUS NOSTRUMS.

Prepared and Issued by the Propaganda Department of the American Medical Association, Fourth Edition, Paper, 142 Pages. Price 20 cents. 1919; American Medical Association, 535 North Dearborn St., Chicago.

"Our national quality of commercial shrewdness fails us when we go into the open market to purchase relief from suffering—Samuel Hopkins Adams", is the observation carried on the front cover of this little publication.

We pay far too little attention to the accurate report of findings of the various committees of our central organization at Chicago. We have grown in the habit of assuming that everyone should know that patent medicines and nostrums are understood by most intelligent people as the physician understands them, when as a matter of fact a few minutes reading of these findings by any physician will, as a rule, shock his urbane satisfaction.

The conclusions are accurate, based on facts, undisputed by the fakirs anywhere, disclose the heartlessness and meanness of the manufacturer and profitor and should be in the hands of the people rather than physicians. A copy of this little work on the reception room table may do a great deal of good. It should be accessible to all in reading rooms and libraries.

WHAT WE KNOW ABOUT CANCER.

A Handbook for the Medical Profession, Prepared by a special Committee of the American Society for the Control of Cancer, Consisting of Dr. R. B. Greenough, Director, Harvard Cancer Commission, Boston, Mass.; Dr. James Ewing, Director of Cancer Research, Memorial Hospital, New York; and Dr. J. M. Wainwright, Chairman, Cancer Commission. Pennsylvania State Medical Society, Scranton, Pa.

Published in Co-operation with the Council on Health and Public Instruction, American Medical Association.

This is an important communication containing a condensed opinion on various phases of cancer by this committee. It should be read by every physician, for the subject interests all without reference to the special work engaged in. It is authoritative, not tiresome and of great value.

A MANUAL OF OBSTETRICS.

By John Cooke Hirst, M. D., Associate in Gynecology, University of Pennsylvania; Obstetrican and Gynecologist to the Philadelphia General Hospital. 12mo. of 516 pages with 216 illustrations. Philadelphia and London: W. B. Saunders Company, 1919. Cloth $3.00 net.

This manual is prepared for the use of the student, busy practitioner and nurse. It is finely illustrated, contains compact information and necessarily is limited in scope, which insures the elimination of theoretical discussion found in larger works on obstetrics. The methods of treatment and technic are those which have been tested and found satisfactory in actual practice.

1918 COLLECTED PAPERS OF THE MAYO CLINIC, ROCHESTER, MINN.

Octavo of 1196 pages, 442 illustrations. Philadelphia and London: W. B. Saunders Company, 1919. Cloth $8.50 net.

This is a collection of papers read, clinical observation, operative procedure, and every other phase of the work of the Mayo Clinic during 1918. Forty-eight members of the staff are contributors to the work. It is, as usual, ably and beautifully edited and arranged by Mrs. M. H. Mellish who has had charge of similar work for the Mayo Clinic for many years past.

THE SURGICAL CLINICS OF CHICAGO. Volume III., Number 5, (October; 1919). Octavo of 258 pages, 91 illustrations. Philadelphia and London: W. B. Saunders Company, 1919. Published Bi-Monthly: Price, per year; Paper $10.00; Cloth $14.00.

INDEX TO CONTENTS, VOLUME XII

CONTRIBUTED ARTICLES.

SHORT SUBJECTS.

NEW BOOKS.

INDEX TO AUTHORS.

OFFICERS OF COUNTY SOCIETIES, 1919

County	President	Secretary
Adair	D. P. Chambers, Stilwell	J. A. Patton, Stilwell
Alfalfa	E. L. Frazier, Jet	J. M. Tucker, Carmen
Atoka		
Beaver		
Beckham		J. E. Standifer, Elk City
Blaine	W F Griffin, Greenfield	J. A. Norris, Okeene
Bryan	H. B. Fuston, Bokchito	D. Armstrong, Durant
Caddo	P. H. Anderson, Anadarko	C. R. Hume, Anadarko
Canadian		W. J. Murzy, El Reno
Carter	A G Cowles, Ardmore	Robert H Henry, Ardmore
Choctaw	C. H. Hale, Boswell	J. D. Moore, Hugo
Cleveland		D. W. Griffin, Norman.
Cherokee		
Comanche	A. H. Stewart, Lawton	E. B. Mitchell, Lawton
Coal	F. E. Sadler, Coalgate	W. T. Blount, Tupelo
Cotton		
Craig	C. B. Bell, Welch	F. M. Adams, Vinita
Creek		H. S. Garland, Sapulpa.
Custer	K D Gossam, Custer	O H Parker, Custer
Dewey		
Ellis		
Garfield	G. A. Boyle, Enid.	L. W. Cotton, Enid.
Garvin		N. H. Lindsey, Pauls Valley.
Grady	Martha Bledsoe, Chickasha	J. C. Ambrister, Chickasha.
Grant		
Greer	Ney Neel, Mangum	Fowler Border, Mangum
Harmon		
Haskell	T B Turner, Stigler	R. F. Terrell, Stigler.
Hughes		Hugh Scott, Holdenville
Jackson	J. S. Stults, Olustee	J. B. Hix, Altus
Jefferson	D B Collins, Sugden	W M Browning, Waurika
Johnston		H. B. Kniseley, Tishomingo
Kay	G. H. Nieman, Ponca City	D Walker, Blackwell
Kingfisher	Frank Scott, Kingfisher	C. W. Fisk, Kingfisher.
Kiowa		A. T. Dobson, Hobart.
Latimer	E. L. Evias, Wilburton	C. R. Morrison, Wilburton
Le Flore	C. H. Mahar, Spiro	Harrell Hardy, Poteau
Lincoln		C. M. Morgan, Chandler
Logan		O. E. Barker, Guthrie.
Love		
Mayes	J. L. Adams, Pryor	L. C. White, Adair.
Major		
Marshall	J E Reed, Madill	J L Holland, Madill
McClain	J. W. West, Purcell	O. O. Dawson, Wayne
McCurtain	A W Clarkson, Valliant	W B McCaskill, Idabel
McIntosh	S. W. Minor, Hitchita	W. A. Tolleson, Eufaula
Murray	A P Brown, Davis	W. H. Powell, Sulphur.
Muskogee	J. L. Blakemore, Muskogee	H C. Rogers, Muskogee
Noble		B. A. Owen, Perry.
Nowata	J. E. Brookshire, Nowata	J. R. Collins, Nowata
Okfuskee	C. C. Bombarger, Paden	H. A. May, Okemah.
Oklahoma	W. J. Wallace, Oklahoma City	J. N. Alford, Oklahoma City
Okmulgee	Harry Breese, Henryetta	W. B. Pigg, Okmulgee
Ottawa	A. M. Cooter, Miami	G. Pinnell, Miami
Osage	A. J. Smith, Pawhuska	Benj. Skinner, Pawhuska
Pawnee		E. T. Robinson, Cleveland
Payne		J. B. Murphy, Stillwater
Pittsburg	L. C. Kuyrkendall, McAlester	T. H. McCarley, McAlester.
Pottawatomie	E. E. Rice, Shawnee	G. S. Baxter, Shawnee.
Pontotoc	I. M. Overton, Fitzhugh	S. P. Ross, Ada
Pushmataha	H. C. Johnson, Antlers	Edw. Guinn, Antlers
Rogers	J H Haley, Chelsea.	F A Anderson, Claremore
Roger Mills		
Seminole	W. T. Huddleston, Konawa	W. L. Knight, Wewoka.
Sequoyah	V W Hudson, Salisaw	S A McKeel, Sallisaw
Stephens	J. W. Nieweg, Duncan	J. O. Wharton, Duncan.
Texas	W. H. Langston, Guymon	R. B. Hays, Guymon
Tulsa	G. A. Wall, Tulsa	A. W. Pigford, Tulsa
Tillman		J. E. Arrington, Frederick.
Wagoner	C E Haywood, Wagoner	C E Martin, Wagoner
Washita		A. S. Neal, Cordell.
Washington	O. S. Somerville, Bartlesville	J G Smith, Bartlesville
Woods		O. E. Templin, Alva.
Woodward	R. A. Workman, Woodward	C. W. Tedrowe, Woodward

OFFICERS OF OKLAHOMA STATE MEDICAL ASSOCIATION.

President—Dr. L. J. Moorman, Oklahoma City.
President-elect—Dr. John W. Duke, Guthrie.
1st Vice-President—Dr. Jackson Broshears, Lawton.
2nd Vice-President—Dr. G. Pinnell, Miami.
3rd Vice-President—Dr. J. A. Hatchett, El Reno.
Secretary-Treasurer-Editor—Dr. Claude Thompson, Muskogee.
Assistant Editor and Councilor Representative—Dr. C. W. Heitzman, Muskogee.
Delegates to A. M. A.—1920, Dr. LeRoy Long, Oklahoma City. 1920-1921, Dr. L. S. Willour, McAlester.
Meeting place, Oklahoma City, May, 1920.

COUNCILOR DISTRICTS.

District No. 1. Texas, Beaver, Cimarron, Harper, Ellis, Woods, Woodward, Alfalfa, Major, Grant, Garfield, Noble and Kay. G. A. Boyle, Enid.

District No. 2. Dewey, Roger Mills, Custer, Beckham, Washita, Greer, Kiowa, Harmon, Jackson and Tillman. Ellis Lamb, Clinton.

District No. 3. Blaine, Kingfisher, Canadian, Logan, Payne, Lincoln, Oklahoma, Cleveland, Pottawatomie, Seminole and McClain. M. E. Stout, Oklahoma City.

District No. 4. Caddo, Grady, Comanche, Cotton, Stephens, Jefferson, Garvin, Murray, Carter, and Love. J. T. Slover, Sulphur.

District No. 5. Pontotoc, Coal, Johnston, Atoka, Marshall, Bryan, Choctaw, Pushmataha and McCurtain. J. L. Austin, Durant.

District No. 6. Okfuskee, Hughes, Pittsburg, Latimer, LeFlore, Haskell and Sequoyah. L. C. Kurkendall, McAlester.

District No. 7. Pawnee, Osage, Washington, Tulsa, Creek, Nowata and Rogers. N. W. Mayginnis, Tulsa.

District No. 8. Craig, Ottawa, Delaware, Mayes, Wagoner, Cherokee, Adair, Okmulgee, Muskogee and McIntosh. C. W. Heitzman, Muskogee.

CHAIRMEN OF SCIENTIFIC SECTIONS.

Surgery and Gynecology—Chairman, Dr. Ralph V. Smith, Tulsa; Secretary-Vice Chairman, Dr. Ross Grosshart, Wright Building, Tulsa.

Pediatrics and Obstetrics—Chairman, Dr. C. V. Rice, Barnes Building, Muskogee; Secretary-Vice Chairman, Dr. J. Raymond Burdick, Ketchum Hotel, Tulsa.

Eye, Ear, Nose and Throat—Dr. L. C. Kuyrkendall, McAlester.

General Medicine, Nervous and Mental Diseases—Dr. Jas. T. Riley, El Reno.

Genitourinary, Skin and Radiology—Dr. J. Hoy Sanford, Muskogee.

Necrology Committee—Drs. C. W. Heitzman, Muskogee; John W. Duke, Guthrie; L. C. Kurykendall, McAlester.

Legislative Committee—Dr. Millington Smith, Oklahoma City; Dr. J. M. Byrum, Shawnee; Dr. J. C. Mahr, Oklahoma City.

For the Study and Control of Cancer—Drs. LeRoy Long, Oklahoma City; Gayfree Ellison, Norman; D. A. Myers, Lawton.

For the Study and Control of Pellagra—Drs. A. A. Thurlow, Norman; L. A. Mitchell, Frederick; J. C. Watkins, Checotah.

For the Study of Venereal Diseases—Drs. Wm. J. Wallace, Oklahoma City; Ross Grosshart, Tulsa; J. E. Bercaw, Okmulgee.

Tuberculosis—Drs. H. T. Price, Tulsa; C. W. Heitzman, Muskogee; Leila E Andrews, Oklahoma City.

Conservation of Vision—Drs. L. A. Newton, Oklanoma City; L. Haynes Buxton, Oklahoma City; G. E. Hartshorne, Shawnee.

Hospital Committee—F. S. Clinton, Tulsa; M. Smith, Oklahoma City; C. A. Thompson, Muskogee.

Committee on Medical Education—Drs. A. L. Blesh; A. K. West; A. W. White, Oklahoma City.

State Commissioner of Health—Dr. A. R. Lewis, Oklahoma City..

STATE BOARD OF MEDICAL EXAMINERS.

W. E. Sanderson, Altus; W. T. Ray, Gould; O. N. Windle, Sayre; J. E. Farber, Cordell; D. W. Miller, Blackwell; J. M. Byrum, Shawnee, Secretary; J. E. Emanuel, Chickasha; H. C. Montague, Muskogee.

Oklahoma reciprocates with Georgia, Kentucky, Mississippi, Nevada, North Carolina, Wisconsin, Kansas, Arkansas, Virginia, West Virginia, Nebraska, New Mexico, Tennessee, Iowa, Ohio, California, Colorado, Indiana, Missouri, New Jersey, Vermont, Texas, Michigan.

Meetings held on first Tuesday of January, April, July and October, Oklahoma City. Address all communications to the Secretary, Dr. J. M. Byrum, Shawnee.

www.ingramcontent.com/pod-product-compliance
Lightning Source LLC
Chambersburg PA
CBHW071359050326
40689CB00010B/1700